Engineering and Characterisation of Novel Nanomedicine Formulations

Engineering and Characterisation of Novel Nanomedicine Formulations

Editors

Raquel Fernández García
Francisco Bolás-Fernández
Ana Isabel Fraguas-Sánchez

MDPI

Basel • Beijing • Wuhan • Barcelona • Belgrade • Novi Sad • Cluj • Manchester

Editors
Raquel Fernández García
School of Pharmacy
University of Nottingham
Nottingham
United Kingdom

Francisco Bolás-Fernández
Department of Microbiology
and Parasitology
Complutense University of
Madrid
Madrid
Spain

Ana Isabel Fraguas-Sánchez
Department of Pharmaceutics
and Food Technology
Complutense University of
Madrid
Madrid
Spain

Editorial Office
MDPI
St. Alban-Anlage 66
4052 Basel, Switzerland

This is a reprint of articles from the Special Issue published online in the open access journal *Pharmaceutics* (ISSN 1999-4923) (available at: www.mdpi.com/journal/pharmaceutics/special_issues/novel_nanomedicine).

For citation purposes, cite each article independently as indicated on the article page online and as indicated below:

Lastname, A.A.; Lastname, B.B. Article Title. *Journal Name* **Year**, *Volume Number*, Page Range.

ISBN 978-3-7258-1096-3 (Hbk)
ISBN 978-3-7258-1095-6 (PDF)
doi.org/10.3390/books978-3-7258-1095-6

Contents

About the Editors vii

Raquel Fernández-García, Francisco Bolás-Fernández and Ana Isabel Fraguas-Sánchez
Editorial for Special Issue 'Engineering and Characterisation of Novel Nanomedicine Formulations'
Reprinted from: *Pharmaceutics* **2024**, *16*, 585, doi:10.3390/pharmaceutics16050585 1

Nilesh R. Rarokar, Sunil S. Menghani, Deweshri R. Kerzare, Pramod B. Khedekar, Ashish P. Bharne, Abdulhakeem S. Alamri, et al.
Preparation of Terbinafin-Encapsulated Solid Lipid Nanoparticles Containing Antifungal Carbopol® Hydrogel with Improved Efficacy: In Vitro, Ex Vivo and In Vivo Study
Reprinted from: *Pharmaceutics* **2022**, *14*, 1393, doi:10.3390/pharmaceutics14071393 5

Kampanart Huanbutta, Napapat Rattanachitthawat, Kunlathida Luangpraditkun, Pornsak Sriamornsak, Vivek Puri, Inderbir Singh and Tanikan Sangnim
Development and Evaluation of Ethosomes Loaded with *Zingiber zerumbet* Linn Rhizome Extract for Antifungal Skin Infection in Deep Layer Skin
Reprinted from: *Pharmaceutics* **2022**, *14*, 2765, doi:10.3390/pharmaceutics14122765 24

Laura E. Swart, Marcel H. A. M. Fens, Anita van Oort, Piotr Waranecki, L. Daniel Mata Casimiro, David Tuk, et al.
Increased Bone Marrow Uptake and Accumulation of Very-Late Antigen-4 Targeted Lipid Nanoparticles
Reprinted from: *Pharmaceutics* **2023**, *15*, 1603, doi:10.3390/pharmaceutics15061603 36

Eliza Rocha Gomes, Fernanda Rezende Souza, Geovanni Dantas Cassali, Adriano de Paula Sabino, André Luis Branco de Barros and Mônica Cristina Oliveira
Investigation of the Antitumor Activity and Toxicity of Tumor-Derived Exosomes Fused with Long-Circulating and pH-Sensitive Liposomes Containing Doxorubicin
Reprinted from: *Pharmaceutics* **2022**, *14*, 2256, doi:10.3390/pharmaceutics14112256 52

Omkar Bhatavdekar, Inês Godet, Daniele Gilkes and Stavroula Sofou
The Rate of Cisplatin Dosing Affects the Resistance and Metastatic Potential of Triple Negative Breast Cancer Cells, Independent of Hypoxia
Reprinted from: *Pharmaceutics* **2022**, *14*, 2184, doi:10.3390/pharmaceutics14102184 77

Jaqueline Aparecida Duarte, Eliza Rocha Gomes, André Luis Branco De Barros and Elaine Amaral Leite
Co-Encapsulation of Simvastatin and Doxorubicin into pH-Sensitive Liposomes Enhances Antitumoral Activity in Breast Cancer Cell Lines
Reprinted from: *Pharmaceutics* **2023**, *15*, 369, doi:10.3390/pharmaceutics15020369 96

Shengzhuang Tang, Jesse Chen, Jayme Cannon, Mona Chekuri, Mohammad Farazuddin, James R. Baker, Jr. and Su He Wang
Delicate Hybrid Laponite–Cyclic Poly(ethylene glycol) Nanoparticles as a Potential Drug Delivery System
Reprinted from: *Pharmaceutics* **2023**, *15*, 1998, doi:10.3390/pharmaceutics15071998 114

José Garcés-Garcés, Marta Redrado, Ángela Sastre-Santos, María Concepción Gimeno and Fernando Fernández-Lázaro
Synthesis of Dipyridylaminoperylenediimide–Metal Complexes and Their Cytotoxicity Studies
Reprinted from: *Pharmaceutics* **2022**, *14*, 2616, doi:10.3390/pharmaceutics14122616 129

Ming Xia, Pengwei Huang and Ming Tan
A Pseudovirus Nanoparticle-Based Trivalent Rotavirus Vaccine Candidate Elicits High and Cross P Type Immune Response
Reprinted from: *Pharmaceutics* **2022**, *14*, 1597, doi:10.3390/pharmaceutics14081597 . . . . **144**

Valentina Marassi, Ilaria Zanoni, Simona Ortelli, Stefano Giordani, Pierluigi Reschiglian, Barbara Roda, et al.
Native Study of the Behaviour of Magnetite Nanoparticles for Hyperthermia Treatment during the Initial Moments of Intravenous Administration
Reprinted from: *Pharmaceutics* **2022**, *14*, 2810, doi:10.3390/pharmaceutics14122810 . . . . **162**

Saghir Akhtar, Fawzi Babiker, Usman A. Akhtar and Ibrahim F. Benter
Mitigating Cardiotoxicity of Dendrimers: Angiotensin-(1-7) via Its Mas Receptor Ameliorates PAMAM-Induced Cardiac Dysfunction in the Isolated Mammalian Heart
Reprinted from: *Pharmaceutics* **2022**, *14*, 2673, doi:10.3390/pharmaceutics14122673 . . . . **179**

Diego Alejandro Dri, Elisa Gaucci, Ilaria Torrieri, Maria Carafa, Carlotta Marianecci and Donatella Gramaglia
Critical Analysis and Quality Assessment of Nanomedicines and Nanocarriers in Clinical Trials: Three Years of Activity at the Clinical Trials Office
Reprinted from: *Pharmaceutics* **2022**, *14*, 1438, doi:10.3390/pharmaceutics14071438 . . . . **196**

Karim Osouli-Bostanabad, Sara Puliga, Dolores R. Serrano, Andrea Bucchi, Gavin Halbert and Aikaterini Lalatsa
Microfluidic Manufacture of Lipid-Based Nanomedicines
Reprinted from: *Pharmaceutics* **2022**, *14*, 1940, doi:10.3390/pharmaceutics14091940 . . . . **215**

About the Editors

Raquel Fernández García

Raquel Fernández García was awarded a PhD in Pharmacy from the Complutense University of Madrid in 2020, where she focused her research on developing novel oral and topical treatments for infectious diseases. Her thesis was awarded an international distinction and the 'Folch Foundation award' in 2021. After her graduation, Raquel started a new position as a postdoctoral research associate at the School of Pharmacy, the University of Nottingham, where she has been working on two main topics: the development of formulations based on viral vectors and the use of nanotechnology in tree propagation. She is the author of 14 peer-reviewed articles and 1 book chapter. During her career, she has completed several predoctoral and postdoctoral research placements (Trinity College Dublin, University of Barcelona, University of East Anglia and University College London).

Francisco Bolás-Fernández

Francisco Bolás Fernández earned his PhD in Pharmacy from the Complutense University of Madrid in 1981, where he focused on the anthelmintic activity of benzimidazole-carbamates in Trichinella spiralis. After his graduation, Francisco was awarded a Fleming fellowship which allowed him to continue his research career at the Department of Zoology at the University of Nottingham, where he applied humoral and cellular immune responses to characterize the antigens of Trichinella species of different geographical origins. This allowed him to return to the Complutense University of Madrid as a full-time professor, where he established his research group focusing on the investigation of the immunological fundaments of the application of Trichuris and Trichinella sp. in the treatment of autoimmune diseases. Apart from that, he extended his research interest to the development of novel treatments for leishmaniasis. Francisco is the author of 130 publications and has contributed to more than 150 scientific conferences. He has also been part of 33 research projects funded by public institutions and related companies.

Ana Isabel Fraguas-Sánchez

Ana Isabel is an Assistant Professor of Pharmaceutics, Biopharmacy and Pharmacokinetics at the Complutense University of Madrid. She has participated in 19 research projects funded by Spanish public institutions, as well as pharmaceutical and related companies (five of them as the principal investigator). She is the author of 33 peer-reviewed articles and 6 book chapters. She has participated in 42 scientific conferences, with 3 of them as an invited speaker. Her PhD thesis has been awarded the "Doctorate Extraordinary Award 2019" from the Faculty of Pharmacy of the Complutense University and the "Juan Abello I" prize from the Doctor Academy of Spain. She also received the "Juan Abello 2019 prize" of the Spanish Royal Academy of Pharmacy for her scientific research. She is an evaluator of research projects for institutions in Poland and a member of the board of directors of the Spanish Society of Industrial and Galenic Pharmacy. She has completed several predoctoral and postdoctoral research placements (Italy, Switzerland, Finland, and Greece). Her research group is focused on the development, optimization and preclinical evaluation of novel controlled drug delivery systems (with an emphasis on implants, micro- and nanoparticles) for the treatment of cancer, inflammatory and infectious diseases.

pharmaceutics

MDPI

Editorial

Editorial for Special Issue 'Engineering and Characterisation of Novel Nanomedicine Formulations'

Raquel Fernández-García [1,*], Francisco Bolás-Fernández [2] and Ana Isabel Fraguas-Sánchez [3,4,*]

1 School of Pharmacy, University of Nottingham, University Park, Nottingham NG7 2RD, UK
2 Department of Microbiology and Parasitology, Faculty of Pharmacy, Complutense University, 28040 Madrid, Spain; francisb@ucm.es
3 Department of Pharmaceutics and Food Technology, Faculty of Pharmacy, Complutense University, 28040 Madrid, Spain
4 Institute of Industrial Pharmacy, Complutense University, 28040 Madrid, Spain
* Correspondence: raquel.fernandezgarcia@nottingham.ac.uk (R.F.-G.); aifraguas@ucm.es (A.I.F.-S.)

Nanomedicine is the application of nanotechnology to achieve innovations in healthcare and involves the engineering of systems at the nanoscale (particle size < 1000 nm) with the aim of improving drug delivery. These systems can modify the release profile of drugs but also encapsulate poorly soluble drugs and modify their biodistribution, thus achieving the selective targeting of tissues and minimising adverse effects. The encapsulation of drugs within nanosystems also protects the drug from degradation, with it being suitable for sensitive substances, such as proteins or RNA.

This Special Issue entitled 'Engineering and Characterisation of Novel Nanomedicine Formulations' highlights the latest findings in the development of these systems. We are deeply grateful for the 13 articles covering a variety of interesting achievements. The articles cover multiple nanosystems, including nanoparticles (polymeric, lipid and magnetic), ethosomes, liposomes, exosomes, dendrimers and metal complexes.

It is well known that lipid formulations have demonstrated their usefulness in increasing drug permeation through the skin [1]. Rarokar et al. (contribution 1) developed solid lipid nanoparticles (SLNs) loaded with terbinafin hydrochloride, an antifungal drug with a high hepatic first pass metabolism and oral bioavailability of 30–40% [2]. These nanoparticles were incorporated into a carbopol-based hydrogel for their topical application. This hydrogel showed a better skin deposition and higher in vitro antifungal activity than marketed formulations of this drug. Huanbutta et al. (contribution 2) developed ethosomes as a strategy to improve the permeation of Zingiber zerumbet Linn Rhizome Extract that has demonstrated its antifungal properties, for example, against *Candida albicans*. Its encapsulation significantly enhanced the permeation and retention compared to the non-encapsulated extract.

Lipid nanoparticles have also been shown to be useful in delivering oligonucleotides, including siRNAs, due to their high encapsulation efficiency, improved circulation times and reduced immunogenicity [3]. siRNAs are being exploited as therapeutics in a broad range of conditions, including cancer disease [4]. They are highly useful in the treatment of acute myeloid leukaemia. Most haematological diseases, including leukaemia, tend to originate in the bone marrow. In this context, lipid nanoparticles encapsulating siRNAs and accumulated in this tissue could represent a promising nanoformulation for the treatment of this neoplasm. To achieve this selective accumulation in the bone marrow, Swart et al. (contribution 3) developed lipid nanoparticles targeting very late antigen-4 (VLA-4), which is highly expressed in the bone marrow [5]. These researchers prepared lipid nanoparticles functionalised with the tripeptide Leu-Asp-Val, which binds VLA-4 receptors. The functionalised formulation showed a higher accumulation and retention in the bone marrow than their counterparts, resulting in an excellent strategy for improving the treatment of leukaemia.

Citation: Fernández-García, R.; Bolás-Fernández, F.; Fraguas-Sánchez, A.I. Editorial for Special Issue 'Engineering and Characterisation of Novel Nanomedicine Formulations'. *Pharmaceutics* **2024**, *16*, 585. https://doi.org/10.3390/pharmaceutics16050585

Received: 18 April 2024
Accepted: 24 April 2024
Published: 26 April 2024

It is well known that the use of nanocarriers is also an excellent strategy to increase the efficacy and decrease the adverse effects of antineoplastics in solid tumours [6]. Nanoformulations facilitate targeted drug localisation, specifically at the tumour site. For example, Rocha-Gomes et al. (contribution 4) developed pH-sensitive liposomes encapsulating doxorubicin to improve the efficacy of this drug in triple-negative breast cancer, a difficult-to-treat and invasive carcinoma, the treatment of which remains an unmet need worldwide. This formulation exhibited a lower toxicity compared to free drugs. Moreover, it exhibited a tumour-suppressive effect and a lower incidence of metastatic foci in the lungs in a 4T1 breast cancer model developed in mice. On the other hand, it has been demonstrated that the hypoxic tumour microenvironment contributes to the appearance of resistances and metastases and, consequently, to a poor prognosis. Bhatavdekar et al. (contribution 5) demonstrated that nanomedicine could help to overcome this complication. They showed that pH-sensitive nanoparticles loaded with cisplatin allow for a fast and uniform exposure of tumour cells to this drug, inhibiting the population of hypoxia-affected cells and their metastatic potential. The use of nanoencapsulated cisplatin was more effective than free drugs.

It should be noted that nanocarriers also offer the capability to encapsulate multiple drugs simultaneously. This presents a compelling prospect in tumour therapy, as it enables the coordinated release of these agents in the tumour microenvironment, potentially augmenting their synergistic therapeutic effects. Duarte et al. (contribution 6) used this strategy. These researchers developed pH-sensitive liposomes encapsulating both simvastatin and doxorubicin. In TNBC, a higher cytotoxic effect was observed with this formulation compared to the administration of the free drugs in combination. For example, while the combination of doxorubicin and simvastatin at molar ratios of 1:1 and 1:2 showed IC50 values of around 0.96 and 0.71 μM, respectively, the nanoencapsulated drugs showed values of around 0.47 and 0.35 μM at the same ratios, respectively.

Tang et al. (contribution 7) evaluated the efficacy of nanoencapsulated doxorubicin in lung cancer, which is the leading cause of cancer death worldwide [7]. They developed nanoformulations using laponite and linear or cyclic poly(ethylene glycol) (PEG). However, these nanosystems did not exert a significantly higher antiproliferative effect in A549 than free doxorubicin. This cytotoxic effect washigher in the formulations developed with cyclic poly(ethylene glycol). Moreover, these formulations also exerted a higher apoptotic activity in primary lung epithelial cells. These results suggest that nanosystems elaborated with laponite and cyclic-PEG could represent an interesting strategy to administer doxorubicin in cancer therapy.

Garcés-Garcés et al. (contribution 8) synthesised a novel group of silver and copper complexes based on perylenediimide that showed an antiproliferative effect in cervical cancer cells (HeLa cells). While the free perylenediimide ligands displayed moderate cytotoxicity, coordination with silver or copper notably augmented the activity, suggesting a synergistic interplay between these compounds.

Vaccine development is another therapeutic area where nanoparticles show a great potential. For example, Xia et al. (contribution 9) developed S60-VP8* pseudovirus nanoparticles as a parenteral vaccine candidate for the most prevalent rotavirus infections. It was a trivalent vaccine with the glycan receptor binding VP8* domains of rotavirus spike proteins, and it exerted a high and broad immunogenicity in mice when administered intramuscularly, resulting in a promising candidate for this disease that causes vomiting, severe watery diarrhoea, abdominal pain and/or fever usually in infants and young children.

It is imperative to evaluate the potential toxicity and interaction with biological structures of nanocarriers [8]. For example, magnetic nanoparticles (MNPs) exhibit exceptional characteristics, rendering them suitable for application as therapeutic agents in hyperthermia, as well as in adjuvant local anticancer therapy that involves elevating temperatures beyond the physiologically optimal range, typically from 40 to 43 °C. In this context, it is essential to study the interaction mechanisms experienced by MNPs upon intravenous administration, as upon introduction into the bloodstream, MNPs transition from a synthetic identity to a biological one. The study by Marassi et al. (contribution 10) aimed to study this aspect. These researchers employed a dynamic methodology utilising flow field-flow fractionation and showed that, within a dynamic biological environment and subsequent to interactions with serum albumin, MNPs maintain their colloidal properties. This supports their safety profile for intravenous administration and use in hyperthermia.

Dendrimers are nanoscale molecules characterised by symmetrical structures, wherein a central atom or group of atoms is enveloped by branching units referred to as dendrons with potential application as drug delivery carriers [9]. Akhtar et al. (contribution 11) evaluated the impact of physiochemical attributes of dendrimer nanoparticles on cardiac contractility and hemodynamics. Specifically, these researchers examined the influence of polyamidoamine (PAMAM) dendrimer generation (G7, G6, G5, G4 and G3) and surface chemistry (–NH2, –COOH and –OH). This study revealed that cardiac function impairment diminished with decreasing dendrimer generation, with G3 exhibiting minimal or no cardiotoxicity. Cationic PAMAMs (–NH2) were more toxic than anionic (–COOH), while neutral PAMAMs (–OH) displayed the least cardiotoxicity. Cationic G7 PAMAM-induced cardiac dysfunction was significantly ameliorated by Ang-(1-7) administration.

As discussed by Dri et al. (contribution 12), although nanoparticulate technology has revolutionised the treatment of many pathologies such as infectious disease, cancer and neurological disorders, among others, the clinical translation of nanomedicines is extremely complex. One of the main challenges is to find elaboration methods that can be applied on a large scale and allow for the production of nanomedicines that preserve their original features and show a low batch-to-batch variability. In this context, microfluidics has emerged as a new and excellent strategy for the industrial manufacturing of nanomedicines. This strategy allows for the obtention of highly tuneable and reproducible strategies. All these aspects were discussed by Osouli-Bostanabad et al. (contribution 13) in their review paper.

Author Contributions: Conceptualization: A.I.F.-S. and R.F.-G.; Writing—original draft preparation: A.I.F.-S. and R.F.-G.; Writing—review and editing: A.I.F.-S., R.F.-G. and F.B.-F. All authors have read and agreed to the published version of the manuscript.

Conflicts of Interest: The authors declare no conflict of interest.

List of Contributions

1. Rarokar, N.R.; Menghani, S.S.; Kerzare, D.R.; Khedekar, P.B.; Bharne, A.P.; Alamri, A.S.; Alsanie, W.F.; Alhomrani, M.; Sreeharsha, N.; Asdaq, S.M.B. Preparation of Terbinafin-Encapsulated Solid Lipid Nanoparticles Containing Antifungal Carbopol® Hydrogel with Improved Efficacy: In Vitro, Ex Vivo and In Vivo Study. *Pharmaceutic* **2022**, *14*, 1393.
2. Huanbutta, K.; Rattanachitthawat, N.; Luangpraditkun, K.; Sriamornsak, P.; Puri, V.; Singh, I.; Sangnim, T. Development and Evaluation of Ethosomes Loaded with Zingiber zerumbet Linn Rhizome Extract for Antifungal Skin Infection in Deep Layer Skin. *Pharmaceutics* **2022**, *14*, 2765. https://doi.org/10.3390/pharmaceutics14122765.
3. Swart, L.E.; Fens, M.H.A.M.; van Oort, A.; Waranecki, P.; Mata Casimiro, L.D.; Tuk, D.; Hendriksen, M.; van den Brink, L.; Schweighart, E.; Seinen, C.; et al. Increased Bone Marrow Uptake and Accumulation of Very-Late Antigen-4 Targeted Lipid Nanoparticles. *Pharmaceutics* **2023**, *15*, 1603.
4. Gomes, E.R.; Souza, F.R.; Cassali, G.D.; Sabino, A.D.; Barros, A.L.; Oliveira, M.C. Investigation of the Antitumor Activity and Toxicity of Tumor-Derived Exosomes Fused with Long-Circulating and pH-Sensitive Liposomes Containing Doxorubicin. *Pharmaceutics* **2022**, *14*, 2256. https://doi.org/10.3390/pharmaceutics14112256.
5. Bhatavdekar, O.; Godet, I.; Gilkes, D.; Sofou, S. The Rate of Cisplatin Dosing Affects the Resistance and Metastatic Potential of Triple Negative Breast Cancer Cells, Independent of Hypoxia. *Pharmaceutics* **2022**, *14*, 2184. https://doi.org/10.3390/pharmaceutics14102184.
6. Duarte, J.A.; Gomes, E.R.; De Barros, A.L.; Leite, E.A. Co-Encapsulation of Simvastatin and Doxorubicin into pH-Sensitive Liposomes Enhances Antitumoral Activity in Breast Cancer Cell Lines. *Pharmaceutics* **2023**, *15*, 369. https://doi.org/10.3390/pharmaceutics15020369.

7. Tang, S.; Chen, J.; Cannon, J.; Chekuri, M.; Farazuddin, M.; Baker, J.R.; Wang, S.H. Delicate Hybrid Laponite–Cyclic Poly(ethylene glycol) Nanoparticles as a Potential Drug Delivery System. *Pharmaceutics* **2023**, *15*, 1998. https://doi.org/10.3390/pharmaceutics15071998.
8. Garcés-Garcés, J.; Redrado, M.; Sastre-Santos, Á.; Gimeno, M.C.; Fernández-Lázaro, F. Synthesis of Dipyridylaminoperylenediimide–Metal Complexes and Their Cytotoxicity Studies. *Pharmaceutics* **2022**, *14*, 2616.
9. Xia, M.; Huang, P.; Tan, M. A Pseudovirus Nanoparticle-Based Trivalent Rotavirus Vaccine Candidate Elicits High and Cross P Type Immune Response. *Pharmaceutics* **2022**, *14*, 1597.
10. Marassi, V.; Zanoni, I.; Ortelli, S.; Giordani, S.; Reschiglian, P.; Roda, B.; Zattoni, A.; Ravagli, C.; Cappiello, L.; Baldi, G.; et al. Native Study of the Behaviour of Magnetite Nanoparticles for Hyperthermia Treatment during the Initial Moments of Intravenous Administration. *Pharmaceutics* **2022**, *14*, 2810. https://doi.org/10.3390/pharmaceutics14122810.
11. Akhtar, S.; Babiker, F.; Akhtar, U.A.; Benter, I.F. Mitigating Cardiotoxicity of Dendrimers: Angiotensin-(1-7) via Its Mas Receptor Ameliorates PAMAM-Induced Cardiac Dysfunction in the Isolated Mammalian Heart. *Pharmaceutics* **2022**, *14*, 2673. https://doi.org/10.3390/pharmaceutics14122673.
12. Dri, D.A.; Gaucci, E.; Torrieri, I.; Carafa, M.; Marianecci, C.; Gramaglia, D. Critical Analysis and Quality Assessment of Nanomedicines and Nanocarriers in Clinical Trials: Three Years of Activity at the Clinical Trials Office. *Pharmaceutics* **2022**, *14*, 1438.
13. Osouli-Bostanabad, K.; Puliga, S.; Serrano, D.R.; Bucchi, A.; Halbert, G.; Lalatsa, A. Microfluidic Manufacture of Lipid-Based Nanomedicines. *Pharmaceutics* **2022**, *14*, 1940.

References

1. Akombaetwa, N.; Ilangala, A.B.; Thom, L.; Memvanga, P.B.; Witika, B.A.; Buya, A.B. Current Advances in Lipid Nanosystems Intended for Topical and Transdermal Drug Delivery Applications. *Pharmaceutics* **2023**, *15*, 656. [CrossRef] [PubMed]
2. Wang, A.; Ding, H.; Liu, Y.; Gao, Y.; Zeng, Z. Single dose pharmacokinetics of terbinafine in cats. *J. Feline Med. Surg.* **2012**, *14*, 540–544. [CrossRef] [PubMed]
3. Paunovska, K.; Loughrey, D.; Dahlman, J.E. Drug delivery systems for RNA therapeutics. *Nat. Rev. Genet.* **2022**, *23*, 265–280. [CrossRef] [PubMed]
4. Friedrich, M.; Aigner, A. Therapeutic siRNA: State-of-the-Art and Future Perspectives. *BioDrugs* **2022**, *36*, 549–571. [CrossRef] [PubMed]
5. Avemaria, F.; Gur-Cohen, S.; Avci, S.; Lapidot, T. VLA-4 Affinity Assay for Murine Bone Marrow-derived Hematopoietic Stem Cells. *Bio-Protoc. J.* **2017**, *7*, e2134. [CrossRef]
6. Alsaab, H.O.; Alghamdi, M.S.; Alotaibi, A.S.; Alzhrani, R.; Alwuthaynani, F.; Althobaiti, Y.S.; Almalki, A.H.; Sau, S.; Iyer, A.K. Progress in clinical trials of photodynamic therapy for solid tumors and the role of nanomedicine. *Cancers* **2020**, *12*, 2793. [CrossRef] [PubMed]
7. Bray, F.; Laversanne, M.; Sung, H.; Ferlay, J.; Siegel, R.L.; Soerjomataram, I.; Jemal, A. Global cancer statistics 2022: GLOBOCAN estimates of incidence and mortality worldwide for 36 cancers in 185 countries. *CA Cancer J. Clin.* **2024**. [CrossRef]
8. Demir, E. A review on nanotoxicity and nanogenotoxicity of different shapes of nanomaterials. *J. Appl. Toxicol.* **2021**, *41*, 118–147. [CrossRef] [PubMed]
9. Mittal, P.; Saharan, A.; Verma, R.; Altalbawy, F.M.A.; Alfaidi, M.A.; Batiha, G.E.; Akter, W.; Gautam, R.K.; Uddin, M.S.; Rahman, M.S. Dendrimers: A New Race of Pharmaceutical Nanocarriers. *Biomed. Res. Int.* **2021**, *2021*, 8844030. [CrossRef]

pharmaceutics

MDPI

Article

Preparation of Terbinafin-Encapsulated Solid Lipid Nanoparticles Containing Antifungal Carbopol® Hydrogel with Improved Efficacy: In Vitro, Ex Vivo and In Vivo Study

Nilesh R. Rarokar [1], Sunil S. Menghani [2,*], Deweshri R. Kerzare [3], Pramod B. Khedekar [1], Ashish P. Bharne [1], Abdulhakeem S. Alamri [4,5], Walaa F. Alsanie [4,5], Majid Alhomrani [4,5], Nagaraja Sreeharsha [6,7] and Syed Mohammed Basheeruddin Asdaq [8,*]

[1] Computer Aided Drug Design Laboratory, Department of Pharmaceutical Sciences, Mahatma Jyotiba Fuley Shaikshanik Parisar, Rashtrasant Tukadoji Maharaj Nagpur University, Amravati Road, Nagpur 440033, India; nileshrarokar@outlook.com (N.R.R.); pbkhedekarudps@gmail.com (P.B.K.); ashishbharne2@gmail.com (A.P.B.)
[2] Department of Pharmaceutical Chemistry, Krupanidhi College of Pharmacy, Bangalore 560035, India
[3] Department of Pharmaceutical Chemistry, Dadasaheb Balpande College of Pharmacy, Nagpur 440037, India; kerzarepritee@gmail.com
[4] Department of Clinical Laboratory Sciences, The Faculty of Applied Medical Sciences, Taif University, Taif 21944, Saudi Arabia; a.alamri@tu.edu.sa (A.S.A.); w.alsanie@tu.edu.sa (W.F.A.); m.alhomrani@tu.edu.sa (M.A.)
[5] Centre of Biomedical Sciences Research (CBSR), Deanship of Scientific Research, Taif University, Taif 21944, Saudi Arabia
[6] Department of Pharmaceutical Sciences, College of Clinical Pharmacy, King Faisal University, Al-Ahsa 31982, Saudi Arabia; sharsha@kfu.edu.sa
[7] Department of Pharmaceutics, Vidya Siri College of Pharmacy, Off Sarjapura Road, Bangalore 560035, India
[8] Department of Pharmacy Practice, College of Pharmacy, AlMaarefa University, Dariyah, Riyadh 13713, Saudi Arabia
* Correspondence: sunil_sunmegh@rediffmail.com (S.S.M.); sasdaq@gmail.com or sasdag@mcst.edu.sa (S.M.B.A.)

Citation: Rarokar, N.R.; Menghani, S.S.; Kerzare, D.R.; Khedekar, P.B.; Bharne, A.P.; Alamri, A.S.; Alsanie, W.F.; Alhomrani, M.; Sreeharsha, N.; Asdaq, S.M.B. Preparation of Terbinafin-Encapsulated Solid Lipid Nanoparticles Containing Antifungal Carbopol® Hydrogel with Improved Efficacy: In Vitro, Ex Vivo and In Vivo Study. *Pharmaceutics* **2022**, *14*, 1393. https://doi.org/10.3390/pharmaceutics14071393

Academic Editors: Ana Isabel Fraguas-Sánchez, Raquel Fernández García and Francisco Bolás-Fernández

Received: 6 June 2022
Accepted: 27 June 2022
Published: 30 June 2022

Publisher's Note: MDPI stays neutral with regard to jurisdictional claims in published maps and institutional affiliations.

Abstract: The present research was aimed to develop a terbinafin hydrochloride (TH)-encapsulated solid lipid nanoparticles (SLNs) hydrogel for improved antifungal efficacy. TH-loaded SLNs were obtained from glyceryl monostearate (lipid) and Pluronic® F68 (surfactant) employing high-pressure homogenization. The ratio of drug with respect to lipid was optimized, considering factors such as desired particle size and highest percent encapsulation efficiency. Lyophilized SLNs were then incorporated in the hydrogel prepared from 0.2–1.0% *w/v* carbopol 934P and further evaluated for rheological parameters. The z-average, zeta potential and polydispersity index were found to be 241.3 nm, −15.2 mV and 0.415, respectively. The SLNs show a higher entrapment efficiency of about 98.36%, with 2.12 to 6.3602% drug loading. SEM images, XRD and the results of the DSC, FTIR show successful preparation of SLNs after freeze drying. The TH-loaded SLNs hydrogel showed sustained drug release (95.47 ± 1.45%) over a period of 24 h. The results reported in this study show a significant effect on the zone of inhibition than the marketed formulation and pure drug in *Candida albicans* cultures, with better physical stability at cooler temperatures. It helped to enhance skin deposition inthe ex vivostudy and improved, in vitro and in vivo, the antifungal activity.

Keywords: solid lipid nanoparticles; hydrogel; antifungal; terbinafin; *Candida albicans*

1. Introduction

Fungal infections of the skin, scalp, or nails are treated by oral and topical antifungal agents. Terbinafin hydrochloride is a widely used drug for the treatment of fungal infections of the skin, and it has been well tolerated by oral or topical administration [1]. However, insufficient bioavailability and hepatic first pass metabolism (about 40%) made the topical route more suitable for drug administration [2]. It offers and enables a reduction in the systemic load as well as systemic side effects of the active pharmaceutical ingredients (API) [3]. Controlled drug delivery systems are one of the best approaches that have the potential to cure disease conditions by targeting specific cells in the body [4]. Thus, site specificity and time specificity are the advantages of nanotechnology, a novel drug delivery system [5]. Nanoparticles have proven their potential to target the cells or receptors at the site of action. Hence, this can be helpful to overcome the pharmacokinetic drawbacks of drugs [2].

Solid lipid nanoparticles act as a carrier for the delivery of therapeutic agents. SLNs are generally fabricated by the incorporation of a solid form of lipid into the o/w type of emulsion with the help of a stabilizer, which results in the easier entrapment of API. SLNs are composed of physiological supermolecules, and hence the pathways for lipid transportation and metabolism are already gifted within the body to confirm thein vivofate of the carrier. These are stable for an extended period and straight forward to rescale compared to different mixture systems, so they are also vital for several modes of targeting. SLNs contain a variety of drugs from various pharmacological categories, such as steroids, vitamins, cancer-fighting agents, and antifungals [6–12]. Since SLNs are speculated to deliver drugs to the site of action [13], they are also widely used for topical applications. These SLN formulations additionally supply higher localization, occlusiveness, controlled unleash, and skin association for higher effectivity [14].

Previously, Vaghasiyaet al.prepared TH-loaded SLNs by the solvent-injection method, but the SLNs with the desired entrapment efficiency and lower particle size were not obtained [15]. Then the SLNs were supplied in carbopol gel, which shows improved skin retention ability upon topical application to the abdominal skin. In another study, Chenet al.manufactured SLNs by the microemulsion technique using glyceryle monostearate (GMS) and glyceryle behenate. The combination of both these lipids enhanced the skin penetration of TH across the dermal layers and resolved the practical problem of a longer administration period [16]. All this literature revealed that incorporation of GMS as a lipid for SLNs preparation helps to improve the skin penetration, whereas SLNs incorporation in carbopol gel enhances the skin retention on the skin. Hence, the present study was designed to prepare a TH-loaded SLNs carbopol gel to enhance the skin retention with improved skin penetration upon topical application for the treatment of fungal infection. Terbinafine is a standard agent that structurally belongs to the allylamine category and pharmacologically acts by selective inhibition of plant life squalene epoxidase. It is a broad-spectrum agent having associated activity against yeast, fungi, molds, and dermatophytes [17]. The formulation of TH is difficult on the bench, since it is very lipophilic (log *p* value of 3.3) and nearly insoluble in water. Topical application of TH has the advantages of direct distribution and targeting ability to the affected area of the skin, as well as low dose requirements and minimal toxicities [18].

2. Material and Methods

2.1. Drug and Chemicals

Terbinafine hydrochloride was obtained from FDC LIMITED, (Waluj, Aurangabad India) as a gift sample. Colorcon Asia Pvt. Ltd., (Verna, Goa, India) provided glyceryl monostearate (GMS), Compritol 888 ATO, and Precirol ATO5. The Hi-Media Lab. Pvt. Ltd., Mumbai, (India) provided sabouraud dextrose agar (SDA), chitosan, and pluronic F68. Using a Milli-Q system, pure water was obtained (Millipore, Billerica, MA, USA). All of the other compounds were of the analytical variety.

2.2. Drug and Excipient Compatibility Studies

2.2.1. Thermal Analysis

Differential scanning calorimetry (DSC) was used to examine the drug, polymers, and their physical mixture with TH. DSC measurements were carried out in open pans using a DSC Q20 (Mettler-Toledo, Zurich, Switzerland) with a sample size of approximately 5 mg, weighed in each aluminum pan. From 0 to 400 °C, samples were gradually heated at a rate of 10 °C per minute. Nitrogen was supplied at a flow rate of 40 mL/min as a purging gas. Universal Analysis software version 4.5 A, build 4.5.0.5, was used to examine the data and dates acquired (TA Instruments, Inc., New Castle, DE, USA). The procedure was repeated for the freeze-dried SLNs.

2.2.2. Fourier Transform Infrared (FTIR) Spectroscopy

The possible interaction of a physical mixture of drug and polymer was investigated using the FTIR spectroscopy technique. The samples were dried for 2 h in a hot air oven at 50 °C. The samples were crushed and completely mixed with potassium bromide at a ratio of 1:100 (Sample:KBr), and circular KBr discs were formed at a pressure of 10 t/nm^2 by compression The IR spectra obtained were compared and studied to detect, the physical interactions between the drug and the polymers, if any.

2.3. Preparation of Solid Lipid Nanoparticles (SLNs)

Solid lipid nanoparticles (SLNs) containing TH were prepared by the hot high-pressure homogenization method reported previously [19]. In brief, glyceryl monostearate (GMS) used as a lipid phase was melted by heating in a water bath at 80 °C. About 1.0–3.0% *w/w* TH was added to the molten lipid phase simultaneously. The aqueous solution of pluronic F68 was prepared separately and was dispersed in the previously prepared molten lipid phase at 80 °C with continuous stirring on a magnetic stirrer (Remi Instruments Ltd., Mumbai, India) at 400 RPM for 30 min to get a pre-emulsion. The prepared pre-emulsion was subjected to homogenization using a high-pressure homogenizer (PANDA 2K, Niro Soavi, Parma, Italy) at 500 bar pressure for up to 5 cycles to form the SLN dispersion. The prepared SLN dispersion was allowed to cool at normal conditions and was subject to characterization.

2.4. Characterization of SLNs

2.4.1. Particle Size, Polydispersity Index and Zeta Potential Measurement

Photon correlation spectroscopy (PCS) was used to determine the particle size of the blank and TH-loaded SLNs using dynamic light scattering on a Zetasizer® nano (Model: Zen 3600, Malvern Instruments, Malvern, UK) aided by a 5-mW helium neon laser (wavelength output of 633 nm). The experiment was carried out at a temperature of 25 °C and a 173° angle [20]. On the instrument, a run time of at least 40–80 s was set. As a dispersion medium, water was used. The polydispersity index was also used to investigate the nanoparticle dispersion. Smoluchowski's equation was used to calculate the zeta potential from the electrophoretic mobility using a previously described approach [21]. All results were obtained in triplicate.

2.4.2. Percent Drug Loading

About 1 mL of the SLN dispersion was taken into pre-weighed vials, allowed to freeze dry, and then dissolved in methanol [22]. The concentration of TH present in the solution was estimated by spectrophotometry at 283 nm. The below formulae were applied to calculate the drug-loading capacity (DL):

$$\%\ Drug\ Loading = \frac{Mass\ of\ drug\ in\ SLNs}{Mass\ of\ SLNs\ containing\ drug} \times 100$$

2.4.3. Entrapment Efficiency

The entrapment efficiency (EE), or the amount of TH contained in SLNs, was assessed using a variety of methods previously described [23]. One milliliter of SLNs containing TH was put into a Centricon® reservoir (Model: YM-100, Amicon, Millipore, Bedford, MA, USA). The dispersion of SLNs was centrifuged at 15,000× *g* rpm for 40 min. Filtration was used to eliminate the free TH component. Dilution with wood spirit (methanol) was carried out for the dispersed filtrate, followed by TH content determination using HPLC to compute the total concentration of TH (C_t) and the concentration of TH retained in the filtrate post centrifugation (C_f). The entrapment efficiency was determined using the following equation:

$$\%\ EE = \frac{Amount\ of\ drug\ (C_t) - Amont\ of\ drug\ in\ supernatant\ (C_f)}{Amount\ of\ drug\ added} \times 100$$

2.5. Preparation of Lyophilized SLNs

The SLN dispersions were rapidly frozen at −75 °C along with the mannitol as a cryoprotectant in varying concentrations, such as 2, 4, 6, 8 and 10% *w/v* in a deep-freezer for 1 h. The mannitol-containing SLN dispersions were then freeze dried (Freeze Drier, VirTis Benchtop SP Industries, Warminster, PA, USA) for 72 h by applying a vacuum at 100 mTorr. Freeze-dried SLN powder was then collected and used for further analysis.

2.6. Characterization of Lyophilized SLNs

2.6.1. Scanning Electron Microscopy (SEM)

SEM (JSM-6390LV, JEOL, Tokyo, Japan) was used to examine the morphological structures of the TH and optimized freeze-dried SLNs formulation [24]. A freeze-dried SLNs formulation that had been optimized was put on double-sided carbon tape and placed on a brass stub. Using the auto fine coater, a thin layer of metal palladium was applied to the surface powder (Model: JFC1600, Jeol Ltd., Tokyo, Japan). A scanning electron microscope (Model: JSM-6390LV, Jeol Ltd., Tokyo, Japan) attenuated with a digital camera was used to examine the metal-coated samples at a 10 kilovolt accelerating voltage.

2.6.2. X-ray Diffraction Analysis (XRD)

The changes in polymorphic form and crystalline nature of the drugs after the formation of SLNs were studied by an XRD. The XRD patterns of the samples (API, physical mixture of API and lipid, freeze-dried SLNs formulation) were estimated by an X-ray diffractometer (BruckerAxs, D8 Advance, Karlsruhe, Germany) provided with a source of radiation, a Cu-Kα line, operated at a 40 kV voltage and a current of 30 mA. Each sample was analyzed in the 2θ angle range between 100 and 600. The estimation was carried out at a scanning rate of 30/min and a step size of 0.020 was maintained.

2.7. Formulation of the TH-Loaded SLNs Hydrogel

The hydrogel of TH-loaded SLNs was prepared by using different gelling agents, such ascarbopol 934P, chitosan, and pluronic F127 [25]. The result of a preliminary study shows that carbopol 934P (0.2–1.0% *w*/*v*) and chitosan (0.5–2.0% *w*/*v*) were found to be compatible with TH-loaded lyophilized SLNs. Carbopol 934P showed greater ease of spreadability than chitosan. Hence, carbopol 934P was used for the preparation of the gel and chitosan was used as gelling agent to improve the gel strength. Different concentrations of carbopol 934P were dispersed using a mechanical stirrer at a speed of 800 rpm for a 3 h duration in order to improve the stiffness of the gel with optimum viscosity. Triethanolamine (0.05% *w*/*w*) was added with the aid of a magnetic stirrer to neutralize the gelling system. Phenyl mercuric nitrate (0.02% *v*/*v*) was added as a preservative to prevent it from microbial contamination.

2.8. Characterization of the TH-Loaded SLN-Based Hydrogel

2.8.1. Measurement of Viscosity and pH

The apparent viscosity and rheological behavior of the TH-loaded SLN-based gel was measured using a Brookfield Viscometer provided with spindle no. 5 at 10 to100 rpm [26]. A pH meter (Elico Pvt Ltd., Hydrabad, India) was used to measure the pH of the gel formulations by dissolving one gram of the TH-loaded SLN-based gel in 100 mL of distilled water. The pH meter was calibrated with buffered solutions of pH 4.0 and 7.0 before measuring the pH of the samples.

2.8.2. Extrudability and Spreadability

The formulations were crammed in the collapsible tubes. The extrudability of the formulation was estimated, which is explained in terms of weights in grams required to extrude a 0.5 cm ribbon of gel in 10 s.

The spreadability represents the extent of area to which a gel readily spreads, once applied on the affected part. The spreadability confines the therapeutic efficacy of a formulation. The Wooden block and glass slide apparatus was employed to check the spreadability of the TH-loaded SLN-based gel [27]. This is expressed in terms of the time (seconds) taken by the two slides to slip off from the gel and be placed in between the slides under the direction of a certain load. Separation of the two slides shall be in the minimum time and as low as possible, which is better for a good spreadability of the gel. About 95 g of gel was placed to the pan and the time required to separate the upper slide (movable) completely from the fixed slides was noted. It was calculated by using the formula $S = M \times L/T$, where M is the weight tied to upper slide, L is the length of glass slides, and T is the time taken to separate the slides.

2.8.3. Determination of Gel Strength

The gel strength test was performed using the gel strength apparatuses, using a modified method previously reported by Yong et al. [28]. About 50 g of TH-loaded SLN-based gel was transferred into a 100 mL measuring cylinder and a piston (weighing about 35 g) was then placed onto the surface of the gel. The gel strength was measured as the time (seconds) required for moving the piston by 5 cm through the gel. If necessary, various weights were placed when more than 5 min were taken to drop the apparatus into the gel

2.9. Determination of Drug Content

A 100 mL volumetric flask [29] was used to properly weigh 200 mg of TH-loaded SLN-based hydrogel before dilution with methanol and 45 min of sonication. Following sonication, 5 mL was pipetted out and diluted with methanol once more, this time up to 50 mL. Finally, the average values of three separate measurements of absorbance at 283 nm were calculated.

2.10. In Vitro Drug Release

An in vitro drug release study of the TH-loaded SLN-based hydrogel was performed using Franz diffusion [30]. The dialysis membrane (Himedia® Pvt. Ltd., Mumbai, India) has a cut-off molecular weight of 12,000–16,000 Dalton and a pore size of 2.4 nm and is placed between the donor and receptor compartments. This membrane allows passage of drugs to the receptor compartment from the donor compartment. Phosphate-buffered saline (PBS), pH 7.4, was filled in the receptor compartment. The whole assembly was shaken on a magnetic stirrer at a speed of 100 rpm and a temperature of 37 $\pm$ 0.5 °C. Samples were periodically withdrawn from the receptor compartment and absorbance was measured at 283 nm. The volume of sample withdrawn was replenished each time with the same volume of fresh PBS. The results were taken in triplicates and the cumulative percent drug release was calculated and plotted against the time.

2.11. ExVivo Skin Permeation Study

The exvivo permeation study of the TH-loaded SLN-based gel was carried out on abdominal skin of Sprague-Dawley rats using the procedure reported previously [31]. The hair and subcutaneous tissues were removed using a shaving razor. The dermis side was wiped with isopropyl alcohol to get rid of the residual fat material, washed with distilled water, and stored under pH 7.4 PBS in a freezer till further use. The Franz diffusion cell with an efficient and effective diffusion area of 3.14 cm^2 was used for this study. The skin was placed over the diffusion cell along with the dermal side to bear with the receptor phase. Diffusion medium of 40 mL (pH 7.4 PBS) was filled in the receptor compartment and was then subjected to pausing to be stirred less, at 100 rpm, using a magnetic stirrer. The equilibrium of the system was allowed to sustain at 37 $\pm$ 0.5 °C using a water bath. About 100 mg of gel was applied and spread over the diffusion area on the skin. The sample solution, for estimation, was taken out at predetermined time intervals (0.5 to 14 and 24 h) from the receptor compartment and replenished with the fresh buffer medium. Every study was continued for a day (24 h) and the percent drug released across the skin was calculated.

2.12. Evaluation of Antifungal Efficacy of Formulation

2.12.1. In Vitro Antifungal Activity

In vitro antifungal activity was measured by the "cup plate method" by using Sabouraud dextrose agar (SDA), a medium for the cultivation of *Candida albicans*, and the previously sterilized antifungal assay agar medium. In brief, a quantity of fungal culture equal to 1 mL was inoculated and thoroughly mixed with the antifungal assay agar media. The agar medium was left to solidify in the Petridish and 4 holes were made by a cork borer having a diameter of 1 cm. A quantity of gel formulation equal to 30 mg was poured into 2 holes, and the remaining 2 holes were sampled with a marketed gel formulation. It was subjected to diffuse at 25–27 degrees Celsius for an hour. The plates were placed in an incubator at 25 °C. The diameters of the growth zones of inhibition were measured every 24 h for 3 days.

2.12.2. In Vivo Antifungal Activity

The in vivo antifungal activity of the produced mixture was determined using a *C. albicans*-induced mycosis model in Wistar albino rats (100–150 g) [32]. The entire protocol was followed with the agreement of the Institutional Animal Ethics Committee. To begin, the rat's hair was removed using a hair removal treatment (depilation). The skin was marked on a 2- to 3-cm^2 region, and then the skin was scraped out somewhat the next day using sandpaper. A glass rod was used to apply a previously prepared *C. albicans* inoculums. Three groups of Wistar albino rats were formed, each with five animals. The first group was designated as a control group that received no therapy. A commercially available terbinafine gel was provided to the second group. The third set of animals received the test formulation. Except for the first group, animals were treated for 6 days after infection. Animals were observed for any obvious morphological alterations. After six days, the animal skin was cleaned with a cotton swab. Skin was removed from the treatment area and homogenized in a tissue homogenizer with 5 mL saline. After streaking on a solid yeast extract–peptone–dextrose medium, the homogenate was incubated at 25 °C for 4 days. The number of colony-forming units (CFUs) on the agar plate was counted, and the logarithm of the number of CFUs per infected site was determined. A positive animal was defined as one that had more than one fungal colony.

2.13. Stability Study

The lyophilized SLNs and TH-loaded SLN-based gel were stored in airtight containers and further subjected to evaluation of physical stability during storage conditions according to International Conference on Harmonization (ICH) Q1A (R2) guidelines (FDA, 2003). The particle size as well as percentage of drug content were also determined periodically to check the physical stability of the formulations.

An accelerated stability study for the TH-loaded SLN-based gel was also carried out for 3 months. In the first test, the TH-loaded SLN-based gel was packed in a collapsible aluminum tube and kept at 25 °C and a humidity of 60%. Secondly, another sample of the formulation was kept at a freezing temperature (Remi Instruments Ltd., Mumbai, India). After a predetermined time interval, the TH-loaded SLN-based gel was evaluated by measuring the pH and determining the drug content.

2.14. Statistical Analysis

The mean and standard deviation were used to express all of the data (SD). GraphPad® Prism® software version 5.03, Dr. Harvey Motulsky, San Diego, USA, was used to conduct the statistical analysis, which included a two-way analysis of variance (ANOVA) and a Bonferroni post-test (San Diego, CA, USA). If the p value was less than 0.05, the differences between the means were judged to be significant.

3. Results and Discussion

3.1. Drug and Excipient Compatibility Study

3.1.1. Thermal Analysis

The DSC thermograms of pure TH (A), glyceryl monostearate (B), physical mixture of TH, as well as GMS (C) and lyophilized SLNs (D) are represented in Figure 1. TH showed a characteristic crystalline form melting peak at about 209.26 °C and the DSC curve of glyceryl monostearate reflected one endothermic peak at 60.93 °C. The SLNs dispersion showed a small endothermic peak around 230.31 °C. The DSC curve of TH showed a characteristic crystalline form melting peak at about 209.26 °C and the DSC curve of glyceryl monostearate showed one endothermic peak at 60.93 °C. These results revealed the absence of an interaction between the drug and lipid excipient. Previous research [33] interpreted similar types of findings [33]. The SLNs dispersion showed a small endothermic peak around 230.31 °C. This change in melting point is indicative of the transformation of the crystalline form to the amorphous form of a drug.

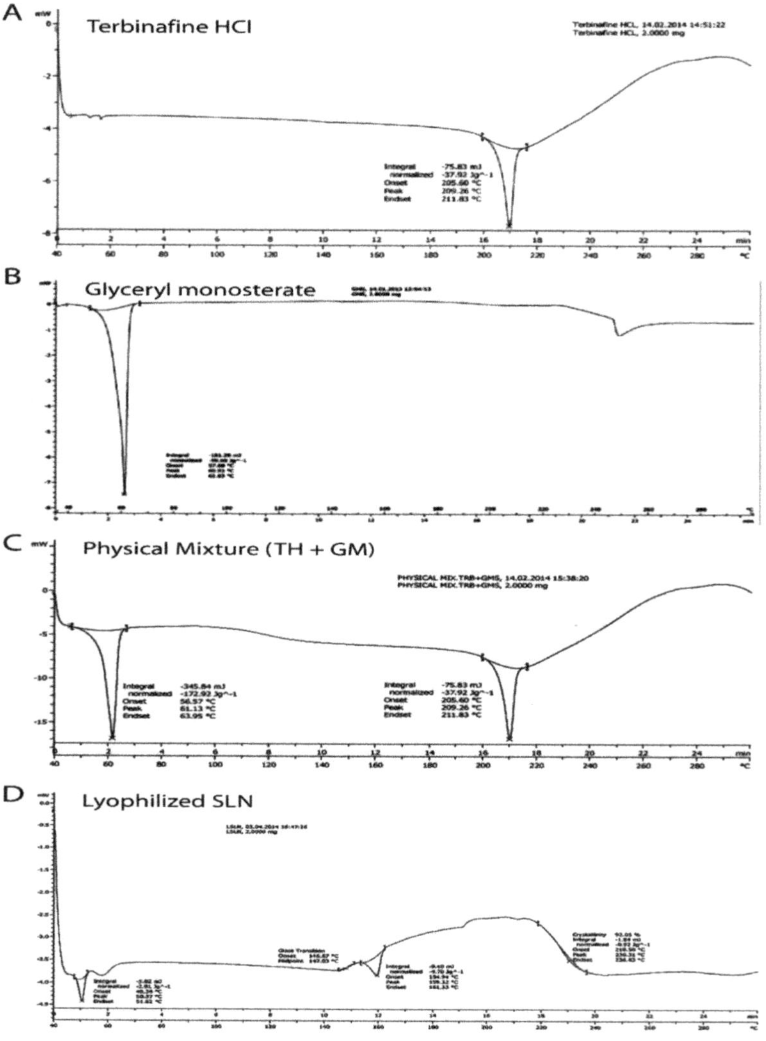

Figure 1. Differentialscanning calorimetric thermograms showing the endothermic peak of terbinafin hydrochloride (**A**); glyceryle monostearate (**B**); physical mixture of terbinafin hydrochloride (TH) and glyceryle monostearate (GM) (**C**); and lyophilized solid lipid nanoparticles (**D**).

3.1.2. Fourier Transform Infrared (FTIR) Spectroscopy

Figure 2 illustrates the FTIR spectrum of pure TH (A), glyceryl monostearate (B), physical mixture of TH, GMS (C), and lyophilized SLNs (D). All the characteristic peaks obtained at wave numbers 2400, 1700, 1400, and 850 cm^{-1} were fromthe drugs and are present in the spectrum of a formulation similar to that of TH. The peaks found in the physical mixture of TH and GMS were present at the same wave number as those of the individual peaks of TH and GMS. Thus, no interaction of the drug with a lipid can be concluded.

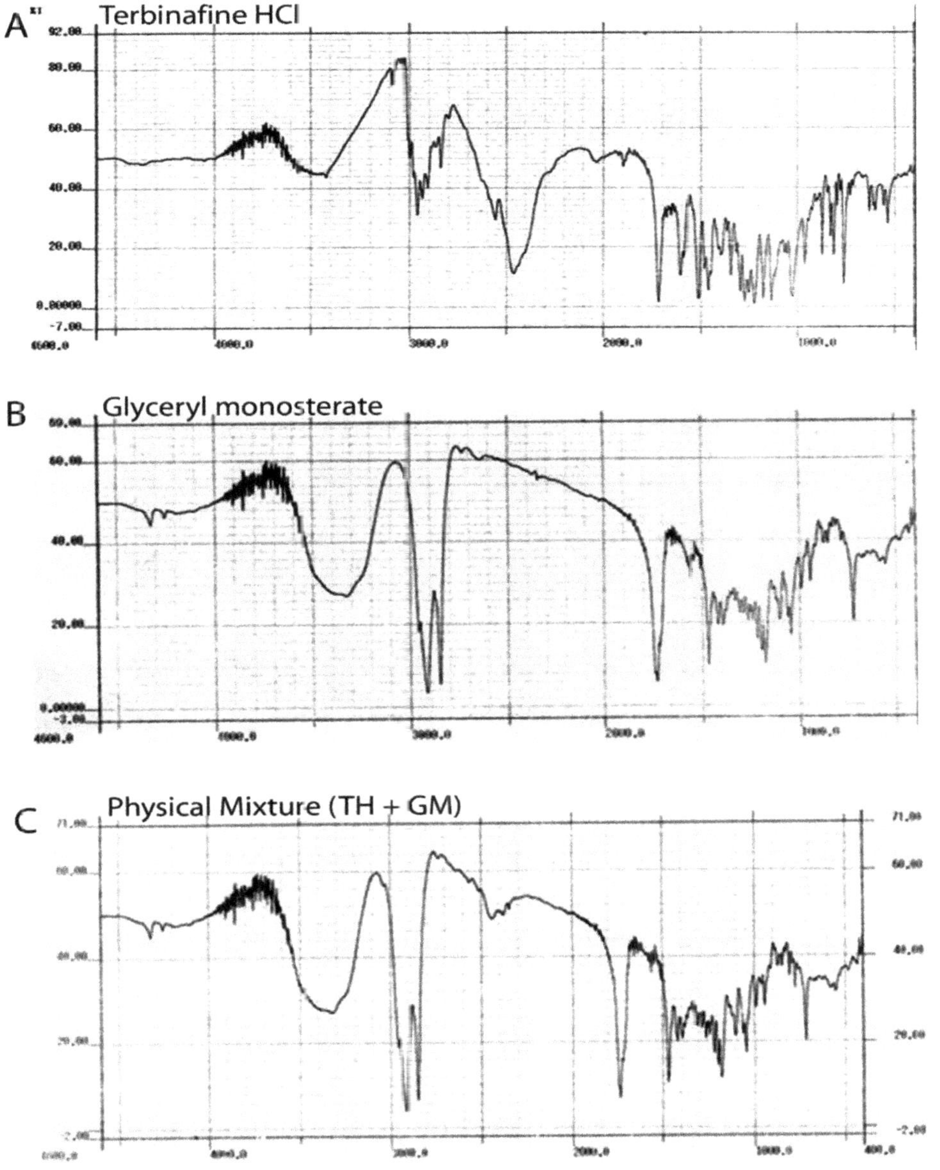

Figure 2. FTIR spectrum of pure TH (**A**), glyceryl monostearate (**B**), physical mixture of TH and GMS (**C**).

3.2. Characterization of SLNs

3.2.1. Particle Size, Polydispersity Index, and Zeta Potential

The data are presented in Table 1. The particle size of the SLNs was found to be in the range of 241.3 to 321.8 nm. Particle size analysis revealed that the increase in the size of the particles is directly proportional to the increase in the amount of lipid [34].

Table 1. Characterization of the formulated SLNs.

Formulation Code	Particle Size (nm)	Zeta Potential (mV)	Polydispersity Index	% Drug Loading	% Encapsulation Efficiency
P F 1	241.3	−15.2	0.415	6.3602	98.36
P F 2	248.7	−18.1	0.47	4.2192	97.84
P F 3	274.7	−19.4	0.542	3.1652	97.49
P F 4	302.4	−20.2	0.577	2.5322	96.89
P F 5	321.8	−24.8	0.543	2.12	95.39

The polydispersity index was found in the range of 0.415 to 0.577. The lower values of the polydispersity index correspond to the wide distribution of particles.

The zeta potential values of all batches were found within the range of −15.2 mV to −24.8 mV. The value of the zeta potential from −15.0 mV to −30.0 mV indicates that the dispersions remain deflocculated owing to electrostatic repulsion between the particles and are physically stable over time [35,36]. The zeta potential was influenced by the anionic property of the lipid matrix and thus reflects the physical stability of the SLNs [37].

3.2.2. Percent Drug Loading and Encapsulation Efficiency

The data are presented in Table 1. The drug-loading percentage was found in the range of 2.12 to 6.3602. The TH-loaded lyophilized SLNs prepared using the high-pressure homogenization technique showed a higher entrapment efficiency, which is about 98.36%. A similar type of result was reported previously [38].

3.3. Characterization of Lyophilized SLNs

3.3.1. Scanning Electron Microscopy

Scanning electron microscopy photographs of TH and the optimized batch of SLNs (PF1) are presented in Figure 3. The hexagonal crystalline form of TH (Figure 3A) was observed on the scanning electron microscope images, with varying size of particles. Figure 3B illustrates the longitudinal amorphous structures, which confirm the formation of SLNs.

The varying particle size was obtained during the preparation of the SLNs, as the previous literature reported the increased in particle size while usingcompritol and pluronic f68 as a surfactant, and there were almost a 4-fold increase in particle size observed. This increase in particle size leads to the increased viscosity of the lipid matrix. On the other hand, the incorporation of a higher amount of drugs could be the reason for the significant increase in viscosity, which directly relates to the increase in particle size of the SLNs [39–41]. However, the size shown in the figure is the dimension of the particles and it is not considered as an average mean diameter of the particles. The mean diameter of the SLNs was found in the range of 241.3 to 321.8 nm.

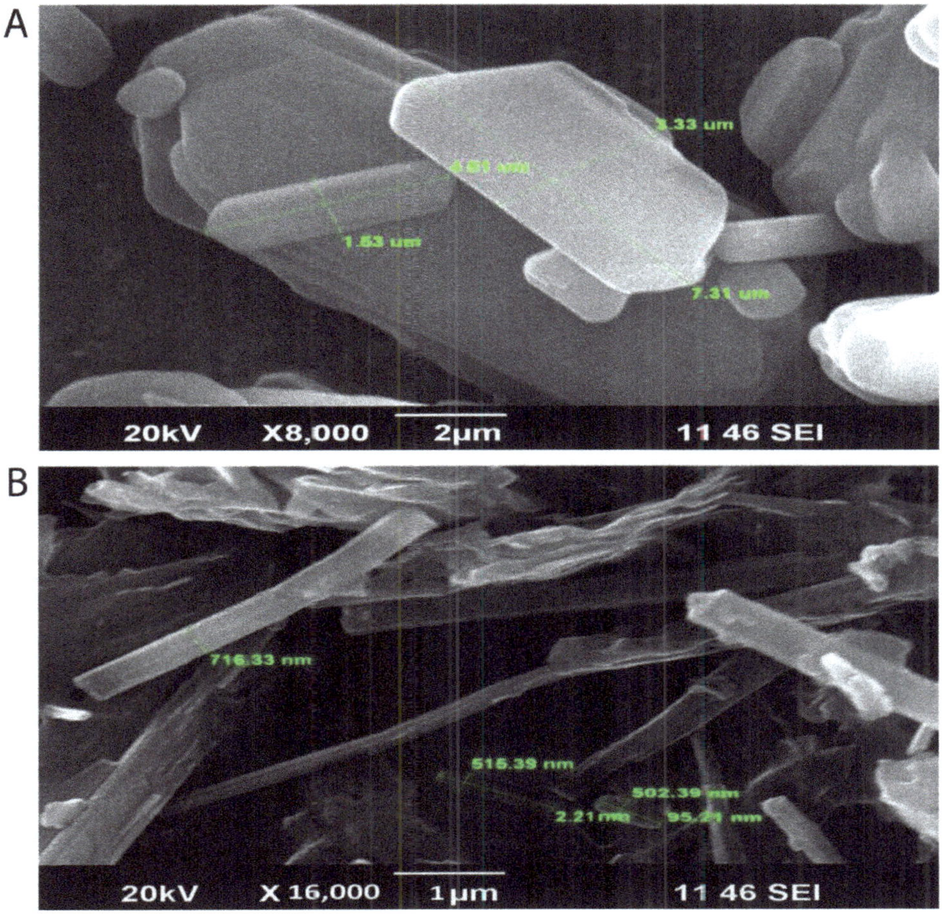

Figure 3. Scanning electron microscopy images showing the hexagonal crystalline form of TH (**A**) with varying sizes of particles and longitudinal amorphous structures, which confirm the formation of SLNs (**B**).

3.3.2. X-ray Diffraction Studies

In Figure 4, X-ray diffraction patterns of TH, physical mixture bearing the TH along with the glyceryl monostearate, and the freeze-dried SLNs preparation are presented. The X-ray diffractogram of TH shows sharp peaks at diffraction angles (2θ) of 19.656°, 20.914°, 23.750°, 25.032°, 29.948°, 30.688°, 35.508°, 37.780°, 42.921°, 53.747°, and 56.013°, which confirms the typical crystalline pattern. However, all the major characteristic crystalline peaks become visible in the diffractogram of the nanoparticulate system but with low intensity. Thus, it confirms that some amount of the drug is converted into its amorphous form.

The results of the X-ray diffractometry analysis were supported by FTIR and DSC studies.

These results collectively indicated that the crystallinity of the drug decreased when formulated as the SLNs using lipids.

Further, they suggested the conversion of TH from crystalline to molecular form.

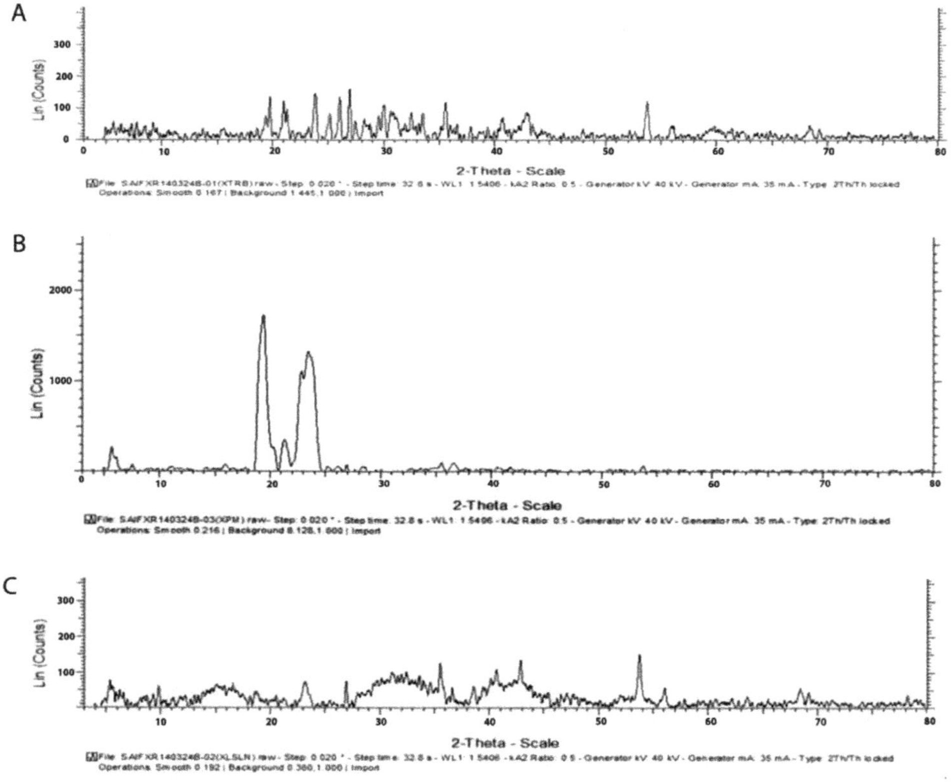

Figure 4. X-ray diffractogram of TH shows sharp peaks at diffraction angles (2θ) with the typical crystalline pattern (**A**), csrystalline pattern of physical Mixture of glyceryl monosterate (**B**) and Freezed Dried SLNs preparation (**C**).

3.4. Characterization of the TH-Loaded SLN-Based Hydrogel

3.4.1. Rheological Behavior

The formulation showed pseudo-plastic flow behavior as results revealed in Figure 5. The SLN-loaded hydrogel revealed a distinct up and down curve; that is, the samples were non-Newtonian in nature, with a thixotropic behavior. The formulated hydrogel takes time to come back to its original viscosity state after application of shear stress but during this process it maintained its structural properties associated with the gel network [42]. Rheological and texture analyses showed that the TH-loaded SLN-based gel had satisfied the ideal rheological and texture properties in order to assist its topical application.

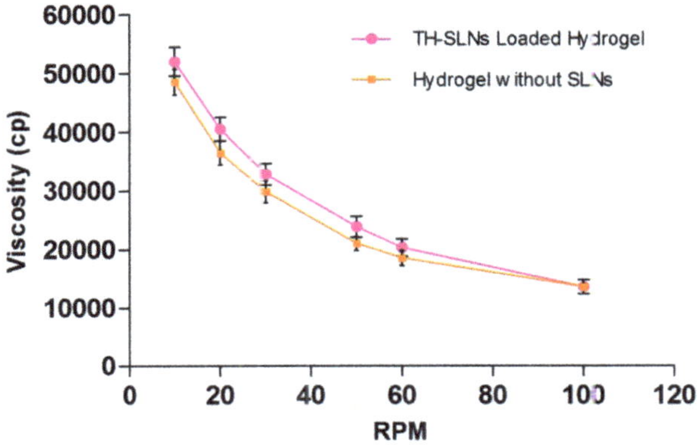

Figure 5. Formulations showed pseudo-plastic flow behavior. Rheological behaviors of the TH-loaded SLNs containing the carbopol hydrogel, showing no coincidence of the up curve with the down curve, indicating non-Newtonian thixotropic behavior.

3.4.2. Determination of Viscosity, pH, Gel Strength, Spreadability, Extrudability and Drug Content

These gel formulation characteristics reflect improved patient compliance for topical application. The formulation was subjected to the determination of these values ($n = 6$), and the mean ± SEM for the viscosity of the TH-loaded SLN hydrogel is presented in Table 2.

Table 2. Rheological behavior of the TH-loaded SLNs hydrogel.

Viscosity(Cp)	RPM	Viscosity(Cp)	RPM
52,000	10	13,570	100
40,460	20	18,500	60
32,800	30	21,000	50
23,890	50	29,800	30
20,320	60	36,400	20
13,570	100	48,500	10

It was free from any particles, easily spreadable, extrudable, and followed a pseudo-plastic flow. The optimized SLNs were then incorporated into the Carbopol 934P gel base with tri-ethanolamine as a neutralizer and phenylmercuric nitrate as a preservative. The formulated gel appeared white in color and was acceptable. The pH of the formulated gel was found within the normal pH range of the skin (pH~5.5 to 6.5), which is under the range (pH 3–9) essentially required for treatment of skin infections [43].

Gel strength is an important parameter for topical gels. It indicates suitability for easy application and skin retention without leakage after application. Our formulation showed better gel strength, and that was achieved with 0.6% Carbopol 934P. Spreadability dictates the ease of application of a gel onto the skin's surface [44]. The formulated gel showed spreadability in the range of 30.46 ± 0.25 to 36.23 ± 0.61 g cm/s.

The viscosity and consistency are both correlative properties ofgel formulation. Consistency is inversely proportional to the rate of shear. Non-Newtonian flow (shear thinning) is generally preferred, when applied under high shear conditions, as low resistance was observed. Further, the pseudoplastic nature also reduces viscosity decreases, as observed in the formulation. This characteristic property, in turn, defines high spreadability due to the decrease in viscosity and resistance to flow.

3.5. *In Vitro Release Study*

The in vitro release pattern was determined using a Franz diffusion cell with a dialysis membrane with diffusion media, a phosphate buffer (pH 7.4). It is observed that 50% of the drug was found to release within the initial first 2 h, while, approximately, about 80% of the drug from the TH-loaded SLN-based gel was released upto 12 h (Figure 6A). The SLN-loaded gel showed a 95.47 ± 1.45% cumulative drug release over the period of 24 h (n = 6). When compared to conventional marketed TH cream, the SLN-based gel exhibited greater antifungal activity, even at a lower concentration. A Higuchi model of the drug release patternshowed a sustained released pattern of the drug found in the SLN-based gel, over a prolonged period. We observed that approximately 60% of the drug was released over the period of 12 h. The rest of the drug remained in the cutaneous layer of the skin. These studies revealed that SLNs as drug carriers were found to deposit in the corneocytes and thus prolongedthe release of the drug [38].

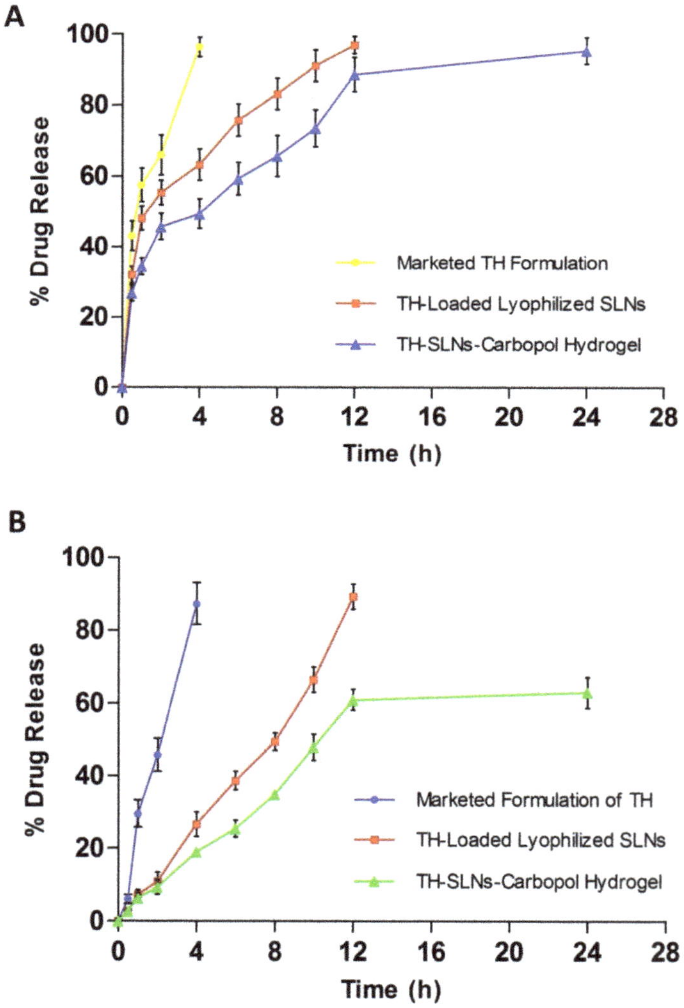

Figure 6. Sustained release of the drug from lyophilized SLNs (**A**) and the TH-loaded carbopol hydrogel over a period of 24 h (**B**).

3.6. Ex Vivo Skin Permeation Studied

We measured the cumulative drug release using rat skin (Figure 6B). We discovered that approximately 60% of the drug was released over a 12-h period. The rest of the drug remained in the cutaneous layer of the skin. The ex vivo drug release data conclude that the SLN-based gel might target the drug to the skin, thus reducing the systemic access of the drug. Ultimately, the systemic side effects can be reduced.

3.7. In Vitro Antifungal Activity

In the *Candida albicans* culture, the TH-loaded SLNs gel (0.6%) showed a significant effect on the zone of inhibition when compared with the marketed formulation (Figure 7). The zones of inhibition for the test formulation and conventional marketed formulation were measured to be 34.5 ± 0.69 mm and 27.9 ± 0.49 mm, respectively (n = 6). It proves the fungicidal activity of the TH-loaded SLNs gel is comparable to the marketed formulation. The TH shows significant antifungal activity against a broad range of fungi, as stated in previous literature [45]. Whereas when we incorporated TH in the SLN-loaded hydrogel, thein vitroantifungal activity of TH was improved due to the sustained release of TH. The alteration in the release of TH after loading into SLNs leads to its enhanced activity [15].

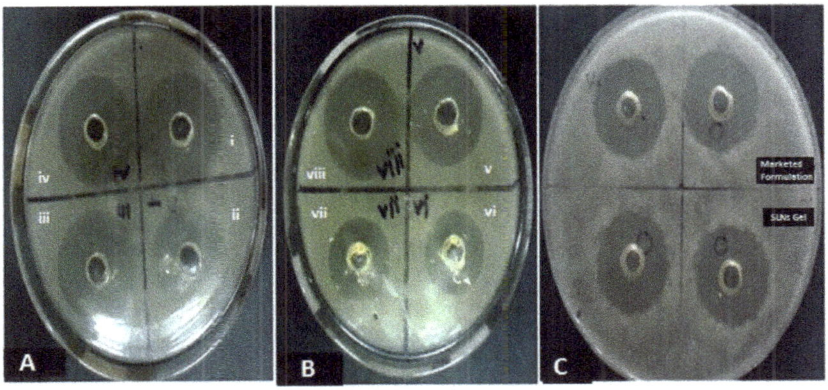

Figure 7. The in vitro antifungal activity of the TH-loaded SLNs carbopol hydrogel, showing significant effect on zone of inhibition compared to the marketed formulation in *Candida albicans* at different time intervals of 24 h on consecutive days for 3 days (**A**–**C**).

3.8. In Vivo Efficacy of the SLN Hydrogel against C. albicans-Induced Dermal Mycosis in Rats

In vivoefficacy of the test formulation was assessed by the *C. albicans*-induced rat mycosis model. Table 3 showed the number of animals with a positive culture out of seven animals included per group and the log CFU per infected site on rat skin. Isolates of *Candida* were scrapped from the skin and a viability test was carried out. In the TH-loaded SLN hydrogel-treated group, only 2 out of 7 animals exhibited a positive culture test. While 7 out of 7 and 6 out of 7 were found in the control (base formulation) and TH in the ethanol solution group, respectively. In the marketed conventional terbinafine formulation-treated group, only 1 animal showed a positive culture test out of 7. Rapid recovery of infection was observed with marketed conventional terbinafin and TH-loaded SLNs hydrogel formulation-treated groups. The marketed conventional formulation was applied twice a day on the infected site. This topical application of the commercial gel leads to the fast recovery of the infected animals, which may be due to the higher dosing of TH. However, the drawback of the marketed conventional formulations is that they should be applied from time to time; hence, the minimum effective concentration needs to be maintained during the whole therapy. However, the SLN-loaded hydrogel acts as a sustained release system and was successfully used to avoid multiple dosing but shows slower recovery than the marketed conventional topical formulation. Statistical significance of the latter was checked by one-way ANOVA and Dunnett's multiple comparison test. Significant efficacy of the TH-loaded SLNs hydrogel formulation in treating *Candida* infections when compared to the base formulation (control $p < 0.05$) or TH solution prepared in ethanol ($p < 0.05$) was noted. This result is comparable with that of the marketed conventional terbinafine formulation-treated group, which also showed a significant reduction in log CFU per infected site on rat skin ($p < 0.01$).

Table 3. Colony-forming unit of *Candida albicans* on skin (dermal mycosis) of rats after treatment with the TH-loaded SLN-based hydrogel.

Treatment	No. of Animals with Positive Culture/Total No. of Animals	Log CFU/Infected Sites
Control (Base formulation)	7/7	5.69 ± 0.45
TH solution in ethanol	6/7	4.01 ± 0.33
TH-loaded SLN-based hydrogel	2/7	2.23 ± 0.19 $^{*,\#}$
Conventional marketed formulation of TH	1/7	1.46 ± 0.15 **

* $p < 0.05$, ** $p < 0.01$ vs. control group; $^{\#}$ $p < 0.05$ vs. group received TH solution in ethanol.

3.9. Stability Study

The stability study of the optimized lyophilized SLNs showed a slight change in the drug content from 99.7± 0.6 to 98.0 ± 0.4 at room temperature, whereas from 99.8 ± 0.2 to 99.0 ± 0.2 at freezing temperature, as shown in Table 4. Drug leaching from the solid lipid nanoparticles may be the possible reason [46]. This leaching was lower at the freezing temperature than at the room temperature. Particle size analysis also indicated an increase in the size of the nanoparticles from 241 nm to 269 nm over the period of 3 months during the stability study.

Table 4. Stability of the terbinafine hydrochloride-loaded SLNs.

	Drug Content		Particle Size
	Room Temperature	Refrigerator Temperature	Room Temperature
Initial	100.0	100.0	241 nm
After 1 month	99.7 ± 0.6	99.8 ± 0.2	248 nm
After 2 months	99.4 ± 0.4	99.7 ± 0.5	250 nm
After 3 months	99.1 ± 0.2	99.5 ± 0.6	269 nm

The prepared TH-loaded SLNs hydrogel shows a decrease in the drug content after an observation period of 3 months during the stability study. The drug content was found to be 97.1 ± 0.3 and 98.6 ± 0.4 at room and freezing temperatures, respectively, after 3 months, as shown in Table 5. This indicates the preparation being more stable at a cooling temperature than at room temperature. Again, the pH of the TH-loaded SLNs gel was found to decrease over the period from 6.5 to 6.4 ± 0.1.

Table 5. Stability of the gel containing terbinafine hydrochloride-loaded SLNs.

	Drug content		pH
	Room Temperature	Refrigerator Temperature	Room Temperature
Initial	100.0	100.0	6.5
After 1 month	99.7 ± 0.5	99.8 ± 0.1	6.6 ± 0.1
After 2 months	98.6 ± 0.7	98.9 ± 0.8	6.7 ± 0.0
After 3 months	97.1 ± 0.3	98.6 ± 0.4	6.4 ± 0.1

4. Conclusions

The aim of the study was to formulate an SLN-based gel for topical delivery of TH to decrease the dose, dosing regimen, and side effects associated with oral drug delivery. A high-pressure homogenization technique was employed to prepare the TH-loaded SLNs, prepared with the help of glyceryl monostearate as a lipid matrix, Pluronic® F68, a surfactant, and distilled water as a dispersion medium. The drug-to-lipid ratio was optimized to obtain the desired particle size with the highest percent encapsulation efficiency. Desirable results were obtained while preparing the systemic formulation, such as time saving and a reduction in the number of experiments. Cost effectiveness is also important. In this work, an optimized SLN formulation is offered as an alternative to standard formulations for topical treatment of fungal infections, with an improved permeability and reduced dosing regimen and side effects. In comparison to the commercial formulation, the SLN-based gel showed better skin deposition and in vitro antifungal efficacy. This improved TH–SLN-based gel will improve antifungal therapy's safety, affordability, and tolerance. As a result, developing a topical TH–SLN-based gel could be a unique, industrially scalable, and successful alternative to currently available conventional dosage forms.

Author Contributions: Conceptualization, N.R.R. and D.R.K.; Data curation, S.S.M.; Formal analysis, N.R.R. and D.R.K.; Funding acquisition, P.B.K.; Investigation, P.B.K.; Methodology, A.S.A.; Resources, N.S.; Writing—original draft, A.P.B. and W.F.A.; Writing—review & editing, M.A. and S.M.B.A. All authors have read and agreed to the published version of the manuscript.

Funding: Abdulhakeem S. Alamri would like to acknowledge Taif University for support No. TURSP (2020/288). Syed Mohammed Basheeruddin Asdaq would like to thank AlMaarefa University, Riyadh, Saudi Arabia, for extending financial support (TUMA-2021-1) to do this research.

Institutional Review Board Statement: The research proposal of this study was approved by institutional ethical committee with reference number IAEC/UDPS/2015/22, 12/08/2018.

Informed Consent Statement: Not Applicable.

Data Availability Statement: Data is contained within the article.

Acknowledgments: The authors are thankful to Punjab University for providing the NMR and mass spectra. The authors are also thankful to AlMaarefa University for their support.

Conflicts of Interest: The authors declare no conflict of interest. The company had no role in thedesign of the study; in the collection, analyses, or interpretation of data; in the writing of the manuscript; or in the decision to publish the results.

References

1. Trombino, S.; Mellace, S.; Cassano, R. Solid lipid nanoparticles for antifungal drugs delivery for topical applica-tions. *Ther. Deliv.* **2016**, *7*, 639–647. [CrossRef] [PubMed]
2. Leppert, W.; Malec-Milewska, M.; Zajaczkowska, R.; Wordliczek, J. Transdermal and Topical Drug Administration in the Treatment of Pain. *Molecules* **2018**, *23*, 681. [CrossRef] [PubMed]
3. Scorzoni, L.; de Paula, E.S.A.C.; Marcos, C.M.; Assato, P.A.; de Melo, W.C.; de Oliveira, H.C.; Costa-Orlandi, C.B.; Mendes-Giannini, M.J.; Fusco-Almeida, A.M. Antifungal Therapy: New Advances in the Understanding and Treatment of Mycosis. *Front. Microbiol.* **2017**, *8*, 36. [CrossRef] [PubMed]

4. Ud Din, F.; Aman, W.; Ullah, I.; Qureshi, O.S.; Mustapha, O.; Shafique, S.; Zeb, A. Effective use of nanocarriers as drug delivery systems for the treatment of selected tumors. *Int. J. Nanomed.* **2017**, *12*, 7291–7309. [CrossRef] [PubMed]
5. Patra, J.K.; Das, G.; Fraceto, L.F.; Campos, E.V.R.; del Pilar Rodriguez-Torres, M.; Acosta-Torres, L.S.; Diaz-Torres, L.A.; Grillo, R.; Swamy, M.K.; Sharma, S.; et al. Nano based drug delivery systems: Recent developments and future prospects. *J. Nanobiotechnol.* **2018**, *16*, 71. [CrossRef]
6. Jain, S.K.; Chourasia, M.K.; Masuriha, R.; Soni, V.; Jain, A.; Jain, N.K.; Gupta, Y. Solid Lipid Nanoparticles Bearing Flurbiprofen for Transdermal Delivery. *Drug Deliv.* **2005**, *12*, 207–215. [CrossRef]
7. Maia, C.; Mehnert, W.; Schäfer-Korting, M. Solid lipid nanoparticles as drug carriers for topical glucocorticoids. *Int. J. Pharm.* **2000**, *196*, 165–167. [CrossRef]
8. Liu, J.; Hu, W.; Chen, H.; Ni, Q.; Xu, H.; Yang, X. Isotretinoin-loaded solid lipid nanoparticles with skin targeting for topical delivery. *Int. J. Pharm.* **2007**, *328*, 191–195. [CrossRef]
9. Mei, Z.; Wu, Q.; Hu, S.; Lib, X.; Yang, X. Triptolide Loaded Solid Lipid Nanoparticle Hydrogel for Topical Application. *Drug Dev. Ind. Pharm.* **2005**, *31*, 161–168. [CrossRef]
10. Pople, P.V.; Singh, K.K. Development and evaluation of topical formulation containing solid lipid nanoparticles of vitamin A. *AAPS PharmSciTech* **2006**, *7*, E63–E69. [CrossRef]
11. Souto, E.; Anselmi, C.; Centini, M.; Müller, R. Preparation and characterization of n-dodecyl-ferulate-loaded solid lipid nanoparticles (SLN®). *Int. J. Pharm.* **2005**, *295*, 261–268. [CrossRef]
12. Souto, E.B.; Müller, R.H. The use of SLN and NLC as topical particulate carriers for imidazole antifungal agents. *Pharm.-Int. J. Pharm. Sci.* **2006**, *61*, 431–437.
13. Chen, H.; Chang, X.; Du, D.; Liu, W.; Liu, J.; Weng, T.; Yang, Y.; Xu, H.; Yang, X. Podophyllotoxin-loaded solid lipid nanoparticles for epidermal targeting. *J. Control. Release* **2006**, *110*, 296–306. [CrossRef]
14. Liu, B.; Han, L.; Liu, J.; Han, S.; Chen, Z.; Jiang, L. Co-delivery of paclitaxel and TOS-cisplatin via TAT-targeted solid lipid nanoparticles with synergistic antitumor activity against cervical cancer. *Int. J. Nanomed.* **2017**, *12*, 955–968. [CrossRef]
15. Vaghasiya, H.; Kumar, A.; Sawant, K. Development of solid lipid nanoparticles based controlled release system for topical de-livery of terbinafine hydrochloride. *Eur. J. Pharm. Sci.* **2013**, *4*, 311–322. [CrossRef]
16. Sheu, M.-T.; Chen, Y.-C.; Liu, D.-Z.; Chang, T.-W.; Ho, H.-O. Development of terbinafine solid lipid nanoparticles as a topical delivery system. *Int. J. Nanomed.* **2012**, *7*, 4409–4418. [CrossRef]
17. Khanna, D.; Bharti, S. Luliconazole for the treatment of fungal infections: An evidence-based review. *Core Évid.* **2014**, *9*, 113–124. [CrossRef]
18. Sudaxshina, M. Drug delivery to the nail following topical application. *Int. J. Pharm.* **2004**, *226*, 1–26.
19. Rarokar, N.R.; Khedekar, P.B.; Bharne, A.P.; Umekar, M.J. Development of self-assembled nanocarriers to enhance antitumor efficacy of docetaxel trihydrate in MDA-MB-231 cell line. *Int. J. Biol. Macromol.* **2019**, *125*, 1056–1068. [CrossRef]
20. Silva, A.; Gonzalez, E.; García, M.L.; Egea, M.; Fonseca, J.; Silva, R.; Santos, D.; Souto, E.; Ferreira, D. Preparation, characterization and biocompatibility studies on risperidone-loaded solid lipid nanoparticles (SLN): High pressure homogenization versus ultrasound. *Colloids Surf. B Biointerfaces* **2011**, *86*, 158–165. [CrossRef]
21. Sze, A.; Erickson, D.; Ren, L.; Li, D. Zeta-potential measurement using the Smoluchowski equation and the slope of the cur-rent-time relationship in electroosmotic flow. *J. Colloid Interface Sci.* **2003**, *261*, 402–410. [CrossRef]
22. Rarokar, N.R.; Saoji, S.D.; Raut, N.A.; Taksande, J.B.; Khedekar, P.B.; Dave, V.S. Nanostructured Cubosomes in a Thermoresponsive Depot System: An Alternative Approach for the Controlled Delivery of Docetaxel. *AAPS PharmSciTech* **2015**, *17*, 436–445. [CrossRef]
23. Novelli, F.; De Santis, S.; Diociaiuti, M.; Giordano, C.; Morosetti, S.; Punzi, P.; Sciubba, F.; Viali, V.; Masci, G.; Scipioni, A. Curcumin loaded nanocarriers obtained by self-assembly of a linear d,loctapeptide-poly(ethylene glycol) conjugate. *Eur. Polym. J.* **2018**, *98*, 28–38. [CrossRef]
24. Saoji, S.D.; Raut, N.A.; Dhore, P.W.; Borkar, C.D.; Popielarczyk, M.; Dave, V.S. Preparation and Evaluation of Phospholipid-Based Complex of Standardized Centella Extract (SCE) for the Enhanced Deliv-ery of Phytoconstituents. *AAPS J.* **2016**, *18*, 102–114. [CrossRef]
25. Silva, A.C.; Amaral, M.H.; González-Mira, E.; Santos, D.; Ferreira, D. Solid lipid nanoparticles (SLN)-based hydrogels as potential carriers for oral transmucosal delivery of risperidone: Preparation and characterization studies. *Colloids Surf. B Biointerfaces* **2012**, *93*, 241–248. [CrossRef]
26. Benoit, S.; Afizah, M.N.; Ruttarattanamongkol, K.; Rizvi, S. Effect of pH and Temperature on the Viscosity of Texturized and Commercial Whey Protein Dispersions. *Int. J. Food Prop.* **2013**, *16*, 322–330. [CrossRef]
27. Harish, N.M.; Prabhu, P.; Charyulu, R.N.; Gulzar, M.A.; Subrahmanyam, E.V. Formulation and Evaluation of in situ Gels Containing Clotrimazole for Oral Candidiasis. *Indian J. Pharm. Sci.* **2009**, *71*, 421–427. [CrossRef]
28. Yong, C.S.; Choi, J.S.; Quan, Q.-Z.; Rhee, J.-D.; Kim, C.-K.; Lim, S.-J.; Kim, K.-M.; Oh, P.-S.; Choi, H.-G. Effect of sodium chloride on the gelation temperature, gel strength and bioadhesive force of poloxamer gels containing diclofenac sodium. *Int. J. Pharm.* **2001**, *226*, 195–205. [CrossRef]
29. Jenning, V.; Schäfer-Korting, M.; Gohla, S. Vitamin A-loaded solid lipid nanoparticles for topical use: Drug release properties. *J. Control. Release* **2000**, *66*, 115–126. [CrossRef]

30. Ankola, D.D.; Durbin, E.W.; Buxton, G.A.; Schäfer, J.; Bakowsky, U.; Kumar, M.R. Preparation, characterization and in silico mod-eling of biodegradable nanoparticles containing cyclosporine A and coenzyme Q10. *Nanotechnology* **2010**, *21*, 065104. [CrossRef] [PubMed]
31. Sanna, V.; Gavini, E.; Cossu, M.; Rassu, G.; Giunchedi, P. Solid lipid nanoparticles (SLN) as carriers for the topical de-livery of econazole nitrate: In-vitro characterization, ex-vivo and in-vivo studies. *J. Pharm. Pharmacol.* **2007**, *59*, 1057–1064. [CrossRef] [PubMed]
32. Ganeshpurkar, A.; Vaishya, P.; Jain, S.; Pandey, V.; Bansal, D.; Dubey, N. Delivery of amphotericin B for effective treatment of Candida albicans induced dermal mycosis in rats via emulgel system: Formulation and evaluation. *Indian J. Dermatol.* **2014**, *59*, 369–374. [CrossRef] [PubMed]
33. Deshkar, S.S.; Bhalerao, S.G.; Jadhav, M.S.; Shirolkar, S.V. Formulation and Optimization of Topical Solid Lipid Nanoparticles based Gel of Dapsone Using Design of Experiment. *Pharm. Nanotechnol.* **2018**, *6*, 264–275. [CrossRef] [PubMed]
34. Madan, J.; Dua, K.; Khude, P. Development and evaluation of solid lipid nanoparticles of mometasone furoate for topical delivery. *Int. J. Pharm. Investig.* **2014**, *4*, 60–64. [CrossRef]
35. Freitas, C.; Muller, R.H. Effect of light and temperature on zeta potential and physical stability in solid lipid nanoparticle (SLN™) dispersions. *Int. J. Pharm.* **1998**, *168*, 221–229. [CrossRef]
36. Oehlke, K.; Behsnilian, D.; Mayer-Miebach, E.; Weidler, P.G.; Greiner, R. Edible solid lipid nanoparticles (SLN) as carrier system for antioxidants of different lipophilicity. *PLoS ONE* **2017**, *12*, e0171662. [CrossRef]
37. Guo, D.; Dou, D.; Li, X.; Zhang, Q.; Bhutto, Z.A.; Wang, L. Ivermection-loaded solid lipid nanoparticles: Preparation, characterisa-tion, stability and transdermal behaviour. *Artif. Cells Nanomed. Biotechnol.* **2018**, *46*, 255–262. [CrossRef]
38. Padhye, S.G.; Nagarsenker, M.S. Simvastatin Solid Lipid Nanoparticles for Oral Delivery: Formulation Development and In vivo Evaluation. *Indian J. Pharm. Sci.* **2013**, *75*, 591–598.
39. Andreozzi, E.; Seo, J.W.; Ferrara, K.; Louie, A. Novel Method to Label Solid Lipid Nanoparticles with ^{64}Cu for Positron Emission Tomography Imaging. *Bioconjugate Chem.* **2011**, *22*, 808–818. [CrossRef]
40. Danaei, M.; Dehghankhold, M.; Ataei, S.; Hasanzadeh Davarani, F.; Javanmard, R.; Dokhani, A.; Khorasani, S.; Mozafari, M.R. Im-pact of particle size and polydispersity index on the clinical applications of lipidic nanocarrier systems. *Pharmaceutics* **2018**, *10*, 57. [CrossRef]
41. Gupta, B.; Poudel, B.K.; Pathak, S.; Tak, J.W.; Lee, H.H.; Jeong, J.-H.; Choi, H.-G.; Yong, C.S.; Kim, J.O. Effects of Formulation Variables on the Particle Size and Drug Encapsulation of Imatinib-Loaded Solid Lipid Nanoparticles. *AAPS PharmSciTech* **2016**, *17*, 652–662. [CrossRef]
42. El-Housiny, S.; Shams Eldeen, M.A.; El-Attar, Y.A.; Salem, H.A.; Attia, D.; Bendas, E.R.; El-Nabarawi, M.A. Bendas and Mohamed A. El-Nabarawi. Fluconazole-loaded solid lipid nanoparticles topical gel for treatment of pityriasis versicolor: For-mulation and clinical study. *Drug Deliv.* **2018**, *25*, 78–90. [CrossRef]
43. Molan, P. The role of honey in the management of wounds. *J. Wound Care* **1999**, *8*, 415–418. [CrossRef]
44. Janga, K.Y.; Tatke, A.; Balguri, S.P.; Lamichanne, S.P.; Ibrahim, M.M.; Maria, D.N.; Jablonski, M.M.; Majumdar, S. Ion-sensitive in situ hydrogels of natamycin bilosomes for enhanced and prolonged ocular pharmacotherapy: In vitro permeability, cytotoxicity and in vivo evaluation. *Artif. Cells NanomedBiotechnol.* **2018**, *46* (Suppl. 1), 1039–1050. [CrossRef]
45. Jessup, C.J.; Ghannoum, M.A.; Ryder, N.S. An evaluation of the in vitro activity of terbinafine. *Med. Mycology.* **2000**, *38*, 155–159. [CrossRef]
46. Rarokar, N.R.; Saoji, S.D.; Khedekar, P.B. Investigation of effectiveness of some extensively used polymers on thermoreversible properties of Pluronic® tri-block copolymers. *J. Drug Deliv. Sci. Technol.* **2018**, *44*, 220–230. [CrossRef]

pharmaceutics

MDPI

Article

Development and Evaluation of Ethosomes Loaded with *Zingiber zerumbet* Linn Rhizome Extract for Antifungal Skin Infection in Deep Layer Skin

Kampanart Huanbutta [1], Napapat Rattanachitthawat [2], Kunlathida Luangpraditkun [2], Pornsak Sriamornsak [3], Vivek Puri [4], Inderbir Singh [5] and Tanikan Sangnim [2,*]

[1] School of Pharmacy, Eastern Asia University, Thanyaburi 12110, Thailand
[2] Faculty of Pharmaceutical Sciences, Burapha University, Chonburi 20131, Thailand
[3] Department of Pharmaceutical Technology, Faculty of Pharmacy, Silpakorn University, Nakhon Pathom 73000, Thailand
[4] School of Pharmacy, Chitkara University, Baddi 174103, India
[5] Chitkara College of Pharmacy, Chitkara University, Rajpura 140401, India
* Correspondence: tanikan@go.buu.ac.th

Abstract: Skin fungal infection is still a serious public health problem due to the high number of cases. Even though medicines are available for this disease, drug resistance among patients has increased. Moreover, access to medicine is restricted in some areas. One of the therapeutic options is herbal medicine. This study aims to develop an ethosome formulation loaded with *Zingiber zerumbet* (L.) Smith. rhizome extract for enhanced antifungal activity in deep layer skin, which is difficult to cure. Ethosomes were successfully prepared by the cold method, and the optimized formulation was composed of 1% (*w*/*v*) phosphatidylcholine and 40% (*v*/*v*) ethanol. Transmission electron microscope (TEM) images revealed that the ethosomes had a vesicle shape with a diameter of 205.6–368.5 nm. The entrapment of ethosomes was 31.58% and could inhibit the growth of *Candida albicans* at a concentration of 312.5 μg/mL. Finally, the ethosome system significantly enhanced the skin penetration and retention of the active compound (zerumbone) compared with the liquid extract. This study showed that *Z. zerumbet* (L.) rhizome extract could be loaded into ethosomes. The findings could be carried over to the next step for clinical application by conducting further in vivo penetration and permeation tests.

Keywords: ethosome; *Zingiber zerumbet* Linn; antifungal; skin permeation; fungal infection

Citation: Huanbutta, K.; Rattanachitthawat, N.; Luangpraditkun, K.; Sriamornsak, P.; Puri, V.; Singh, I.; Sangnim, T. Development and Evaluation of Ethosomes Loaded with *Zingiber zerumbet* Linn Rhizome Extract for Antifungal Skin Infection in Deep Layer Skin. *Pharmaceutics* **2022**, *14*, 2765. https://doi.org/10.3390/pharmaceutics14122765

Academic Editors: Ana Isabel Fraguas-Sánchez, Raquel Fernández García and Francisco Bolás-Fernández

Received: 22 October 2022
Accepted: 8 December 2022
Published: 9 December 2022

1. Introduction

Nearly a billion people worldwide suffer from skin, nail, and hair fungal infections. The most common fungal diseases are fungal nail infections, ringworm, vaginal candidiasis, and *Candida* infections of the gastrointestinal tract [1]. *Candida*, *Cryptococcus*, and *Aspergillus* are the most prevalent organisms responsible for life-threatening fungal infections in humans [2]. Despite the accessibility of drugs for fungal infection, the increase in morbidity and mortality associated with invasive fungal infections is due to the increasing number of antifungals with a small safety margin. Furthermore, certain fungi are growing resistant to treatment, making the infections difficult to treat [3]. Hence, the development of a new antifungal agent is critical to provide a treatment option for this disease.

Skin fungal infections can be classified as either superficial or deep. Superficial fungal infections, including dermatophytes, have an affinity for keratin and therefore are typically limited to either the epidermis or adnexal structures. Deep fungal infections affect deep structures, including internal organs, and continue to be an important cause of morbidity and mortality, especially in transplant recipients and other immunosuppressed patients. These diseases are extremely difficult to cure because the antifungal drugs must penetrate the stratum corneum, which is challenging due to the limited solubility of the drugs used to treat this disease and the difficulty in penetrating the skin [4].

Antifungal drug resistance and deep skin fungal infections can be remedied by discovering natural products or extracts and distributing them with an appropriate drug delivery system. Among various herbal plants, *Zingiber zerumbet* (L.) Smith. exhibits antifungal, antioxidant, and anti-inflammatory properties, all of which are essential for treating skin fungal infections [5]. *Z. zerumbet* (L.) is a ginger species with leafy stems and reaches a height of around 1.2 m [6]. Although it originated in Asia, it is now found in a variety of tropical nations. Our previous study found that the minimum bactericidal and fungicidal concentrations of hexane and dichloromethane extracts against *Staphylococcus epidermidis* and *Candida albicans* were 31.25 and 62.5 µg/mL, respectively [5]. Moreover, the ethanol extract outperformed the dichloromethane and hexane extracts in terms of antioxidant activity as measured by ABTS and DPPH assays and showed anti-inflammatory properties as determined by protein denaturation test.

Even though the activity of *Z. zerumbet* (L.) rhizome is considerable, the extremely low solubility of its extract limits its application. Therefore, advanced topical formulations that significantly enhance skin penetration are required to improve the therapeutic efficacy of the extract. Ethosome is a soft and malleable vesicle primarily composed of phospholipids, ethanol, and water. The increased flexibility of vesicular membranes due to the addition of ethanol enables the elastic vesicles to squeeze through pores with diameters smaller than their own. Ethosomal systems are significantly superior to conventional liposomes and hydroalcoholic solutions for the delivery of substances to the skin in terms of quantity and depth [7–9].

This study aims to develop and evaluate ethosomes containing *Z. zerumbet* (L.) rhizome extract for the treatment of antifungal skin infections in deep layer skin. The rhizome of *Z. zerumbet* (L.) was extracted with hexane, and ethosomes containing this extract were prepared using the cold method. The ethosomes' size, size distribution, zeta potential, and morphology were investigated, and the percentage of extract loading and antifungal activities of the prepared ethosomes were analyzed. Finally, the efficiency of ethosome penetration in pig skin was evaluated.

2. Materials and Methods

2.1. Materials

Ethanol (batch no. 20060068) and hexane (batch no. 21070007) were purchased from RCI Labscan, Thailand. Phosphatidylcholine from soya lecithin (batch no. MM3D32) and polyethylene glycol 4000 (PEG 4000) (batch no. J7F3RW) were acquired from MySkin-Recipes, Thailand. Zerumbone (batch no. S00321110, purity $\geq$ 98%) were obtained from ChemFaces (Wuhan, China). All other chemicals and reagents were of analytical grade.

2.2. Methods

2.2.1. *Z. zerumbet* (L.) Extract

The *Z. zerumbet* (L.) rhizomes were identified by Dr. Boonyadist Vongsak, Faculty of Pharmaceutical Sciences, Burapha University, Thailand. The voucher specimens (KM No. 0415001, KM No. 0415002, and KM No. 0415003) were deposited at the Faculty of Pharmaceutical Sciences, Burapha University, Thailand.

Fresh rhizomes of *Z. zerumbet* (L.) were collected in Chantaburi Province last February 2022 and then cleaned with water. The rhizomes were milled and then dried at 50 °C for 48 h. For extraction, *Z. zerumbet* (L.) rhizomes were soaked with hexane for 24 h. The extract was then filtered, evaporated using a rotary vacuum evaporator (R-100, Buchi, Taito, Japan), and stored at 2 °C–8 °C for further ethosome preparation.

2.2.2. Ethosome Preparation

Ethosomes were prepared using the cold method. Soya lecithin, PEG 4000, and *Z. zerumbet* (L.) rhizome extract were dissolved in ethanol, and the volume of the prepared ethosome was adjusted by adding purified water. The mixture was then stirred at 30 °C to allow ethosome formation. The obtained ethosomes were sonicated for 15 min. To prevent structural damage to the ethosome, the applied sonication duration was 5 min per round for 15 min of sonication (Ultrasonic Sonicator, GT-SONIC-20, PASTEL, Shenzhen, China). Variable amounts of soya lecithin, PEG 4000, and ethanol were used, as shown in Table 1, and the effect of sonication time was also evaluated. The optimized blank ethosome formulation was selected for the loading of *Z. zerumbet* (L.) rhizome extract at a concentration range of 2.5–125 mg/20 mL.

Table 1. Formulation of blank ethosome.

Ingredients	Formulations							
	SL100	**SL200**	**SL300**	**SL400**	**E5**	**E6**	**E8**	**E9**
Soya lecithin (mg)	100	200	300	400	200	200	200	200
Ethanol (mL)	7	7	7	7	5	6	8	9
Polyethylene glycol 4000 (mg)	100	100	100	100	100	100	100	100
Water qs (mL)	20	20	20	20	20	20	20	20

2.2.3. Physical Evaluation of Ethosomes

- Vesicle size, size distribution, and zeta potential

The vesicle size, size distribution, and zeta potential of blank and extract-loaded ethosomes were monitored by Zetasizer (MAL1070387, Malvern, UK). The samples were diluted to 0.5% *w*/*v* using deionized water as a solvent and then agitated for 3 min before measurement. The average and standard deviation of the measurements for three batches of samples were reported.

- Morphology

The surface morphology was determined by transmission electron microscopy (TEM; Tecnai 20, Philips, Eindhoven, The Netherlands). For TEM examination, a drop of the sample was placed on a carbon-coated copper grid and then negatively stained with 1% aqueous solution of phosphotungstic acid after 15 min. The grid was air dried thoroughly, and the samples were viewed on a TEM.

2.2.4. Entrapment Efficiency (EE) of Ethosomes

Zerumbone, which is the major constituent of *Z. zerumbet* (L.) rhizome extract was used as an active substance marker to indirectly determine the EE of the ethosome system. First, the free zerumbone was separated from the ethosome dispersion by 90 min of centrifugation (Centrifuge, MPW-260R, MPW MED Instruments, Warsaw, Poland) at 15,000 rpm and 4 °C. After that, 900 µL of ethanol were added to 100 µL of the supernatant containing unentrapped zerumbone. Then, the unentrapped zerumbone in the sample was examined by high-performance liquid chromatography (HPLC; SPD-M20A, Shimadzu, Nakagyo, Japan) and quantified using a slightly modified, previously validated method with the limit of quantification (LoQ) of 2.5 µg/mL [5,10]. A stainless steel analytical symmetry column (ACE5C18 V17-1586, Avantor®, Lutterworth, UK) with 5 µm particle size (4.6 mm internal diameter × 250 mm length) packed with a dimethyl octylsilyl (C18)-bonded amorphous silica stationary phase was used. The mobile phase was a binary mixture of HPLC-grade acetonitrile and purified water at gradient ratio of 65:35–75:25% (*v*/*v*) that was blended within 26 min, freshly prepared for each run, and degassed before use. The injection volume was 10 µL, and the flow rate was 1 mL/min. The samples were estimated by ultraviolet detection at a wavelength of 250 nm. The EE percentage was calculated by Equation (1):

$$EE\% = \frac{\text{zerumbone in extract added to the formulation} - \text{zerumbone amount in supernatant}}{\text{zerumbone in extract added to the formulation}} \times 100. \quad (1)$$

2.2.5. Antifungal Activities of Ethosomes Loaded with *Z. zerumbet* (L.) Rhizome Extract

The antifungal activities of the ethosomes loaded with different concentrations of *Z. zerumbet* (L.) rhizome extract were examined. The loaded *Z. zerumbet* (L.) rhizome extract was varied at 0.1, 0.25, 0.5, 1, 1.5, 2.5, and 5X the minimum fungicidal concentration (MFC; 62.5 μg/mL) of *Z. zerumbet* (L.) rhizome hexane extract, which was discovered in our previous study [5]. Broth dilution was used to test the sensitivity of *Candida albicans* for the ethosomes loaded with different concentrations of *Z. zerumbet* (L.) rhizome extract. For this process, Sabouraud dextrose broth (SDB) was prepared and diluted with purified water to achieve a turbidity level equivalent to the 0.5 McFarland standard at about 1×10^8 CFU/mL *C. albicans*. The prepared SDB was then mixed with the ethosomes loaded with different concentrations of *Z. zerumbet* (L.) rhizome extract (6.25–312.5 μg/mL) in test tubes and kept in a 37 °C incubator for 24 h. The turbidity of the samples was determined and compared with that of the control. The lowest concentration of ethosome loaded with the extract that can inhibit microorganism growth was defined as the minimum inhibition concentration (MIC) [11].

The MFC of the ethosome loaded with extract was determined by streaking the turbid mixture from the MIC test onto the surface of Sabouraud dextrose agar (SDA), which was then incubated at 37 °C for 20–24 h. The lowest concentration of the ethosome loaded with extract that can inhibit the formation of fungal colonies on the SDA plate was defined as the MFC [11].

2.2.6. In Vitro Skin Penetration Studies of Ethosomes Loaded with *Z. zerumbet* (L.) Rhizome Extract

In vitro skin penetration studies were conducted using vertical Franz diffusion cells. Neonatal porcine skin from piglets that died of natural causes and provided by a local pig farm in Chonburi province, Thailand, was used as the barrier membrane. Subcutaneous fat was removed using surgical blades and scissors. Prior to the experiment, the skin was washed with phosphate-buffered saline to remove any contaminants. Then the skin was cut to the Franz diffusion cell mount size, wrapped by aluminum foil, and stored at −10 °C before further experimentation. In order to set up the experiment, piglet skin was mounted between the donor and receptor chambers of diffusion cells. The stratum corneum was turned to face the donor side [12]. Phosphate buffer (pH 7.4)–ethanol (80:20) was applied as the medium. The in vitro experiment was run for 24 h at controlled temperature of 32 °C with agitation by a magnetic stirrer. The *Z. zerumbet* (L.) rhizome liquid extract (62.5 and 312.5 μg) or the ethosomes loaded with the extract (62.5 and 312.5 μg) was poured at the donor sides and covered by Parafilm. The diffused substance was sampled at 1 mL from the receptor side at 15, 30 min, 1 2, 3, 4, 6, 12, and 24 h. The zerumbone from the sample was analyzed by HPLC as mentioned in the EE method.

2.2.7. In Vitro Skin Retention Studies of Ethosomes Loaded with *Z. zerumbet* (L.) Rhizome Extract

Following the in vitro skin penetration test, the used pig skin (n = 3) [13–15] was washed three times with deionized water for 15 s each and then wiped with a paper tissue. The stratum corneum layers were removed from the treated skin using the tape strip method [12]. The stratum corneum was peeled 30 times using a 24 mm wide pressure-sensitive adhesive tape (Scotch® Transparent Tape 500, 3M Co., Ltd., Bangkok, Thailand). All of the stripped tapes were placed in glass vials containing 5 mL of ethanol and sonicated for 15 min. Afterward, 1 mL of the ethanol solution was drawn and centrifuged at 10,000 rpm at 25 °C for 30 min. Zerumbone was quantified by HPLC.

After the stratum corneum was removed, the remaining skin was sliced into small fragments and placed in a glass vial containing 3 mL of ethanol for 24 h. In brief, 1 mL of the collected ethanol was pipetted into a centrifuge tube and centrifuged at 10,000 rpm and 25 °C for 15 min. The zerumbone concentration in the resulting supernatant was determined using HPLC. The quantity of zerumbone in the viable epidermis and dermis was measured using Equation (2):

$$\text{Drug amount in the viable epidermis and dermis } \left(\mu g/cm^2\right) = \frac{R_v}{S} \quad (2)$$

where R_v is the amount of zerumbone in the viable epidermis and dermis (μg), and S is the skin penetration area (cm^2).

The enhancement ratio (ER) was calculated using Equation (3):

$$ER = \frac{\text{Drug amount in the viable epidermis and dermis of ethosomal formulation}}{\text{Drug amount in the viable epidermis and dermis of extracts}} \quad (3)$$

2.2.8. Statistical Analysis

Data were statistically analyzed using one-way ANOVA, followed by Tukey's honest significant difference post hoc test for the data from three independent experiments.

3. Results and Discussion

3.1. Vesicle Size, Size Distribution, and Zeta Potential

The vesicle size, size distribution, and zeta potential of blank ethosomes are depicted in bar chart format and presented in Figure 1a–c, respectively. Most of the sizes ranged between 140.8 and 184.1 nm (Figure 1a), except for E9 formulation whose size was 280.9 nm. An excessive amount of ethanol in the ethosome structure may result in an unstable membrane because phospholipids dissolve rapidly in ethanol, causing the vesicles to enlarge significantly [16]. SL200 formulation produced the smallest vesicle size. The addition of 300 and 400 mg of soy lecithin considerably enlarged the vesicles, and this finding is consistent with previous research stating that an increasing phospholipid concentration slightly or moderately increases the vesicle size [17–19]. The recommended amount of phospholipids that should be included in an ethosomal formulation is between 0.5% and 5% [20], which was applied in our formulation. As shown in Figure 1b, all the polydispersity index (PDI) values were between 0.245 and 0.453 nm. The formulations of SL300, E8, and E9 yielded PDI values below 0.280, showing that the preparation and formulations in this study were able to generate particles with low size dispersion [21].

Vesicular charge is a crucial characteristic that can affect vesicular features, such as stability and vesicle–skin contact. Therefore, the zeta potential of the entire ethosome formulation was measured. The zeta potential of the blank ethosomes was negative and in the range of −31.57 to −27.73 mV (Figure 1c). This high negative charge could stabilize the nanoparticle/vesicle system [22]. The phosphate group in soy lecithin was responsible for the negative charge on the ethosome's surface [23,24]. The zeta potential was unaffected by soy lecithin at a portion ranging from 100 mg to 400 mg. Finally, a high ethanol concentration in the formulation resulted in a low negative charge.

Owing to its small vesicle size, low PDI, and zeta potential lower than −30 mV, the ethosome with E8 formulation was chosen for further development through sonication. The effect of sonication period during preparation on the vesicle size, size distribution, and zeta potential of ethosomes is exhibited in Figure 2a–c, respectively. Sonication time reduced the vesicle size from 255.6 nm to 218.5 nm. At 15 min (5 min for three rounds), sonication slightly increased the PDI because this process breaks coarse drops into nanodroplets, hence producing ethosomes with a small, highly variable particle size [25]. The zeta potential altered with the length of time spent sonicating, which is consistent with the findings of another study regarding the effects of sonication on drug release, zeta potential, and pH [25].

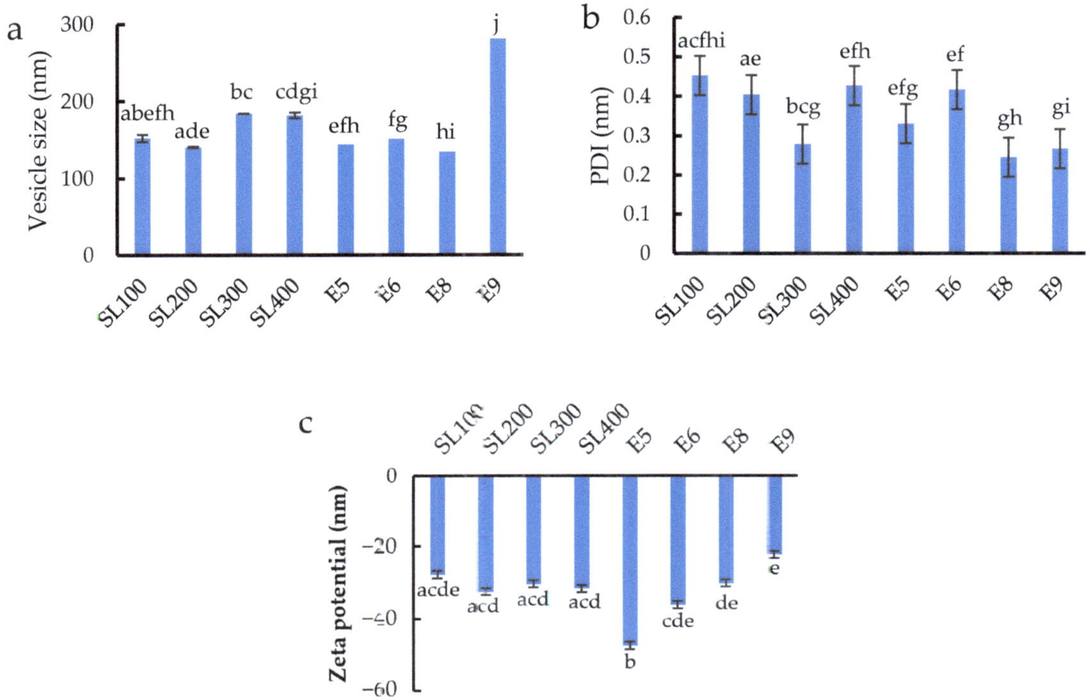

Figure 1. (**a**) Vesicle size, (**b**) size distribution, and (**c**) zeta potential of different formulations of blank ethosomes. Different letters above the error bars indicate significant differences at the 0.05 level (ANOVA and post hoc test).

The E8 formulation with 15 min of sonication (5 min for three rounds) was chosen for loading with the active ingredient, *Z. zerumbet* (L.) rhizome extract (6.25–312.5 µg/mL). The vesicle size, size distribution, and zeta potential of ethosomes loaded with the extract are presented in Figure 3a–c, respectively. The size of ethosomes varied between 134.5 and 184.1 nm, and the PDI ranged from 0.118 to 0.253. The high extract concentration reduced the PDI, indicating that the loading of 6.25–312.5 µg/mL *Z. zerumbet* (L.) rhizome extract did not alter the physical properties of the ethosome.

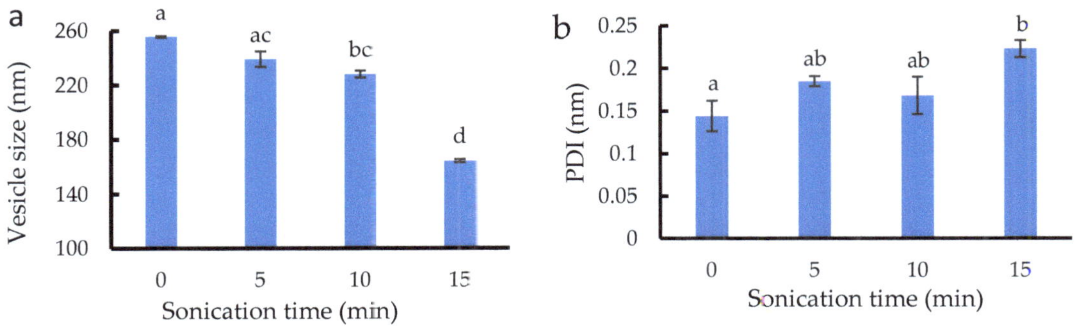

Figure 2. *Cont.*

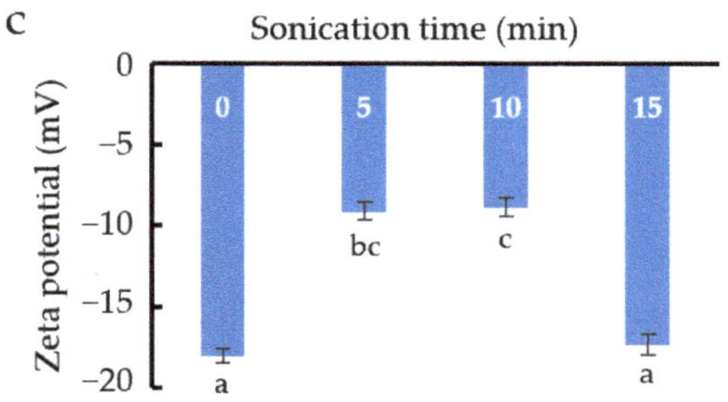

Figure 2. (**a**) Vesicle size, (**b**) size distribution, and (**c**) zeta potential of blank ethosomes treated by different sonication times. Different letters above the error bars indicate significant differences at the 0.05 level (ANOVA and post hoc test).

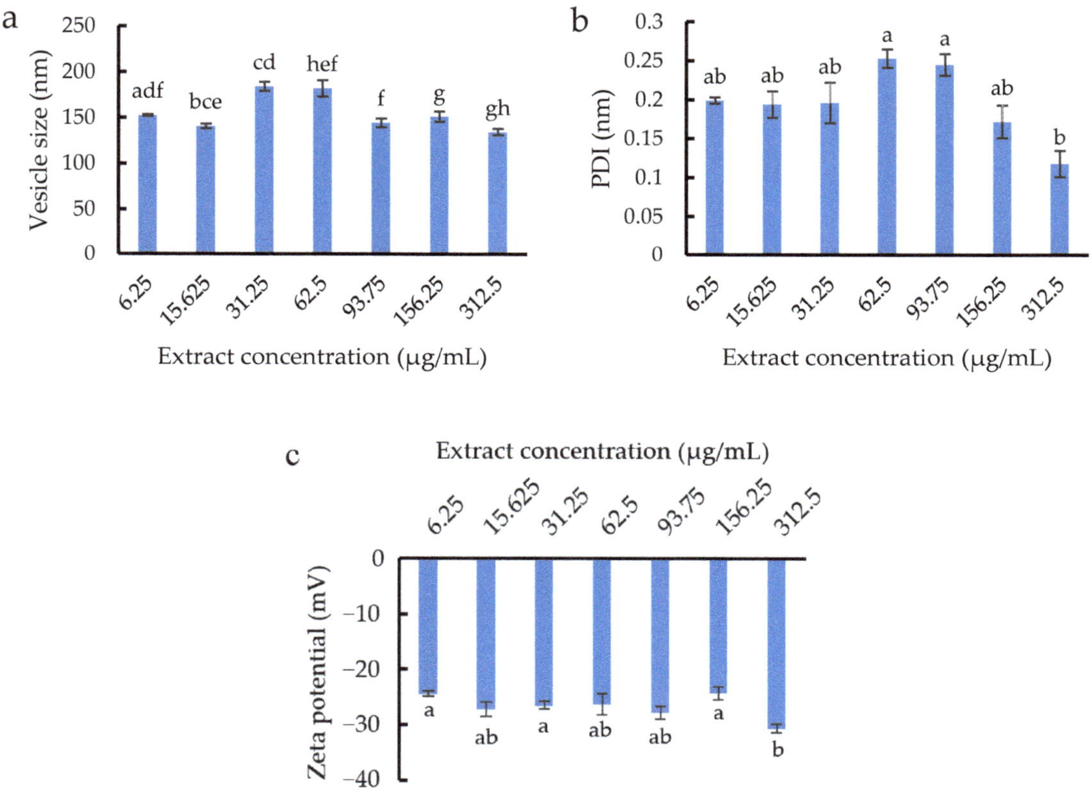

Figure 3. (**a**) Vesicle size, (**b**) size distribution, and (**c**) zeta potential of ethosomes loaded with different concentrations of *Z. zerumbet* (L.) rhizome extract. Different letters above the error bars indicate significant differences at the 0.05 level (ANOVA and post hoc test).

3.2. Morphology

The TEM images of the blank and extract-loaded ethosomes are shown in Figure 4a,b, respectively. The blank ethosomes had an irregular shape with an average diameter size of 200–400 nm. The vesicles shrunk and did not aggregate. Meanwhile, the morphology of extract-loaded ethosomes was spherical with gnarled surface. The vesicles were packed together, and their average size was around 150–400 nm. The TEM results for vesicle size were comparable with those from the vesicle size analyzer (Zetasizer), which measures particle size using dynamic light scattering. These results demonstrated that the ethosomes were generated using the cold procedure and subsequently filled with the *Z. zerumbet* (L.) rhizome extract.

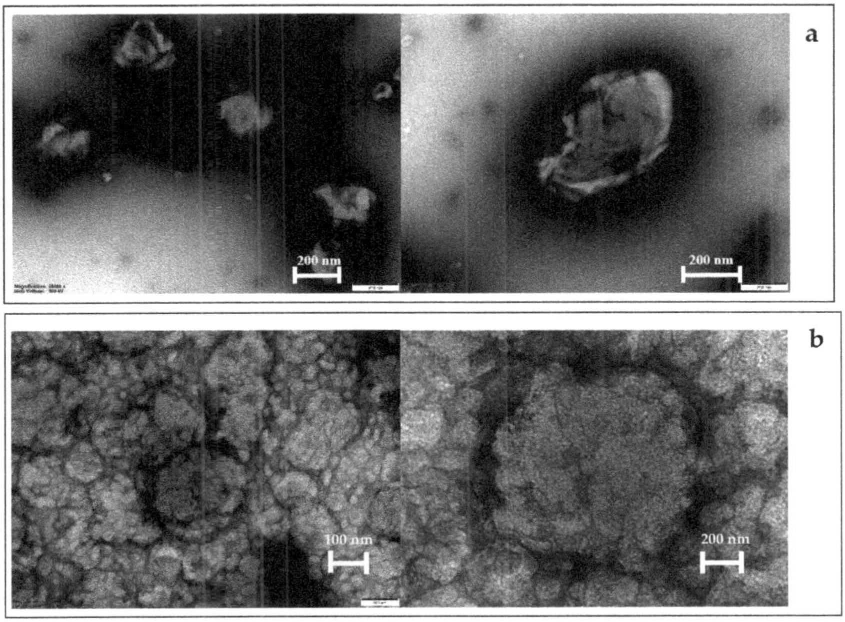

Figure 4. TEM of (**a**) blank ethosomes and (**b**) extract-loaded ethosomes.

3.3. Entrapment Efficiency of Ethosomes

The zerumbone in *Z. zerumbet* (L.) rhizome extract was quantified by HPLC and then monitored to evaluate the EE of the ethosomes as presented in Table 2. The herbal extract was added at two concentrations (156.25 and 312.5 μg/mL) to the E8 formulation. The EE percentage ranged from 24.42% to 31.58%, indicating that the developed ethosome was incapable of completely entrapping zerumbone. One possible reason is the high solubility of the active ingredient (zerumbone) in ethanol [26], leading to its dissolution in the solvent during the preparing of the ethosome. Moreover, the sonication process can significantly reduce the size of ethosomes. However, it might also affect the entrapment efficiency of the system [27]. Furthermore, some zerumbone may leak during centrifugation in the EE determination process [28]. These reasons can make the EE% slightly lower than in the previous study.

Table 2. Entrapment efficiency of the ethosomes loaded with *Z. zerumbet* (L.) rhizome extract.

***Z. zerumbet* (L.) Rhizome Extract Concentration (μg/mL)**	**AUC**	**%Zerumbone Entrapment**
156.25	1,375,327	24.42 ± 0.04
312.5	2,435,877	31.58 ± 0.05

3.4. Antifungal Activities of Ethosomes Loaded with Z. zerumbet (L.) Rhizome Extract

Broth dilution was applied to determine the MIC of ethosomes loaded with *Z. zerumbet* (L.) rhizome extract against *C. albicans* (Figure 5a). The tested concentrations of *Z. zerumbet* (L.) rhizome extract loaded onto ethosome were between 6.25 and 312.5 μg/mL.

The MIC of ethosomes loaded with *Z. zerumbet* (L.) rhizome extract was 312.5 µg/mL, which is five times higher than that of *Z. zerumbet* (L.) rhizome extract as reported previously [5]. As shown in Figure 5b, all incubated dilutions were then streaked on SDA plates to detect MFC. The MFC was discovered to be similar to the MIC, which has a concentration of 312.5 µg/mL, or five times that of the MFC hexane liquid extract. Compared with that in the liquid extract, the ability of *Z. zerumbet* (L.) rhizome extract in the ethosome to inhibit *C. albicans* growth was lower because a portion of the extract was not entrapped during ethosome preparation. Moreover, some active compounds entrapped inside the ethosome could retard the release or dissolution of the active ingredient to inhibit the growth of *C. albicans* [29].

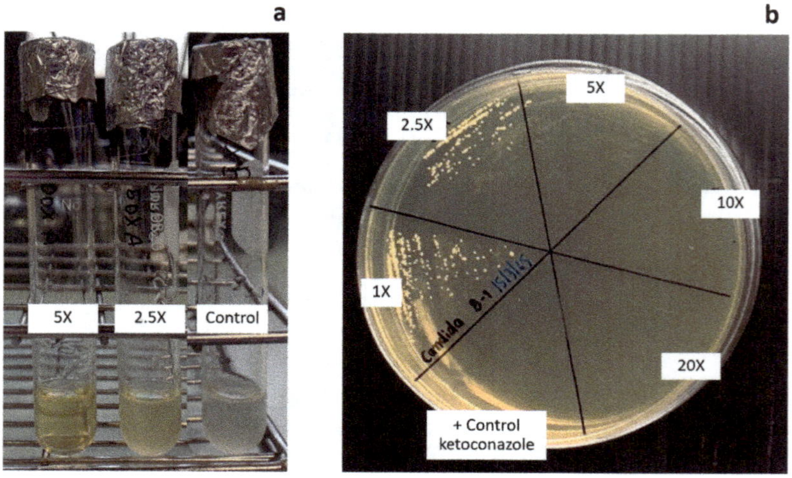

Figure 5. Antifungal test result of the ethosome loaded with different concentration of *Z. zerumbet* (L.) rhizome extract from (**a**) broth dilution technique test and (**b**) streaking onto the surface of Sabouraud dextrose agar.

3.5. In Vitro Skin Penetration Studies of Ethosomes Loaded with Z. zerumbet (L.) Rhizome Extract

Figure 6 illustrates the skin penetration ability of zerumbone from the liquid extract and the ethosome containing *Z. zerumbet* (L.) rhizome extract at a concentration of 312.5 µg/mL. During the initial 12 h, the penetration of zerumbone from both dosage forms was around 5%. After 24 h, the ethosomes significantly increased zerumbone's penetration compared with the liquid extract.

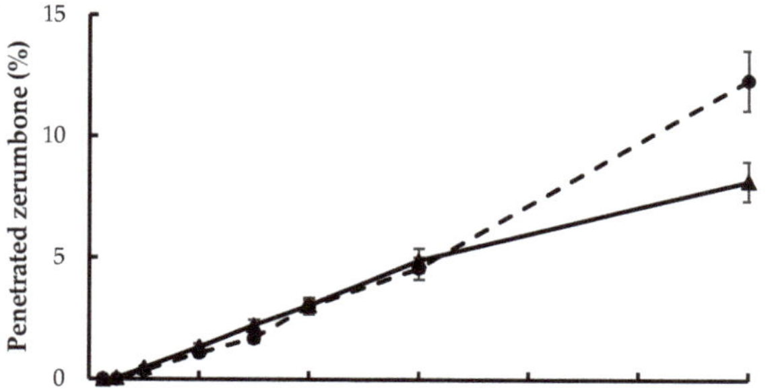

Figure 6. Time-integrated skin penetration percentage of zerumbone from the liquid extract (solid line) and the ethosomes loaded with *Z. zerumbet* (L.) rhizome extract (dash line) at 312.5 µg/mL.

3.6. In Vitro Skin Retention Studies of Ethosomes Loaded with Z. zerumbet (L.) Rhizome Extract

The retention ratio of zerumbone in the stratum corneum, epidermis, dermis, and deeper layers of the skin was measured from the adhesive tape, small fragments of skin, and the medium (phosphate buffer) from the receptor chamber. After 24 h, the majority of zerumbone from the liquid extract and ethosome had penetrated through the porcine skin as illustrated in Figure 7. Owing to its chemical structure with low polarity [30], zerumbone can penetrate the medium after 24 h of testing. However, 30.48% of zerumbone was still present in the stratum corneum treated with the liquid extract. Meanwhile, the stratum corneum treated with the ethosome contained only 6.08% of zerumbone. This finding suggested that the ethosome can greatly increase zerumbone's skin penetration into the deep layer skin of porcine models by interacting with the stratum corneum and disrupting its structure. According to one study, ethosomes with an average diameter of more than 600 nm were unable to reach the deep skin layers and stayed predominantly on the stratum corneum's surface, and those with an average diameter of 300 nm were able to go further into the skin layers [31]. This finding was in agreement with the ethosome size in the current work at 134.5–184.1 nm, which is lower than 300 nm. Finally, the ER of the ethosome was 1.51, indicating that the zerumbone content in the viable epidermis and dermis was higher after the treatment of ethosome than after the treatment with the liquid extract. This finding confirmed the permeation-enhancing ability of the ethosome.

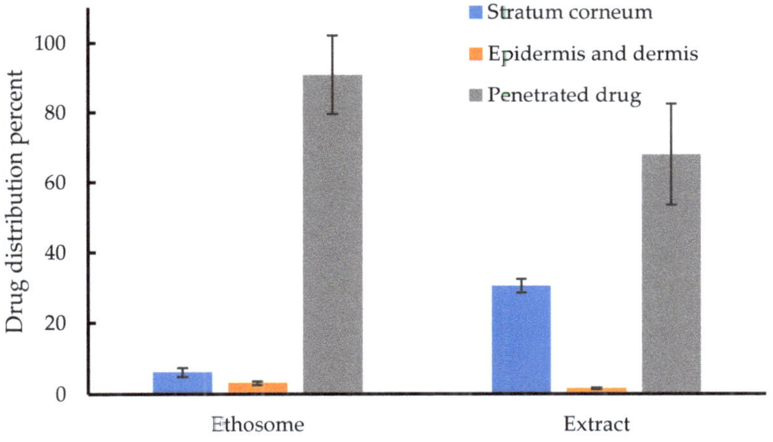

Figure 7. Retained ratio of zerumbone from the in vitro skin retention investigation in various skin layers.

4. Conclusions

In this study, *Z. zerumbet* (L.) rhizome extract was successfully loaded onto ethosome systems. TEM and light scattering analysis showed that the ethosome size was less than 200 nm, making it an excellent candidate as permeation enhancer for drugs or active ingredients. Size distribution and zeta potential analysis suggested that the ethosome production method and formulation were stable and consistent. In addition, the ethosome loaded with *Z. zerumbet* (L.) rhizome extract prevented the growth of *C. albicans* and considerably improved the skin penetration and retention of zerumbone, the major compound of *Z. zerumbet* (L.) rhizome extract. This finding demonstrates the potential utilization of the ethosome loaded with *Z. zerumbet* (L.) rhizome extract in the treatment of deep skin fungal infections.

Author Contributions: Conceptualization, T.S. and K.H.; methodology, K.H. and V.P.; investigation, T.S., N.R., and K.L.; writing—original draft preparation, T.S. and K.H.; writing—review and editing, K.H., I.S. and P.S.; supervision, V.P., P.S. and I.S.; funding acquisition, T.S. All authors have read and agreed to the published version of the manuscript.

Funding: This research was funded by Faculty of Pharmaceutical Sciences, Burapha University, grant number Rx2/2564.

Institutional Review Board Statement: Not applicable.

Informed Consent Statement: Not applicable.

Data Availability Statement: Not applicable.

Acknowledgments: We are grateful to the Faculty of Pharmaceutical Sciences at Burapha University for the laboratory equipment and financial support. We appreciate Wipada Siritanyong, Kritchaon Nantasopa, Chanya Thaiutid, and Supawee Jarassrichoung's assistance with laboratory work.

Conflicts of Interest: The authors declare no conflict of interest.

References

1. Centers for Disease Control and Prevention. Fungal Diseases. 2018. Available online: http://www.cdc.gov/ncezid/dfwed/mycotics (accessed on 16 January 2022).
2. Boral, H.; Metin, B.; Döğen, A.; Seyedmousavi, S.; Ilkit, M. Overview of selected virulence attributes in Aspergillus fumigatus, Candida albicans, Cryptococcus neoformans, Trichophyton rubrum, and Exophiala dermatitidis. *Fungal Genet. Biol.* **2018**, *111*, 92–107. [CrossRef] [PubMed]
3. Bouz, G.; Doležal, M. Advances in Antifungal Drug Development: An Up-To-Date Mini Review. *Pharmaceuticals* **2021**, *14*, 1312. [CrossRef]
4. Felton, T.; Troke, P.F.; Hope, W.W. Tissue penetration of antifungal agents. *Clin. Microbiol. Rev.* **2014**, *27*, 68–88. [CrossRef] [PubMed]
5. Rattanachitthawat, N.; Sriamornsak, P.; Puri, V.; Singh, I.; Huanbutta, K.; Sangnim, T. Bioactivity assessment of *Zingiber zerumbet* Linn rhizome extract for topical treatment of skin diseases. *J. Appl. Pharm. Sci.* **2022**. [CrossRef]
6. Roskov, Y.; Orrell, T.; Abucay, L.; Paglinawan, L.; Culham, A.; Bailly, N.; Kirk, P.; Bourgoin, T.; Baillargeon, G.; Decock, W.; et al. (Eds.) *Species 2000 & ITIS Catalogue of Life, 2014 Annual Checklist*; Naturalis: Leiden, The Netherlands, 2000. Available online: www.catalogueoflife.org/annual-checklist/2014 (accessed on 3 February 2022).
7. Verma, P.; Pathak, K. Therapeutic and cosmeceutical potential of ethosomes: An overview. *J. Adv. Pharm. Technol. Res.* **2010**, *1*, 274. [CrossRef] [PubMed]
8. Paolino, D.; Mancuso, A.; Cristiano, M.C.; Froiio, F.; Lammari, N.; Celia, C.; Fresta, M. Nanonutraceuticals: The New Frontier of Supplementary Food. *Nanomaterials* **2021**, *11*, 792. [CrossRef] [PubMed]
9. Natsheh, H.; Vettorato, E.; Touitou, E. Ethosomes for dermal administration of natural active molecules. *Curr. Pharm. Des.* **2019**, *25*, 2338–2348. [CrossRef]
10. Rahman, H.S.; Rasedee, A.; How, C.W.; Abdul, A.B.; Zeenathul, N.A.; Othman, H.H.; Saeed, M.I.; Yeap, S.K. Zerumbone-loaded nanostructured lipid carriers: Preparation, characterization, and antileukemic effect. *Int. J. Nanomed.* **2013**, *8*, 2769. [CrossRef]
11. Anyanwu, C. Investigation of in vitro antifungal activity of honey. *J. Med. Plants Res.* **2012**, *6*, 3512–3516. [CrossRef]
12. Subongkot, T.; Sirirak, T. Development and skin penetration pathway evaluation of microemulsions for enhancing the dermal delivery of celecoxib. *Colloids Surf. B Biointerfaces* **2020**, *193*, 111103. [CrossRef]
13. Barbosa, A.I.; Lima, S.A.C.; Reis, S. Development of methotrexate loaded fucoidan/chitosan nanoparticles with anti-inflammatory potential and enhanced skin permeation. *Int. J. Biol. Macromol.* **2019**, *124*, 1115–1122. [CrossRef]
14. Duangjit, S.; Pamornpathomkul, B.; Opanasopit, P.; Rojanarata, T.; Obata, Y.; Takayama, K.; Ngawhirunpat, T. Role of the charge, carbon chain length, and content of surfactant on the skin penetration of meloxicam-loaded liposomes. *Int. J. Nanomed.* **2014**, *9*, 2005. [CrossRef]
15. Subongkot, T.; Ngawhirunpat, T.; Opanasopit, P. Development of ultradeformable liposomes with fatty acids for enhanced dermal rosmarinic acid delivery. *Pharmaceutics* **2021**, *13*, 404. [CrossRef]
16. Abdulbaqi, I.M.; Darwis, Y.; Khan, N.A.K.; Abou Assi, R.; Khan, A.A. Ethosomal nanocarriers: The impact of constituents and formulation techniques on ethosomal properties, in vivo studies, and clinical trials. *Int. J. Nanomed.* **2016**, *11*, 2279. [CrossRef]
17. Puri, R.; Jain, S. Ethogel topical formulation for increasing the local bioavailability of 5-fluorouracil: A mechanistic study. *Anti-Cancer Drugs* **2012**, *23*, 923–934. [CrossRef]
18. Liu, X.; Liu, H.; Liu, J.; He, Z.; Ding, C.; Huang, G.; Zhou, W.; Zhou, L. Preparation of a ligustrazine ethosome patch and its evaluation in vitro and in vivo. *Int. J. Nanomed.* **2011**, *6*, 241. [CrossRef]
19. Paolino, D.; Lucania, G.; Mardente, D.; Alhaique, F.; Fresta, M. Ethosomes for skin delivery of ammonium glycyrrhizinate: In vitro percutaneous permeation through human skin and in vivo anti-inflammatory activity on human volunteers. *J. Control. Release* **2005**, *106*, 99–110. [CrossRef]

20. Limsuwan, T.; Amnuaikit, T. Development of ethosomes containing mycophenolic acid. *Procedia Chem.* **2012**, *4*, 328–335. [CrossRef]
21. Bhattacharjee, S. DLS and zeta potential—what they are and what they are not? *J. Control. Release* **2016**, *235*, 337–351. [CrossRef]
22. Shah, R.; Eldridge, D.; Palombo, E.; Harding, I. Optimisation and stability assessment of solid lipid nanoparticles using particle size and zeta potential. *J. Phys. Sci.* **2014**, *25*, 59–75.
23. Paolino, D.; Ventura, C.A.; Nistico, S.; Puglisi, G.; Fresta, M. Lecithin microemulsions for the topical administration of ketoprofen: Percutaneous adsorption through human skin and in vivo human skin tolerability. *Int. J. Pharm.* **2002**, *244*, 21–31. [CrossRef]
24. Chen, W.; Soucie, W. Modification of surface charges of soy protein by phospholipids. *J. Am. Oil Chem. Soc.* **1985**, *62*, 1686–1689. [CrossRef]
25. Tiwari, R.; Tiwari, G.; Wal, P.; Wal, A.; Maurya, P. Development, characterization and transdermal delivery of dapsone and an antibiotic entrapped in ethanolic liposomal gel for the treatment of lapromatous leprosy. *Open Nanomed. J.* **2018**, *5*, 1–15. [CrossRef]
26. Rahman, H.S.; Rasedee, A.; Yeap, S.K.; Othman, H.H.; Chartrand, M.S.; Namvar, F.; Abdul, A.B.; How, C.W. Biomedical properties of a natural dietary plant metabolite, zerumbone, in cancer therapy and chemoprevention trials. *BioMed Res. Int.* **2014**, *2014*, 920742. [CrossRef]
27. Iizhar, S.A.; Syed, I.A.; Satar, R.; Ansari, S.A. In vitro assessment of pharmaceutical potential of ethosomes entrapped with terbinafine hydrochloride. *J. Adv. Res.* **2016**, *7*, 453–461. [CrossRef]
28. Lin, M.; Qi, X.-R. Purification method of drug-loaded liposome. In *Liposome-Based Drug Delivery Systems*; Springer Berlin/Heidelberg, Germany, 2021; pp. 111–121. [CrossRef]
29. Samad, A.; Sultana, Y.; Aqil, M. Liposomal drug delivery systems: An update review. *Curr. Drug Deliv.* **2007**, *4*, 297–305. [CrossRef]
30. Kesharwani, S.S.; Bhat, G.J. Formulation and Nanotechnology-Based Approaches for Solubility and Bioavailability Enhancement of Zerumbone. *Medicina* **2020**, *56*, 557. [CrossRef]
31. Choi, M.; Maibach, H. Liposomes and niosomes as topical drug delivery systems. *Ski. Pharmacol. Physiol.* **2005**, *18*, 209–219. [CrossRef]

pharmaceutics

MDPI

Article

Increased Bone Marrow Uptake and Accumulation of Very-Late Antigen-4 Targeted Lipid Nanoparticles

Laura E. Swart [1], Marcel H. A. M. Fens [2], Anita van Oort [1], Piotr Waranecki [1], L. Daniel Mata Casimiro [1], David Tuk [1], Martijn Hendriksen [1], Luca van den Brink [1], Elizabeth Schweighart [1], Cor Seinen [3], Ryan Nelson [1], Anja Krippner-Heidenreich [1], Tom O'Toole [1], Raymond M. Schiffelers [3], Sander Kooijmans [3] and Olaf Heidenreich [1,4,*]

1 Princess Máxima Center for Pediatric Oncology, Heidelberglaan 25, 3584 CS Utrecht, The Netherlands
2 Department of Pharmaceutics, Utrecht Institute for Pharmaceutical Sciences, Utrecht University, 3584 CG Utrecht, The Netherlands
3 CDL Research, University Medical Center Utrecht, Heidelberglaan 100, 3584 CX Utrecht, The Netherlands
4 Wolfson Childhood Cancer Research Centre, Newcastle University, Newcastle upon Tyne NE1 7RY, UK
* Correspondence: o.t.heidenreich@prinsesmaximacentrum.nl

Abstract: Lipid nanoparticles (LNPs) have evolved rapidly as promising delivery systems for oligonucleotides, including siRNAs. However, current clinical LNP formulations show high liver accumulation after systemic administration, which is unfavorable for the treatment of extrahepatic diseases, such as hematological disorders. Here we describe the specific targeting of LNPs to hematopoietic progenitor cells in the bone marrow. Functionalization of the LNPs with a modified Leu-Asp-Val tripeptide, a specific ligand for the very-late antigen 4 resulted in an improved uptake and functional siRNA delivery in patient-derived leukemia cells when compared to their non-targeted counterparts. Moreover, surface-modified LNPs displayed significantly improved bone-marrow accumulation and retention. These were associated with increased LNP uptake by immature hematopoietic progenitor cells, also suggesting similarly improved uptake by leukemic stem cells. In summary, we describe an LNP formulation that successfully targets the bone marrow including leukemic stem cells. Our results thereby support the further development of LNPs for targeted therapeutic interventions for leukemia and other hematological disorders.

Keywords: acute myeloid leukemia; targeted delivery; siRNA lipid nanoparticles (LNPs); very-late antigen-4 (VLA-4); bone marrow targeting

Citation: Swart, L.E.; Fens, M.H.A.M.; van Oort, A.; Waranecki, P.; Mata Casimiro, L.D.; Tuk, D.; Hendriksen, M.; van den Brink, L.; Schweighart, E.; Seinen, C.; et al. Increased Bone Marrow Uptake and Accumulation of Very-Late Antigen-4 Targeted Lipid Nanoparticles. *Pharmaceutics* **2023**, *15*, 1603. https://doi.org/10.3390/pharmaceutics15061603

Academic Editors: Ana Isabel Fraguas-Sánchez, Raquel Fernández García and Francisco Bolás-Fernández

Received: 26 April 2023
Revised: 17 May 2023
Accepted: 25 May 2023
Published: 27 May 2023

1. Introduction

Chromosomal rearrangements are a hallmark of pediatric acute myeloid leukemias (AMLs). These rearrangements give rise to leukemic fusion genes that initiate and drive leukemia. Therefore, they present ideal therapeutic targets; however, targeting fusion genes using conventional drug molecules has proven challenging. A promising alternative is to target fusion transcripts by RNA interference [1–5]. Because of the poor pharmacokinetic properties of siRNAs, caused by low stability, poor uptake by cells, fast clearance and induction of immunogenic responses, delivery vehicles such as micelles, liposomes, nanoplexes, or lipid nanoparticles (LNPs) are required [6–15]. LNPs are currently amongst the most promising non-viral delivery systems used for the delivery of siRNAs because of their high encapsulation efficiency combined with reduced immunogenicity and improved circulation times [14]. Commonly, LNPs consist of a cationic ionizable lipid such as D_{lin}-MC_3-DMA or C12-200, together with helper lipids distearoylphosphatidylcholine (DSPC) and cholesterol. To provide stealth properties, lipids conjugated to polyethylene glycol (PEG) are added to the formulation, such as 1,2-dimyristoyl-rac-glycero-3-methoxyPEG-2000 (DMG-PEG_{2000}) or 1,2-Distearoyl-sn-glycero-3-phosphoethanolamine-PEG-2000 ($DSPE$-PEG_{2000}).

The majority of systemically administered LNPs accumulate in the liver due to the liver's large size, functionalized vascular structure and, for some LNP types, surface-absorbed apolipoprotein-E-mediated uptake by the hepatocytes [16–18]. The resultant liver accumulation is widely exploited to effectively modulate therapeutic targets in this organ. Targeting other organs and tissues has proven to be more challenging [17,19,20]. The bone marrow, for instance, is the site where most hematological diseases, including leukemia, originate. In principle, the bone marrow is accessible for LNPs as it is well vascularized with sinusoids that have highly fenestrated endothelial layers required for the facile migration of mature cells into the bloodstream [21]. Consequently, these sinusoids might also allow access by lipid nanocarriers. However, current retention times of LNPs in the bone marrow are too low to reach therapeutically effective doses for therapeutic oligonucleotides. To increase tissue retention, the physicochemical properties of the LNPs can be modified, which is also known as passive targeting. For drug delivery, functionalizing LNPs with chemical or biological moieties can significantly increase LNP cellular specificity [22–26]. The targeting moiety should ideally bind to a receptor that is disease-specific, highly expressed on target cells and induce receptor-mediated endocytosis of the LNPs after binding.

Integrin receptors display all these qualities. These heterodimeric cell adhesion receptors are involved in cell–cell and cell–extracellular matrix interactions. Several integrin dimers such as the very-late antigen-4 (VLA-4) receptor, the lymphocyte function-associated antigen-1 and the Lymphocyte Peyer patch adhesion molecule have been explored for targeting hematological malignancies [27–34]. VLA-4 is expressed on all leukocytes and plays a key role in mediating homing to and retention of hematopoietic stem and progenitor cells (HSPC) in the bone marrow [32,35]. It is a heterodimer of integrin α4 (CD49d) and β1 (CD29b) and binds to vascular cell adhesion molecule-1 (VCAM-1) present on endothelial cells and fibronectin. Because of its crucial role in the pathophysiology of many diseases, this receptor is a strong candidate as a therapeutic target. The tripeptide Leu-Asp-Val (LDV) was identified as the smallest sequence of fibronectin necessary to bind the VLA-4 receptor [36]. The terminal amino acid of this tripeptide is chemically modified with a benzyloxycarbamido phenylurea group to increase the binding potency, offer protection for enzymatic hydrolysis and aid in T cell adhesion inhibition [37–39].

We hypothesized that targeting the VLA-4 receptor using LDV-functionalized LNPs potentially leads to increased uptake and retention of LNPs in the bone marrow by interacting with resident leukocytes. We, therefore, investigated the uptake and efficacy of LDV-LNPs in patient-derived xenotransplants (PDX) and their biodistribution in mice. LDV-LNPs showed improved cellular uptake and efficacious siRNA delivery in PDX, in contrast to their non-targeted counterparts. In vivo, LDV-LNPs displayed a significantly higher accumulation in the bone marrow compared to non-targeted LNPs and an increased association of LDV-LNPs with both immature and mature hematopoietic bone marrow cells. These data provide proof of concept for the delivery of siRNA to the bone marrow through VLA-4 targeting, which could be used to treat a broad range of hematological disorders, including leukemia.

2. Material and Methods

2.1. siRNA LNPs Preparation

LNPs were prepared as described previously [40]. Briefly, a 25 mM lipid mix was prepared by dissolving D_{Lin}-MC3-DMA:DSPC:Cholesterol:DMG-PEG_{2000} in absolute ethanol at molar ratios of 50:10:38.5:1.5. To specifically target the leukemic fusion gene *RUNX1/ETO*, we designed an siRNA homologous to the fusion site of the *RUNX1/ETO* transcript: siRE-mod. As a mismatch control, we used siMM-mod, where two nucleotides in the siRE sequence have been swapped [5,41]. siRNAs were dissolved in a hybridization buffer (25 mM HEPES, 100 mM NaCl, pH 7.5) to a final concentration of 100 µM. To generate LNPs with an optimal nitrogen/phosphate ratio of 4 [42], siRNAs were diluted to a concentration of 26 µM in 25 mM acetic acid pH 4. The siRNA sequences are included in

Supplementary Table S1. For ex vivo visualization, 0.1% molar ratio Cy3-DBCO-DSPE-PEG_{2000} was post-inserted into preformed LNPs. For in vivo visualization, 50% or 30% of the siRE-mod was replaced by siRE-mod-Cy7 (Axolabs, Kulmbach, Germany), conjugated to the sense strand and 0.2% molar ratio DSPE-Cy5.5 was added as a lipid label. siRNA LNPs were prepared using microfluidic mixing in a NanoAssemblr Benchtop Instrument (Precision Nanosystems, Vancouver, Canada) with a total flow rate of 4 mL/min and 1:3 lipid:siRNA volume ratio. Ethanol and acetic acid were removed by overnight dialysis against phosphate-buffered saline (PBS) at 4 °C using sterile 10 kDa molecular weight cut-off (MWCO) Slide-A-Lyzers (Thermofisher Scientific™, Waltham, MA, USA) with PBS replacements after one and three hours. After dialysis, the LNPs were concentrated using Amicon®Ultra-4 Centrifugal Filter Units with 10 kDa MWCO cellulose membrane (Amicon®, Merck, Rahway, NJ, USA) according to the supplier's protocol.

2.2. Particle Size Determination by Dynamic Light Scattering (DLS)

The hydrodynamic diameter and polydispersity index (PDI) of 1:10 diluted samples in Dulbecco's phosphate-buffered saline (DPBS) were measured before and after post-insertion of ligand-conjugates using the Zetasizer Nano Series ZS (Malvern Instruments, Malvern Panalytical, Malvern, UK). Samples were measured in three runs over 5 min at 25 °C, with backscatter set at 173° and attenuator set at 7. Hydrodynamic diameters and PDI values were averaged from three runs.

2.3. Zeta Potential Determination

The zeta potential of the LNPs was determined using the Zetasizer Nano Series ZS. LNPs were diluted 1:100 in 10 mM HEPES (pH = 7.4) prior to analysis. Each sample was measured three times.

2.4. Particle Size Determination by Cryo-Electron Microscopy (cryoEM)

The LNPs were characterized by cryoEM as previously described [40].

2.5. siRNA Concentration and Encapsulation Efficiency

Total siRNA amount loaded into the LNPs was determined using the Quant-It™ Ribogreen microRNA Assay kit (Thermofisher Scientific™) in the presence of 0.5% Triton X-100, whereas the free/unencapsulated siRNA amount was determined in DPBS. The encapsulation efficiency was calculated by the following formula $(([siRNA_{triton}] - [siRNA_{DBPS}])/[siRNA_{triton}]) \times 100\%$.

2.6. Click Chemistry Conjugation and Functionalization of LNPs

Functionalized LNPs were prepared following the protocol we previously established [40]. In brief, Cyanine 3-azide (Cy3) or LDV-azide was first conjugated to the ring-constrained alkyne dibenzocyclooctyne (DBCO), which is covalently linked to DSPE-PEG_{2000}, overnight at room temperate at a 1:3 molar ratio. The conjugated product was immediately post-inserted at a 0.1% molar ratio into preformed LNPs for 30 min at 45 °C [40]. Functionalized LNPs were kept at 4 °C protected from light for up to 7 days.

2.7. Cell Culture

Kasumi-1 (DSMZ no. ACC 220) cell line was obtained from the DSMZ (LGC Standards GmbH, Wesel, Germany) and cultured in Roswell Park Memorial Institute Medium 1640 supplemented with Glutamax (Gibco, Thermofisher Scientific™) 10% fetal bovine serum (FBS, Bodinco, Alkmaar, The Netherlands). Cells were regularly authenticated and tested negative for mycoplasma. Mesenchymal stem cells (MSCs) were obtained from healthy human bone marrow and cultured in Dulbecco's Modified Eagle Medium low glucose (Gibco) supplemented with 1% L-glutamine, 8 ng/mL recombinant human fibroblast growth factor-basic (Peptrotech, Rocky Hill, CT, USA), 20% FBS and 100 U/mL penicillin–streptomycin (P/S) at a density of 7500 cells/cm^2 one day prior to PDX seeding [43].

Bone marrow and ascites PDX expressing the *RUNX1/ETO* fusion were co-cultured on MSCs feeders and cultured in serum-free AML expansion medium (Serum-Free Expansion Medium II (Stemcell, Vancouver, Canada) supplemented with 150 ng/mL stem cell factor, 100 ng/mL thrombopoietin, 10 ng/mL Fms-related tyrosine kinase 3 ligand and 1.35 μM UM729, 750 nM StemRegenin 1 (Biogeme, Lausanne, Switzerland), 10 ng/mL interleukin-3, 10 ng/mL granulocyte-macrophage colony-stimulating factor; all cytokines have been purchased from PeproTech) and 100 u/mL P/S. All patients gave written consent for the use of their material for research purposes. All cells were cultured at 37 °C in a humidified atmosphere containing 5% CO_2.

2.8. LNP Treatment

Leukemia blasts were seeded at a density of 10^6 cells/mL in AML expansion medium on MSC feeders and treated with 4 ug/mL LNPs or LDV-LNPs for 24 h followed by dilution to a density of 5×10^5 cell/mL allowing expansion. Leukemic cells were collected after 3 days for analysis.

2.9. LNP Uptake and Internal ETO Visualization

Cells were seeded at a density of 5×10^5 cells/mL and 100 μL/well in a flat-bottom 96-well plate. Cy3-labeled siRE LNPs with and without LDV-ligand were added to the wells to a final siRNA concentration of 2 (cell lines) or 4 (blasts) μg/mL followed by incubation for up to 24 h at 37 °C and 5% CO_2. Cells were collected after indicated time points for microscopy and flow cytometry analysis and washed once in sterile FACS buffer (PBS containing 0.025% bovine serum albumin, 0.02% sodium azide and 1% FBS) followed by centrifugation for 4 min at × 350 g (cell lines) or 4 min × 500 g (blasts). Cell pellets were resuspended in 150 μL FACS buffer and washed once with acetic acid buffer (0.5 M NaCl, 0.2 M acetic acid, pH 4) to remove membrane-bound LNPs and sterile PBS. To visualize the uptake via flow cytometry, leukemia blasts were stained with 1:50 huCD90-BV421 (clone 5E10, cat #562556, BD Biosciences, San Jose, CA, USA), 1:50 huCD34-APC (clone 8G12, cat #345804, BD Biosciences, San Jose, CA, USA) and 1:25 hu-IgG in FACS buffer, fixed at least overnight using 2% paraformaldehyde in PBS and fluorescence acquired on a Cytoflex LX. To visualize the uptake and internal ETO expression via microscopy, cells and blasts were spun on coverslips using a Thermofisher Scientific™ Cytospin 4 Centrifuge at program 1 (680 rpm for 7 min) with low acceleration. Subsequently, cells and blasts were permeabilized using 0.1% Triton X-100 for 15 min and counterstained with 4′,6-diamidino-2-phenylindole (DAPI) for 5 min or 1:250 polyclonal anti-RUNX1T1 (cat #PA5-79943, Thermofisher Scientific™) for 1 h followed by 1:2000 gt-anti-rb-IgG-AF555 antibody incubation (cat #405324, Biolegend, San Diego, CA, USA) for 1 h. LNP uptake and internal ETO stain were then determined using a DM6 widefield microscope (Leica Microsystems, Wetzlar, Germany) or an SP8 confocal microscope (Leica Microsystems, Wetzlar, Germany).

2.10. RNA Extraction, cDNA Synthesis and qPCR

Total RNA was extracted using the RNeasy Mini Kit (Qiagen, CA, USA) following the supplier's protocol. A total of 500 ng cDNA was prepared using the RevertAid H Minus First Strand cDNA Synthesis Kit (Thermofisher Scientific™) according to the manufacturer's protocol. The qPCR primers are provided in Supplementary Table S2. cDNA samples were diluted to 15 ng input/well prior to qPCR analysis with RNase-free H_2O. The SSoAdvanced™ Universal SYBR® Green Supermix (Bio-rad, Berkeley, CA, USA) was used according to the supplier's protocol.

2.11. Protein Extraction and Western Blot for RUNX1/ETO

Proteins were isolated simultaneously with the RNA by precipitating the RNeasy Mini Kit flow-through with 2 volumes of cold acetone and incubation for 2 h at −80 °C. The protein pellets were then dissolved in 9 M Urea buffer (4% CHAPs and 1% dithiothreitol) at a concentration of 5×10^4 cells per μL. Western blotting was carried out as previously described [5]. Polyclonal Rb-anti-RUNX1 (1:250, cat #4334S, Cell Signaling) and 1:10,000 polyclonal m-anti-GAPDH (cat #AM4300, Invitrogen, Carlsbad, CA, USA) were used as primary antibodies. Goat-anti-mouse (1:10,000, cat #P0447, Agilent, Santa Clara, CA, USA) or anti-rb (1:10,000, cat #sc-2004, Santa Cruz Biotechnology, Dallas, TX, USA) polyclonal IgG HRP-conjugates were used as secondary antibodies.

2.12. Animal Experiments

All animal experiments were performed with the permission of the Animal Welfare Body Utrecht and complied with the Dutch Experiments on Animals Act (WOD) under license AVD10800202115026. The experiment was carried out in accordance with the Guide for the Care and Use of Laboratory Animals. Animals received ad libitum standard chow and water and were housed under standard conditions with 12 h light/dark cycles until experimental procedures.

2.13. In Vivo Biodistribution of LDV-LNPs and LNPs

The biodistribution of LDV-LNPs and LNPs was assessed in female C57/Bl6J (n = 8, weight between 18 and 22 g, 11 weeks old, Charles River, Leiden, the Netherlands) upon tail vein injection of LNPs loaded with Cy7-labelled siRNA (50% of total siRNA content). Animals were randomized into groups of three mice receiving either 50 μg LDV-LNPs or undecorated LNPs. Two control mice received PBS. After 2, 4 and 24 h the animals were live-imaged under isoflurane anesthesia.

2.14. In Vivo Circulation Time and Uptake of LDV-LNPs and LNPs by Bone Marrow Cell Populations

The biodistribution and uptake of LDV-LNPs and LNPs in bone marrow cell populations were assessed in female BALB/c AnNCrl mice (n = 16, weight between 18 and 22 g, 11 weeks old, Charles River, Leiden, the Netherlands) upon intravenous (i.v.) injection of Cy5.5-labelled LNPs (containing a 0.2% molar ratio of DSPE-Cy5.5) loaded with Cy7-labelled siRNA (30% of total siRNA content). Animals were randomized into groups of six mice receiving either LDV-LNPs or non-targeted LNPs. Four control mice received PBS. Either 50 μg of LNPs in 100 μL or an equal volume of vehicle were administered via the tail vein. Blood was collected after 1 min and 1, 2, 4 and 24 h via vena saphena puncture (1 min and 1 and 2 h), submandibular puncture (4 h) and retro-orbital puncture (endpoints) and collected in EDTA anti-coagulated capillaries (1 min and 1 and 2 h) and tubes (endpoints). Blood samples were centrifuged at 2000× g for 10 min at 4 °C. Plasma was collected and stored at −80 °C until further analysis.

After 4 (n = 4 for LDV-LNPs and LNPs or n = 2 for PBS) or 24 h (n = 2 for all groups), mice received an intraperitoneal injection of 100 mg/kg of ketamine and 10 mg/kg of xylazine followed by perfusion with PBS via the left ventricular cavity of the heart. Organs (brain, liver, spleen, kidneys, lungs, heart, femora and tibiae) were collected. Next, whole organ tissue distribution of the LNPs was measured using a Pearl Impulse Imager (Li-Cor Biosciences, Lincoln, NE, USA). Fluorescence in plasma samples was measured on a Spectramax ID3 plate reader (Molecular Devices, San Jose, CA, USA) at excitation/emission wavelengths of 680/720 (Cy5.5) and 750/790 (Cy7). Plasma samples were first diluted 1:1 with pooled control mouse plasma (t = 1 min and 1 h) and subsequently diluted 1:1 with DPBS. Diluted plasma samples (20 μL) were transferred to a clear-bottom black 384-well plate in duplicates and fluorescence was measured. Data are expressed as a percentage of the fluorescence signal obtained at t = 1 min (100% of injected dose).

2.15. Flow Cytometry

To study the association of LNPs with femur cells, we isolated single cells from the femur. Briefly, femora were sterilized with 70% ethanol and washed twice with PBS. Both epiphyses were removed and 1 mL of Iscove's Modified Dulbecco's Medium (IMDM, Gibco, Carlsbad, CA, USA) was slowly flushed through the length of the bone marrow at each end.

Harvested cells were re-suspended and transferred through a 70 µM cell strainer, followed by a wash with 5 mL IMDM.

For staining, single cell suspensions were spun for 5 min at 500× g and subsequently re-suspended in 1 mL of Hybri-Max Red Blood Cell (RBC) Lysis Buffer (cat #11814389001, Sigma Aldrich, St. Louis, MO, USA). The suspension was gently mixed for 1 min at room temperature after which 20 mL of PBS was added to deactivate the RBC lysis buffer. Next, cells were pipetted through a 70 µM cell strainer, washed with 10 mL PBS and re-suspended in 5 mL PBS. Cells were counted 1:1 with 0.4% Trypan Blue and seeded at a density of 0.2×10^6–1×10^6 cells/well in a V-bottom 96-well plate, blocked for non-specific binding of immunoglobulin to the Fc receptors on ice for 10 min with Trustain FcX (1:250 in PBS; clone 93, cat# 101319 and spun for 5 min at 500× g. The following antibody cocktail was added: 1:200 mCD45-PacificBlue (clone S18009F, cat# 157211), 1:50 mCD34-PE (clone SA376A4, cat# 152203), 1:200 mCD49d-APC (clone R1-2, cat# 103621) and 1:100 Zombie Green™ Fixable Viability Kit (cat# 423111) in 50 µL Trustain FcX 1:250 in PBS; all antibodies were obtained from BioLegend. After incubation for 45 min on ice, cells were washed twice with FACS buffer and then fixed in 100 µL 2% PFA in PBS. Samples were stored in the dark at 4 °C for 1–2 days.

Samples were analyzed with a Cytoflex LX (Beckman Coulter, Brea, CA, USA). Data were analyzed using FlowJo.v10.7.1. Cell populations were identified according to the gating strategies shown in Supplementary Figure S1.

2.16. Statistical Analysis

Data were analyzed with GraphPad Prism 8 (GraphPad Software, Inc., San Diego, CA, USA) using a two-sided unpaired or paired Student's t-test. Differences with p values < 0.05 were considered statistically significant.

3. Results

3.1. Characterization of LNPs and LDV-LNPs

For siRNA delivery to leukemic cells, we packaged modified siRNAs into LNPs containing the cationic ionizable lipid Dlin-MC3-DMA by microfluidic mixing (Figure 1a1). To improve uptake in leukemia cells, we conjugated LDV-azide to DSPE-PEG_{2000} by click-chemistry followed by post-insertion of the LDV-DSPE-PEG_{2000} conjugate into preformed LNPs (Figure 1a2) [40]. The LDV-peptide binds with high affinity to the VLA-4 receptor expressed on the cell surface of hematopoietic and leukemic cells (Figure 1a3), upon uptake of the cargo *RUNX1/ETO* target mRNA in leukemic cells is degraded by RNAi (Figure 1a4). To monitor the biodistribution, we incorporated DSPE-Cy5.5 in LNPs and loaded them with 30% siRNA-Cy7. Both LDV-conjugate post-inserted LNPs or LNPs containing fluorescent-labeled siRNA and DSPE-Cy5.5 displayed similar physicochemical characteristics with a hydrodynamic diameter <100 nm (Table 1), PDI of 0.2 and slightly negative zeta potential (Table 1). CryoEM imaging confirmed that the LNPs and LDV-LNPs are uniformly sized (Figure 2b).

3.2. In Vitro Cell Specificity and Delivery Efficacy of LDV-LNPs

To investigate the uptake kinetics of LDV-LNPs in AML cells, we labeled LNPs with Cy3 conjugated to DSPE-PEG_{2000} and monitored the uptake by fluorescence microscopy and flow cytometry. Incorporation of the LDV peptide in LNPs increased their uptake 10-fold in VLA-4-expressing AML cell lines over 24 h (Figure 1c) [40]. Next, we examined the uptake of LDV-LNPs in a more complex cellular environment where *RUNX1/ETO*-expressing PDX are cultivated on MSCs (Figure 1d). The uptake of LDV-LNPs by *RUNX1/ETO*-expressing PDX was increased 10-fold compared to untargeted LNPs within 24 h and led to a twofold reduction of the *RUNX1/ETO* transcript and a complete loss of the fusion protein in different PDX samples after 3 days compared to the controls (Figure 1e–g, Supplementary Figure S2) The knockdown of RUNX1/ETO on protein level after LDV-LNPs treatment in *RUNX1/ETO*-positive PDX was confirmed by imaging upon intracellular staining of ETO (Figure 1h). An overlay of the DAPI and ETO channels shows nuclear localization of the ETO protein in the control PDX. This fluorescence signal was lost in the treated PDX, indicative of substantial loss of the RUNX1/ETO fusion protein.

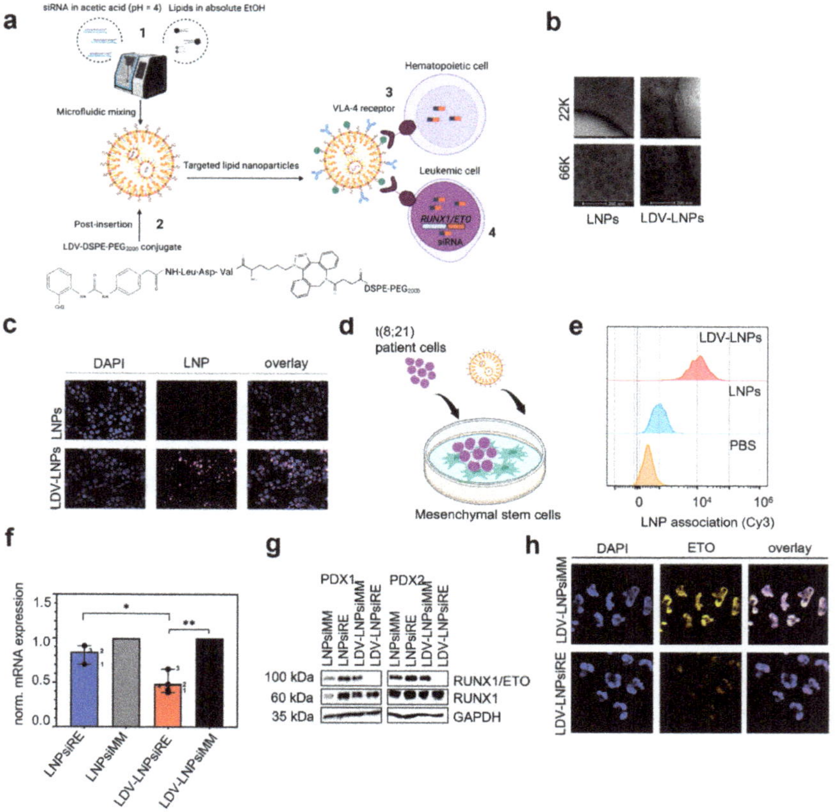

Figure 1. Characterization and siRNA delivery efficacy of lipid nanoparticles in patient-derived leukemia cells. (**a**) Schematic illustration of LDV-LNP production using microfluidic mixing (1), where the LDV-DSPE-PEG_{2000} conjugate is post-inserted into preformed LNPs (2). The LDV-LNPs bind with high affinity to the VLA-4 receptor present on all hematopoietic and leukemic cells (3). In leukemic cells, the active siRNA, siRE-mod, binds to the target mRNA and induces degradation via RNAi (4). (**b**) CryoEM analysis of LNPs (**left**) or LDV-LNPs (**right**) morphology at 22,000× magnification. The bottom panel shows 3-times-enlarged details of the top images. (**c**,**e**–**h**) RUNX1/ETO-expressing AML cells were incubated for 24 h with 2 µg/mL (cell lines) or 4 µg/mL (PDX) siRNA LNPs. (**c**) Uptake of fluorescently labeled LNPs (cyan) without (**top**) and with (**bottom**) LDV-ligand was measured by widefield fluorescence microscopy. Cells were counterstained with DAPI (blue). (**d**) Schematic illustration of the co-culture platform with MSCs feeder layer and RUNX1/ETO-expressing PDX on top. (**e**) LNP Cy3 signal in RUNX1/ETO-expressing PDX after 6 h for LDV-LNPs (red, **top**), LNPs (blue, **middle**) and PBS (orange, **bottom**) as measured by flow cytometry. (**f**,**g**) Reduction of the RUNX1/ETO fusion transcript (**f**) and protein (**g**) of siRNA-LNP-treated PDX detected by qPCR or Western blotting after 3 days of LNP addition. (**h**) Intracellular ETO expression (yellow) was measured by confocal microscopy in RUNX1/ETO-expressing PDX incubated with siMM-mod LDV-LNPs (**top** images) or siRE-mod LDV-LNPs (**bottom** images) Cell were counterstained with DAPI (blue). (**g**) Mean + ranges are displayed. Significance was tested by paired Student's *t*-test * $p < 0.05$, ** $p < 0.001$, $n = 4$. [1] PDX2 bone marrow, [2] PDX1 bone marrow, [3] PDX2 ascites and [4] PDX2 ascites.

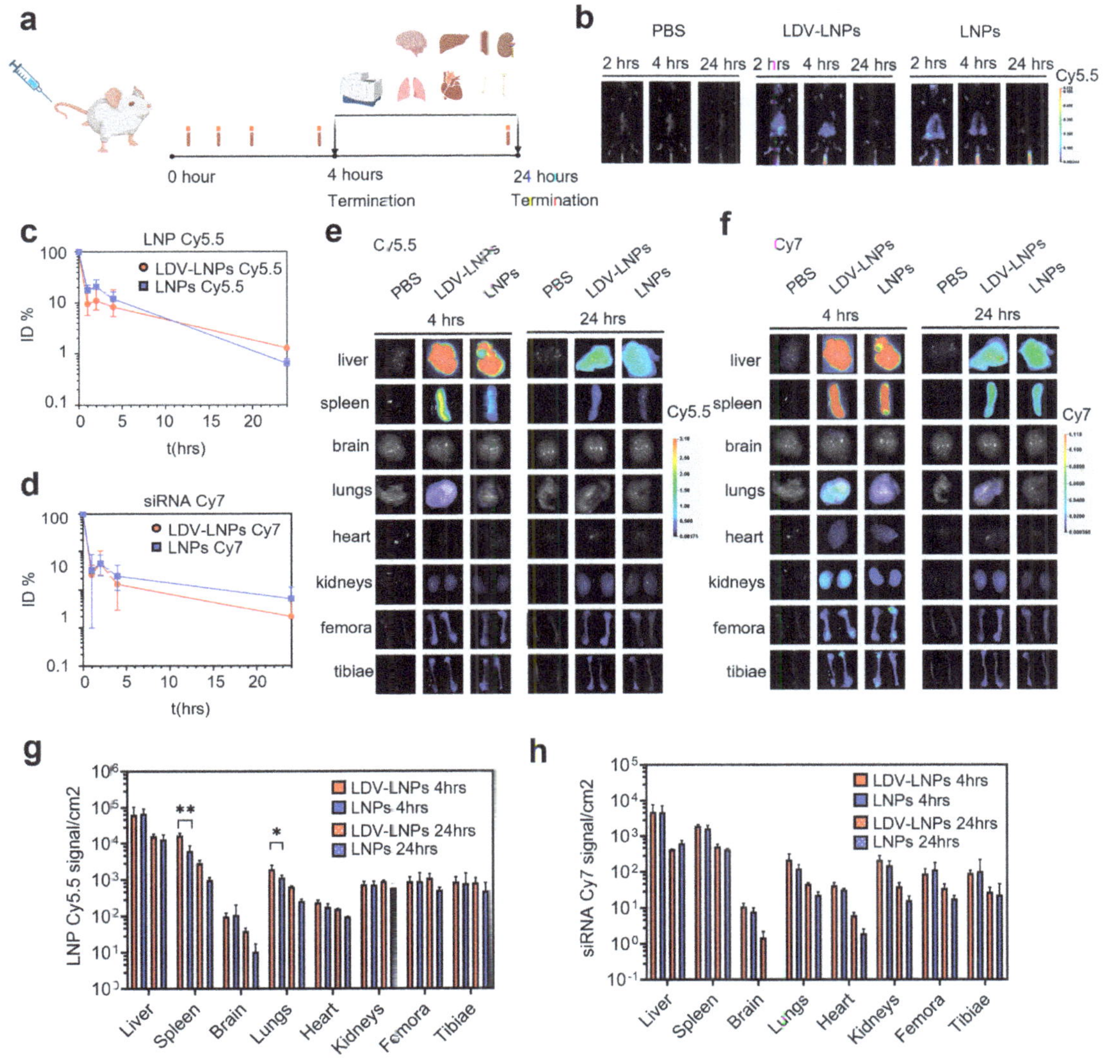

Figure 2. Biodistribution of LDV-LNPs and LNPs after systemic administration. LDV-LNPs or LNPs were administered intravenously at a total dose of 50 ug siRNA per mouse. Mice were live-imaged after 2, 4 and 24 h (**b**) or killed after 4 or 24 h (**c**–**h**). (**a**) Experimental design of the biodistribution study. (**b**) In vivo imaging of LNP-treated mice after 2, 4 and 24 h showing the fluorescent siRNA Cy7 signal in PBS control group (**left**), LDV-LNPs group (**middle**) and LNPs group (**right**). (**c**,**d**) Circulation time of LNPs on a log10 scale. Plasma concentration is expressed as a percentage of the plasma Cy5.5 (**c**) or Cy7 (**d**) fluorescence measured directly after injection ($t = 1$ min). (**e**,**f**) Biodistribution of fluorescently labeled LDV-LNPs and LNPs was measured by whole-organ fluorescence spectroscopy. The image shows the representative LNP Cy5.5 (**e**) fluorescence/white overlay or siRNA Cy7 (**f**) fluorescence/white overlay images of the resected organs 4 and 24 h after injection. (**g**,**h**) Bar graphs showing LNP Cy5.5 (**g**) or siRNA Cy7 (**h**) quantification in whole organs shown in panels e and f using fluorescence spectroscopy. Significance was tested by unpaired Student's *t*-test * $p < 0.05$, ** $p < 0.001$. (**c**,**d**,**g**,**h**) Mean + ranges are displayed. $n = 2$–6.

Table 1. Characteristics of LNPs used in this study. DLS measurement of LNPs. mean +/− range is displayed (n = 3). For LNP and LDV-LNP, three independent batches of LNPs have been prepared. For LNP-Cy7 and LDV-LNP-Cy7, the displayed ranges indicate technical triplicates.

Formulation	Components	Particle Size (nm)	PDI	Zeta Potential (mV)	Encapsulation Efficiency (%)
LNP	Dlin-MC3-DMA/DSPC/Cholesterol/DMG-PEG_{2000} = 50/10/38.5/1.5	66 (57, 83)	0.14 (0.12, 0.16)	−2.5 (−4.2, −1.0)	94 (93, 95)
LDV-LNP	Dlin-MC3-DMA/DSPC/Cholesterol/DMG-PEG_{2000}/LDV-azide-DBCO-DSPE-PEG_{2000} = 50/10/38.5/1.5/0.1	94 (87, 105)	0.26 (0.20, 0.35)	−4.1 (−6.3, −2.3)	93 (91, 94)
LNP-Cy7	Dlin-MC3-DMA/DSPC/Cholesterol/DMG-PEG_{2000}/DBCO-DSPE-PEG_{2000} = 50/10/38.5/1.5/0.1	69 (68, 70)	0.08 (0.07, 0.09)	−0.3 (−0.2, −0.3)	97
LDV-LNP-Cy7	Dlin-MC3-DMA/DSPC/Cholesterol/DMG-PEG_{2000}/LDV-azide-DBCO-DSPE-PEG_{2000} = 50/10/38.5/1.5/0.1	74 (73, 75)	0.08 (0.07, 0.09)	−3.1 (−2.7, −3.7)	97

3.3. Pharmacokinetics and In Vivo Biodistribution of LDV-LNPs and LNPs

Our data demonstrate the benefit of LDV-functionalization for LNP uptake and siRNA delivery efficacy ex vivo. To gain insight into the pharmacokinetics and biodistribution of the LNPs in vivo, we prepared dual fluorescently labeled LNPs containing Cy7-siRNA and DSPE-Cy5.5. LNPs were injected into the tail vein of wild-type C57/Bl6J or BALB/cAnNCrl mice. Next, we performed in vivo imaging and quantified the tissue distribution of both LNP vehicles and siRNA cargo by fluorescent imaging of blood samples and organs (Figure 2a). Treatment did not cause any adverse effect in either mouse strain during the observation times of up to 2 days. In vivo imaging of C57Bl/6J mice showed the highest siRNA Cy7 fluorescent signal in the liver region after 4 h, with a strong reduction in the signal after 24 h (Figure 2b). This was in line with the circulation time of the LNPs, which was analyzed in plasma samples at various time points in BALB/c mice. Both LNPs displayed circulation half-lives of 45 min, with less than 10% of the injected dose still present in the circulation 5 h after injection (Figure 2c,d). No difference in circulation time was observed between the two fluorophores, indicating that the particles remained intact. Moreover, the circulation kinetics did not significantly differ between the LDV-LNPs and LNPs, nor between individual mice (Supplementary Figure S3). Thus, surface modification of the LNPs with LDV did not affect their circulation time.

We then investigated in which tissues the LNPs accumulated. To that end, we quantified the fluorescence of LNP Cy5.5 and siRNA Cy7 in organs by fluorescence spectroscopy after 4 (n = 4) and 24 h (n =2) (Figure 2e–h). LNP- and siRNA-associated fluorescence was found in several organs, including the liver and spleen, and to a smaller extent, in the lungs, heart, kidneys, femora and tibiae. We detected a significantly higher LNPs Cy5.5 signal in the spleen and lungs in animals treated with the LDV-LNPs compared with untargeted LNPs after 4 h (Figure 2e,g). This could be explained by an increased association of LDV-LNPs with VLA-4-positive lymphocytes and macrophages present in these organs [32,44]. In all organs, the overall tissue fluorescence decreased after 24 h. Co-localization of the LNPs Cy5.5 and siRNA Cy7 signal show that the observed biodistribution pattern is unlikely to be caused by Cy7-siRNA leaked from the LNPs, as this would have caused mainly accumulation in the kidneys due to the small size of siRNA (<50 kDa) [45–47]. Instead, these data demonstrate LNP-mediated delivery of siRNA to tissues and long bones.

3.4. LDV-Decoration Improves LNP Uptake via VLA-4 in Hematopoietic Bone Marrow Cells

To further explore LNPs association with hematopoietic bone marrow cells, we examined the LNP Cy5.5 and Cy7 signal in long bones by whole organ fluorescence spectroscopy and on a single cell level. We observed a high accumulation of both LNPs and siRNA in the femora and tibiae 4 h after injection based on Cy5.5 and Cy7 fluorescence, respectively

(Figure 3a, adjusted scaling for the femora and tibiae alone). Although the overall signal decreased over 24 h, the LDV-LNPs were still detectable and were equally distributed along the length of the femora and in the epiphyses of the tibiae (Figure 3b). A significant twofold increase in median LNP Cy5.5 fluorescent signal in single cell suspensions of the bone marrow was observed after 4 and 24 h in the animals treated with LDV-LNPs compared to animals treated with LNPs, indicative of improved accumulation and retention of LNPs in the bone marrow (Figure 3b,c). LNP uptake in the hematopoietic bone marrow cells appeared to be VLA-4-dependent as cells with higher VLA-4 expression showed a significantly higher LNP uptake (Figure 3d,e).

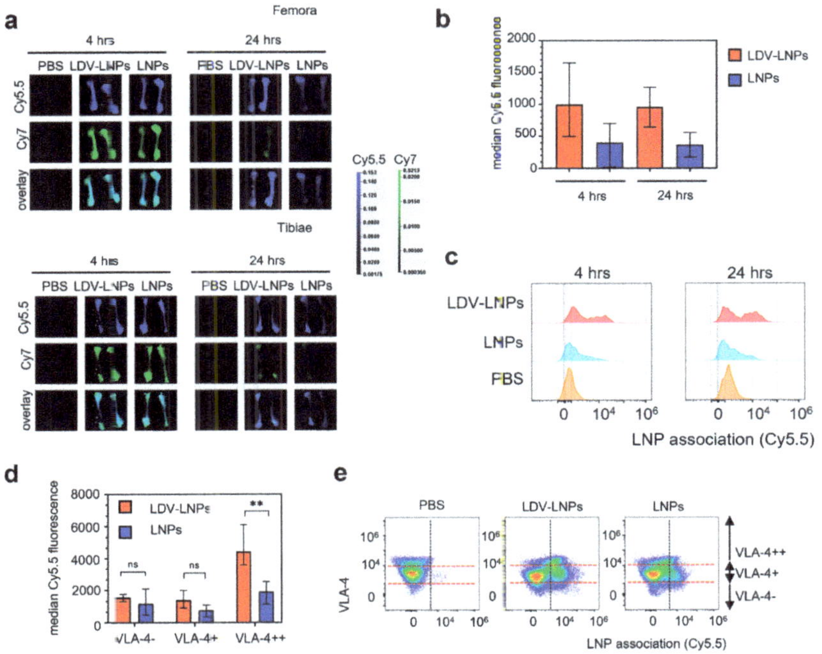

Figure 3. LDV-LNPs and LNPs accumulate in the femora and tibiae. Accumulation of fluorescently labeled LDV-LNPs and LNPs in the femur and tibia was measured at the whole-organ and single-cell levels. (**a**) The LNP Cy5.5 fluorescence/siRNA Cy7/white overlay images for the femora (**top** figure) and tibiae (**bottom** figure) 4 and 24 h after injection. The scale of both channels has been adjusted for the long bones alone. (**b**) Median Cy5.5 fluorescence (minus the Cy5.5 fluorescence signal in control PBS) in the bulk single femur cells as determined by flow cytometry. (**c**) LNP signal in bulk single femur cells after 4 (**left**) or 24 h (**right**) for LDV-LNPs (red, **top**), LNPs (blue, **middle**) and PBS (orange, **bottom**) as measured by flow cytometry. (**d**) Median Cy5.5 fluorescence in VLA-4-positive femur cells after 4 h as determined by flow cytometry. (**e**) Scatter plots showing the VLA-4 expression and LNP Cy5.5 accumulation in single femur cells after 4 h for PBS, LDV-LNPs and LNPs as determined by multiparameter flow analysis. The red dotted lines indicate gating for VLA-4-, VLA-4+ and VLA-4++ cells. (**b**,**d**) Mean + ranges are displayed. $n = 4$ (4 h) $n = 2$ (24 h). Significance was tested by two-tailed unpaired Student's *t*-test, ** $p < 0.001$, ns = not significant, unpaired two-tailed Student's *t*-test.

3.5. LDV-LNPs Target VLA-4-Positive Immature Myeloid Cells in the Bone Marrow

Leukemia is characterized by the uncontrolled proliferation of immature malignant hematopoietic progenitor-like cells (HSPCs). To investigate whether more immature, progenitor cells can be targeted with the LDV-LNPs and LNPs, we examined LNP uptake and retention in the bone marrow in HSPCs subpopulations. We therefore stained single cells isolated from the bone marrow with antibodies specific for hematopoietic markers such as CD45, CD49d (VLA-4 receptor) and CD34 (expressed by immature myeloid cells). 54% of immature HSPCs (CD45+/VLA-4+/CD34+) were LNP-positive in LDV-LNP-treated mice after 4 and 24 h of injection, as compared to 29% in the LNPs group (Figure 4a–c and Supplementary Figure S4a–c). Notably, more mature hematopoietic cells (CD34-CD45+CD49d+) also showed enhanced uptake of LDV-LNPs compared to untargeted LNPs (Figure 4b,c: left). Both immature and mature hematopoietic bone marrow cells also showed significant twofold-higher LNP Cy5.5 fluorescence in the LDV-LNPs group compared to the LNPs group, indicating that the improved LDV-LNP uptake is dependent on the expression of the ligand VLA-4 (Figure 4d and Supplementary Figure S4d).

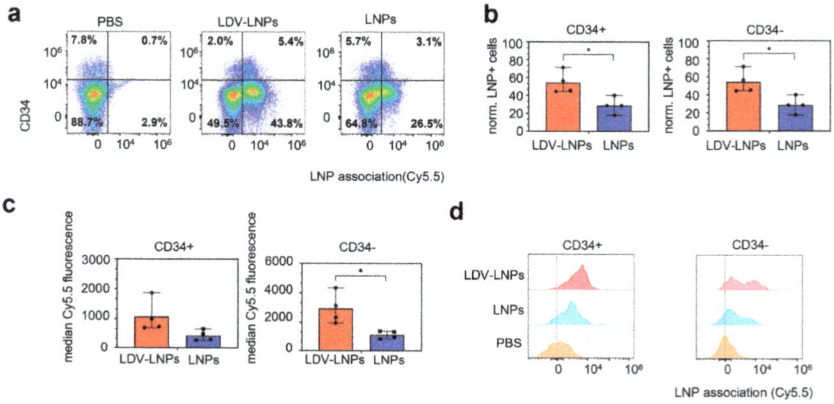

Figure 4. Increased uptake of LDV-LNPs in HPSC in the bone marrow. (**a**) Scatter plots showing CD34 expression and LNP association with CD45+/VLA-4+ cells in the bone marrow after 4 h after administration of PBS, LDV-LNPs, or LNPs as determined by multiparameter flow analysis. (**b**) Bar graphs showing the percentage of LNP+ cells in CD45+/VLA-4+/CD34+ (**left**) or CD45+/VLA-4+/CD34- (**right**) bone marrow cells as determined by multiparameter flow analysis after 4 h. (**c**,**d**) LNP Cy5.5 association with CD34+ (**left**) and CD34- (**right**) bone marrow cells after 4 h displayed in bar graphs (**c**) and histograms (**d**) where LDV-LNPs is red, LNPs blue and control PBS orange. (**b**,**c**) Means + ranges are displayed. Significance was tested by two-tailed unpaired Student's *t*-test * $p < 0.05$, unpaired two-tailed Student's *t*-test. $n = 4$.

These results clearly show that LDV-LNPs associate with both VLA-4-positive immature and mature HSPCs resulting in higher LNP accumulation and longer retention in the bone marrow. Consequently, these findings strongly support the concept of augmented retain and improved uptake in leukemic cells including leukemic stem cells in vivo.

4. Discussion

RNA interference represents a highly attractive alternative to current treatment regimens, however, extrahepatic delivery of siRNA using LNPs has proven difficult due to high liver accumulation. Modification of the LNP surface with targeting ligands could potentially improve LNP uptake beyond the liver. Here we show that targeting the VLA-4 receptor using the LDV motif on the surface of LNPs improved the cellular uptake of LNPs in HSPCs ex vivo and in vivo. These combined data thereby provide evidence for the use of LDV-LNPs for the treatment of hematological disorders.

High liver accumulation is commonly reported for both liposomes and LNP-based therapies. Both LNPs, targeting and non-targeting, used in this study displayed a short circulation time of 45 min. However, longer circulation times are desired as this will improve the passive accumulation of LNPs in extrahepatic tissues [48]. The circulation time is dictated by the lipid components of the nanoparticle formulation and can be finetuned by modifying the length of the PEG-lipid chain, as longer lipid chains will increase the circulation time [49,50]. Since longer circulation times of PEG usually result in reduced endosomal release and will also increase the chances of evoking an anti-PEG immune response [51], PEG does not seem to possess ideal characteristics for being incorporated in LNPs for in vivo usage. As an alternative, PEG could be replaced with polysaccharides, naturally occurring membrane lipids, or stealth-providing compounds such as polysarcosine to shield the nanoparticle from rapid removal by opsonization [52–56]. Additionally, an attractive concept is passive targeting by changing the lipid formulation, however, little is known about the optimal lipid composition for bone marrow targeting [57–59]. For liposomes, it is reported that cholesterol aids in bone marrow uptake by phagocytic cells via selective opsonization such as C3 complement protein—an interesting point for future studies on targeting the bone marrow with LNPs [60,61].

Whereas the use of higher dosages to saturate the liver will also improve accumulation in other tissues including the bone marrow, ionizable lipids including D_{lin}-MC_3-DMA show dose-limiting toxicity at higher doses [62,63]. The first FDA- and EMA-approved siRNA LNP treatment, Onpattro, is given at a dose of 0.3 mg/kg body weight once every three weeks. Converting this human dose to the equivalent mouse dose, this is almost double the dose of 2 mg/kg body weight used in this study [64]. Since we already observe a high bone marrow accumulation and retention of the LDV-LNPs at 2 mg/kg body weight, we might already achieve therapeutic effects of the LDV-LNPs in the bone marrow at a clinically safe dose. Thus, efficacy studies in a leukemia disease model would be of high interest. For multiple myeloma, VLA-4-targeting nanoparticles containing chemotherapeutic agents have proven successful in reducing leukemic burden in vivo [31,65]. These studies used immunodeficient mice, which might exhibit longer nanoparticle circulation times due to the lack of immune-related clearance [66–68]. In contrast, our model provides evidence that LNPs can reach hematopoietic target cells in the bone marrow even in the presence of a fully functional immune system. Thus, in a murine leukemia model, we expect to observe increased bone marrow accumulation of LDV-LNPs due to improved bone marrow permeability [67,68]. Future studies will uncover whether this is sufficient to reach therapeutically relevant siRNA concentrations in leukemic cells of the bone marrow.

5. Conclusions

In summary, we here demonstrate that bone-marrow targeting using LDV-ligand-functionalized LNPs results in substantially enhanced LNP uptake by immature and mature hematopoietic progenitor cells, cell compartments also shown to harbor leukemic stem cells. This study thereby supports the further development of targeted therapeutic interventions for the treatment of leukemia and other hematological disorders.

Supplementary Materials: The following supporting information can be downloaded at: https://www.mdpi.com/article/10.3390/pharmaceutics15061603/s1, Figure S1: Gating strategy for single bone marrow cells; Figure S2: Reduction of RUNX1/ETO transcript in PDX; Figure S3: Biodistribution of LDV-LNPs and LNPs in BALB/cAnNCrl mice; Figure S4: Improved accumulation of LDV-LNPs in HPSC in the bone marrow; Table S1: siRNA sequences and their chemical modifications. F, 2′-fluoronucleoside; OMe, 2′-methoxynucleoside; d, 2′-deoxynucleoside; PS, phosphorothioate-. For in vivo visualization the sense strand of the siRNA was modified with Cy7 linked via an NHS ester bond. The two swapped nucleotides in the mismatch siRNA control are displayed bold; Table S2: qPCR primer sequences.

Author Contributions: Conceptualization, L.E.S., M.H.A.M.F., R.M.S., S.K. and O.H.; Methodology, L.E.S., A.K.-H., A.v.O., P.W., D.T., R.N., L.v.d.B., E.S., C.S., T.O. and O.H.; Investigation, L.E.S., M.H.A.M.F., A.v.O., P.W., L.D.M.C., D.T., M.H., L.v.d.B., R.N., M.H., E.S. and C.S.; Data analysis and interpretation, L.E.S., A.v.O., P.W., M.H.A.M.F., R.M.S., S.K., T.O., O.H.; Resources, A.K.-H., R.N., D.T., C.S., L.v.d.B., R.M.S. and O.H.; Validation, L.D.M.C., M.H.; Writing—Original Draft Preparation, L.E.S. and O.H.; Writing—Review & Editing, L.E.S., M.H.A.M.F., E.S., A.K.-H., S.K. and O.H.; Supervision, M.H.A.M.F., S.K. and O.H.; Funding Acquisition, O.H. All authors have read and agreed to the published version of the manuscript.

Funding: This research was supported by KiKa program grant 329 to O.H.

Institutional Review Board Statement: The animal study protocol was approved by the Animal Welfare Body Utrecht and complied with the Dutch Experiments on Animals Act (WOD) under license AVD10800202115026.

Informed Consent Statement: Informed consent was obtained from all subjects in this study.

Data Availability Statement: All created data is available in this manuscript and the Supplementary Material.

Acknowledgments: We would like to thank Nicky van Kronenburg for providing the material to test and setup the antibody panels, Nina van der Wilt for acting as courier to transport samples from the animal facility to the research lab and Martijn Evers for providing the necessary protocols for bone marrow cell isolation.

Conflicts of Interest: The authors declare the following financial interests/personal relationships which may be considered as potential competing interests: Olaf Heidenreich and Laura Swart are inventors on a patent for Targeted lipid nanoparticle formulations pending to Princess Máxima Center for Pediatric Oncology.

References

1. Rothdiener, M.; Müller, D.; Castro, P.G.; Scholz, A.; Schwemmlein, M.; Fey, G.; Heidenreich, O.; Kontermann, R.E. Targeted delivery of SiRNA to CD33-positive tumor cells with liposomal carrier systems. *J. Control. Release* **2010**, *144*, 251–258. [CrossRef]
2. Gavrilov, K.; Seo, Y.-E.; Tietjen, G.T.; Cui, J.; Cheng, C.J.; Saltzman, W.M. Enhancing potency of siRNA targeting fusion genes by optimization outside of target sequence. *Proc. Natl. Acad. Sci. USA* **2015**, *112*, E6597–E6605. [CrossRef] [PubMed]
3. Jyotsana, N.; Sharma, A.; Chaturvedi, A.; Budida, R.; Scherr, M.; Kuchenbauer, F.; Lindner, R.; Noyan, F.; Sühs, K.-W.; Stangel, M.; et al. Lipid nanoparticle-mediated siRNA delivery for safe targeting of human CML in vivo. *Ann. Hematol.* **2019**, *98*, 1905–1918. [CrossRef]
4. Mohanty, S.; Jyotsana, N.; Sharma, A.; Kloos, A.; Gabdoulline, R.; Othman, B.; Lai, C.K.; Schottmann, R.; Mandhania, M.; Schmoellerl, J.; et al. Targeted Inhibition of the NUP98-NSD1 Fusion Oncogene in Acute Myeloid Leukemia. *Cancers* **2020**, *12*, 2766. [CrossRef] [PubMed]
5. Issa, H.; Swart, L.E.; Rasouli, M.; Ashtiani, M.; Nakjang, S.; Jyotsana, N.; Schuschel, K.; Heuser, M.; Blair, H.; Heidenreich, O. Nanoparticle-mediated targeting of the fusion gene RUNX1/ETO in t(8;21)-positive acute myeloid leukaemia. *Leukemia* **2023**, *37*, 820–834. [CrossRef]
6. Jackson, A.L.; Burchard, J.; Leake, D.; Reynolds, A.; Schelter, J.; Guo, J.; Johnson, J.M.; Lim, L.; Karpilow, J.; Nichols, K.; et al. Position-specific chemical modification of siRNAs reduces "off-target" transcript silencing. *RNA* **2006**, *12*, 1197–1205. [CrossRef]
7. Soutschek, J.; Akinc, A.; Bramlage, B.; Charisse, K.; Constien, R.; Donoghue, M.; Elbashir, S.; Geick, A.; Hadwiger, P.; Harborth, J.; et al. Therapeutic silencing of an endogenous gene by systemic administration of modified siRNAs. *Nature* **2004**, *432*, 173–178. [CrossRef] [PubMed]
8. Marques, J.T.; Williams, B.R.G. Activation of the mammalian immune system by siRNAs. *Nat. Biotechnol.* **2005**, *23*, 1399–1405. [CrossRef]
9. Kim, D.H.; Rossi, J.J. Strategies for silencing human disease using RNA interference. *Nat. Rev. Genet.* **2007**, *8*, 173–184. [CrossRef]
10. Aigner, A. Nonviral in vivo delivery of therapeutic small interfering RNAs. *Curr. Opin. Mol. Ther.* **2007**, *9*, 345–352.
11. Lee, S.J.; Son, S.; Yhee, J.Y.; Choi, K.; Kwon, I.C.; Kim, S.H.; Kim, K. Structural modification of siRNA for efficient gene silencing. *Biotechnol. Adv.* **2013**, *31*, 491–503. [CrossRef]
12. Liu, P.; Chen, G.; Zhang, J. A Review of Liposomes as a Drug Delivery System: Current Status of Approved Products, Regulatory Environments, and Future Perspectives. *Molecules* **2022**, *27*, 1372. [CrossRef] [PubMed]
13. Ahmad, Z.; Shah, A.; Siddiq, M.; Kraatz, H.-B. Polymeric micelles as drug delivery vehicles. *RSC Adv.* **2014**, *4*, 17028–17038. [CrossRef]
14. Paunovska, K.; Loughrey, D.; Dahlman, J.E. Drug delivery systems for RNA therapeutics. *Nat. Rev. Genet.* **2022**, *23*, 265–280. [CrossRef] [PubMed]
15. Yan, Y.; Liu, X.-Y.; Lu, A.; Wang, X.-Y.; Jiang, L.-X.; Wang, J.-C. Non-viral vectors for RNA delivery. *J. Control. Release* **2022**, *342*, 241–279. [CrossRef]
16. Sato, Y.; Kinami, Y.; Hashiba, K.; Harashima, H. Different kinetics for the hepatic uptake of lipid nanoparticles between the apolipoprotein E/low density lipoprotein receptor and the N-acetyl-d-galactosamine/asialoglycoprotein receptor pathway. *J. Control. Release* **2020**, *322*, 217–226. [CrossRef] [PubMed]
17. Akinc, A.; Querbes, W.; De, S.; Qin, J.; Frank-Kamenetsky, M.; Jayaprakash, K.N.; Jayaraman, M.; Rajeev, K.G.; Cantley, W.L.; Dorkin, J.R.; et al. Targeted Delivery of RNAi Therapeutics With Endogenous and Exogenous Ligand-Based Mechanisms. *Mol. Ther.* **2010**, *18*, 1357–1364. [CrossRef] [PubMed]

18. Yan, X.; Kuipers, F.; Havekes, L.M.; Havinga, R.; Dontje, B.; Poelstra, K.; Scherphof, G.L.; Kamps, J.A. The role of apolipoprotein E in the elimination of liposomes from blood by hepatocytes in the mouse. *Biochem. Biophys. Res. Commun.* **2005**, *328*, 57–62. [CrossRef]
19. Zhang, X.; Goel, V.; Attarwala, H.; Sweetser, M.T.; Clausen, V.A.; Robbie, G.J. Patisiran Pharmacokinetics, Pharmacodynamics, and Exposure-Response Analyses in the Phase 3 APOLLO Trial in Patients With Hereditary Transthyretin-Mediated (hATTR) Amyloidosis. *J. Clin. Pharmacol.* **2020**, *60*, 37–49. [CrossRef]
20. Adams, D.; Gonzalez-Duarte, A.; O'Riordan, W.D.; Yang, C.C.; Ueda, M.; Kristen, A.V.; Tournev, I.; Schmidt, H.H.; Coelho, T.; Berk, J.L.; et al. Patisiran, an RNAi Therapeutic, for Hereditary Transthyretin Amyloidosis. *N. Engl. J. Med.* **2018**, *379*, 11–21. [CrossRef]
21. Sweetenham, J.; Masek, L. *Endothelial Cell Culture*; Bicknell, R., Ed.; Cambridge University Press: Cambridge, UK, 1996; pp. 23–35.
22. Lorenzer, C.; Dirin, M.; Winkler, A.-M.; Baumann, V.; Winkler, J. Going beyond the liver: Progress and challenges of targeted delivery of siRNA therapeutics. *J. Control. Release* **2015**, *203*, 1–15. [CrossRef] [PubMed]
23. Huang, B.; Abraham, W.D.; Zheng, Y.; López, S.C.B.; Luo, S.S.; Irvine, D.J. Active targeting of chemotherapy to disseminated tumors using nanoparticle-carrying T cells. *Sci. Transl. Med.* **2015**, *7*, 291ra94. [CrossRef] [PubMed]
24. Shi, J.; Xiao, Z.; Kamaly, N.; Farokhzad, O.C. Self-Assembled Targeted Nanoparticles: Evolution of Technologies and Bench to Bedside Translation. *Accounts Chem. Res.* **2011**, *44*, 1123–1134. [CrossRef] [PubMed]
25. Bertrand, N.; Wu, J.; Xu, X.; Kamaly, N.; Farokhzad, O.C. Cancer nanotechnology: The impact of passive and active targeting in the era of modern cancer biology. *Adv. Drug Deliv. Rev.* **2014**, *66*, 2–25. [CrossRef]
26. Peer, D.; Margalit, R. Tumor-Targeted Hyaluronan Nanoliposomes Increase the Antitumor Activity of Liposomal Doxorubicin in Syngeneic and Human Xenograft Mouse Tumor Models. *Neoplasia* **2004**, *6*, 343–353. [CrossRef]
27. Dammes, N.; Goldsmith, M.; Ramishetti, S.; Dearling, J.L.J.; Veiga, N.; Packard, A.B.; Peer, D. Conformation-sensitive targeting of lipid nanoparticles for RNA therapeutics. *Nat. Nanotechnol.* **2021**, *16*, 1030–1038. [CrossRef]
28. Li, H.; Huang, S.Y.; Shi, F.H.; Gu, Z.C.; Zhang, S.G.; Wei, J.F. α(4)β(7) integrin inhibitors: A patent review. *Expert Opin. Ther. Pat.* **2018**, *28*, 903–917. [CrossRef]
29. Petrovic, A.; Alpdogan, O.; Willis, L.M.; Eng, J.M.; Greenberg, A.S.; Kappel, B.J.; Liu, C.; Murphy, G.J.; Heller, G.; Van Den Brink, M.R. LPAM (α4β7 integrin) is an important homing integrin on alloreactive T cells in the development of intestinal graft-versus-host disease. *Blood* **2004**, *103*, 1542–1547. [CrossRef] [PubMed]
30. de la Puente, P.; Azab, A.K. Nanoparticle delivery systems, general approaches, and their implementation in multiple myeloma. *Eur. J. Haematol.* **2017**, *98*, 529–541. [CrossRef]
31. Kiziltepe, T.; Ashley, J.D.; Stefanick, J.F.; Qi, Y.M.; Alves, N.J.; Handlogten, M.W.; Suckow, M.A.; Navari, R.M.; Bilgicer, B. Rationally engineered nanoparticles target multiple myeloma cells, overcome cell-adhesion-mediated drug resistance, and show enhanced efficacy in vivo. *Blood Cancer J.* **2012**, *2*, e64. [CrossRef]
32. Hemler, M.E.; Elices, M.J.; Parker, C.; Takada, Y. Structure of the Integrin VLA-4 and its Cell-Cell and Cell-Matrix Adhesion Functions. *Immunol. Rev.* **1990**, *114*, 45–65. [CrossRef] [PubMed]
33. Härzschel, A.; Zucchetto, A.; Gattei, V.; Hartmann, T.N. VLA-4 Expression and Activation in B Cell Malignancies: Functional and Clinical Aspects. *Int. J. Mol. Sci.* **2020**, *21*, 2206. [CrossRef]
34. Deshantri, A.K.; Fens, M.H.; Ruiter, R.W.; Metselaar, J.M.; Storm, G.; van Bloois, L.; Varela-Moreira, A.; Mandhane, S.N.; Mutis, T.; Martens, A.C.; et al. Liposomal dexamethasone inhibits tumor growth in an advanced human-mouse hybrid model of multiple myeloma. *J. Control. Release* **2019**, *296*, 232–240. [CrossRef] [PubMed]
35. Hemler, M.E. VLA proteins in the integrin family: Structures, functions, and their role on leukocytes. *Annu. Rev. Immunol.* **1990**, *8*, 365–400. [CrossRef]
36. Komoriya, A.; Green, L.; Mervic, M.; Yamada, S.; Yamada, K.; Humphries, M. The minimal essential sequence for a major cell type-specific adhesion site (CS1) within the alternatively spliced type III connecting segment domain of fibronectin is leucine-aspartic acid-valine. *J. Biol. Chem.* **1991**, *266*, 15075–15079. [CrossRef]
37. Baiula, M.; Spampinato, S.; Gentilucci, L.; Tolomelli, A. Novel Ligands Targeting α4β1 Integrin: Therapeutic Applications and Perspectives. *Front Chem* **2019**, *7*, 489. [CrossRef]
38. Lin, K.C.; Ateeq, H.S.; Hsiung, S.H.; Chong, L.T.; Zimmerman, C.N.; Castro, A.; Lee, W.C.; Hammond, C.E.; Kalkunte, S.; Chen, L.L.; et al. Selective, tight-binding inhibitors of integrin alpha4beta1 that inhibit allergic airway responses. *J. Med. Chem.* **1999**, *42*, 920–934. [CrossRef] [PubMed]
39. Gérard, E.; Meulle, A.; Feron, O.; Marchand-Brynaert, J. LDV peptidomimetics equipped with biotinylated spacer-arms: Synthesis and biological evaluation on CCRF-CEM cell line. *Bioorg. Med. Chem. Lett.* **2012**, *22*, 586–590. [CrossRef]
40. Swart, L.E.; Koekman, C.; Seinen, C.; Issa, H.; Rasouli, M.; Schiffelers, R.; Heidenreich, O. A robust post-insertion method for the preparation of targeted siRNA LNPs. *Int. J. Pharm.* **2022**, *620*, 121741. [CrossRef]
41. Heidenreich, O.; Krauter, J.; Riehle, H.; Hadwiger, P.; John, M.; Heil, G.; Vornlocher, H.P.; Nordheim, A. AML1/MTG8 oncogene suppression by small interfering RNAs supports myeloid differentiation of t(8;21)-positive leukemic cells. *Blood* **2003**, *101*, 3157–3163. [CrossRef] [PubMed]

42. Chen, S.; Tam, Y.Y.C.; Lin, P.J.; Sung, M.M.; Tam, Y.K.; Cullis, P.R. Influence of particle size on the in vivo potency of lipid nanoparticle formulations of siRNA. *J. Control. Release* **2016**, *235*, 236–244. [CrossRef]
43. Pal, D.; Blair, H.J.; Elder, A.; Dormon, K.; Rennie, K.J.; Coleman, D.J.L.; Weiland, J.; Rankin, K.S.; Filby, A.; Heidenreich, O.; et al. Long-term in vitro maintenance of clonal abundance and leukaemia-initiating potential in acute lymphoblastic leukaemia. *Leukemia* **2016**, *30*, 1691–1700. [CrossRef] [PubMed]
44. Lobb, R.R.; Hemler, M.E. The pathophysiologic role of alpha 4 integrins in vivo. *J. Clin. Investig.* **1994**, *94*, 1722–1728. [CrossRef] [PubMed]
45. van de Water, F.M.; Boerman, O.C.; Wouterse, A.C.; Peters, J.G.; Russel, F.G.; Masereeuw, R. Intravenously administered short interfering RNA accumulates in the kidney and selectively suppresses gene function in renal proximal tubules. *Drug Metab. Dispos.* **2006**, *34*, 1393–1397. [CrossRef]
46. Bumcrot, D.; Manoharan, M.; Koteliansky, V.; Sah, D.W.Y. RNAi therapeutics: A potential new class of pharmaceutical drugs. *Nat. Chem. Biol.* **2006**, *2*, 711–719. [CrossRef] [PubMed]
47. Santel, A.; Aleku, M.; Keil, O.; Endruschat, J.; Esche, V.; Fisch, G.; Dames, S.; Löffler, K.; Fechtner, M.; Arnold, W.; et al. A novel siRNA-lipoplex technology for RNA interference in the mouse vascular endothelium. *Gene Ther.* **2006**, *13*, 1222–1234. [CrossRef]
48. Sou, K.; Klipper, R.; Goins, B.; Tsuchida, E.; Phillips, W.T. Circulation Kinetics and Organ Distribution of Hb-Vesicles Developed as a Red Blood Cell Substitute. *Experiment* **2005**, *312*, 702–709. [CrossRef]
49. Miteva, M.; Kirkbride, K.C.; Kilchrist, K.V.; Werfel, T.A.; Li, H.; Nelson, C.E.; Gupta, M.K.; Giorgio, T.D.; Duvall, C.L. Tuning PEGylation of mixed micelles to overcome intracellular and systemic siRNA delivery barriers. *Biomaterials* **2015**, *38*, 97–107. [CrossRef]
50. Suk, J.S.; Xu, Q.; Kim, N.; Hanes, J.; Ensign, L.M. PEGylation as a strategy for improving nanoparticle-based drug and gene delivery. *Adv. Drug Deliv. Rev.* **2016**, *99*, 28–51. [CrossRef]
51. Zalba, S.; Hagen, T.L.M.T.; Burgui, C.; Garrido, M.J. Stealth nanoparticles in oncology: Facing the PEG dilemma. *J. Control. Release* **2022**, *351*, 22–36. [CrossRef]
52. Curcio, M.; Brindisi, M.; Cirillo, G.; Frattaruolo, L.; Leggio, A.; Rago, V.; Nicoletta, F.P.; Cappello, A.R.; Iemma, F. Smart Lipid–Polysaccharide Nanoparticles for Targeted Delivery of Doxorubicin to Breast Cancer Cells. *Int. J. Mol. Sci.* **2022**, *23*, 2386. [CrossRef] [PubMed]
53. De Leo, V.; Milano, F.; Agostiano, A.; Catucci, L. Recent Advancements in Polymer/Liposome Assembly for Drug Delivery: From Surface Modifications to Hybrid Vesicles. *Polymers* **2021**, *13*, 1027. [CrossRef] [PubMed]
54. LoPresti, S.T.; Arral, M.L.; Chaudhary, N.; Whitehead, K.A. The replacement of helper lipids with charged alternatives in lipid nanoparticles facilitates targeted mRNA delivery to the spleen and lungs. *J. Control. Release* **2022**, *345*, 819–831. [CrossRef] [PubMed]
55. Weber, B.; Seidl, C.; Schwiertz, D.; Scherer, M.; Bleher, S.; Süss, R.; Barz, M. Polysarcosine-Based Lipids: From Lipopolypeptoid Micelles to Stealth-Like Lipids in Langmuir Blodgett Monolayers. *Polymers* **2016**, *8*, 427. [CrossRef]
56. Hu, Y.; Hou, Y.; Wang, H.; Lu, H. Polysarcosine as an Alternative to PEG for Therapeutic Protein Conjugation. *Bioconjugate Chem.* **2018**, *29*, 2232–2238. [CrossRef]
57. Wang, X.; Liu, S.; Sun, Y.; Yu, X.; Lee, S.M.; Cheng, Q.; Wei, T.; Gong, J.; Robinson, J.; Di Zhang, D.; et al. Preparation of selective organ-targeting (SORT) lipid nanoparticles (LNPs) using multiple technical methods for tissue-specific mRNA delivery. *Nat. Protoc.* **2023**, *18*, 265–291. [CrossRef]
58. Dilliard, S.A.; Cheng, Q.; Siegwart, D.J. On the mechanism of tissue-specific mRNA delivery by selective organ targeting nanoparticles. *Proc. Natl. Acad. Sci. USA* **2021**, *118*, e2109256118. [CrossRef]
59. Dahlman, J.E.; Kauffman, K.J.; Xing, Y.; Shaw, T.E.; Mir, F.F.; Dlott, C.C.; Langer, R.; Anderson, D.G.; Wang, E.T. Barcoded nanoparticles for high throughput in vivo discovery of targeted therapeutics. *Proc. Natl. Acad. Sci. USA* **2017**, *114*, 2060–2065. [CrossRef]
60. Moghimi, S.M.; Patel, H.M. Opsonophagocytosis of liposomes by peritoneal macrophages and bone marrow reticuloendothelial cells. *Biochim. Biophys. Acta (BBA) Mol. Cell Res.* **1992**, *1135*, 269–274. [CrossRef]
61. Nagayasu, A.; Uchiyama, K.; Nishida, T.; Yamagiwa, Y.; Kawai, Y.; Kiwada, H. Is control of distribution of liposomes between tumors and bone marrow possible? *Biochim. Biophys. Acta* **1996**, *1278*, 29–34. [CrossRef]
62. Ouyang, B.; Poon, W.; Zhang, Y.-N.; Lin, Z.P.; Kingston, B.R.; Tavares, A.J.; Zhang, Y.; Chen, J.; Valic, M.S.; Syed, A.M.; et al. The dose threshold for nanoparticle tumour delivery. *Nat. Mater.* **2020**, *19*, 1362–1371. [CrossRef] [PubMed]
63. Biscans, A.; Ly, S.; McHugh, N.; Cooper, D.A.; Khvorova, A. Engineered ionizable lipid siRNA conjugates enhance endosomal escape but induce toxicity in vivo. *J. Control. Release* **2022**, *349*, 831–843. [CrossRef] [PubMed]
64. Nair, A.B.; Jacob, S. A simple practice guide for dose conversion between animals and human. *J. Basic Clin. Pharm.* **2016**, *7*, 27–31. [CrossRef] [PubMed]
65. Ashley, J.D.; Stefanick, J.F.; Schroeder, V.A.; Suckow, M.A.; Alves, N.J.; Suzuki, R.; Kikuchi, S.; Hideshima, T.; Anderson, K.C.; Kiziltepe, T.; et al. Liposomal carfilzomib nanoparticles effectively target multiple myeloma cells and demonstrate enhanced efficacy in vivo. *J. Control. Release* **2014**, *196*, 113–121. [CrossRef] [PubMed]

66. Varela-Moreira, A.; van Straten, D.; van Leur, H.F.; Ruiter, R.W.; Deshantri, A.K.; Hennink, W.E.; Fens, M.H.; Groen, R.W.; Schiffelers, R.M. Polymeric micelles loaded with carfilzomib increase tolerability in a humanized bone marrow-like scaffold mouse model. *Int. J. Pharm. X* **2020**, *2*, 100049. [CrossRef]
67. Mitroulis, I.; Kalafati, L.; Bornhäuser, M.; Hajishengallis, G.; Chavakis, T. Regulation of the Bone Marrow Niche by Inflammation. *Front. Immunol.* **2020**, *11*, 1540. [CrossRef]
68. Leimkuhler, N.B.; Schneider, R.K. Inflammatory bone marrow microenvironment. *Hematol. Am. Soc. Hematol. Educ. Program* **2019**, *2019*, 294–302. [CrossRef]

pharmaceutics

Article

Investigation of the Antitumor Activity and Toxicity of Tumor-Derived Exosomes Fused with Long-Circulating and pH-Sensitive Liposomes Containing Doxorubicin

Eliza Rocha Gomes [1,*], Fernanda Rezende Souza [2], Geovanni Dantas Cassali [2], Adriano de Paula Sabino [3], André Luis Branco de Barros [1,3] and Mônica Cristina Oliveira [1,*]

1 Department of Pharmaceutical Products, Faculty of Pharmacy, Universidade Federal de Minas Gerais, Av. Antônio Carlos, 6627, Belo Horizonte 31270-901, Minas Gerais, Brazil
2 Department of General Pathology, Institute of Biological Sciences, Universidade Federal de Minas Gerais, Av. Antônio Carlos, 6627, Belo Horizonte 31270-901, Minas Gerais, Brazil
3 Department of Clinical and Toxicological Analysis, Faculty of Pharmacy, Universidade Federal de Minas Gerais, Av. Antônio Carlos, 6627, Belo Horizonte 31270-901, Minas Gerais, Brazil
* Correspondence: elizagomes2009@ufmg.br or elizarochagomes@gmail.com (E.R.G.); monicacristina@ufmg.br or itabra2001@yahoo.com.br (M.C.O.)

Abstract: Exosome–liposome hybrid nanocarriers containing chemotherapeutic agents have been developed to enhance drug delivery, improve the efficacy of the treatment of metastatic cancer, and overcome chemoresistance in cancer therapy. Thus, the objectives of this study were to investigate the toxicological profiles of exosomes fused with long-circulating and pH-sensitive liposomes containing doxorubicin (ExoSpHL-DOX) in healthy mice and the antitumor activity of ExoSpHL-DOX in Balb/c female mice bearing 4T1 breast tumors. The acute toxicity was determined by evaluating the mortality and morbidity of the animals and conducting hematological, biochemical, and histopathological analyses after a single intravenous administration of ExoSpHL-DOX. The results of the study indicated that the ExoSpHL-DOX treatment is less toxic than the free doxorubicin (DOX) treatment. ExoSpHL-DOX showed no signs of nephrotoxicity, even at the highest dose of DOX, indicating that the hybrid nanosystem may alter the distribution of DOX and reduce the kidney damage. Regarding the antitumor activity, ExoSpHL-DOX showed an antitumor effect compared to the control group. Furthermore, the hybrid nanocarrier of tumor-derived exosomes fused with long-circulating and pH-sensitive liposomes reduced the number of metastatic foci in the lungs. These results indicate that ExoSpHL-DOX may be a promising nanocarrier for the treatment of breast cancer, reducing toxicity and inhibiting metastasis, mainly in the lungs.

Keywords: acute toxicity; breast cancer; metastasis; exosomes; liposomes; doxorubicin

Citation: Gomes, E.R.; Souza, F.R.; Cassali, G.D.; Sabino, A.d.P.; Barros, A.L.B.d.; Oliveira, M.C. Investigation of the Antitumor Activity and Toxicity of Tumor-Derived Exosomes Fused with Long-Circulating and pH-Sensitive Liposomes Containing Doxorubicin. *Pharmaceutics* **2022**, *14*, 2256. https://doi.org/10.3390/pharmaceutics14112256

Academic Editors: Raquel Fernández García, Francisco Bolás-Fernández and Ana Isabel Fraguas-Sánchez

Received: 20 September 2022
Accepted: 20 October 2022
Published: 22 October 2022

1. Introduction

Cancer is one of the leading causes of death and an important barrier to efforts to increase life expectancy across the world. Annually, more than 19 million people develop cancer and approximately 10 million people die from the disease. Breast cancer is the most commonly diagnosed cancer in women, with 2.3 million new cases [1]. Doxorubicin (DOX) is a chemotherapeutic drug used as the first-line treatment for breast cancer. However, this drug causes serious toxic effects, mainly dose-dependent cardiotoxicity, which limits its clinical use [2,3]. To minimize the adverse effects caused by DOX, liposomes have been used in the treatment of patients [2,4]. However, there is no increase in the therapeutic efficacy of liposomal formulations, mainly in DOX-resistant cancer, compared to conventional DOX [2]. In order to improve the therapeutic efficacy of DOX, liposomes can be fused with exosomes released by breast cancer cells. Tetraspanins and integrins, which are present on the surface of exosomes, can facilitate fusion and membrane interactions, achieving a greater cell uptake of fused vesicles [5,6]. Considering the potential strategy of liposome and exosome fusion, Gomes and coworkers [7] developed and characterized a hybrid nanocarrier of tumor-derived exosomes fused with long-circulating and pH-sensitive liposomes containing DOX (ExoSpHL-DOX) for the treatment of breast cancer. The mean diameter of the developed formulation was equal to 100.8 ± 7.8 nm, the polydispersity index (PDI) was 0.122 ± 0.004, and the encapsulated DOX content was equal to 83.5 ± 2.5%. ExoSpHL-DOX was shown to be stable at 4 °C for 60 days. The study of the release of DOX from ExoSpHL-DOX in dilution media with different pH values confirmed the pH sensitivity that is characteristic of the nanosystem, and the cytotoxic study of the 4T1 murine breast cancer cell line demonstrated that the ExoSpHL-DOX treatment significantly reduced the cancer cell viability. Herein, we investigated the toxicological profile of ExoSpHL-DOX in healthy mice and the antitumor activity of ExoSpHL-DOX in Balb/c female mice bearing 4T1 breast tumors.

2. Materials and Methods

2.1. Chemicals

1,2-Dioleoyl-sn-glycero-3-phosphoethanolamine (DOPE) and 1,2-distearoyl-sn-glycero-3-phosphoethanolamine-N-[amino(polyethyleneglycol)-2000 ($DSPE\text{-}PEG_{2000}$) were supplied by Lipoid GmbH (Ludwigshafen, Germany). Cholesterol hemisuccinate (CHEMS), DOX, phosphate-buffered saline (PBS), sodium hydroxide, 4-(2-hydroxyethyl)piperazine-1-ethanesulfonic acid (HEPES), and sodium bicarbonate were obtained from Sigma-Aldrich (St. Louis, MO, USA). Total exosome isolation reagent was obtained from Thermo Fisher Scientific (Waltham, MA, USA).

2.2. Cells

The 4T1 murine breast cancer cells were purchased from the American Type Culture Collection (ATCC) (Manassas, VA, USA). Roswell Park Memorial Institute (RPMI) 1640 Medium and fetal bovine serum (FBS) were obtained from Gibco Life Technologies (Carlsbad, CA, USA). Trypsin was obtained from Sigma-Aldrich (St. Louis, MO, USA). A mycoplasma test using Hoechst fluorescence staining was performed on the cell line.

2.3. Isolation of Exosomes

The 4T1 cells were grown in RPMI-1640 supplemented with 10% of ultracentrifuged FBS and maintained at 37 °C and 5% CO_2 in a humidified atmosphere. When the 4T1 cells reached an approximate confluence of 80%, the supernatant was removed from the cell culture flask T-75. The exosome isolation reagent was added to the supernatant (1:2 v/v ratio, respectively) and kept in a refrigerator for 15 h. After that time, the mixture was centrifuged at 10,000× g for 1 h at 4 °C using a centrifuge from Thermo Scientific, model Heraeus Multifuge X 1R. The pellet was dissolved in a mixture of chloroform and methanol (1:1 v/v ratio).

2.4. Preparation of ExoSpHL-DOX

ExoSpHL-DOX was prepared using the Bangham method [8] followed by extrusion for the size calibration. Chloroform aliquots of DOPE, CHEMS, and $DSPE\text{-}PEG_{2000}$ (5.7:3.8:0.5 molar ratio, respectively) and exosomes in a mixture of chloroform and methanol were added to a round-bottomed flask to obtain a lipid film. For each mL of liposome, we added an exosome pellet obtained from 2 mL of cell supernatant (concentration of 3.6×10^{10} particles/mL). After the evaporation of the solvents, NaOH 0.228 M solution was added to ionize the CHEMS molecules and, subsequently, promote the formation of vesicles. The hydration of the lipid film was carried out under agitation with an ammonium sulfate solution (300 mM, pH 7.4). The vesicles obtained were calibrated by extrusion using the Lipex Biomembranes extruder, Model T001 (Vancouver, BC, Canada) [9]. The external ammonium sulfate was removed by ultracentrifugation (Ultracentrifuge Optima® L-80XP, Beckman Coulter, Brea, CA, USA) at 150,000× g, 4 °C, for 120 min. The pellet was resuspended with HEPES buffered saline (HBS). The vesicles were incubated with a DOX solution for 2 h in the dark at room temperature. The non-encapsulated DOX was removed by ultracentrifugation using the same method as that described above. The final pellet was resuspended with HBS. Blank breast-tumor-derived exosomes fused with long-circulating and pH-sensitive liposomes (ExoSpHL) and long-circulating and pH-sensitive liposomes containing DOX (SpHL-DOX) were prepared in the same way without the addition of DOX and exosomes, respectively.

2.5. ExoSpHL-DOX Characterization

2.5.1. Determination of the Diameter, Polydispersity Index, and Zeta Potential

The mean diameter and the polydispersity index (PDI) of ExoSpHL-DOX were measured by dynamic light scattering (DLS). The zeta potential value was determined by DLS combined with electrophoretic mobility. To perform both analyses, 50 μL of ExoSpHL-DOX was diluted in 1 mL of HBS, and the Zetasizer Nano ZS90 equipment was used (Malvern Instruments Ltd., Worcestershire, UK).

2.5.2. Determination of the Content of DOX

The DOX content was measured by high-performance liquid chromatography (HPLC). The mobile phase consisted of methanol:phosphate buffer pH 3.0 (65:35 v/v). Samples were injected (20 μL), and the separation was performed with an ACE® C8 column, 25 cm × 4.6 mm, 5 μm (Merck, Darmstadt, Germany), at a flow rate of 1.0 mL/min. The detection was performed in the model 2475 fluorescence mode (Waters Instruments, Milford, MA, USA), with excitation and emission wavelengths of 470 nm and 555 nm, respectively [10]. The ExoSpHL-DOX was opened with isopropyl alcohol (1:2 v/v, respectively) and diluted in the mobile phase. The encapsulation percentage (EP) of DOX in ExoSpHL-DOX was calculated according to the following equation:

$$\text{DOX encapsulation percentage } (\%) = \frac{[\text{DOX}] \text{ in purified vesicles}}{[\text{DOX}] \text{ in non} - \text{purified vesicles}} \times 100$$

2.6. Animals

Healthy female Balb/c mice aged 8–10 weeks and approximately 18 g in weight were obtained from Central Biotery, Universidade Federal de Minas Gerais (UFMG, Belo Horizonte, Brazil). The mice were kept in plastic cages with free access to food and water and under standardized light/dark cycle conditions. All protocols were approved by the Ethics Committee for Animal Experiments from the Universidade Federal de Minas Gerais (CEUA/UFMG—protocol number 265/2019).

2.7. Acute Toxicity

The acute toxicity was assessed according to the recommendations of the Organization for Economic Cooperation and Development (OECD) 423 [11], adapted for intravenous administration, as previously performed by our research group [12]. The animals were divided into five groups. Each group intravenously received a single dose of HBS, ExoSpHL, free DOX, SpHL-DOX, or ExoSpHL-DOX. The mice were observed for 14 days in terms of their behavior, weight, and mortality. After the observation period, the animals were intraperitoneally anesthetized with a mixture of xylazine (15 mg/kg) and ketamine (80 mg/kg). The blood was collected by puncture of the brachial plexus for hematological and biochemical analyses. The organs were collected for histopathological analyses. In previous studies, our research group evaluated the toxicity of 10 mg/kg and 15 mg/kg of free DOX and SpHL-DOX in mice. A weight loss of around 5%, prostration, and intense piloerection were observed in the animals treated with free DOX (15 mg/kg). No significant signs of toxicity were observed in the animals treated with SpHL-DOX (15 mg/kg). Based on the findings of this study, the initial doses proposed in this study were 10 mg/kg of free DOX and 15 mg/kg of SpHL-DOX and ExoSpHL-DOX [12]. According to the OECD guideline [11], initially, each treatment group was composed of 3 animals. If the dose tested was capable of causing the death of 2 or more animals in the group, the dosing of 3 additional animals at the previous lowest dose level was required. However, if the tested dose was able to cause one or no death, the next step was the dosing of 3 additional animals with the same dose. In the case of the confirmation of the results of one or no death, it was necessary to administer the following higher dose level to 3 additional animals. The dose scheme used to assess the median lethal dose (LD50) after the treatments with the free DOX and formulations (SpHL-DOX and ExoSpHL-DOX) is presented in Appendix A (Figures A1 and A2, respectively). LD50 refers to the single dose of DOX that was required to cause death in 50 percent of the animals tested.

2.7.1. Hematology and Biochemistry Analyses

For the hematological analysis, the blood was collected in tubes containing anticoagulant (EDTA 0.1 M) and inserted into the automated hematological analyzer HEMOVET 2300 (Hemovet, São Paulo, Brazil). Hematological parameters related to red and white blood cells were evaluated for each treatment group. For the biochemical analysis, the blood was centrifuged (3000 rpm, 15 min), and the plasma obtained was collected. The tests were performed with the Bioplus BIO-2000 semiautomatic analyzer (Bioplus, São Paulo, Brazil) using commercial kits (Labtest, Lagoa Santa, Brazil). The renal, liver, and cardiac functions were evaluated for each treatment group.

2.7.2. Histopathological Analysis

The liver, kidneys, spleen, and heart were harvested and fixed in formalin (10% *w*/*v* in phosphate-buffered saline (PBS), pH 7.4) and incorporated in paraffin blocks. Consecutive histological sections were prepared and stained by the hematoxylin and eosin routine method. The slides were evaluated by trained pathologists, and images of histological sections were captured using a digital camera connected to an optical microscope, Olympus BX-40 (Olympus, Tokyo, Japan).

2.8. Evaluation of the Antitumor Activity

The 4T1 breast cancer cells were injected into the right flank of the female Balb/c mice (1.0×10^6 cells in 100 μL PBS). When the tumor volume reached approximately 100 mm^3, the animals were randomly divided into five treatment groups, each containing six animals. Each group intravenously received five administrations of HBS, ExoSpHL, free DOX, SpHL-DOX, or ExoSpHL-DOX. The cumulative dose of DOX was 25 mg/kg. The dose used in this study was based on a previous study of our research group [13]. The antitumor activity was evaluated based on the tumor volume (TV), calculated as previously described [14], where TV = $0.52 \times (d1 \times d2^2)$, d1 and d2 being the largest and the smallest perpendicular diameters, respectively. Six measurements of the diameters of the tumors were carried out during ten days of treatment using a caliper MIP/E-103 (Mitutoyo, Suzano, São Paulo, Brazil). The TV at day 0 was considered as 100%, and changes in the TV were determined every two days by calculating the percentages of the TV increase or decrease. The relative tumor volume (RTV) and inhibition percentage of tumor growth (TGI) were calculated according to the following equations:

$$RTV = \frac{\text{TV on day 10}}{\text{TV on day 0}}$$

$$TGI = 1 - \frac{\text{RTV of each treatment}}{\text{RTV of the control group}} \times 100$$

On day 10, the animals were intraperitoneally anesthetized with a mixture of xylazine (15 mg/kg) and ketamine (80 mg/kg). The liver, spleen, lungs, heart, and tumor were collected for the histopathological analysis.

2.9. Statistical Analyses

To confirm the normality and homoscedasticity of variance, D'Agostino and Shapiro–Wilk tests were applied, respectively. The differences between the experimental groups were tested by analysis of variance (one-way ANOVA followed by Tukey's test). If the data were not normal or homoscedastic, the Kruskal–Wallis test with Dunn's post-test was used for the same purpose. The two-way ANOVA test with Tukey's post-test was also used to relate two different independent variables with respect to one dependent variable. Values of $p < 0.05$ were considered significant. The analyses were performed using the GraphPad Prism software (version 6.00, La Jolla, CA, USA).

3. Results

3.1. ExoSpHL-DOX Characterization

ExoSpHL-DOX presented a mean diameter of 105.4 ± 2.9 nm and a PDI value of 0.132 ± 0.010, indicating the presence of monodisperse vesicles. The zeta potential value was near neutrality (−6.4 ± 1.2 mV), as expected for vesicles that contain PEG in their composition. The encapsulation percentage of DOX was 88.5 ± 2.4%, achieved by using the ammonium sulfate gradient method.

3.2. Acute Toxicity Study

3.2.1. Evaluation of Animal Mortality and Morbidity

The HBS and ExoSpHL treatments did not show significant differences in relation to the mortality and morbidity. These findings indicate the lack of toxicity of the treatments applied to the mice in the control groups. The LD50 assessment of animals treated with free DOX started with 10 mg/kg and with 15 mg/kg for both formulations (SpHL-DOX and ExoSpHL-DOX). For the free DOX treatment, the 10 mg/kg dose showed no significant signs of toxicity in the first three animals tested. Thus, the next step was the dosing of three additional animals with the same dose. The results remained the same in all animals; therefore, the following higher dose level was injected into three animals. After 8 days of application of 12.5 mg/kg of DOX, piloerection and ascites in the animals were observed. It is worth mentioning that the most notable result was a weight loss of 13%, observed at day 12 post-administration. However, no deaths were observed. Therefore, the next step was the dosing of three additional animals with the same dose. The previous observations were confirmed, and there was one death on day 13. According to Appendix A (Figure A2), the next step was the dosing of three additional animals at the following higher dose level (15 mg/kg). For the first three mice evaluated, there was one death on day 10 and one death on day 12 of the study. In addition, intense piloerection was observed in all animals. Additionally, we observed a loss of weight in the animals ranging between 7% and 20% during the days after treatment. Therefore, according to the OECD 423 guideline [11], the LD50 value for free DOX treatment is between 12.5 and 15 mg/kg for this experimental model. Thus, 15 mg/kg was the last dose tested for the treatment with the free drug.

The studies carried out using the SpHL-DOX and ExoSpHL-DOX treatments started with a dose of 15 mg/kg. For both treatments, there was no death or weight loss in all of the six animals tested. After treatment with a dose of 17.5 mg/kg, no deaths were observed. However, there was a 5% weight loss in the animals. According to these results, we repeated the experiments for the groups treated with SpHL-DOX and ExoSpHL-DOX at a dose of 17.5, using three more animals per treatment, and the previous observations were confirmed. We followed the treatment scheme (Appendix A, Figure A1), increasing the dose to 20 mg/kg for the SpHL-DOX and ExoSpHL-DOX treatments. After treatments with the 20 mg/kg dose, we observed two deaths on day 6 and one death on day 8 in the SpHL-DOX treatment group. In the ExoSpHL-DOX treatment group, one death on day 6, one death on day 8, and one death on day 10 occurred. In addition, during the days after treatment, the animals treated with ExoSpHL-DOX and SpHL-DOX had weight losses of 10% and 20%, respectively. Therefore, according to the OECD 423 guideline [11], the LD50 value for the SpHL-DOX and ExoSpHL-DOX treatments is between 17.5 and 20 mg/kg for this experimental model. Thus, 20 mg/kg was the last dose tested for both formulations.

3.2.2. Hematological Analysis

The hematological parameters of the mice treated with DOX, SpHL-DOX, and ExoSpHL-DOX are shown in Table 1. The HBS and ExoSpHL treatment groups showed no significant difference; therefore, only the HBS treatment group was expressed as a control. The evaluation of white blood cells (WBC) showed that there was an increase in the WBC count after treatment with DOX at a dose of 12.5 mg/kg when compared to the control group (HBS). The other treatments did not change the WBC count when compared to HBS. The same increase was observed in the granulocytes (neutrophils, eosinophils and basophils) and agranulocytes (lymphocytes and monocytes) in the group treated with DOX at a dose of 12.5 mg/kg when compared to HBS. The other treatments did not change the granulocyte and agranulocyte count when compared to HBS. Regarding the red blood cells, the number of red blood cells (RBC), amount of hemoglobin (HGB), and hematocrit (HCT) showed a decrease in the mice treated with DOX at a dose of 12.5 mg/kg and did not change among the other treatments when compared to the control. The platelet count showed no difference between all the treatments.

Table 1. Hematological parameters for healthy Balb/c mice treated with different doses of free DOX, SpHL-DOX, or ExoSpHL-DOX.

Blood Components	Control	Free DOX		SpHL-DOX		ExoSpHL-DOX	
		10 mg/kg	12.5 mg/kg	15 mg/kg	17.5 mg/kg	15 mg/kg	17.5 mg/kg
WBC ($10^3/mm^3$)	4.95 ± 1.13	4.55 ± 1.62 [b]	9.53 ± 2.12 [a]	4.20 ± 1.18 [b]	4.85 ± 0.41 [b]	5.83 ± 1.40 [b]	4.48 ± 0.82 [b]
AGRANULOCYTES ($10^3/mm^3$)	3.68 ± 0.99	3.15 ± 1.25 [b]	7.15 ± 2.58 [a]	2.58 ± 0.95 [b]	2.87 ± 0.30 [b]	3.77 ± 0.97 [b]	3.00 ± 0.60 [b]
GRANULOCYTES ($10^3/mm^3$)	1.27 ± 0.27	1.40 ± 0.41 [b]	2.80 ± 1.05 [a]	1.34 ± 0.46 [b]	1.98 ± 0.36 [b]	2.07 ± 0.59 [b]	1.48 ± 0.26 [b]
RBC ($10^6/mm^3$)	6.26 ± 0.72	5.95 ± 0.45 [b]	4.18 ± 0.36 [a]	6.06 ± 0.25 [b]	5.79 ± 0.18 [b]	5.30 ± 0.26 [b]	6.10 ± 0.14 [b]
HGB (g/dL)	12.68 ± 2.26	11.43 ± 1.06 [b]	8.40 ± 1.35 [a]	11.72 ± 0.64 [b]	11.53 ± 0.45 [b]	10.23 ± 0.43	12.10 ± 0.41 [b]
HCT (%)	30.90 ± 3.47	30.00 ± 2.05 [b]	21.55 ± 1.52 [a]	29.68 ± 1.30 [b]	28.87 ± 1.01 [b]	26.82 ± 2.03 [b]	30.04 ± 0.86 [b]
PLT ($10^3/mm^3$)	338.20 ± 22.66	254.2 ± 24.70	335.50 ± 78.57	351.80 ± 57.90	333.80 ± 61.90	314.20 ± 40.51	314.00 ± 79.53

WBC: white blood cells; RBC: red blood cells; HGB: hemoglobin; HCT: hematocrit; PLT: platelet. The results are presented as mean ± standard deviation from the mean (n = 6, except for free DOX treatment at a dose of 12.5 mg/kg n = 5). [a] Statistical significance compared to control (HBS) ($p < 0.05$). [b] Statistical significance compared to free DOX treatment at a dose of 12.5 mg/kg ($p < 0.05$). Data were evaluated by one-way ANOVA (Tukey's post-test). If the data were abnormal, the Kruskal–Wallis test with Dunn's post-test was used.

3.2.3. Biochemical Analysis

The biochemical parameters of the mice treated with DOX, SpHL-DOX, and ExoSpHL-DOX are shown in Table 2. The HBS and ExoSpHL treatment groups showed no significant difference; therefore, only the HBS treatment group was expressed as a control. The renal function was evaluated by measuring the creatinine and urea. There was no change in the creatinine values in all treatments when compared to the control. For the quantification of the urea, only the DOX treatment at a dose of 12.5 mg/kg presented an increase in relation to the control group. The hepatic function was evaluated by determining the alanine aminotransferase (ALT) and aspartate aminotransferase (AST) activity, and the doses used did not cause liver damage, since there was no significant difference in the serum levels of ALT and AST in all the treatment groups when compared to the control group. Cardiac injury was assessed by measuring the creatine kinase-MB (CK-MB) activity. The DOX treatment at a dose of 12.5 mg/kg and SpHL-DOX and ExoSpHL-DOX treatments at a dose of 17.5 mg/kg showed high levels of CK-MB in relation to the control group. Furthermore, the increase in the CK-MB level due to DOX treatment at a dose of 12.5 mg/kg was greater than that of SpHL-DOX and ExoSpHL-DOX at a dose of 17.5 mg/kg.

Table 2. Biochemical parameters for healthy Balb/c mice treated with different doses of free DOX, SpHL-DOX, or ExoSpHL-DOX.

Biochemical Parameters	Control	Free DOX		SpHL-DOX		ExoSpHL-DOX	
		10 mg/kg	12.5 mg/kg	15 mg/kg	17.5 mg/kg	15 mg/kg	17.5 mg/kg
Creatinine (mg/dL)	0.30 ± 0.09	0.22 ± 0.07	0.29 ± 0.12	0.19 ± 0.04	0.20 ± 0.03	0.31 ± 0.06	0.22 ± 0.04
Urea (mg/dL)	35.54 ± 3.92	40.51 ± 18.06 [b]	149.10 ± 14.89 [a]	34.82 ± 9.91 [b]	39.20 ± 13.33 [b]	31.16 ± 1.73 [b]	30.63 ± 1.37 [b]
ALT (U/L)	44.09 ± 7.34	52.97 ± 15.68	48.01 ± 9.34	45.54 ± 11.21	56.39 ± 10.01	47.72 ± 5.86	51.67 ± 7.71
AST (U/L)	124.30 ± 24.72	93.78 ± 25.79	127.80 ± 10.44	109.20 ± 41.60	128.00 ± 26.19	110.70 ± 30.26	126.30 ± 24.95
CK-MB (U/L)	28.31 ± 6.36	33.46 ± 13.55 [b,c]	89.34 ± 8.03 [a]	33.90 ± 10.33 [b]	52.49 ± 13.51 [a,b]	25.99 ± 7.47 [b,c,d]	49.11 ± 6.58 [a,b]

The results are presented as mean ± standard deviation from the mean (n = 6, except for free DOX treatment at a dose of 12.5 mg/kg n = 5). [a] Statistical significance compared to control group (HBS) ($p < 0.05$). [b] Statistical significance compared to free DOX treatment at a dose of 12.5 mg/kg ($p < 0.05$). [c] Statistical significance compared to SpHL-DOX treatment at a dose of 17.5 mg/kg ($p < 0.05$). [d] Statistical significance compared to ExoSpHL-DOX treatment at a dose of 17.5 mg/kg ($p < 0.05$). Data were evaluated by one-way ANOVA (Tukey's post-test). If they were abnormal, the Kruskal–Wallis test with Dunn's post-test was used.

3.2.4. Histological Analysis

Histological analyses of the different organs were performed at the end of the treatment period. The mice treated with HBS and ExoSpHL presented with the same histopathological profile and, therefore, only the HBS treatment group's photomicrography was presented as the control group. The liver analysis showed no changes in the SpHL-DOX (15 mg/kg) and ExoSpHL-DOX (15 mg/kg) treatment groups compared to the control group (Figure 1A). In contrast, diffuse hydropic degeneration was observed in the animals treated with DOX (10 and 12.5 mg/kg), SpHL-DOX (17.5 mg/kg), and ExoSpHL-DOX (17.5 mg/kg) (Figure 1B). In the splenic analysis, no changes were observed after the treatments with both doses of SpHL-DOX and ExoSpHL-DOX (15 and 17.5 mg/kg) (Figure 1C). In the animals treated with DOX (10 and 12.5 mg/kg), we observed splenic congestion. The red pulp sinusoids had a large number of erythrocytes (Figure 1D).

The histopathological analysis of the kidneys revealed no changes in the case of the SpHL-DOX (15 mg/kg) and ExoSpHL-DOX (15 and 17.5 mg/kg) treatment groups compared to the control group (Figure 2A). Animals treated with DOX (10 and 12.5 mg/kg) and SpHL-DOX (17.5 mg/kg) presented with tubule dilation and hyalinization of the glomeruli (Figure 2B).

The cardiac muscle analysis revealed that, after the DOX treatments, areas of cardiomyocyte vacuolization were observable. Compared to the control group (Figure 3A), the treatment with free DOX (10 and 12.5 mg/kg) (Figure 3B,C, respectively) presented multifocal areas of cardiomyocyte vacuolization. The extent of the lesions was greater in the DOX treatment group at a dose of 12.5 mg/kg. For the SpHL-DOX (15 and 17.5 mg/kg) and ExoSpHL-DOX (15 and 17.5 mg/kg) treatment groups, discrete foci of cardiomyocyte vacuolization were observed (Figure 3D). The analyzed histological sections of all the groups and organs analyzed that showed some difference compared to the control are presented in Appendix B.

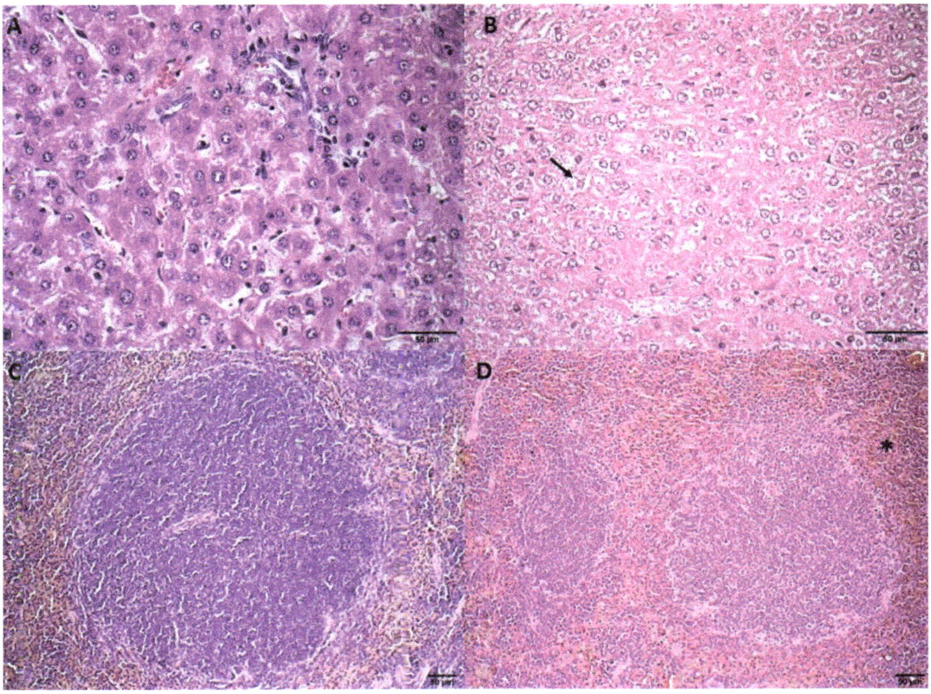

Figure 1. Histological sections of female Balb/c mice liver (**A**,**B**) and spleen (**C**,**D**). (**A**) Represents the control group (HBS) and the groups treated with SpHL-DOX and ExoSpHL-DOX at a dose of 15 mg/kg (**B**) Represents the groups treated with both doses of free DOX (10 and 12.5 mg/kg) and the groups treated with SpHL-DOX and ExoSpHL-DOX at a dose of 17.5 mg/kg. The arrow indicates the regions of diffuse hydropic degeneration. (**C**) Represents the control group (HBS) and the groups treated with both tested doses of SpHL-DOX and ExoSpHL-DOX (15 and 17.5 mg/kg). (**D**) Represents the groups treated with both tested doses of free DOX (10 and 12.5 mg/kg). The asterisk indicates the increase in erythrocytes in the red pulp. HE, scale bar = 50 μm.

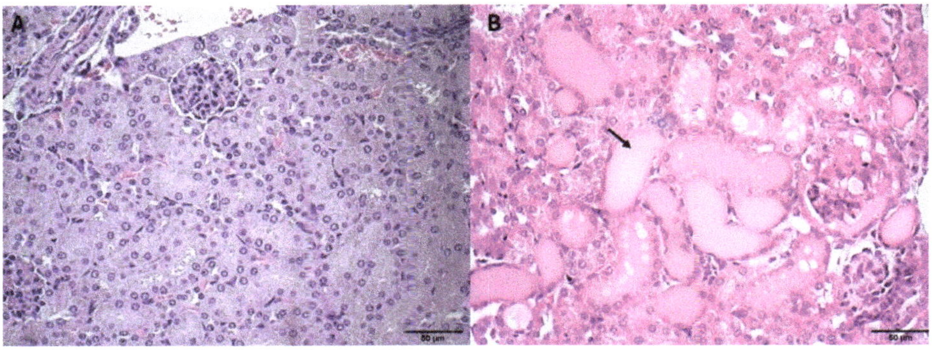

Figure 2. Histological sections of female Balb/c mice kidney. (**A**) Represents the control group (HBS) and the groups treated with both doses of ExoSpHL-DOX (15 and 17.5 mg/kg) and SpHL-DOX at a dose of 15 mg/kg. (**B**) Represents the groups treated with both tested doses of free DOX (10 and 12.5 mg/kg) and SpHL-DOX at a dose of 17.5 mg/kg. The arrow indicates the regions of tubule dilation. HE, scale bar = 50 μm.

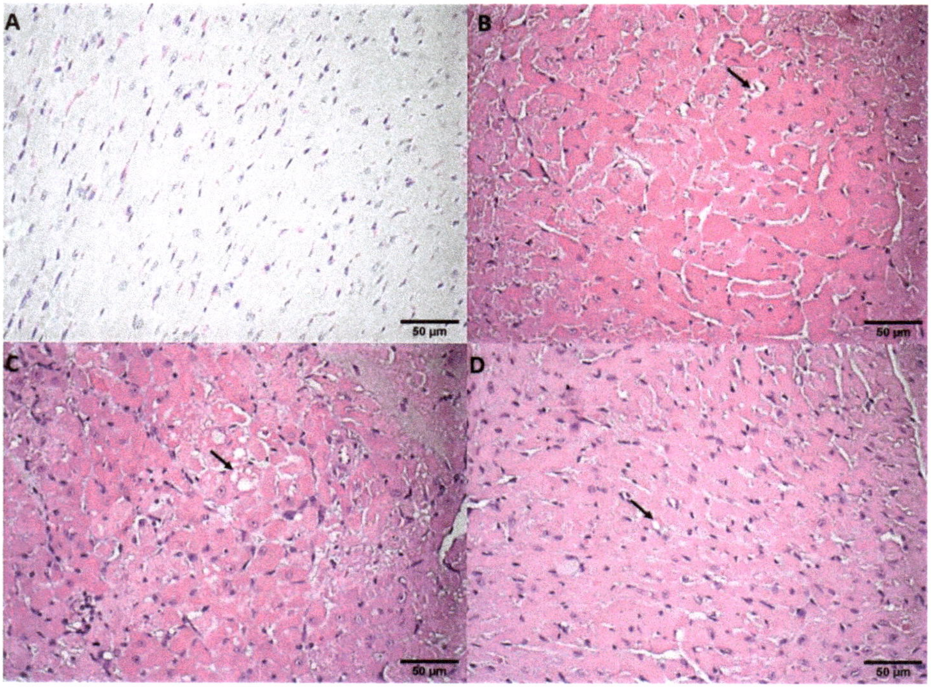

Figure 3. Histological sections of female Balb/c mice heart. (**A**) Represents the control group (HBS). (**B**) Represents the group treated with free DOX at a dose of 10 mg/kg. The arrow indicates the areas of cardiomyocyte vacuolization. (**C**) Represents the group treated with free DOX at a dose of 12.5 mg/kg. The arrow indicates the areas of cardiomyocyte vacuolization that were more intense than (**B**). (**D**) Represents the groups treated with both doses of SpHL-DOX and ExoSpHL-DOX. The arrow indicates the areas of discrete cardiomyocyte vacuolization. HE, scale bar = 50 µm.

3.3. Antitumor Activity Evaluation

The antitumor efficacy of the free DOX, SpHL-DOX, and ExoSpHL-DOX treatments was evaluated in the female Balb/c mice with 4T1 breast tumors by assessing the tumor volume variation over time. The tumor volume in the HBS (control) and ExoSpHL treatment groups increased rapidly over time and showed no significant differences between them. By contrast, significant differences in the tumor volume were observed between the control treatment groups and the groups treated with DOX, SpHL-DOX, and ExoSpHL-DOX at a dose of 5.0 mg/kg (Figure 4A). The tumor volume data were confirmed by the RTV values (Table 3). The treatments with formulations containing DOX significantly decreased the tumor growth compared to the control group. However, there was no significant difference between the DOX, SpHL-DOX, and ExoSpHL-DOX treatments at the cumulative dose of 25.0 mg/kg. In addition, the treatments showed similar TGIs, which were close to 50%, compared to the control group.

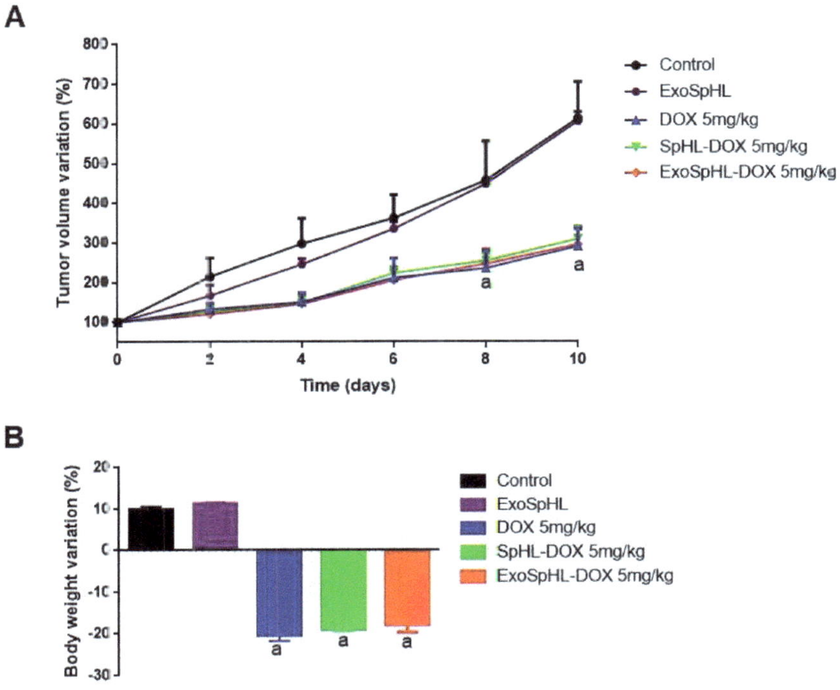

Figure 4. Antitumor efficacy evaluation of female Balb/c mice with 4T1 breast tumors. (**A**) Variation in the mice breast cancer tumor volume after treatment with HBS, ExoSpHL, DOX, SpHL-DOX, and ExoSpHL-DOX. Every 2 days, the animals intravenously received five administrations of HBS (control), ExoSpHL, or DOX at a cumulative dose of 25 mg/kg, SpHL-DOX at a cumulative dose of 25 mg/kg, or ExoSpHL-DOX at a cumulative dose of 25 mg/kg. (**B**) Percentage of body weight variation on day 10 after the administration of HBS (control), ExoSpHL, or DOX at a cumulative dose of 25 mg/kg, SpHL-DOX at a cumulative dose of 25 mg/kg, or ExoSpHL-DOX at a cumulative dose of 25 mg/kg. All data are presented as mean ± SEM, $n = 6$. [a] Statistical significance compared to the control group (HBS) and ExoSpHL ($p < 0.05$). Abbreviations: HBS: HEPES buffered saline; ExoSpHL: tumor-derived exosomes fused with long-circulating and pH-sensitive liposomes; DOX: doxorubicin; SpHL-DOX: long-circulating and pH-sensitive liposomes containing doxorubicin; ExoSpHL-DOX: tumor-derived exosomes fused with long-circulating and pH-sensitive liposomes containing doxorubicin; SEM: standard error of the mean.

Table 3. Relative tumor volume and tumor growth inhibition after the administration of HBS, ExoSpHL, free DOX, SpHL-DOX, and ExoSpHL-DOX by the intravenous route.

Treatment	RTV	TGI (%)
HBS (control)	6.1 ± 0.9	-
ExoSpHL	6.1 ± 0.6	-
Free DOX 5 mg/kg	2.9 ± 0.4 [a]	52.5
SpHL-DOX 5 mg/kg	2.8 ± 0.1 [a]	54.1
ExoSpHL-DOX 5 mg/kg	2.7 ± 0.4 [a]	55.7

The results are presented as mean ± standard error ($n = 6$). [a] Statistical significance compared to the control (HBS) and ExoSpHL ($p < 0.05$).

3.3.1. Evaluation of Body Weight Loss

The body weight loss after the treatments with DOX, SpHL-DOX, and ExoSpHL-DOX was evaluated in the Balb/c female mice with 4T1 breast tumors. The results are presented in Figure 4B. The mice treated with HBS (control) and ExoSpHL presented with similar body weight gain. By contrast, significant differences in the animals' weights were observed between the control treatments and treatments with DOX, SpHL-DOX, and ExoSpHL-DOX. However, there was no significant difference in body weight loss among the animals treated with DOX, SpHL-DOX, and ExoSpHL-DOX at the cumulative dose of 25.0 mg/kg.

3.3.2. Histological Analysis

Histological analyses of the tumors and different organs were performed at the end of the treatment period. The 4T1 tumor cells grow in a solid arrangement. The proliferation of pleomorphic cells and a high mitotic index were observed [15]. The mice treated with HBS or ExoSpHL presented with tumors affected by necrosis only in the central region (Figure 5A). On the other hand, the animals treated with DOX, SpHL-DOX, or ExoSpHL-DOX presented with extensive necrosis and few areas of viable cells due to the DOX-induced cell death (Figure 5B).

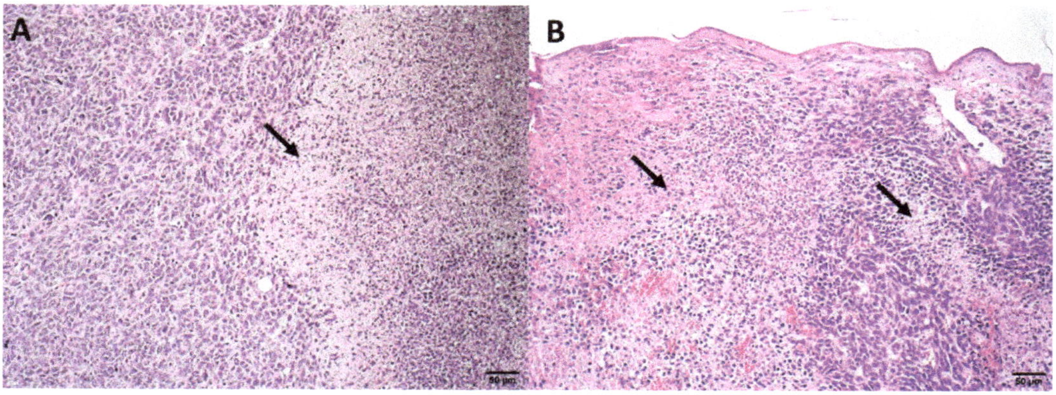

Figure 5. Representative photomicrographs of histological sections of the primary tumors of female Balb/c mice bearing 4T1 breast tumors treated with (**A**) HBS and ExoSpHL. The arrow indicates the central tumor necrosis area. (**B**) DOX, SpHL-DOX, and ExoSpHL-DOX at a cumulative dose of 25 mg/kg. The arrows indicate multiple tumor necrosis areas. HE, scale bar = 50 µm.

The 4T1 murine breast cancer is highly tumorigenic and invasive, wherein metastatic foci are observed in various organs [15]. The lungs and liver are common organs affected by the appearance of 4T1 tumor metastases. Pulmonary histology revealed metastatic foci in the animals in all the treatment groups (Figure 6A). The main difference was related to the number of animals with pulmonary metastasis. In all the animals treated with HBS, metastatic foci were observed. However, in the animals treated with ExoSpHL, free DOX, SpHL-DOX, or ExoSpHL-DOX, few metastatic foci were observed. Additionally, the ExoSpHL-DOX-treated group exhibited fewer metastatic foci in a semi-quantitative comparison with the SpHL-DOX and free DOX treatments (Table 4). Multiple metastatic foci in the liver were observed in the animals treated with HBS or ExoSpHL, with no difference between them. Meanwhile, few metastatic foci were observed in the animals treated with DOX, SpHL-DOX, and ExoSpHL-DOX. However, in the liver, there was no difference between the groups treated with DOX, SpHL-DOX, and ExoSpHL-DOX (Figure 6B).

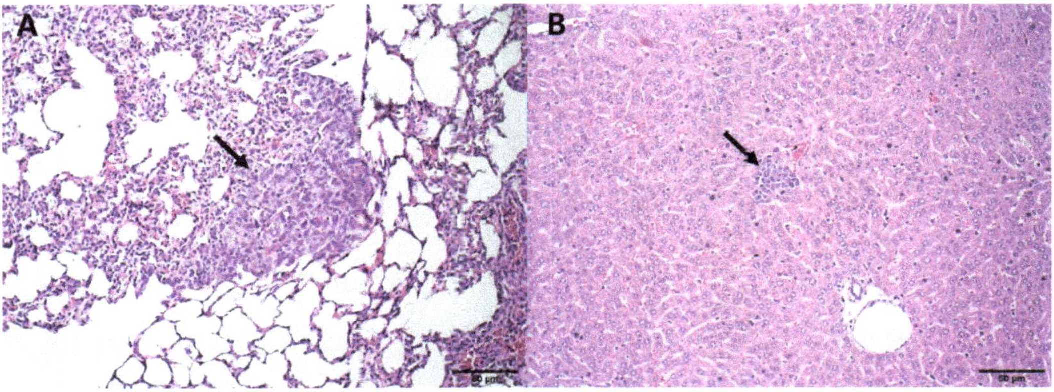

Figure 6. Representative photomicrographs of metastatic foci in the lungs (**A**) and liver (**B**) of female Balb/c mice bearing 4T1 breast tumors treated with HBS (control), ExoSpHL, or DOX at a cumulative dose of 25 mg/kg, SpHL-DOX at a cumulative dose of 25 mg/kg, or ExoSpHL-DOX at a cumulative dose of 25 mg/kg. Arrows indicate tumor metastasis. HE, scale bar = 50 µm.

Table 4. Number of metastatic foci in the lungs of female Balb/c mice bearing 4T1 breast tumors treated with HBS, ExoSpHL, free DOX, SpHL-DOX, or ExoSpHL-DOX. Animals received each treatment intravenously five times at a dose of 5 mg/kg every 2 days.

		HBS	ExoSpHL	DOX	SpHL-DOX	ExoSpHL-DOX
Score	Animal 1	+	+	0	+	0
	Animal 2	++	0	++	0	0
	Animal 3	+	+	+	+	+
	Animal 4	++	0	0	0	0
	Animal 5	++	0	0	+	0

Data are expressed as scores: 0, no metastasis detected; +, 1–3 metastatic foci; ++, 4–7 metastatic foci.

The macroscopic analysis of the spleen showed splenomegaly in the animals treated with HBS or ExoSpHL, which is commonly observed in mice with 4T1 murine breast cancer. In the DOX, SpHL-DOX, and ExoSpHL-DOX treatments groups, the spleen size was normal, indicating that the treatments were able to reverse the splenomegaly. Regarding the histological analysis, the spleen tissue of the animals treated with SpHL-DOX or ExoSpHL-DOX was preserved (Figure 7A). The spleens of the mice treated with HBS, ExoSpHL, or DOX showed white and red pulp hyperplasia (Figure 7B). The cardiac muscle analysis revealed that, compared to the control (Figure 7C), after treatments with free DOX, SpHL-DOX, and ExoSpHL-DOX, there were focal areas of degenerative hyalinization (Figure 7D). Regarding the extent of the lesions, there was no significant difference, and the pattern was similar to that found in the acute toxicity study. Histological sections of all the groups and organs analyzed that showed some difference compared to the control are presented in Appendix C.

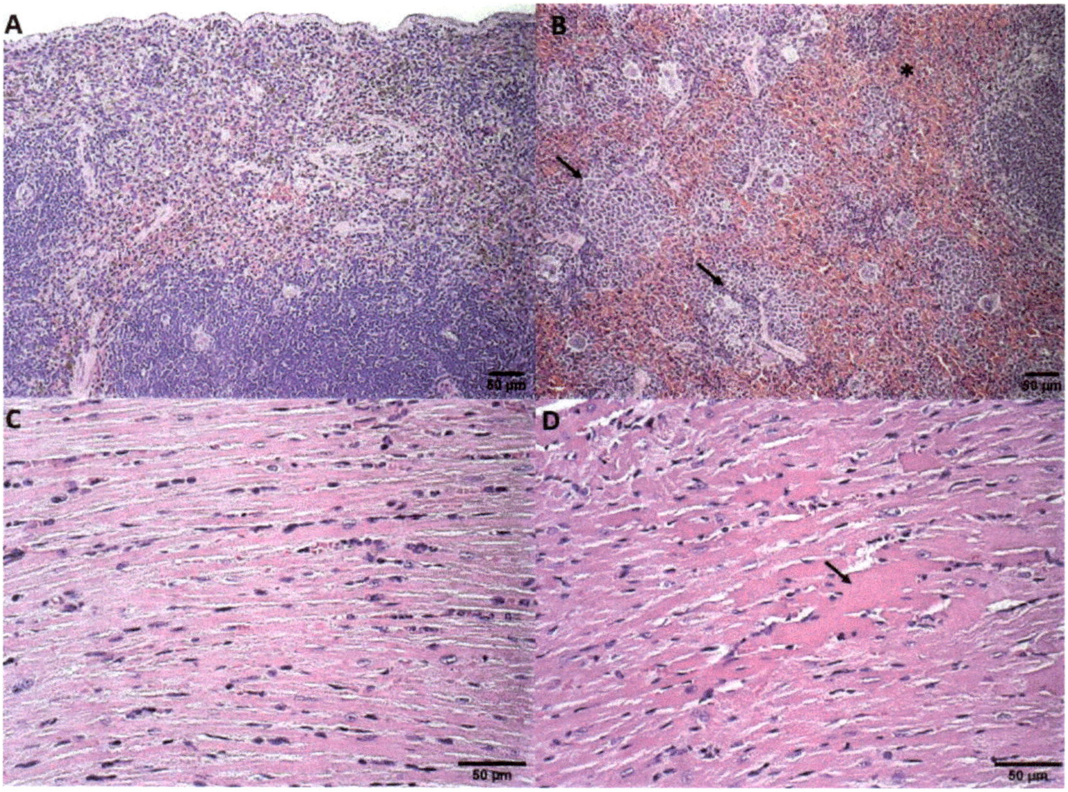

Figure 7. Histological sections of the spleen (**A**,**B**) and heart (**C**,**D**) of female Balb/c mice bearing 4T1 breast tumors. (**A**) Represents the groups treated with SpHL-DOX and ExoSpHL-DOX. Normal spleen. (**B**) Represents the groups treated with HBS, ExoSpHL, and DOX. The asterisk indicates red pulp hyperplasia, and arrows indicate the white pulp hyperplasia of the spleen. (**C**) Represents the groups treated with HBS and ExoSpHL. Normal heart. (**D**) Represents the groups treated with DOX, SpHL-DOX, and ExoSpHL-DOX. The arrow indicates the areas of degenerative hyalinization in the heart. HE, scale bar = 50 µm.

4. Discussion

Tumor-cell-derived exosomes contain proteins and lipids similar to the cells that secrete them and fuse preferentially with their cells of origin, allowing for a higher concentration of drug delivery in the tumor [16]. Exosome–liposome hybrid nanocarriers have been developed to enhance drug delivery, improve the treatment of metastatic cancer, and overcome chemoresistance in cancer [16–19]. Based on these findings, our research group developed a hybrid nanocarrier of tumor-derived exosomes fused with long-circulating and pH-sensitive liposomes containing DOX (ExoSpHL-DOX) for the treatment of breast cancer. Our results showed that the developed formulation was stable for 60 days and presented a high DOX encapsulation percentage and a DOX release that was pH-dependent on the medium. Furthermore, our data showed the cytotoxic potential of ExoSpHL-DOX against 4T1 breast cancer cells [7]. In this study, we investigated the acute toxicity and antitumor efficacy of ExoSpHL-DOX. The data obtained indicated that the LD50 for the free DOX treatment is between 12.5 and 15 mg/kg. Meanwhile, for the SpHL-DOX and ExoSpHL-DOX treatments, the LD50 is between 17.5 and 20 mg/kg. As expected, the LD50 values were higher when DOX encapsulated in liposomes or the exosome–liposome hybrid nanocarrier was administered compared to the free form. Similar results were previously found by our research group, where female Balb/c mice treated with long-circulating and pH-sensitive liposomes containing DOX (SpHL-DOX) at a dose of 15 mg/kg showed a decrease in the morbidity and reduced renal, hepatic, and cardiac toxicity of DOX when compared to free DOX at a dose of 15 mg/kg [12]. Another study of acute toxicity of long-circulating and pH-sensitive liposomes containing paclitaxel (PTX):DOX at a molar ratio of 1:10 administered to female Balb/c mice revealed an LD50 value between 28.9 and 34.7 mg/kg, while the free PTX:DOX treatment at a molar ratio of 1:10 presented an LD50 between 20.8 and 23.1 mg/kg [20]. Even though the three animals died after treatment with SpHL-DOX or ExoSpHL-DOX at a dose of 20 mg/kg, it is worth mentioning that the treatment with SpHL-DOX caused twice as much weight loss as ExoSpHL-DOX. The hematological analysis showed leukocytosis and anemia in the animals treated with free DOX at a dose of 12.5 mg/kg. Anemia is a frequent alteration that presents after chemotherapy treatment [21]. However, the increase in the white blood cells was not expected, since after DOX administration, leukopenia is common [12]. In contrast, no changes were observed after treatment with both doses of SpHL-DOX and ExoSpHL-DOX, indicating no signs of toxicity in the hematological parameters. The biochemical analyses revealed the renal toxicity of the free DOX treatment at a dose of 12.5 mg/kg, with an increase in the plasmatic urea levels. Renal damage was also confirmed by histopathology, which showed tubule dilation and hyalinization of the glomeruli after treatment with both doses of free DOX and SpHL-DOX at a dose of 17.5 mg/kg. On the other hand, animals treated with both doses of ExoSpHL-DOX showed no signs of nephrotoxicity, indicating that the presence of exosomes may alter the distribution of DOX and reduce kidney damage, even at the highest dose of the drug [22]. As an indicator of cardiac injury, the CK-MB level was found to be increased after the treatments with free DOX at a dose of 12.5 mg/kg and SpHL-DOX and ExoSpHL-DOX at a dose of 17.5 mg/kg. The increase in the CK-MB value was greater following the free DOX treatment at a dose of 12.5 mg/kg than that induced by the liposomal and exosome–liposomal formulations at the highest dose. Cardiac damage due to the free DOX treatment was also confirmed by multifocal areas of cardiomyocyte vacuolization observed in the histopathology of the animals treated with both doses of free DOX (10 and 12.5 mg/kg). However, discrete cardiomyocyte vacuolization was observed for both doses of SpHL-DOX and ExoSpHL-DOX. These findings are in agreement with a previous study performed by our research group, where female Balb/c mice were treated with free DOX at doses of 10 and 15 mg/kg and the SpHL-DOX treatment at doses of 10 and 15 mg/kg [12], and they can be explained by the lower accumulation of liposomes and exosomes in the heart, due to juxtaposed blood vessels and well-developed lymphatic system [22,23]. In this study, acute toxicity in the spleen and liver was also investigated. Due to the known uptake of liposomes by the liver and spleen, the monitoring of the toxicity of these organs is very important [24]. Splenic toxicity was observed by histopathology only in the groups treated with free DOX. The histological analysis revealed liver damage in the animals treated with both doses of free DOX and liposomal and exosome–liposomal formulations at a dose of 17.5 mg/kg. However, there was no change in the plasma levels of ALT and AST for all the treatments. The antitumor efficacy of the ExoSpHL-DOX treatment was evaluated in the Balb/c female mice with 4T1 breast tumors. The blank hybrid nanocarrier of tumor-derived exosomes fused with long-circulating and pH-sensitive liposomes did not inhibit the tumor growth and showed no signs of toxicity, as was also the case for the HBS treatment. From the obtained results of the tumor volume growth and inhibition of the tumor volume growth, it was observed that the three treatments with DOX showed a higher antitumor effect compared to the control group. However, in terms of efficacy, there was no superiority of the hybrid nanocarrier of the tumor-derived exosomes fused with long-circulating and pH-sensitive liposomes compared to free DOX. Regarding the body weight of the animals, the three treatments containing DOX caused the same body weight loss, similar to another study performed by our research group, in which female Balb/c mice received treatments of free DOX, SpHL-DOX, and long-circulating and pH-sensitive folate-coated liposomes containing DOX (SpHL-DOX-Fol) at a cumulative dose of 20 mg/kg [9]. To verify the antimetastatic activity of the ExoSpHL-DOX treatment, the organs commonly exhibiting the appearance of 4T1 tumor metastases were analyzed by histopathology. The hybrid nanocarrier of the tumor-derived exosomes fused with long-circulating and pH-sensitive liposomes reduced the number of metastatic foci in the lungs, even when it did not contain DOX. Regarding liver metastasis, few metastatic foci were found after the treatments with the formulations containing DOX, and treatment with the blank hybrid nanocarrier of the tumor-derived exosomes fused with long-circulating and pH-sensitive liposomes did not inhibit the liver metastasis. Recent works in the literature have shown the inhibition of metastasis after exosome treatment, but the reasons are still being explored. The innate organotropism capacity of exosomes, the capture and neutralization of circulating tumor cells, and the miRNA content of exosomes are probably involved in this ability to inhibit metastasis [25,26]. Therefore, the hybrid nanocarrier of tumor-derived exosomes fused with long-circulating and pH-sensitive liposomes could serve as a promising nanocarrier for the inhibition of breast cancer metastases, mainly in the lungs.

5. Conclusions

In conclusion, the results of the present study demonstrated that the toxicity of the ExoSpHL-DOX treatment is lower than the free DOX treatment, proving that exosome–liposome hybrid nanocarriers are capable of delivering higher doses of DOX without causing serious organ and tissue damage and with reduced adverse effects. In terms of the antitumor efficacy, the ExoSpHL-DOX treatment showed a higher antitumor effect compared to the control. Furthermore, ExoSpHL-DOX reduced the number of metastatic foci in the lungs, even when the exosome–liposome hybrid nanocarrier did not contain DOX. These results indicate that ExoSpHL-DOX may be a promising nanocarrier for the treatment of breast cancer, reducing toxicity and inhibiting metastasis, mainly in the lungs.

6. Patents

Oliveira, M.C.; Gomes, E.R.; Sabino, A.P. "Composição farmacêutica contendo doxorrubicina encapsulada em vesículas híbridas de exossomas tumorais e lipossomas pH-sensíveis, processo e uso". Instituto Nacional da Propriedade Industrial, nr. BR 10 2021 024659 6 (2021).

Author Contributions: Conceptualization, E.R.G. and M.C.O.; data curation, E.R.G.; formal analysis, E.R.G. and A.d.P.S.; investigation, E.R.G., F.R.S., G.D.C. and A.L.B.d.B.; methodology, E.R.G., F.R.S., G.D.C. and A.L.B.d.B.; project administration, M.C.O.; resources, M.C.O.; supervision, M.C.O.; writing—original draft, E.R.G.; writing—review and editing, E.R.G. and M.C.O. All authors have read and agreed to the published version of the manuscript.

Funding: This work was supported by the Fundação de Amparo à Pesquisa do Estado de Minas Gerais—FAPEMIG (PPM-00703-18, CDS—APQ-01588-15 and CDS—RED-00007-14, REDE MINEIRA DE PESQUISAS EM NANOBIOTECNOLOGIA) and Conselho Nacional de Desenvolvimento Científico e Tecnológico—CNPq (306197/2014-6 and 307098/2018-4).

Institutional Review Board Statement: The animal study protocol was approved by the Ethics Committee for Animal Experiments of the Universidade Federal de Minas Gerais (CEUA/UFMG—265/2019).

Acknowledgments: We thank Coordenação de Aperfeiçoamento de Pessoal de Nível Superior (CAPES) for the scholarship provided to Eliza Rocha Gomes.

Conflicts of Interest: The authors declare no conflict of interest.

Appendix A

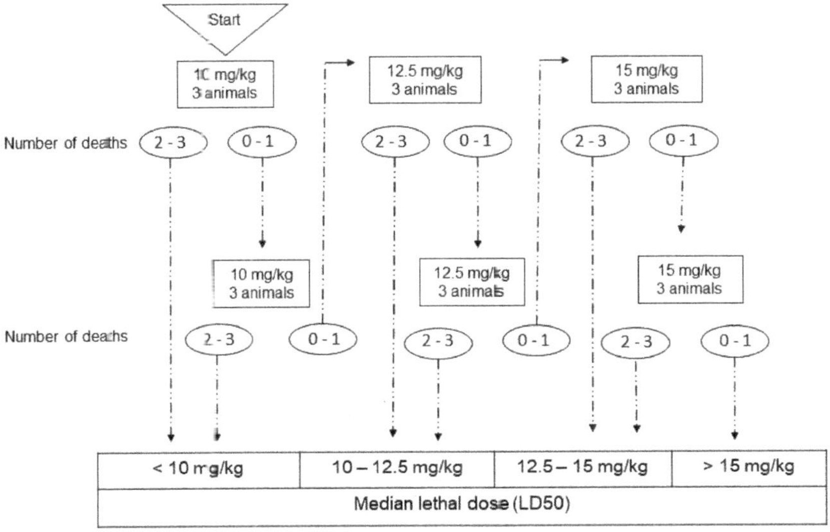

Figure A1. Treatment scheme used to assess the median lethal dose (LD50) after treatment with free DOX.

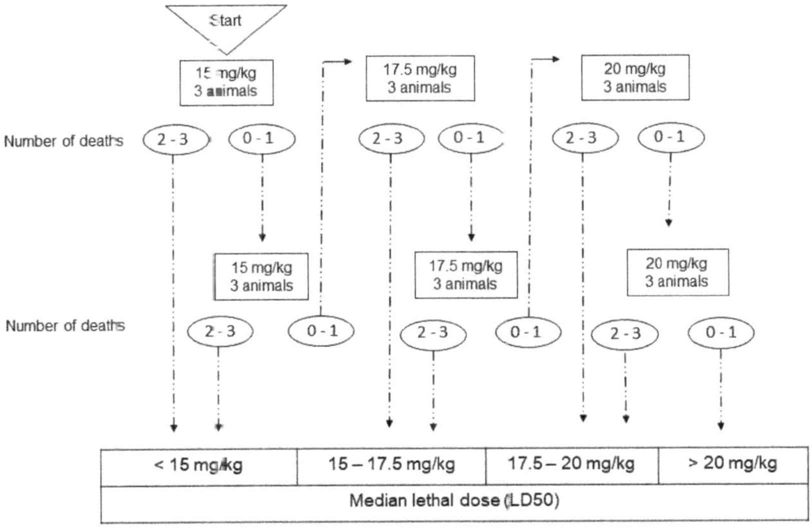

Figure A2. Treatment scheme used to assess the median lethal dose (LD50) after treatment with SpHL-DOX or ExoSpHL-DOX.

Appendix B

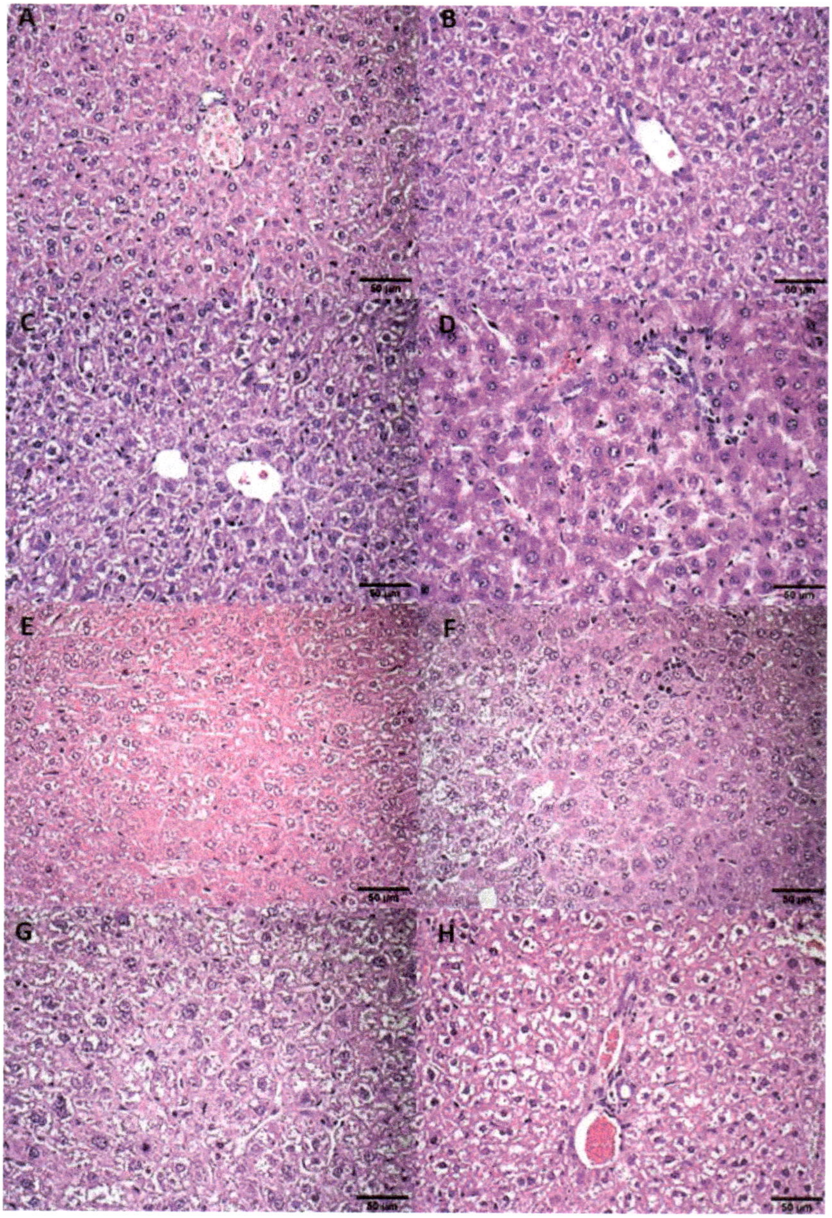

Figure A3. Histological sections of female Balb/c mice liver. (**A**) Control group (HBS), (**B**) ExoSpHL, and (**C**) SpHL-DOX at a dose of 15 mg/kg, (**D**) ExoSpHL-DOX at a dose of 15 mg/kg, (**E**) DOX at a dose of 10 mg/kg, (**F**) DOX at a dose of 12.5 mg/kg, (**G**) SpHL-DOX at a dose of 17.5 mg/kg, (**H**) ExoSpHL-DOX at a dose of 17.5 mg/kg.

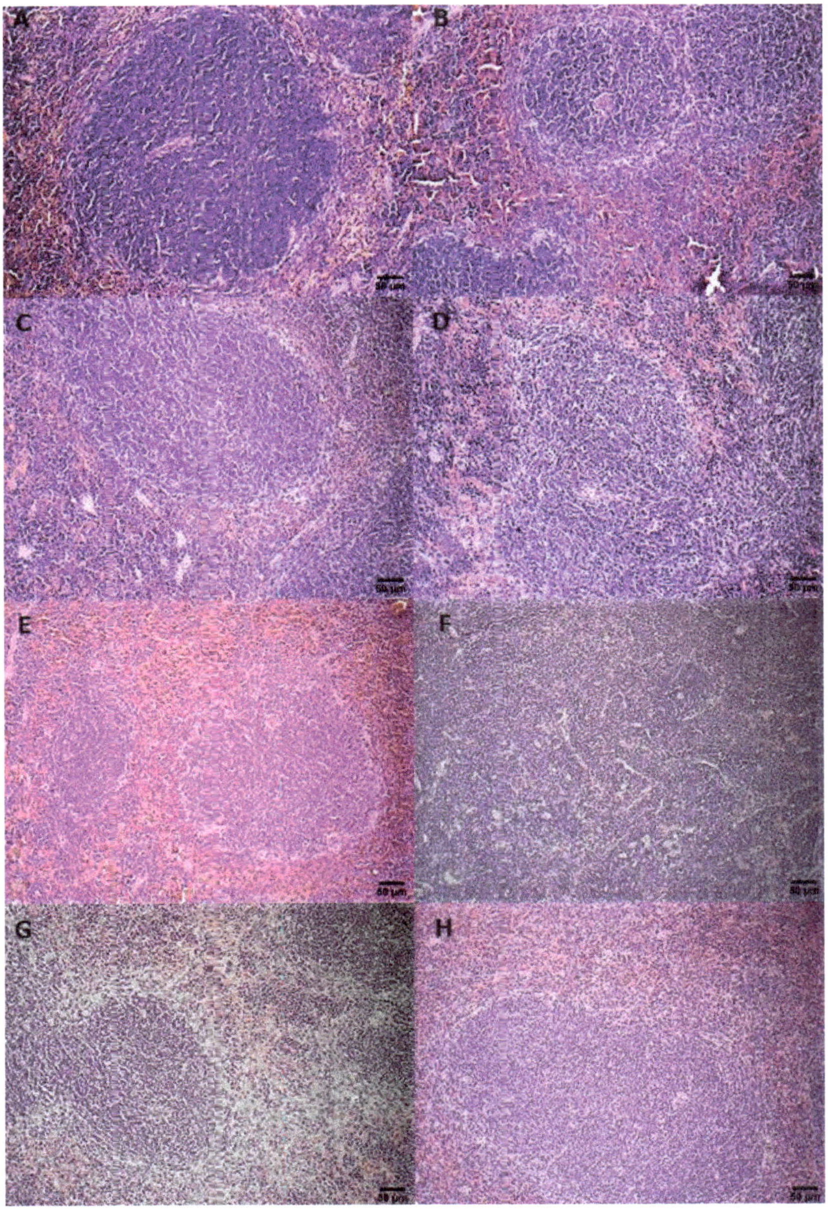

Figure A4. Histological sections of female Balb/c mice spleen. (**A**) Control group (HBS), (**B**) ExoSpHL, and (**C**) SpHL-DOX at a dose of 15 mg/kg, (**D**) SpHL-DOX at a dose of 17.5 mg/kg, (**E**) ExoSpHL-DOX at a dose of 15 mg/kg, (**F**) ExoSpHL-DOX at a dose of 17.5 mg/kg, (**G**) DOX at a dose of 10 mg/kg, (**H**) DOX at a dose of 12.5 mg/kg.

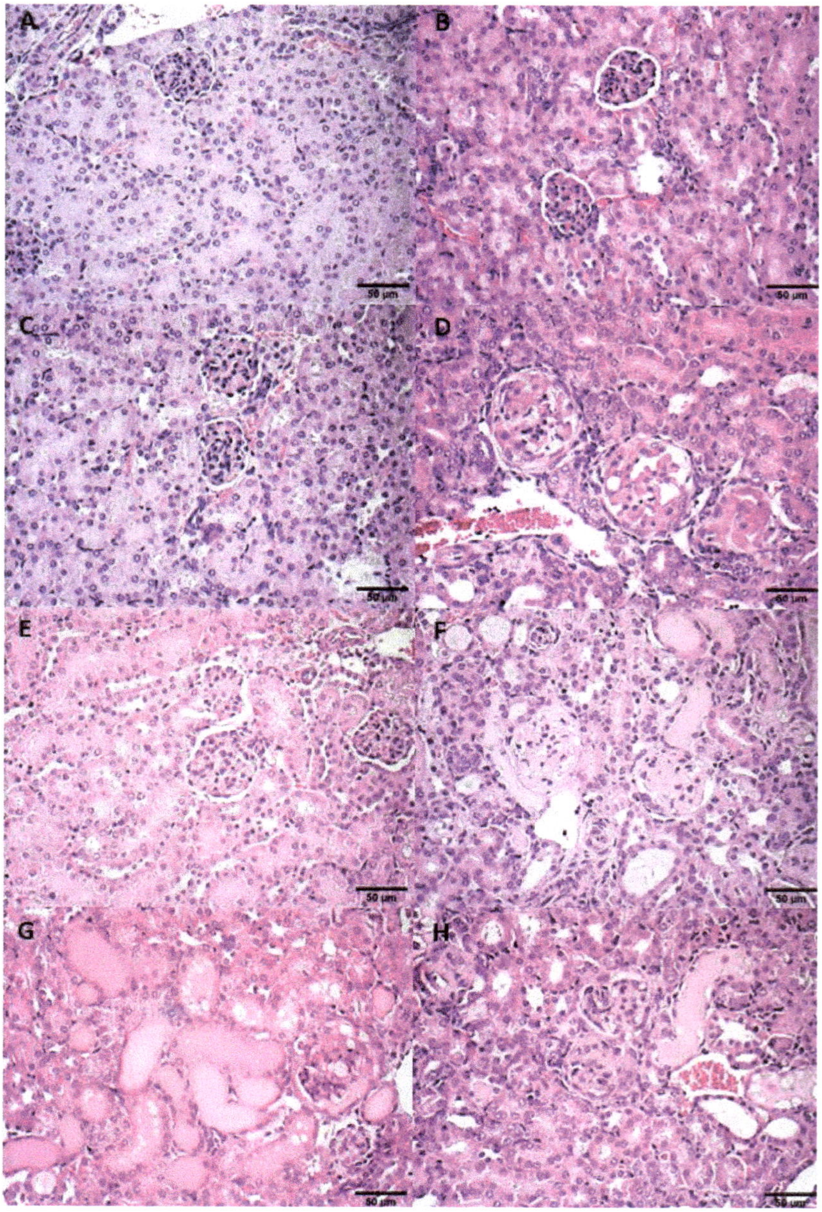

Figure A5. Histological sections of female Balb/c mice kidney. (**A**) Control group (HBS), (**B**) ExoSpHL, and (**C**) SpHL-DOX at a dose of 15 mg/kg, (**D**) ExoSpHL-DOX at a dose of 15 mg/kg, (**E**) ExoSpHL-DOX at a dose of 17.5 mg/kg, (**F**) DOX at a dose of 10 mg/kg, (**G**) DOX at a dose of 12.5 mg/kg, (**H**) SpHL-DOX at a dose of 17.5 mg/kg.

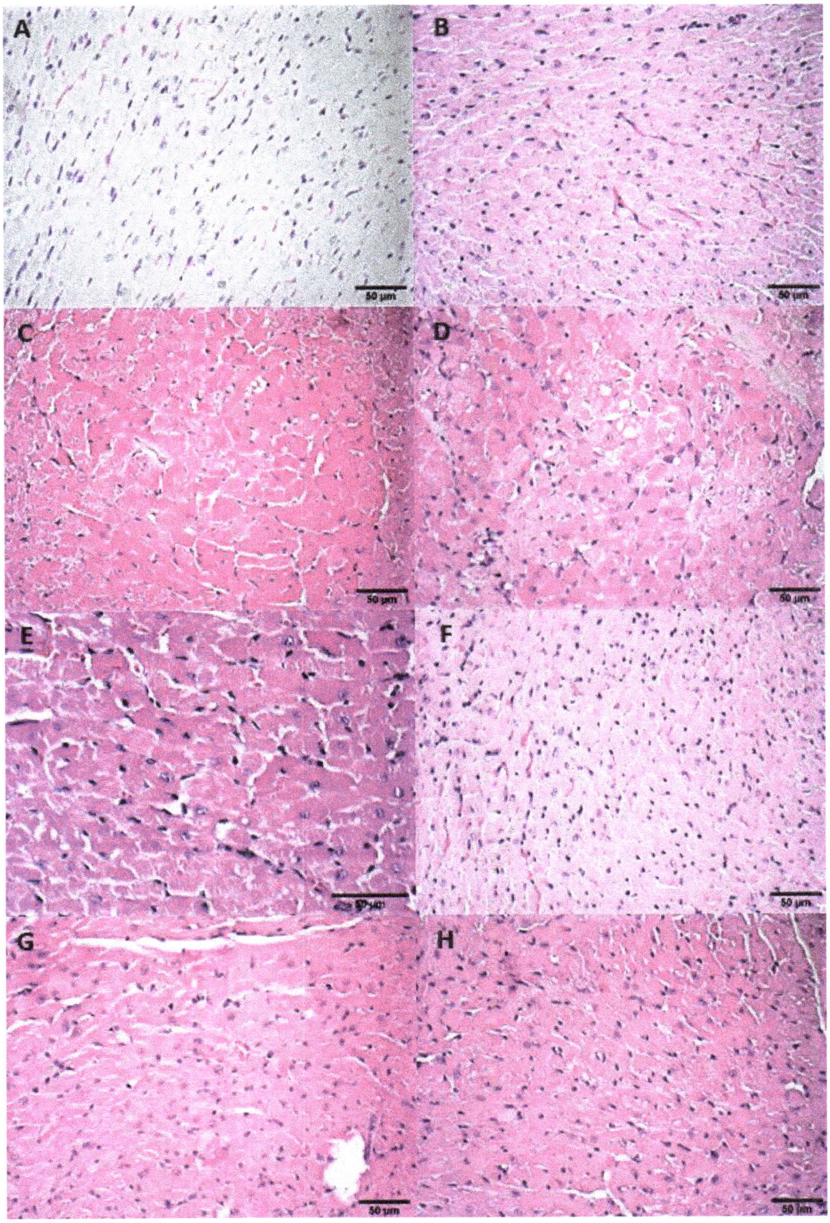

Figure A6. Histological sections of female Balb/c mice heart. (**A**) Control group (HBS), (**B**) ExoSpHL, and (**C**) DOX at a dose of 10 mg/kg, (**D**) DOX at a dose of 12.5 mg/kg, (**E**) SpHL-DOX at a dose of 15 mg/kg, (**F**) ExoSpHL-DOX at a dose of 15 mg/kg, (**G**) SpHL-DOX at a dose of 17.5 mg/kg, (**H**) ExoSpHL-DOX at a dose of 17.5 mg/kg.

Appendix C

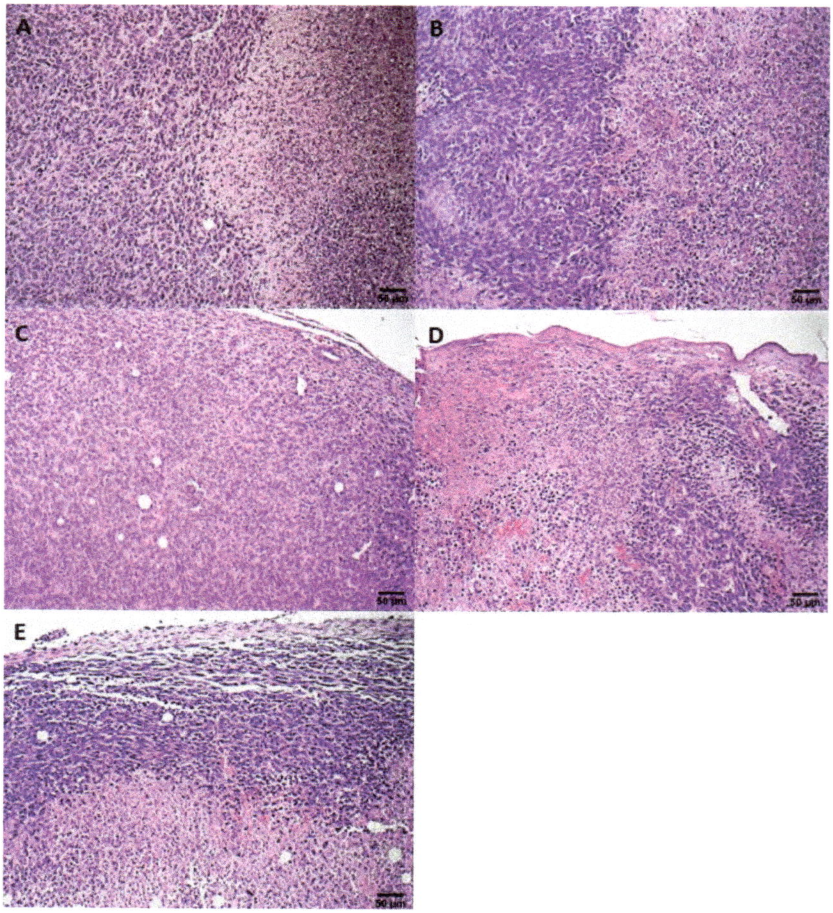

Figure A7. Histological sections of primary tumor of female Balb/c mice bearing 4T1 breast tumors treated with (**A**) control group (HBS), (**B**) ExoSpHL, or (**C**) DOX at a cumulative dose of 25 mg/kg, (**D**) SpHL-DOX at a cumulative dose of 25 mg/kg, (**E**) ExoSpHL-DOX at a cumulative dose of 25 mg/kg.

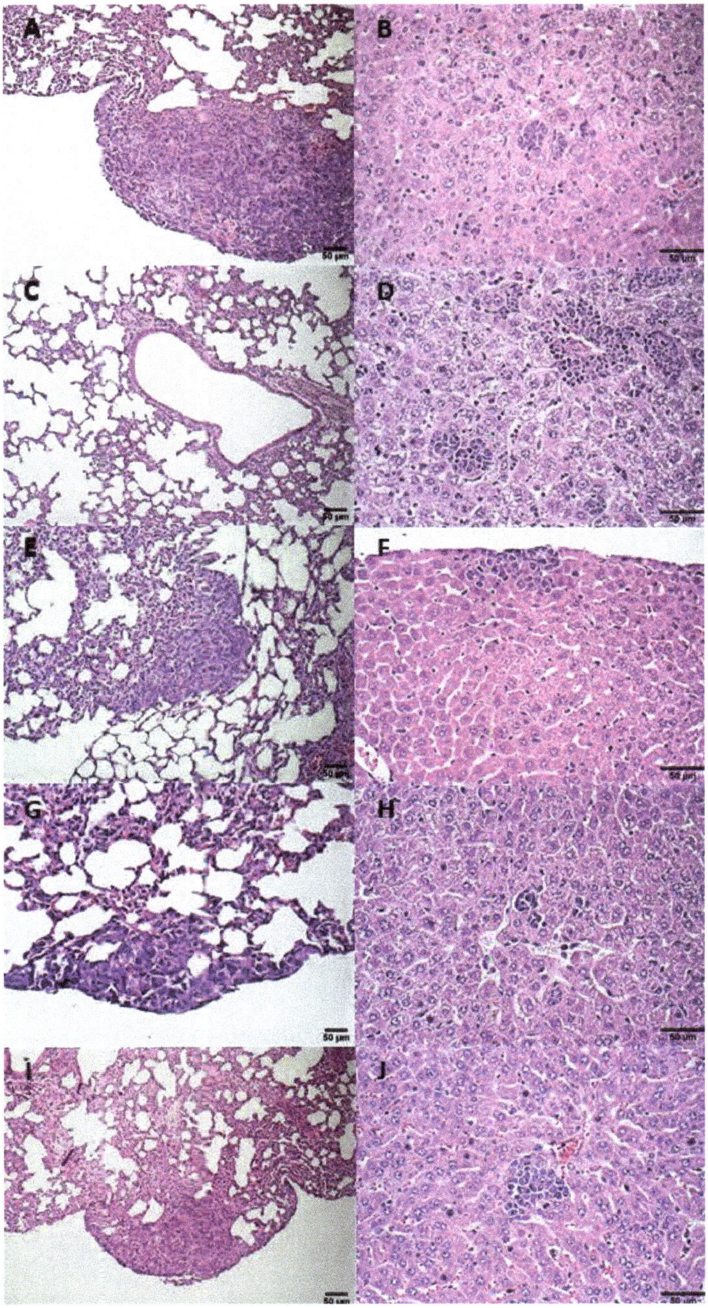

Figure A8. Histological sections of metastatic foci in lungs and liver of female Balb/c mice bearing 4T1 breast tumors treated with HBS (**A**,**B**), ExoSpHL (**C**,**D**), and DOX at a cumulative dose of 25 mg/kg (**E**,**F**), SpHL-DOX at a cumulative dose of 25 mg/kg (**G**,**H**), and ExoSpHL-DOX at a cumulative dose of 25 mg/kg (**I**,**J**).

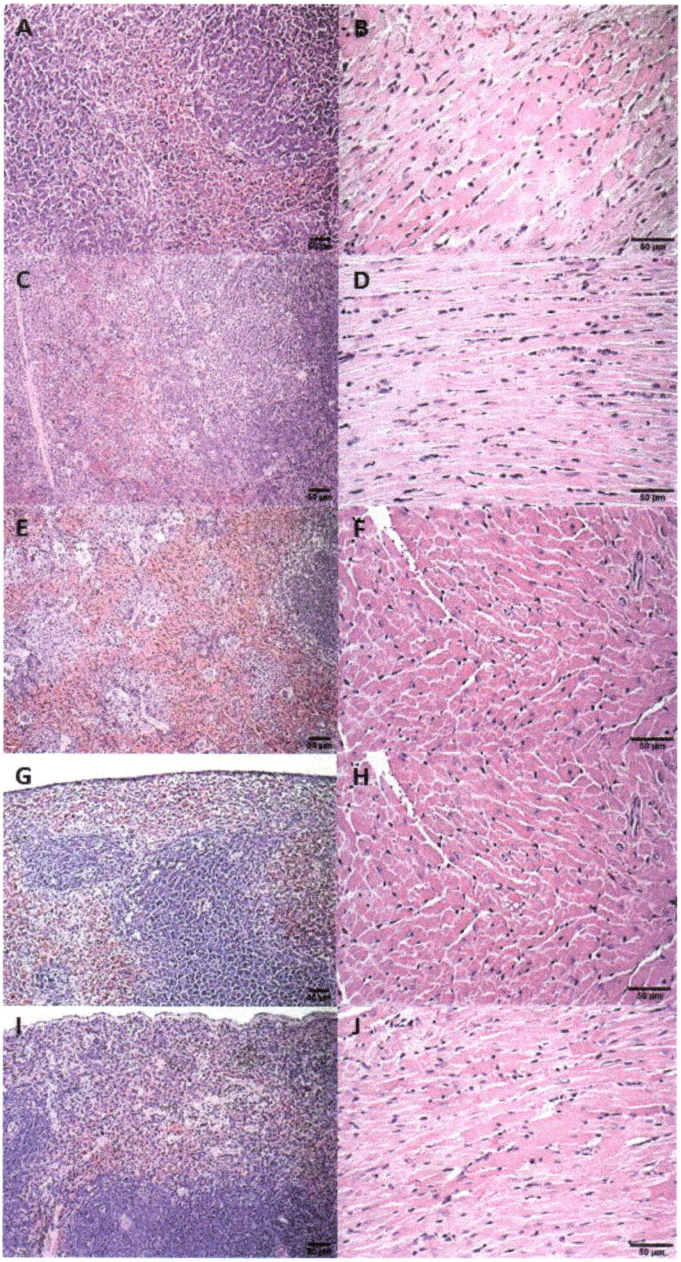

Figure A9. Histological sections of the spleen and heart of female Balb/c mice bearing 4T1 breast tumors treated with HBS (**A**,**B**), ExoSpHL (**C**,**D**), and DOX at a cumulative dose of 25 mg/kg (**E**,**F**), SpHL-DOX at a cumulative dose of 25 mg/kg (**G**,**H**), and ExoSpHL-DOX at a cumulative dose of 25 mg/kg (**I**,**J**).

References

1. Sung, H.; Ferlay, J.; Siegel, R.L.; Laversanne, M.; Soerjomataram, I.; Jemal, A.; Bray, F. Global cancer statistics 2020: GLOBOCAN Estimates of Incidence and Mortality Worldwide for 36 Cancers in 185 Countries. *CA Cancer J. Clin.* **2021**, *71*, 209–249. [CrossRef] [PubMed]
2. Zhao, N.; Woodle, M.C.; Mixson, A.J. Advances in delivery systems for doxorubicin. *J. Nanomed. Nanotechnol.* **2018**, *9*, 519. [CrossRef]
3. Jamialahmadi, K.; Zahedipour, F.; Karimi, G. The role of microRNAs on doxorubicin drug resistance in breast cancer. *J. Pharm. Pharmacol.* **2021**, *73*, 997–1006. [CrossRef] [PubMed]
4. Ngan, Y.H.; Gupta, M. A comparison between liposomal and nonliposomal formulations of doxorubicin in the treatment of cancer: An updated review. *Arch. Pharm. Pract.* **2016**, *7*, 1.
5. Liang, Y.; Duan, L.; Lu, J.; Xia, J. Engineering exosomes for targeted drug delivery. *Theranostics* **2021**, *11*, 3183–3195. [CrossRef]
6. Mukherjee, A.; Bisht, B.; Dutta, S.; Paul, M.K. Current advances in the use of exosomes, liposomes, and bioengineered hybrid nanovesicles in cancer detection and therapy. *Acta Pharmacol. Sin.* **2022**, *43*, 2759–2776. [CrossRef]
7. Gomes, E.R.; Carvalho, A.T.; Barbosa, T.C.; Ferreira, L.L.; Calado, H.D.R.; Sabino, A.P.; Oliveira, M.C. Fusion of tumor-derived exosomes with long-circulating and pH-sensitive liposomes loaded with doxorubicin for the treatment of breast cancer. *AAPS-PharmSciTech* **2022**, *23*, 255. [CrossRef]
8. Bangham, A.D.; Standish, M.M.; Watkins, J.C. Diffusion of univalent ions across the lamellae of swollen phospholipids. *J. Mol. Biol.* **1965**, *13*, 238–252. [CrossRef]
9. Silva, J.O.; Fernandes, R.S.; Oda, C.M.R.; Ferreira, T.H.; Botelho, A.F.M.; Melo, M.M.; de Miranda, M.C.; Gomes, D.A.; Cassali, G.D.; Townsend, D.M.; et al. Folate-coated, long-circulating and pH-sensitive liposomes enhance doxorubicin antitumor effect in a breast cancer animal model. *Biomed. Pharm.* **2019**, *118*, 109323. [CrossRef]
10. Ferreira, D.S.; Faria, S.D.; Lopes, S.C.d.; Teixeira, C.S.; Malachias, A.; Magalhães-Paniago, R.; Filho, J.D.d.; Oliveira, B.L.d.P.; Guimarães, A.R.; Caravan, P.; et al. Development of a bone-targeted pH-sensitive liposomal formulation: Physicochemical characterization, cytotoxicity, and biodistribution evaluation in a mouse model of bone metastasis. *Int. J. Nanomed.* **2016**, *11*, 3737–3751.
11. OECD. Test No. 423: Acute Oral Toxicity—Acute Toxic Class Method. In *OECD Guidelines for the Testing of Chemicals*; Section 4; OECD Publishing: Paris, France, 2002.
12. Silva, J.O.; Miranda, S.E.M.; Leite, E.A.; Sabino, A.P.; Borges, K.B.G.; Cardoso, V.N.; Cassali, G.D.; Guimarães, A.G.; Oliveira, M.C.; Barros, A.L.B.; et al. Toxicological study of a new doxorubicin-loaded pH-sensitive liposome: A preclinical approach. *Toxicol. Appl. Pharmacol.* **2018**, *352*, 162–169. [CrossRef]
13. Lages, E.B.; Fernandes, R.S.; Silva, J.d.; de Souza, Â.M.; Cassali, G.D.; Barros, A.L.B.; Ferreira, L.A.M. Co-delivery of doxorubicin, docosahexaenoic acid, and α-tocopherol succinate by nanostructured lipid carriers has a synergistic effect to enhance antitumor activity and reduce toxicity. *Biomed. Pharm.* **2020**, *132*, 110876. [CrossRef]
14. Rolland, C.L.; Dineen, S.P.; Lynn, K.D.; Sullivan, L.A.; Dellinger, M.T.; Sadegh, L.; Sullivan, J.P.; Shames, D.S.; Brekken, R.A. Inhibition of vascular endothelial growth factor reduces angiogenesis and modulates immune cell infiltration of orthotopic breast cancer xenografts. *Mol. Cancer Ther.* **2009**, *8*, 1761–1771. [CrossRef]
15. Garcia, C.M.; de Araújo, M.R.; Lopes, M.T.P.; Ferreira, M.A.N.D.; Cassali, G.D. Morphological and immunophenotipical characterization of murine mammary carcinoma 4T1. *Braz. J. Vet. Pathol.* **2014**, *7*, 158–165.
16. Qiao, L.; Hu, S.; Huang, K.; Su, T.; Li, Z.; Vandergriff, A.; Cores, J.; Dinh, P.; Allen, T.; Shen, D.; et al. Tumor cell-derived exosomes home to their cells of origin and can be used as Trojan horses to deliver cancer drugs. *Theranostics* **2020**, *10*, 3474–3487. [CrossRef]
17. Sun, L.; Fan, M.; Huang, D.; Li, B.; Xu, R.; Gao, F.; Chen, Y. Clodronate-loaded liposomal and fibroblast-derived exosomal hybrid system for enhanced drug delivery to pulmonary fibrosis. *Biomaterials* **2021**, *271*, 120761. [CrossRef]
18. Li, L.; Di He, D.; Guo, Q.; Zhang, Z.; Ru, D.; Wang, L.; Gong, K.; Liu, F.; Duan, Y.; Li, H. Exosome-liposome hybrid nanoparticle codelivery of TP and miR497 conspicuously overcomes chemoresistant ovarian cancer. *J. Nanobiotechnol.* **2022**, *20*, 50. [CrossRef]
19. Lv, Q.; Cheng, L.; Lu, Y.; Zhang, X.; Wang, Y.; Deng, J.; Zhou, J.; Liu, B.; Liu, J. Thermosensitive exosome-liposome hybrid nanoparticle-mediated chemoimmunotherapy for improved treatment of metastatic peritoneal cancer. *Adv. Sci.* **2020**, *7*, 2000515. [CrossRef]
20. Roque, M.C.; da Silva, C.D.; Lempek, M.R.; Cassali, G.D.; de Barros, A.L.B.; Melo, M.M.; Oliveira, M.C. Preclinical toxicological study of long-circulating and fusogenic liposomes co-encapsulating paclitaxel and doxorubicin in synergic ratio. *Biomed. Pharm.* **2021**, *144*, 112307. [CrossRef]
21. Toblli, J.E.; Rivas, C.; Cao, G.; Giani, J.F.; Funk, F.; Mizzen, L.; Dominici, F.P. Ferric carboxymaltose-mediated attenuation of doxorubicin-induced cardiotoxicity in an iron deficiency rat model. *Chemother. Res. Pract.* **2014**, *2014*, 570241. [CrossRef]
22. Toffoli, G.; Hadla, M.; Corona, G.; Caligiuri, I.; Palazzolo, S.; Semeraro, S.; Gamini, A.; Canzonieri, V.; Rizzolio, F. Exosomal doxorubicin reduces the cardiac toxicity of doxorubicin. *Nanomedicine* **2015**, *10*, 2963–2971. [CrossRef] [PubMed]
23. Dasa, S.S.K.; Suzuki, R.; Mugler, E.; Chen, L.; Jansson-Löfmark, R.; Michaëlsson, E.; Lindfors, L.; Klibanov, A.L.; French, B.A.; Kelly, K.A. Evaluation of pharmacokinetic and pharmacodynamic profiles of liposomes for the cell type-specific delivery of small molecule drugs. *Nanomed. Nanotechnol. Biol. Med.* **2017**, *13*, 2565–2574. [CrossRef] [PubMed]

24. Monteiro, L.O.F.; Fernandes, R.S.; Oda, C.M.R.; Lopes, S.C.; Townsend, D.M.; Cardoso, V.N.; Oliveira, M.C.; Leite, E.A.; Rubello, D.; de Barros, A.L.B. Paclitaxel-loaded folate-coated long circulating and pH-sensitive liposomes as a potential drug delivery system: A biodistribution study. *Biomed. Pharm.* **2018**, *97*, 489–495. [CrossRef]
25. Wang, K.; Ye, H.; Zhang, X.; Wang, X.; Yang, B.; Luo, C.; Zhao, Z.; Zhao, J.; Lu, Q.; Zhang, H.; et al. An exosome-like programmable-bioactivating paclitaxel prodrug nanoplatform for enhanced breast cancer metastasis inhibition. *Biomaterials* **2020**, *257*, 120224. [CrossRef]
26. Nie, H.; Xie, X.; Zhang, D.; Zhou, Y.; Li, B.; Li, F.; Li, F.; Cheng, Y.; Mei, H.; Meng, H.; et al. Use of lung-specific exosomes for miRNA-126 delivery in non-small cell lung cancer. *Nanoscale* **2020**, *12*, 877–887. [CrossRef] [PubMed]

pharmaceutics

MDPI

Article

The Rate of Cisplatin Dosing Affects the Resistance and Metastatic Potential of Triple Negative Breast Cancer Cells, Independent of Hypoxia

Omkar Bhatavdekar [1,2], Inês Godet [1,2,3], Daniele Gilkes [1,2,3,4,5] and Stavroula Sofou [1,2,3,5,*]

1 Department of Chemical and Biomolecular Engineering, The Johns Hopkins University, Baltimore, MD 21218, USA
2 Johns Hopkins Institute for NanoBioTechnology, The Johns Hopkins University, Baltimore, MD 21218, USA
3 Department of Oncology, The Sidney Kimmel Comprehensive Cancer Center, The Johns Hopkins University School of Medicine, Baltimore, MD 21231, USA
4 Cellular and Molecular Medicine Program, The Johns Hopkins University School of Medicine, Baltimore, MD 21231, USA
5 Cancer Invasion and Metastasis Program, The Johns Hopkins University School of Medicine, Baltimore, MD 21231, USA
* Correspondence: ssofou1@jh.edu; Tel.: +1-410-516-0274

Citation: Bhatavdekar, O.; Godet, I.; Gilkes, D.; Sofou, S. The Rate of Cisplatin Dosing Affects the Resistance and Metastatic Potential of Triple Negative Breast Cancer Cells, Independent of Hypoxia. *Pharmaceutics* **2022**, *14*, 2184. https://doi.org/10.3390/pharmaceutics14102184

Academic Editors: Raquel Fernández García, Francisco Bolás-Fernández and Ana Isabel Fraguas-Sánchez

Received: 14 September 2022
Accepted: 10 October 2022
Published: 13 October 2022

Abstract: To best control tumor growth and/or metastasis in triple negative breast cancer (TNBC), it may be useful to understand the effect(s) of chemotherapy delivery (i.e., the rate and pattern of exposure to the drug) on cell sub-populations that have experienced different levels of hypoxia (and/or acidosis). In this spirit, MDA-MB-231 TNBC cells, and their hypoxia-reporter counterparts, were characterized for their sensitivity to cisplatin. When in the form of multicellular spheroids, that capture the diffusion-limited transport that generates hypoxic and acidic subregions within the avascular areas of solid tumors, the effects of the rate and pattern of exposure to cisplatin on cell viability and motility/migration potential were evaluated for each cell sub-population. We demonstrated that cell sensitivity to cisplatin was not dependent on acidosis, but cell resistance increased with exposure to hypoxia. In spheroids, the increase of the rates of cell exposure to cisplatin, at a constant cumulative dose, increased sensitivity to chemotherapy and lowered the cells' metastatic potential, even for cells that had experienced hypoxia. This effect was also shown to be caused by nanocarriers engineered to quickly release cisplatin which deeply penetrated the spheroid interstitium, resulting in the fast and uniform exposure of the TNBC tumors to the agent. This rate and dosing-controlled model may effectively limit growth and/or metastasis, independent of hypoxia. This mode of chemotherapy delivery can be enabled by engineered nanocarriers.

Keywords: triple negative breast cancer; cisplatin; hypoxia; nanoparticle; diffusion; solid tumors; rate of drug release; metastatic potential

1. Introduction

Treatment of advanced triple negative breast cancer (TNBC) remains one of the unmet needs in global healthcare over the last few decades [1,2]. Clinical outcomes for advanced TNBC still remain devastatingly poor with median overall survival ranging from 8 to 13.3 months [3]. Despite the latest advances in immunotherapy [4] and radiotherapy [5], following surgery, chemotherapy [6,7] remains the frontline option for treating both the primary tumors and recurrence in TNBC due to a lack of reliable cell surface markers for molecularly targeted therapies [8]. Therapeutic approaches to treat TNBC have failed due to their inability to reduce the metastatic potential of the disease and/or to effectively handle the induced resistance to chemotherapy.

Cisplatin (CDDP) has been used as a frontline chemotherapeutic for multiple solid tumors including TNBC [9–12]. CDDP's mechanism of action primarily entails the formation of platinum-DNA adducts by binding to the genomic and/or mitochondrial DNA [12] inhibiting DNA replication, which finally leads to apoptosis or necrosis. Although CDDP is extensively used in the clinic, CDDP has major safety considerations, with nephrotoxicity and hepatotoxicity being the primary adverse side-effects [13,14]. These side effects limit the maximum tolerated dose (MTD), which may result in incomplete tumor killing, causing major setbacks on the clinical outcomes. Although there are now second and third generation platinum-based agents, such as carboplatin and oxaliplatin used in the clinic globally, the latter have not been able to markedly improve the therapeutic index [15].

One of the primary reasons for TNBC's lethality is chemoresistance contributing to a poorer prognosis; this has been associated with the prevalence of hypoxia within the established, soft-tissue solid (primary and/or metastatic) tumors. To make the prognosis even worse, the evidence shows that cells that experience hypoxia in the primary tumor have a higher metastatic potential and migrate to distant organs, such as the lungs [16] and/or the brain [17], causing cancer's deadlier recurrence. Although there are a variety of debated mechanisms for how hypoxia affects the tumor landscape, it is well established that hypoxia inducible factor 1 and 2 (HIF-1/2), hypoxia-regulated transcription factors, modulate the expression of hypoxia-inducible genes including, but not limited to, the growth factor regulating genes, tumor survival genes, etc. [18].

Along with metabolic imbalances, hypoxia is accompanied by acidosis [19] which results in a lowered pH in the tumor microenvironment, due to anaerobic glycolysis and a slower clearance of acidic metabolites. This is not just detrimental for the local tumor microenvironment; it has also been hypothesized that acidosis accelerates the late steps in carcinogenesis resulting in the degradation of the extracellular matrix (ECM), potentially increasing the intravasation of tumor cells into the bloodstream and, therefore, contributing to metastasis [20].

The above factors occurring in the solid tumor microenvironment, may promote the development of multiple cancer cell subpopulations, each with a different evolution landscape, resulting in different drug sensitivities, growth patterns and/or migratory potential(s), as shown by Godet et al. [21,22]. Therefore, in order to best therapeutically control tumor growth and metastasis, it may be mechanistically useful also to understand the effect(s) of therapy on these cell sub-populations, so as to ultimately design therapeutic approaches selectively for those types of cancer cells that are most difficult to treat.

Using an orthotopic TNBC mouse model, that developed spontaneous metastases, Stras et al. [23,24] have previously shown that the rate and pattern of cells' exposure to CDDP inhibits at different extents the primary tumor growth and the onset of metastasis. In particular, for the delivery of CDDP, they utilized liposomes with different combinations of two key properties, which essentially affected the levels and rate of exposure of the cancer cells to CDDP that was delivered. They included, first, the release property of CDDP from liposomes when in the tumor interstitium, to increase the CDDP penetration in the tumor; and second, the property of adhesion of liposomes to the tumors' ECM for a slower liposome clearance from the tumors. The systematic interrogation of the combinations of these properties' on liposomes demonstrated that the fastest, most uniform and more prolonged exposure of cancer cells to the delivered chemotherapy (by liposomes with both properties) were most effective in decreasing the tumors' growth rate.

In this study, we aimed to interrogate the role of the rate (and pattern) of exposure of the cancer cells to CDDP on affecting (1) the extent of killing different subpopulations of cancer cells (hypoxic vs. normoxic) and/or (2) the inhibition of the cells' motility, which may impact their metastatic potential. The present study was designed to systematically interrogate these factors on TNBC multicellular spheroids used as surrogates of the solid tumors' avascular regions.

2. Materials and Methods

The lipids 1,2-diarachidoyl-sn-glycero-3-phosphocholine (20PC), 1,2-dipalmitoyl-sn-glycero-3-phospho-L-serine (sodium salt) (DPPS), 1,2-distearoyl-sn-glycero-3-phosphoethan olamine-N-[amino(polyethylene glycol)-2000]-(ammonium salt) (DSPE-PEG(2000)), 1,2-dipalmitoyl-snglycero-3-phosphoethanolamine—N-(lissamine rhodamine B sulfonyl) (ammonium salt) (DPPE-rhodamine), and the custom synthesized 1,2-distearoyl-sn-glycero-3-phosphoethanolamine-N-PEG2000-dimenthylammonium propane (DSPE-PEG(2000)-DAP, the 'adhesion lipid' as previously reported) were purchased from Avanti Polar lipids (Alabaster, AL, USA). Cholesterol, CDDP, and all buffers were purchased from Sigma Aldrich (St. Louis, MO, USA) and cell-related media reagents were purchased from Gibco (Waltham, MA, USA).

2.1. Cell Culture

The MDA-MB-231 TNBC cell line was obtained from the American Type Culture Collection (ATCC, Rockville, MD, USA) and cultured in Dulbecco's modified Eagle's media (DMEM) supplemented with 10% fetal bovine serum (FBS) and 100 units/mL penicillin, 100 mg/mL streptomycin at 37 °C with 5% CO_2. The MDA-MB-231 hypoxia reporter cells (MDA-MB-231HR) were generated, as previously described in Godet et al., 2019 [21]. Briefly, the vectors encoding CMV-loxp-DsRed-loxp-eGFP (Addgene #141148) and 4xHRE-MinTK-CRE-ODD (Addgene #141147) were developed by using Gateway and InFusion cloning strategies, respectively. The final lentiviral vectors were transduced into the MDA-MB-231 cells that were selected and single-cell cloned. The selection and screening process yielded a cell-line that expresses DsRed in normoxic conditions and GFP after the prolonged exposure to hypoxic conditions. The cells were cultured in 20% and 1% O_2 for normoxic and hypoxic conditions, respectively. Hypoxic conditions were achieved by using an InvivO2 hypoxia workstation (Baker, Sanford, ME, USA) with an ICONIC (Baker, Sanford, ME, USA) electronically controlled gas-mixing system maintained at 37 °C and 75% humidity, equilibrated at 1% O_2, 5% CO_2, and 94% N_2.

2.2. NanoParticle (NP) Preparation and CDDP Loading

The compositions of the lipid NPs used in the study were either non-pH responsive or pH-responsive, as previously described in detail [23,24]. The non-pH responsive lipid NP comprised 20PC: cholesterol: DSPE-PEG (2000) at mole ratio 0.72:0.18:0.09. The pH-responsive NP were composed of 20PC: DPPS: cholesterol: DSPE-PEG-DAP at mole ratio 0.60:0.26:0.04:0.09. The pH-responsive release property of the lipid NP was enabled by a lipid membrane comprising a phosphatidylcholine lipid and a titratable anionic lipid, phosphatidylserine, with at least two carbon atoms mismatch in their acyl tail lengths. We have previously demonstrated [25,26] that this lipid bilayer is relatively well mixed at a physiological pH, due to the electrostatic repulsion among the negatively charged phosphatidyl serine lipid headgroups, resulting in the stable retention of the contents by the NP. At acidic pH values, the protonation of the phosphatidyl serine lipid headgroup and the inherent hydrogen bonding between these lipids, results in the attraction of the protonated phosphatidyl serine lipids, while they laterally diffuse on the plane of the lipid bilayer, causing the lipid phase separation and the formation of phosphatidyl serine-rich lipid domains. We have demonstrated that, at the domain boundaries, the transient lipid packing defects spanning the lipid bilayer, due to the difference in the lipid acyl tails and the different intrinsic lipid tilts relative to the plane of the bilayer, result in the increased membrane permeability and the content release from the NP. The property of a pH-triggered adhesion to the tumor ECM was enabled by adding the titratable group dimenthylammonium propane (DAP) at the free end of the PEG chains. The moiety DAP has a pKa of approximately 6.8 [27], which is comparable to the pH in the tumor interstitum [28,29]. Upon the DAP protonation, the cationic charges on the freely undulating PEG chains were shown to not result in significant interactions of the NP with cells, but instead to enable the NP to retain a certain level of adhesion to the negatively charged tumor ECM; this translated into a greater tumor uptake and a slower NP clearance from the tumors in vivo [24]. All lipid nanoparticle compositions were labeled with 0.06 mole % DPPE-rhodamine.

The lipid NPs were prepared using a thin film hydration method [23]. Briefly, a dry lipid film (10−40 µmol total lipid) was hydrated with 1 mL of phosphate-buffered saline (PBS) (10 mM phosphate-buffered saline with 1 mM ethylenediaminetetraacetic acid (EDTA), pH 7.4), and the suspension was annealed at 66 °C for 2 h following the extrusion for 21 times through 100 nm pore-size polycarbonate membranes at 80 °C (10–15 °C above the highest value of the constituent lipid transition temperature). The lipid NPs were passed through a Sepharose 4B column before CDDP was then passively loaded by adding CDDP (17 mg/mL) to the lipid NP suspension (20 mM total lipid) at 80 °C for 4 h under constant mixing. Unencapsulated CDDP was removed from the lipid NP using a Sephadex G50 column, eluted with PBS at pH 7.4. The CDDP content in the lipid NP was analyzed by lysing 100 µL of the NP suspension diluted with 300 µL of 10% HCl with 0.5% Triton X-100, followed by measuring the platinum content using a graphite furnace atomic absorption spectrophotometer (GFAAS) (using a hollow cathode Pt 365.9 nm lamp, Buck Scientific, Norwalk, CT, USA), and was quantified by the comparison of the measured signal to a calibration curve as reported in the supplemental information (Figure S1). Prior to the incubation with the cells, all lipid NPs were filter sterilized (200 µm filters, VWR, Radnor, PA, USA).

2.3. *Characterization of the Lipid NP: ζ-Potential*

The size and ζ-potential of the lipid NP were determined using a Zetasizer Nano ZS 90 (Malvern, UK). The samples were diluted in PBS (10 mM phosphate buffer, 150 mM NaCl, 300 mOsm) for sizing and/or low-salt PBS (10 mM phosphate buffer, 15 mM NaCl, 275 mM sucrose, 300 mOsm) for measuring changes in the ζ-potential as a function of pH.

2.4. *Characterization of the Lipid NP: Release of CDDP from the NP*

To evaluate the retention of CDDP by the NP, 200 µL of the NP suspension was added in 800 µL of a FBS-supplemented cell culture media (10% FBS final concentration), in the presence of cells, in the respective conditions. At the end of the incubation, the released CDDP from the NP was measured by adding 1 mL of the suspension in a Sephadex G50 column, and by collecting the eluted separate fractions that corresponded to the NP and the released CDDP. The content of platinum in the collected fractions was quantified using the GFAAS by diluting 25 µL of the sample with 75 µL of 10% HCl and adding 5 µL Triton-X. The Pt content in these samples was compared to the Pt content at the start of the incubation to determine the % CDDP retained in the lipid NP.

2.5. *Determination of the CDDP IC_{50} Values on the Cell Monolayers*

The cells were plated on 96-well plates at a density of 20,000 cells/well in normoxic and in hypoxic conditions. For the hypoxic conditions, the cells were pre-conditioned to the hypoxic environment for 48 h pre CDDP treatment. Following the required exposure, independent of the condition, the cells were exposed to free or NP containing CDDP for 6 h. For the hypoxic conditions, the experiment was performed at the naturally lowered pH 6.8 whereas for the normoxic conditions, the experiment was performed at pH 7.4 and at pH 6.8, to decouple the effects of pH and hypoxia. Following the completion of the incubation, the cells were washed twice with sterile PBS at the same pH and fresh media was added to the cells. Following two doubling times (2 × 36 h, 2 × 42 h and/or 2 × 41 h, for the cells in the normoxic conditions at pH 7.4 and 6.8, and for the cells in the hypoxic conditions, respectively), the media was removed, washed 1× with PBS and the MTT assay (Promega, Madison, WI, USA) was performed (according to manufacturer's protocol) to assess the cell viability. The cell viability was normalized by the viability of the cells that did not receive any CDDP at the respective oxygen conditions and pH, in triplicate measurements.

2.6. Measurement of the CDDP Cell Uptake

In 6-well plates, 300,000 cells were plated at both normoxic and hypoxic conditions. The cells were exposed to the hypoxic conditions for 48 h prior to the CDDP introduction. The cells were incubated with 200 and 100 μg/mL of CDDP at the respective pH values and oxygen conditions. At different time points, the cells were washed twice with PBS to remove the extracellular CDDP. The cells were then carefully scraped and collected in 1 mL DDI and sonicated for 10 min before measuring the Pt content on a GFAAS, in triplicate measurements.

2.7. Spheroid Formation and the Cell Population Characterization

Spheroids, used as surrogates of the tumors' avascular regions, were formed, as previously reported [23]. Briefly, the MDA-MB-231-HR cell suspension was kept on ice and Matrigel™ (Corning Inc., Corning, NY, USA) and was added at a concentration of 2.5% (*v*/*v*) to promote the spheroid formation. The cells were seeded on U-shaped 96-well plates treated with poly-HEMA (Sigma Aldrich, St. Louis, MO, USA) and centrifuged at 1000 RCF for 10 min at 4 °C.

To image the spatiotemporal distributions of the cells in spheroids, a Leica LSM 780 was used at 488 nm and 514 nm excitation lasers for imaging for the GFP (508–568 nm, detecting hypoxic/post-hypoxic cells) and the RFP (578–660 nm, detecting cells experienced only normoxic conditions), respectively, using 10 μm z-stack optical slices. The spheroids were transferred to a glass bottom 35 mm cell culture dish (VWR, Radnor, PA, USA) and imaged every two days. To quantify the population distributions of the cells in the spheroids of different sizes, first, the spheroids were plated on adherent wells until they reached confluence, and then the cells were lightly trypsinized, washed, and resuspended in ice cold media before they were analyzed using a BD FACS Canto (Franklin Lakes, NJ, USA).

2.8. Spatiotemporal Profiles of the NPs and the Drug Surrogate in the Spheroids

To measure the spatiotemporal distributions of the NPs and of the drug surrogate in the spheroids, the NPs containing 1 mol % DPPE-rhodamine lipid were prepared and loaded with carboxyfluorescein diacetate succinimidyl ester (CFDA-SE) (ex/em: 497/517 nm), which was used as the drug surrogate. The final CFDA-SE concentration in the NP suspension was 200 nM. The extent of the retention, as a function of pH, of CFDA-SE from both types of NPs matched the extent of retention of CDDP from the corresponding NPs (see supporting information, Table S1).

The spheroids were incubated with different concentrations of free CFDA-SE and/or with 1 mM (total lipid concentration) of the lipid NP (containing CFDA-SE) for up to 6 h (to observe the 'uptake' into the spheroids) and then the spheroids were transferred in fresh media (to observe the 'clearance' from the spheroids). At different time points, the spheroids were fished out in 2 μL media and frozen in Cryochrome™gel over dry ice. The spheroids that were not incubated with the NP and/or CFDA-SE were used as background. The equatorial, 20 μm thick spheroid sections were imaged on the Leica LSM 780 microscope. The calibration curves were obtained by imaging, with the same microscope, with the known concentrations of each fluorophore in a quartz cuvette of 20 μm pathlength. At different time points, an in-house eroding code was applied to quantify the radial distributions (using 5 μm concentric rings) of the fluorescence intensities as previously reported [23]. The radially time-integrated profiles were obtained using the trapezoidal rule across the sampled time-points; n = 4–5 spheroid slices were analyzed per time point.

2.9. Spheroid Treatment

The spheroids of approximately 400 μm in diameter were treated with free CDDP and with CDDP delivered by the NP (NP-CDDP) for time periods scaled to their corresponding blood clearance times in mice [30,31], at CDDP concentrations proportional to the corresponding MTD values in mice. Upon completion of the incubation, the spheroids were transferred into fresh media, their size was monitored—by imaging—for 14 days, at which point the size of the non-treated spheroids reached an asymptote, and then each spheroid was plated in a single well on 96-well plates and 6-well plates to evaluate the outgrowth relative to the non-treated spheroids, detailed below, and the population distributions, respectively.

For evaluating the extent of the outgrowth, that was used as a surrogate of recurrence, the following protocol was followed: after the cells from plated, the non-treated spheroids reached confluency, then the cells that were plated from all spheroids (untreated and treated) were trypsinized and counted using trypan blue. The extent of the outgrowth of each condition was defined as the ratio of the cell counts for each condition normalized by the cell counts in the non-treatment condition.

To evaluate the population distributions, the cells from the plated spheroids for each condition, after being allowed to reach confluency in the 6-well plates, were analyzed on a BD FACS Canto, as described above.

2.10. Cell Migration from the Spheroids Embedded in a Matrix

To study the effect of the different treatment conditions on cancer cell migration, after the 400 μm spheroids were treated with free CDDP and NP-CDDP, as described above, the spheroids were then transferred into fresh media for two doubling times (72 h). At that point, the spheroids were then embedded in 2 mg/mL type I collagen gel by modifying the procedure, as described previously by Jimenez et al. [32]. Briefly, each spheroid was fished out in 100 μL of 1:1 (*v*/*v*) complete DMEM media and reconstitution buffer over ice, and was added to the individual wells of a pre-warmed 96-well cover-slip bottom cell culture plate and was immediately transferred to a sterile incubator at 37 °C to facilitate the homogeneous polymerization of the collagen. (The reconstitution buffer was formed by a high density soluble rat-tail collagen I (354,249, Corning Inc., Corning, NY, USA) added to obtain a final collagen I concentration of 2 mg/mL at pH =7.0 that was adjusted with 1 N NaOH). The volume of 100 μL of the warm DMEM was added to each well after 3 h, and spheroids were imaged on a Nikon Ti2 transmission microscope (Minato, Japan) equipped with (GFP and RFP filters) every 20 min for 24 h.

For the different time points, the migration distance for each cell was measured on the NIS elements software (Nikon, Minato, Japan) on both the DsRed (580–680 nm) and GFP (511–561 nm) channels for n = 3 spheroids per condition.

2.11. Statistical Analysis

The results are reported as the arithmetic mean of n independent measurements ± the standard deviation. The significance was evaluated by one-way ANOVA, and the Student's t test with *p*-values less than 0.05, was considered to be significant.

3. Results

3.1. Cell Characterization

Table 1 shows that the two cell lines, the MDA-MB-231 and MDA-MB-231HR (hypoxia reporter), were indistinguishable in terms of the effect of hypoxia and/or extracellular pH on the doubling times of the cells. A comparison of the first column (normoxic/neutral pH) to the second (normoxic/acidic pH) and third columns (hypoxic/naturally acidic pH) suggests that it was the pH of the extracellular environment (acidosis) and not the oxygen levels that delayed the growth rates of cells.

Table 1. Doubling times (in hours) of the TNBC MDA-MB-231 and MDA-MB-231-HR (hypoxia reporter cells) in the normoxic conditions, at pH 7.4 (left column) and 6.8 (middle column), and in the hypoxic conditions (right column), shows that the two cell lines were indistinguishable. Acidosis, and not the oxygen levels, delayed the growth rates of the cells. Values reported as mean ± standard deviation of n = 3 independent runs. * p-value < 0.05.

	Normoxic; pH 7.4 (h) (n = 3)	Normoxic; pH 6.8 (h) (n = 3)	Hypoxic; pH 6.8 (h) (n = 3)
MDA-MB-231	36 ± 1	42 ± 2	41 ± 1
MDA-MB-231-HR (Hypoxia Reporter)	36 ± 1 *	41 ± 2 *	41 ± 2

3.2. NP Characterization

Regardless of the composition, the NP had a size range of 110–130 nm post CDDP loading (Table 2). The pH-responsive NP exhibited less negative ζ-potential with a decreasing pH, due to the protonation of the DSPE-PEG (2000)-DAP moiety, in agreement with our previous reports [24]. The non-pH-responsive NP showed no significant change in the ζ-potential with the changing pH. The CDDP loading in the NP ranged from 3.5 to 3.7%. Only the pH-responsive NP showed a significant decrease in the CDDP retention at pH 6.8, due to the triggered release (75.1% vs. 94.0%). No significant difference in CDDP retention by the NP was measured at pH 6.8 in the normoxic vs. hypoxic conditions (Table S2).

Table 2. Characterization of the CDDP loaded pH-responsive and non-pH-responsive NPs used in this study. (R) stands for release and (A) for the adhesion property. Values reported as mean ± standard deviation of n = 6 independent NP preparations. p-values: * <0.05, ** <0.01.

	Size (nm) (n = 6)	PDI (n = 6)	% CDDP Loading (n = 6)	% Contents Retained at pH 7.4 after 6 h (n = 6)	% Contents Retained at pH 6.8 after 6 h (n = 6)	ζ-Potential (mV) (n = 3)		
						pH 7.4	pH 6.5	pH 6
non-pH-responsive NP (R-A-) (non-responsive NP-CDDP)	115.5 ± 7.1	0.06 ± 0.04	3.7 ± 0.3	93.0 ± 5.1	90.1 ± 8.1	−3.78 ± 2.63	−4.28 ± 2.68	−4.42 ± 2.43
pH-responsive NP (R+A+) (responsive NP-CDDP)	118.6 ± 3.3	0.08 ± 0.06	3.5 ± 0.4	94.0 ± 7.9 *	75.1 ± 6.9 *	−2.66 ± 0.40 **	−0.88 ± 1.03	−0.70 ± 1.20 **

3.3. IC_{50} Values and the Drug Efficacy on the Cell Monolayers

Table 3 (first row) shows that the IC_{50} value of free CDDP increased in the hypoxic conditions relative to the normoxic conditions. This was attributed to the effects of the lower oxygen level and not of acidosis—the latter is naturally occurring in the cell media in the hypoxic chamber (Figure S2)—, and was based on the observation that for free CDDP, the IC_{50} values in the normoxic conditions at a neutral pH (a) and at an acidic pH (b) were not different. The non-pH responsive NP loaded with CDDP (non-responsive NP-CDDP) did not release adequate drug at the incubation conditions to reach 50% of the cell kill. Conversely, the pH-responsive NP loaded with CDDP (responsive NP-CDDP), resulted in measurable IC_{50} values that decreased with the lowering pH (in normoxic (b) and hypoxic (c) conditions), as expected, due to the release of CDDP from the NP in the extracellular media [23,24]. Both NP types used in this study were previously shown to not significantly associate with or become internalized by the cancer cells. The strategy of the drug delivery with these NPs includes the release of free CDDP in the extracellular medium; the delivery strategy is that, ultimately, these NPs are utilized as carriers that deliver their therapeutic cargo in the solid tumor interstitium, where the released, highly diffusing drug may penetrate the tumor, resulting in uniform drug microdistributions and better tumor killing [24,33]. The resistance factor due to hypoxia (shown in column (c)) [34], defined as the ratio of the IC_{50} values in the hypoxic conditions over the IC_{50} values in the normoxic conditions at the same pH, was significant and equal to 2.6, both for the free CDDP and for the responsive NP-CDDP.

Table 3. IC_{50} values (concentrations of CDDP in µg/mL required for achieving 50% killing of the MDA-MB-231 cells) in (a) normoxic conditions at pH 7.4, (b) normoxic conditions at pH 6.8 and (c) hypoxic conditions that naturally develop pH 6.8, incubated as free CDDP, CDDP loaded in the non-pH responsive NP (non-responsive NP-CDDP) and in the pH-responsive NP (responsive NP-CDDP). The resistance factor was evaluated as the ratio of the IC_{50} values in the hypoxic conditions to the IC_{50} values in the normoxic conditions at the same pH of 6.8. Values reported as mean ± standard deviation of n = 3 independent runs. ** p-value < 0.01; NA: 50% cell kill was not reached (dose-effect curves are shown in Figure S3B).

	IC_{50} Normoxic Conditions pH 7.4 (a) (n = 3)	**IC_{50} Normoxic Conditions pH 6.8 (b) (n = 3)**	**IC_{50} Hypoxic Conditions pH 6.8 (c) (n = 3)**	**Resistance Factor (IC_{50} Hypoxic/IC_{50} Normoxic at pH 6.8) (c)/(b)**
free CDDP	9.2 ± 1.2 (10.5 ± 1.4 for HR cells)	10.1 ± 1.6	26.8 ± 2.4	2.6 ± 0.5
non-responsive NP-CDDP	NA	NA	NA	NA
responsive NP-CDDP	230.9 ± 8.2 **	44.9 ± 7.8 **	116.7 ± 9.8 **	2.6 ± 0.5

Both the MDA-MB-231 cell line and the hypoxia reporter derivative, MDA-MB-231HR, exhibited the same IC_{50} value to free CDDP (at pH 7.4, also shown in Figure S3), and, therefore, were considered equivalent for the purpose of this study.

To investigate a potential mechanistic explanation for the observed reduced drug killing in the hypoxic conditions relative to the normoxic conditions, the uptake of free CDDP by the cells was measured in the corresponding conditions (Figure 1). Although the rate of the CDDP uptake remained independent of oxygen levels and/or of the initial extracellular concentration of the drug (Ce) (Table 4), the extent of the drug uptake was lowered in the hypoxic conditions relative to the normoxic conditions (Figure 1a). The extent (and rate, Figure S4) of the free CDDP uptake was not different between the MDA-MB-231 cells and the MDA-MB-231HR cells at both pH 7.4 and 6.8, in the normoxic conditions (Figure 1b).

Table 4. Estimated parameters of the single exponential asymptotic two-parameter growth equation fit $y(t) = a \times (1 - e^{-bt})$ that was applied to obtain the rate and extent of the uptake of free CDDP by the cells shown on Figure 1a. Values reported as mean ± standard deviation of n = 3 independent runs. p-value: *, *# < 0.05.

C_e (µg/mL)	**Condition**	**a (µg/mL)**	**b (h^{-1})**	**ln2/b (h)**
200	Normoxia	0.44 ± 0.01 *	0.38 ± 0.03	1.82 ± 0.13
	Hypoxia	0.36 ± 0.03 *	0.38 ± 0.04	1.85 ± 0.21
100	Normoxia	0.26 ± 0.01 *#	0.32 ± 0.02	2.16 ± 0.11
	Hypoxia	0.18 ± 0.01 *#	0.31 ± 0.04	2.21 ± 0.19

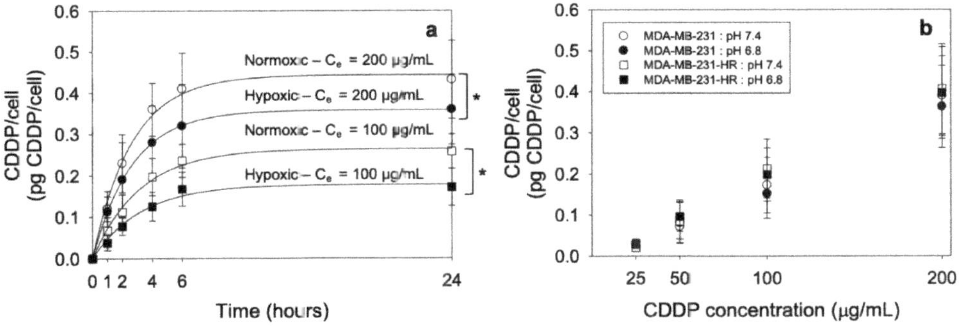

Figure 1. (**a**) Kinetics of the CDDP uptake in the hypoxic (black symbols) and normoxic (white symbols) conditions for 200 μg/mL (circles) and 100 μg/mL (squares) initial free CDDP extracellular concentrations. A single exponential asymptotic two-parameter growth equation was fit to obtain the rate and extent of the uptake. Values reported as mean ± standard deviation of n = 3 independent runs as shown on Table 4. * p-value < 0.05. (**b**) Comparison of the cell-uptake of CDDP for the MDA-MB-231 (circles) and MDA-MB-231HR cells (squares) after 6 h of incubation for the initial extracellular concentrations (Ce) of 25, 50, 100 and 200 μg/mL at pH 7.4 (white symbols) and pH 6.8 (black symbols). Values reported as mean ± standard deviation of n = 3 independent runs.

3.4. Spheroid Characterization

Confocal images of the spheroids formed by the MDA-MB-231HR cells demonstrated heterogeneous spatial distributions of the cells that have experienced hypoxic conditions (green) and the cells that have only experienced normoxic conditions (red) (Figure 2a). As the size of the MDA-MB-231HR spheroids grew from 400 μm to 800 μm in diameter, the cell population distributions evolved. The population of the cells that have experienced hypoxic conditions (Figure 2b, green symbols) grew monotonically after day 4 (spheroid diameter > 573 ± 31 μm, Figure 2c) whereas the population of the cells that never experienced hypoxic conditions decreased (Figure 2, red symbols). The population distribution was unchanged post day 14 (spheroid diameter > 804 ± 67 μm) with >65% of the cells having had experienced hypoxic conditions within the spheroids (green symbols). The flow cytometry results for the selected days are shown in Figure 2d. The observed changes in the population distributions (increasing fraction of hypoxic cells) could be attributed to the increasing formation of the hypoxic regions within the spheroids of increasing size; the relatively slow O_2 transport within the spheroids' interstitium is expected to have contributed to the generation of the heterogeneous O_2 spatiotemporal microdistributions which would become more pronounced as the spheroid size increased over time. One of the reasons of the development of hypoxic and/or of acidic microenvironments within the spheroids (the acidity was demonstrated before, Figure S12 in [23]), is due to the limited diffusivities of oxygen and protons in the spheroid interstitium, relative to the rates of their consumption or production, respectively, by the cells comprising the spheroids.

3.5. Microdistributions in the Spheroids of a Drug Surrogate for the Different Delivery Approaches

In an effort to ultimately compare the effect of the rate of the drug delivered to the cells on cell killing, while keeping the same cumulative delivered dose, we measured and compared the radially integrated spatiotemporal distributions (the area under the curve, AUC) of a drug surrogate (free CFDA-SE) within the spheroids (Figure 3a–c). Figure 3c shows that the AUCs of the free CFDA-SE within the spheroids were identical when the concentration and time of incubation of the free CFDA-SE in the media were adjusted to result in equal products (10 μM × 15 min = 2.5 μM × 60 min).

When the drug surrogate was delivered by the NP, in agreement with previous studies in spheroids [24]—which were shown to capture the diffusion-limited transport in tumor avascular regions—the lipid NP with both pH-responsive properties (i.e., the ECM-adhesion and the interstitial release of contents) shown in Figure 4a, resulted in a greater penetration of the delivered drug surrogate (CFDA-SE fluorophore) and greater values of the time-integrated concentrations (AUC) of the delivered fluorophore, than the extent of penetration and level of the AUC of the same fluorophore when delivered by the NP without these properties (Figure 4b).

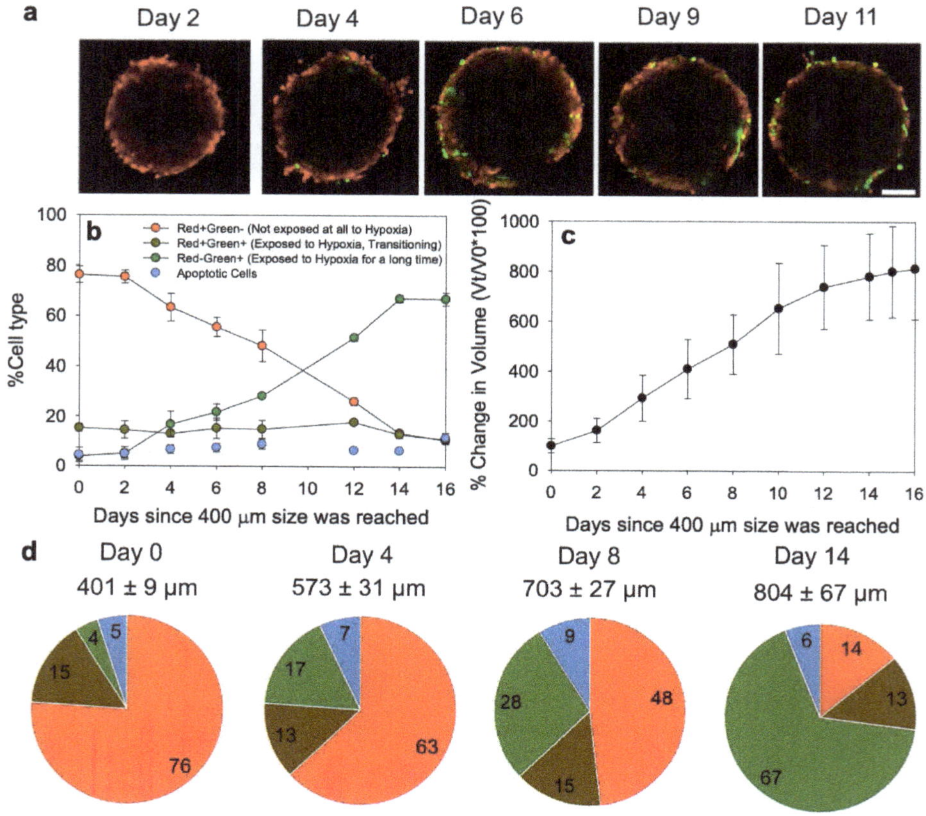

Figure 2. (**a**) Representative confocal microscopy images of the MDA-MB-231HR spheroids, acquired at the longest possible optical depth, where the hypoxic/post-hypoxic cells (green, GFP channel) and the cells that only experienced normoxia (red, in RFP channel) were imaged simultaneously. The optical slices shown were acquired at the spheroids' equator up to the spheroid sizes of approximately 400 μm in diameter. For the larger than 400 μm in diameter spheroids, the optical slices shown indicate the longest working distance within the spheroids at which the photon counts were adequate. Scale bar corresponds to 200 μm. (**b**) Distributions of the cell populations in the spheroids, as measured by flow cytometry, and (**c**) the increase in the spheroid size, over time. (**d**) Pie chart representation of the MDA-MB-231HR TNBC cell populations in the spheroids of different sizes: cells that have not experienced hypoxia (red), cells that were transitioning or partially exposed to the hypoxic conditions (brown), cells that have experienced hypoxic conditions (green) and cells that have undergone apoptosis (cyan) were tracked over time, using flow cytometry, and were plotted as a percentage of the total cell population. Values reported as mean ± standard deviation of n = 6 independent spheroids, per time point.

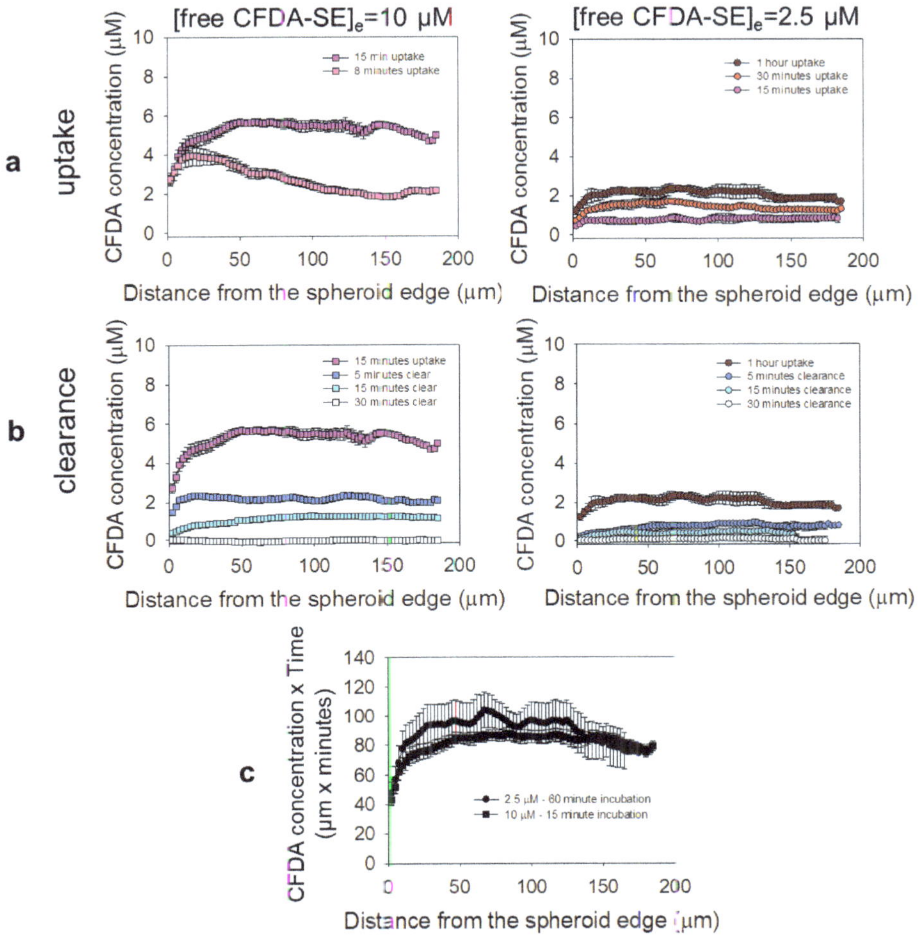

Figure 3. Different rates of exposure at the same 'cumulative dose' of a surrogate of the free drug in the spheroids. Microdistributions in the spheroids of the fluorophore CFDA-SE that was incubated with the spheroids in free form at 10 μM (left column, for up to 15 min) and 2.5 μM (right column, for up to 1 h), and was used as the drug surrogate. (**a**) "Uptake" microdistributions over time, when the spheroids were incubated with the free CFDA-SE in the surrounding media. (**b**) "Clearance" microdistributions over time, when the spheroids were transferred in media without CFDA-SE. (**c**) The time-integrated concentrations of the drug surrogate (AUC) along the spheroid radius for the corresponding incubation conditions indicate similar profiles (cumulative radial doses) within the spheroids. Values reported as mean ± standard deviation of n = 3–4 spheroids imaged per time point.

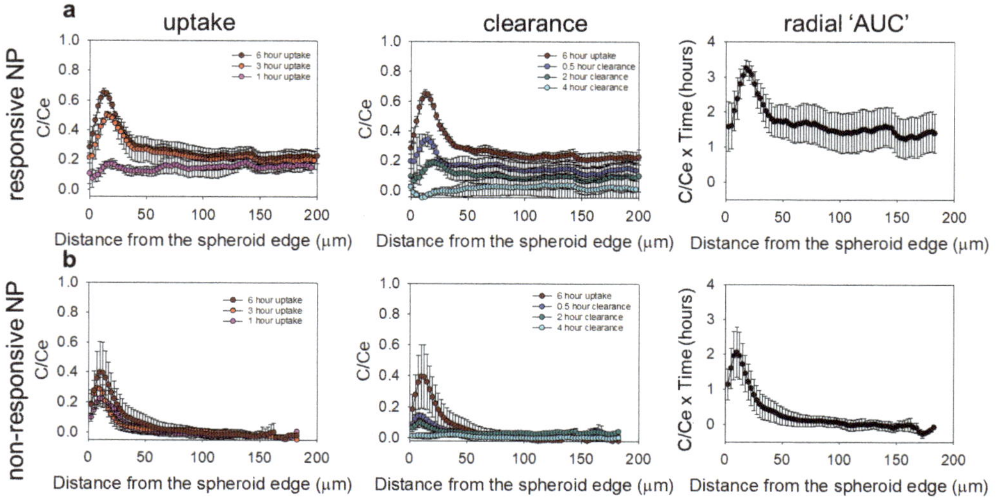

Figure 4. Microdistributions in the spheroids of the fluorophore CFDA-SE delivered by (**a**) responsive NP, and (**b**) non-responsive NP. The first column shows the spatiotemporal microdistributions during the "uptake" (in the presence of the NP), and the second column during the "clearance" (after the removal of the NP from the incubation medium) of the delivered CFDA-SE in the spheroids. The plots on the righthand column show the time-integrated concentrations of the drug surrogate (AUC) along the spheroid radius for the corresponding delivery approaches. Values reported as mean ± standard deviation of n = 3–4 spheroids per time point.

3.6. Effect of the Rate of the Free CDDP Treatment on the Spheroids: Cell Survival

To evaluate the effect of the rate of free CDDP delivered to the cells on cell killing, for the same cumulative delivered dose, the spheroids were incubated with free CDDP (at high, 1.6 μg/mL, and low, 0.4 μg/mL, concentrations) for short (15 min) and long (60 min) periods, respectively. The two treatments of free CDDP were expected to have comparable AUCs within the spheroids, based on the findings of the fluorescent drug surrogate CFDA-SE, shown in Figure 3c. Figure 5a shows that the faster rate of delivery of free CDDP resulted in a significantly better inhibition of the cell growth compared to the same cumulative dose of CDDP that was delivered at a slower rate.

3.7. Effect of the CDDP Delivery Regimens on the Spheroids: Cell Survival

To compare the cell killing efficacy, in the spheroids, of the NP-delivered CDDP and of the free CDDP, the therapeutic treatments were scaled according to the corresponding pharmacokinetic time scales and the reported maximum tolerated doses in mice (MTD). Pharmacokinetically, free CDDP is reported to clear 20–27 times [31] faster than the lipid NP; hence, the spheroids were incubated with free CDDP for 15 min and with the NP-CDDP for 6 h. Regarding the incubation concentrations of CDDP in free vs. NP forms, free CDDP was reported to exhibit MTD values 2.7–3.2 times lower than the MTD values of the liposomal/NP- CDDP [35]. Therefore, the spheroids were incubated with 5 μg/mL and 1.6 μg/mL of CDDP in NP and free form, respectively. In addition, two dosing schedules were designed to compare the efficacy and the population distributions in the spheroids post treatment, as shown in Figures 5b and 6 and Table S3. First, in the single treatment, all of the drug was delivered at day 0, and the incubation time was scaled to the blood clearance kinetics of the respective carrier. Second, in the double treatment, only half of the dose was delivered at day 0, and then a reduced dose of free CDDP was delivered on day seven on all conditions. Overall, the double treatment involved significantly less total concentrations of CDDP (ranging from 20 to 30 % less, compared to the single treatment).

The 6 h treatment with free CDDP was used as a reference of the maximum possible achievable killing effect in vitro, without an in vivo analogue, since free CDDP infused for 6 h at this relative concentration would not be expected to be tolerated well.

Following a single treatment with CDDP (Figure 5b, black bars), the greatest suppression of the cell outgrowth was observed when CDDP was delivered by the responsive NP-CDDP, followed by the treatment with the free agent (for a 15 min incubation), in agreement with previous reports [24]. This order in efficacy was attributed to the corresponding microdistributions of CDDP in the spheroid, and followed the trend of the AUC plots shown in Figures 3 and 4. In the double treatment regimens (Figure 5b, gray bars), the trend in efficacy was unchanged. Importantly, the therapeutic effect was similar to the effect for the single treatment, although the cumulative concentration of CDDP that was incubated with the spheroids was significantly less than the CDDP concentration used in the single treatment approach.

3.8. Effect of the CDDP Delivery Regimens on the Spheroids: Cell Population Progression

Figure 6 shows that the non-treated spheroids had the highest fraction of the hypoxia experienced cells (green), possibly attributed to the greater size of these spheroids over the time-frame of the experiment (as also indicated by Figure 2). When CDDP was delivered by the pH-responsive lipid NP (responsive NP-CDDP) it resulted in the greatest reduction of the hypoxia experienced cells, both after single and double treatments; it also resulted in the maximum apoptotic cell population when compared to other treatments. The double treatment, using the responsive NP-CDDP, not only managed to further lower the overall % outgrowth (Figure 6b) but also further reduced the population of the cells that were hardest to kill (cells in hypoxic conditions shown in green; Figure 6b). Figure S5 shows examples of flow cytometry plots for each treatment.

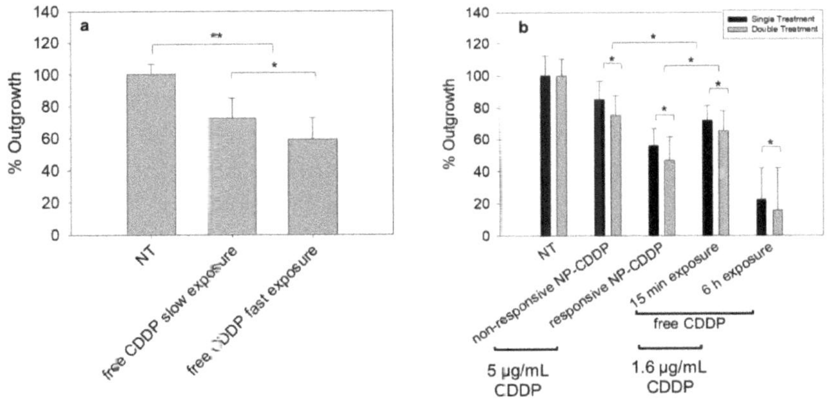

Figure 5. Effect of the CDDP treatment regimen on the extent of the cell outgrowth from the MDA-MB-231HR spheroids. (**a**) Effect of the rate of the spheroid exposure to free CDDP at the same total cumulative dose (demonstrated in Figure 3c). Free CDDP/slow exposure corresponded to 60 min spheroid exposure to 0.4 μg/mL free CDDP. Free CDDP/fast exposure corresponded to 15 min spheroid exposure to 1.6 μg/mL free CDDP. (**b**) In treatment studies of spheroids with NP-CDDP, CDDP concentrations in the incubating medium of 5 μg/mL for a single treatment, and 2.5 μg/mL for a double treatment, followed by 1 μg/mL free CDDP, as shown on Table S3. Percentage outgrowth relative to the non-treatment was calculated as follows: following the exposure to therapy, the spheroid size was monitored until the non-treated spheroids stopped growing in size (14 days post treatment). At that point, each spheroid was plated on a separate adherent well, and when the non-treated condition reached confluency, the number of cells from each treatment were counted and normalized to the number of cells from the non-treated cases. For each treatment, n = 18 spheroids were evaluated across n = 3 independent preparations. p-values: * < 0.05, ** < 0.01.

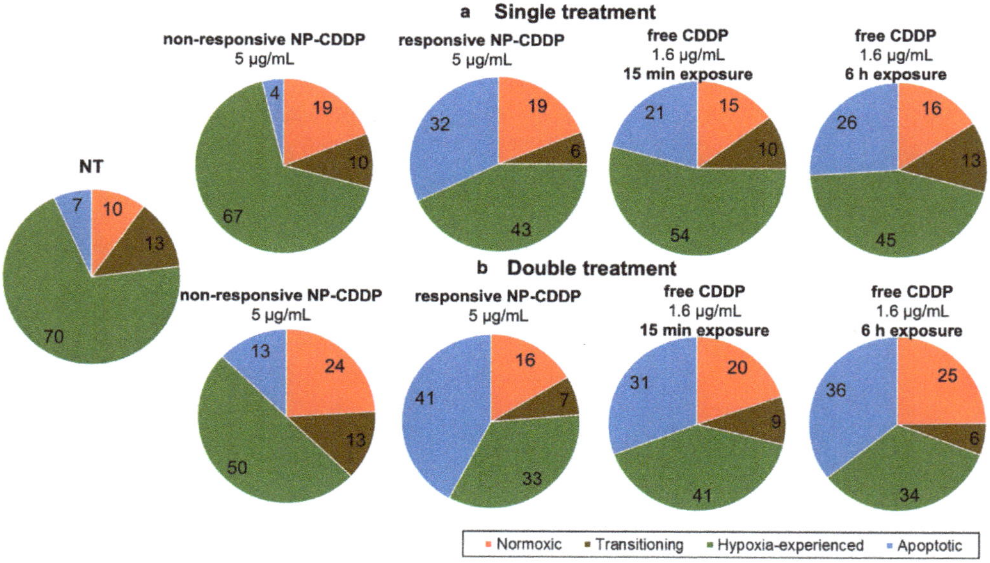

Figure 6. Effect of the type of the CDDP treatment(s) on the progression of the cell populations in the spheroids, evaluated using flow cytometry. Percentage of the cell population of the cells for single (**a**) and double (**b**) treatment with CDDP in different forms. Cells that have not experienced hypoxia (red), cells that were transitioning or partially exposed to hypoxic conditions (brown), cells that have experienced hypoxic conditions (green), and cells that have undergone apoptosis (blue). CDDP concentration was 5 µg/mL in the single treatments, and 2.5 µg/mL in the double treatments (followed by the same dose of free CDDP, as summarized on Table S3). Charts represent the averaged values of n = 3 spheroids per treatment for n = 3 independent treatment preparations/ measurements.

3.9. Effect of the CDDP Delivery Regimens on the Spheroids: Cell Migration

Figure 7 shows that the rate of exposure to CDDP of the cells in the MDA-MB-231HR spheroids affected not only the overall cell survival (as shown in Figure 5) and the progression of the cell populations (as shown in Figure 6), but also the extents of the distances travelled by the cells (cell migration). For treatments with free CDDP, the faster rate of exposure (free CDDP/ fast exposure) resulted in a greater cell kill (Figure 5a) and in shorter distances (Figure 7b) travelled outside the spheroids by fewer cells (Figure 7c,d), compared to the slow rate of the exposure to free CDDP with the same AUC within the spheroids (Figure 3c). Similarly, when delivered by the pH-responsive NP (responsive NP-CDDP), the treatment resulted in the best inhibition of migration, both in terms of the distance travelled by the cells and in terms of the number of cells that travelled the longer distances. As expected [21,36], the cells that have experienced hypoxia (green) travelled longer distances than cells in the normoxic conditions (red) (Figure S6). Interestingly, the faster rate of exposure to CDDP decreased cell migration, independent of the cells being in hypoxic or normoxic environments (Figure 7b,d).

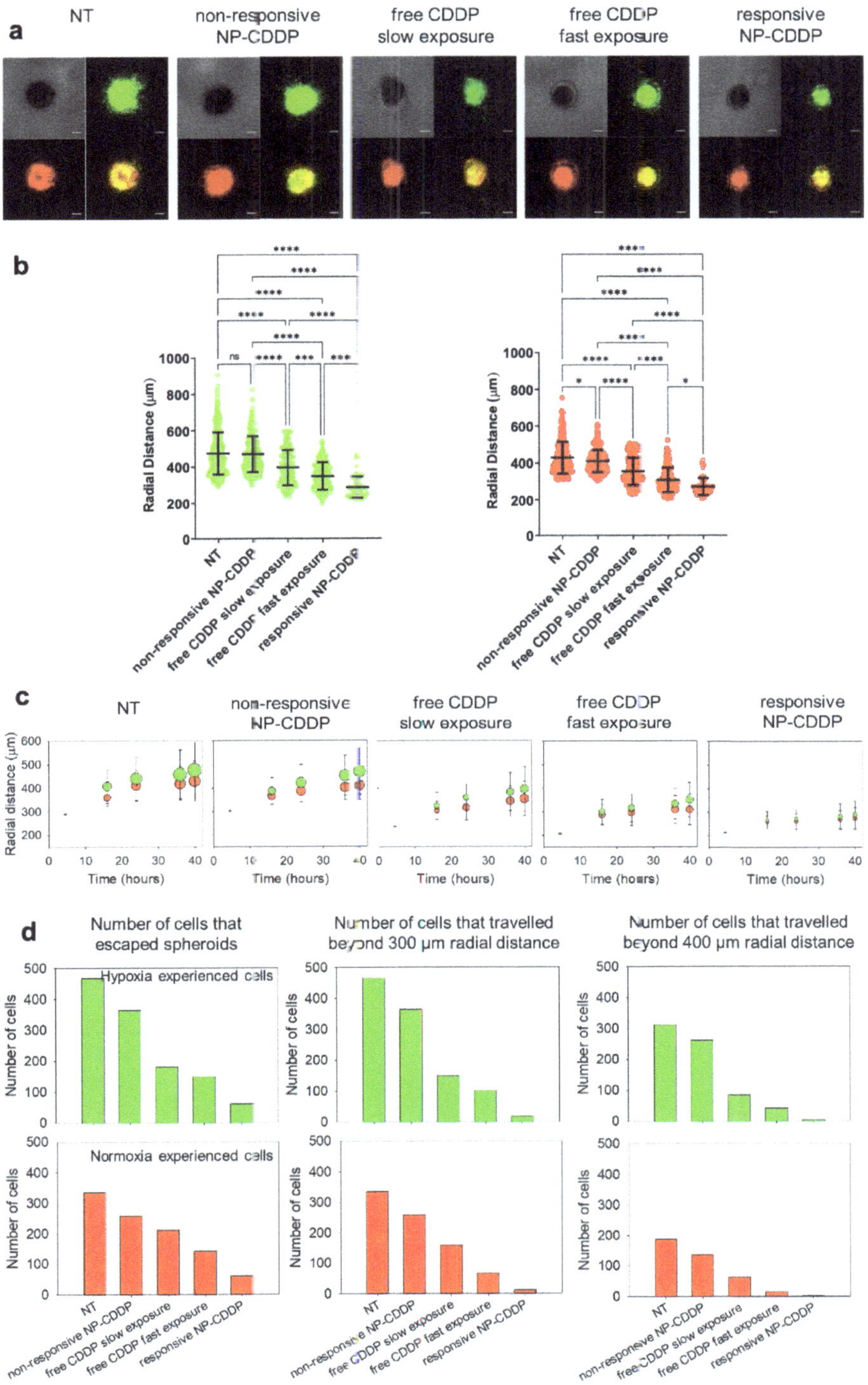

Figure 7. Effect of the different CDDP treatments on the migration of cells from the spheroids

(**a**) Images of the representative spheroids after 40 h post embedment in collagen, following different treatments with CDDP. Images are shown in brightfield, in the GFP (green) channel (showing cells having experienced hypoxic conditions) and the RFP (red) channel (showing cells in the normoxic conditions), and merged. Scale bar corresponds to 200 μm. (**b**) Radial locations of the cells that migrated, from the spheroid into the collagen gel, relative to the spheroid center (migration distance), at the same time point of 40 h as shown in (**a**). Cells in the normoxic conditions are shown in red, and the cells that have experienced hypoxic conditions in green. Data collected from n = 3 spheroids per treatment. Horizonal lines indicate the mean and standard deviation averaged over the entire cell counts. *p*-values: * < 0.05, *** < 0.001, **** < 0.0001. (**c**) Average migration distances over time for the two cell populations: cells in the normoxic conditions (red), and cells that have experienced hypoxic conditions (green). The symbols' area was scaled to the number of cells for each condition. The reported distances correspond to the mean and standard deviation of the distances of all cells migrated from n = 3 spheroids, and quantified as explained in (**b**). (**d**) Number of cells at different distances from the spheroid center at t = 40 h post spheroid embedment in collagen. Free CDDP/slow exposure corresponded to the 60 min spheroid exposure to 0.4 μg/mL free CDDP. Free CDDP/fast exposure corresponded to the 15 min spheroid exposure to 1.6 μg/mL free CDDP. In treatment studies of the spheroids with NP-CDDP, CDDP concentrations in the incubating medium, was 5 μg/mL for a 6 h exposure.

4. Discussion

Although CDDP has shown promising results in the treatment of various cancer types [37], its use in TNBC patients has been limited [38]. This is partly due to the serious adverse effects and the limited responses in patient subpopulations which have narrowed patient compliance [39]. Side effects may, sometimes, be addressed by the formulation of agents in particles, including the lipid nanoparticles (liposomes) [10]. However, although the lipid nanoparticle-delivered chemotherapies, such as Doxil^{TM}, have been used in solid tumor treatments for over two decades, there is still not an FDA approved nanoparticle formulation of CDDP [40–42]. In this study (1) we investigated the effect of the rate of exposure to CDDP on the survival and on migration of TNBC cells, and, based on these findings, (2) we showed that, with an engineered lipid nanoparticle that enabled a fast exposure of the cells to CDDP, we could not only manage to better arrest tumor growth in general, but also to control these cancer cell subpopulations that usually survived post chemotherapy, delivered in a conventional manner, and to limit their migratory potential. The nanoparticles maximized both the rate of the cell exposure to CDDP and the number of cells affected by CDDP, when in the spheroids, which were used as a surrogate of the solid tumors' avascular regions. The findings on the cell migration may have a particular significance in TNBC, which, is characterized by a greater frequency of metastases outside the breast, compared to other types of breast cancer [8].

The development of resistance to chemotherapy has long been a major clinical challenge, and a key determinant of cancer mortality. Enriching information on cancer cell resistance mechanisms to platinum compounds [9,43] enhances our knowledge and understanding of the complexity in molecular pathways affecting drug sensitivity. In addition to this aspect, the evolving intratumoral heterogeneity may also play a role in a solid tumor's response to chemotherapeutics. In particular, we showed in vitro that in addition to transport (drug diffusion) limitations, that decrease bioavailability in the delivered chemotherapeutics, the development of hypoxia within the spheroids may trigger a chemoresistance in TNBC, as demonstrated by the 2–3 fold higher IC_{50} values of free CDDP to hypoxic cells. In agreement with previous studies on elucidating the mechanisms of cell resistance to CDDP [9], we also showed that its lowered efficacy, in the presence of hypoxia, was partly due to the lower CDDP cell uptake compared to the CDDP cell uptake in the normoxic conditions. This can be most likely attributed to HIF-1 regulating the downstream processes of apoptosis, autophagy and necrosis under hypoxia. Acidosis did not seem to affect the cell sensitivity to CDDP.

In addition to hypoxia and the diffusion-limited transport within the spheroids, we investigated the potential role of the rate of exposure of cancer cells to cisplatin on affecting their killing and/or their metastatic potential. We discovered that a faster rate of cell exposure to the same drug (of the same cumulative dose, approximated as the same AUC in the spheroids) caused: (1) more cell killing, and (2) decreased the distances travelled outside the spheroids by fewer cancer cells that survived treatment. Similar results were obtained when CDDP was delivered by the responsive NP-CDDP that were designed to not only release the agents within the tumor interstitium, where the agents may diffuse deeper and reach more cancer cells, but also were designed to bind to the tumor ECM so as to exhibit a delayed tumor clearance and, therefore, to achieve greater tumor delivered doses [24,33]. In all of our studies, the hypoxia reporter TNBC cells were key indicators demonstrating that this cell subpopulation was more difficult to kill, and travelled longer distances, compared to the cells that had only experienced normoxic conditions, in agreement with previous reports [21,22]. The studies presented herein provide a mechanistic explanation of our previous reports on the efficacy of the responsive NP-CDDP to delay the rate of growth of the spontaneous MDA-MB-231 TNBC metastases in a mouse model [24].

Previously, Petr et. al. [44], in an effort to control toxicities, have shown in the clinic that successive low doses of CDDP were non-inferior to a single high dose in inhibiting tumor growth. This was attributed to increased patient compliance as opposed to responses to high-dose regimens. In an effort to investigate treatment schedules of CDDP delivered by the NP, we compared in vitro a single treatment of TNBC spheroids to a double treatment schedule, where the total cumulative CDDP dose was almost half of the dose used in the single treatment. The latter treatment not only showed better efficacy in limiting cell viability, but also further reduced the hypoxia-experienced cell population, compared to single treatment. In the same studies, we showed that the delivery of CDDP by the pH-responsive NP had the best effect on limiting cell survival and migration. Evaluation of the double treatment with the NP in mouse models bearing hypoxia-reporting TNBC cells would be the next step to not only validate the superior efficacy of the responsive NP-CDDP but to also investigate the ability to control the hypoxic cell population. This type of 'fractionated' or multi-dose scheduling may ultimately contribute to lower toxicities in vivo.

5. Conclusions

Hypoxic regions in the tumor microenvironment contribute to a poorer prognosis due to the development of resistance to chemotherapy and/or due to the higher metastatic potential of the cells that have experienced hypoxia. Increasing the rates of cancer cell exposure to cisplatin, while keeping the same total cumulative dose, resulted in a decreased (hypoxic) cell survival and (hypoxic) cell metastatic potential. We demonstrated that the pH-responsive nanoparticles delivering cisplatin to the TNBC multicellular spheroids, used as surrogates of the tumors' avascular regions, (1) fast and uniformly exposed all cells to cisplatin, (2) best inhibited cell survival, (3) lowered the surviving population of hypoxia-experienced cells and (4) decreased their migration potential, compared to conventional NP and to the free drug.

Supplementary Materials: The following supporting information can be downloaded at: https://www.mdpi.com/article/10.3390/pharmaceutics14102184/s1, Figure S1: Calibration curve of the platinum content using AAS; Figure S2: Extracellular pH (pHe) in the normoxic and hypoxic conditions; Figure S3: IC_{50} studies; Figure S4: Kinetics of the CDDP uptake by the cells; Figure S5: Characterization of the cell populations by flow cytometry after treatment; Figure S6: Effect of the treatment(s) on the migration of cells from the spheroids; Table S1: Extent of the retention of CFDA-SE from both types of NPs at different pH conditions; Table S2: Extent of the retention of CDDP from both types of NPs at different pH values in the normoxic and hypoxic conditions; Table S3: Concentrations of CDDP and the treatment duration for the single and double treatment schedules of the spheroids.

Author Contributions: Conceptualization, S.S. and D.G.; methodology, S.S., O.B., I.G. and D.G.; validation, O.B.; formal analysis, O.B. and S.S.; writing—review and editing, S.S., O.B., I.G. and D.G.; supervision, S.S.; funding acquisition, S.S. All authors have read and agreed to the published version of the manuscript.

Funding: This research was funded by a grant from the Elsa U. Pardee Foundation, the Under Armour-Innovation Award, and the W.W. Smith Charitable Trust.

Institutional Review Board Statement: Not applicable.

Informed Consent Statement: Not applicable.

Data Availability Statement: All data are presented within the article and the Supplementary Materials.

Acknowledgments: We are grateful to Hanhvy Bui for her help with the flow cytometry analysis, Michael Bevan for allowing us to use the DLS instrumentation, and Gabriella Russo for her help with optimizing the migration assay.

Conflicts of Interest: The authors declare no conflict of interest.

References

1. Hutchinson, L. Breast cancer: TNBC: Can we treat the untargetable? *Nat. Rev. Clin. Oncol.* **2014**, *11*, 379. [CrossRef] [PubMed]
2. Jain, R.K.; Stylianopoulos, T. Delivering nanomedicine to solid tumors. *Nat. Rev. Clin. Oncol.* **2010**, *7*, 653–664. [CrossRef]
3. Vagia, E.; Mahalingam, D.; Cristofanilli, M. The Landscape of Targeted Therapies in TNBC. *Cancers* **2020**, *12*, 916. [CrossRef]
4. Kwapisz, D. Pembrolizumab and atezolizumab in triple-negative breast cancer. *Cancer Immunol Immun.* **2021**, *70*, 607–617. [CrossRef] [PubMed]
5. He, M.Y.; Rancoule, C.; Rehailia-Blanchard, A.; Espenel, S.; Trone, J.C.; Bernichon, E.; Guillaume, E.; Vallard, A.; Magne, N. Radiotherapy in triple-negative breast cancer: Current situation and upcoming strategies. *Crit. Rev. Oncol. Hematol.* **2018**, *131*, 96–101. [CrossRef]
6. Gupta, G.K.; Collier, A.L.; Lee, D.; Hoefer, R.A.; Zheleva, V.; Siewertsz van Reesema, L.L.; Tang-Tan, A.M.; Guye, M.L.; Chang, D.Z.; Winston, J.S.; et al. Perspectives on Triple-Negative Breast Cancer: Current Treatment Strategies, Unmet Needs, and Potential Targets for Future Therapies. *Cancers* **2020**, *12*, 2392. [CrossRef]
7. Tannock, I.F. Tumor physiology and drug resistance. *Cancer Metastasis Rev.* **2001**, *20*, 123–132. [CrossRef]
8. Dent, R.; Trudeau, M.; Pritchard, K.I.; Hanna, W.M.; Kahn, H.K.; Sawka, C.A.; Lickley, L.A.; Rawlinson, E.; Sun, P.; Narod, S.A. Triple-negative breast cancer: Clinical features and patterns of recurrence. *Clin. Cancer Res.* **2007**, *13*, 4429–4434. [CrossRef]
9. Cohen, S.M.; Lippard, S.J. Cisplatin: From DNA damage to cancer chemotherapy. *Prog. Nucleic Acid Res. Mol. Biol.* **2001**, *67*, 93–130. [CrossRef]
10. Sempkowski, M.; Locke, T.; Stras, S.; Zhu, C.; Sofou, S. Liposome-Based Approaches for Delivery of Mainstream Chemotherapeutics: Preparation Methods, Liposome Designs, Therapeutic Efficacy. *Crit. Rev. Oncog.* **2014**, *19*, 177–221. [CrossRef]
11. Rottenberg, S.; Disler, C.; Perego, P. The rediscovery of platinum-based cancer therapy. *Nat. Rev. Cancer* **2021**, *21*, 37–50. [CrossRef] [PubMed]
12. Vianello, C.; Cocetta, V.; Catanzaro, D.; Dorn, G.W.; De Milito, A.; Rizzolio, F.; Canzonieri, V.; Cecchin, E.; Roncato, R.; Toffoli, G.; et al. Cisplatin resistance can be curtailed by blunting Bnip3-mediated mitochondrial autophagy. *Cell Death Dis.* **2022**, *13*, 398. [CrossRef]
13. Harmers, F.P.; Gispen, W.H.; Neijt, J.P. Neurotoxic side-effects of cisplatin. *Eur. J. Cancer* **1991**, *27*, 372–376. [CrossRef]
14. Duffy, E.A.; Fitzgerald, W.; Boyle, K.; Rohatgi, R. Nephrotoxicity: Evidence in Patients Receiving Cisplatin Therapy. *Clin. J. Oncol. Nurs.* **2018**, *22*, 175–183. [CrossRef]
15. Santana-Davila, R.; Szabo, A.; Arce-Lara, C.; Williams, C.D.; Kelley, M.J.; Whittle, J. Cisplatin versus carboplatin-based regimens for the treatment of patients with metastatic lung cancer. An analysis of Veterans Health Administration data. *J. Thorac. Oncol.* **2014**, *9*, 702–709. [CrossRef]
16. Gilkes, D.M.; Semenza, G.L. Role of hypoxia-inducible factors in breast cancer metastasis. *Future Oncol.* **2013**, *9*, 1623–1636. [CrossRef]
17. Ebright, R.Y.; Zachariah, M.A.; Micalizzi, D.S.; Wittner, B.S.; Niederhoffer, K.L.; Nieman, L.T.; Chirn, B.; Wiley, D.F.; Wesley, B.; Shaw, B.; et al. HIF1A signaling selectively supports proliferation of breast cancer in the brain. *Nat. Commun.* **2020**, *11*, 6311. [CrossRef]
18. Semenza, G.L. Targeting HIF-1 for cancer therapy. *Nat. Rev. Cancer* **2003**, *3*, 721–732. [CrossRef]
19. Damgaci, S.; Ibrahim-Hashim, A.; Enriquez-Navas, P.M.; Pilon-Thomas, S.; Guvenis, A.; Gillies, R.J. Hypoxia and acidosis: Immune suppressors and therapeutic targets. *Immunology* **2018**, *154*, 354–362. [CrossRef]
20. Voss, N.C.S.; Dreyer, T.; Henningsen, M.B.; Vahl, P.; Honoré, B.; Boedtkjer, E. Targeting the Acidic Tumor Microenvironment: Unexpected Pro-Neoplastic Effects of Oral NaHCO3 Therapy in Murine Breast Tissue. *Cancers* **2020**, *12*, 891. [CrossRef]
21. Godet, I.; Shin, Y.J.; Ju, J.A.; Ye, I.C.; Wang, G.; Gilkes, D.M. Fate-mapping post-hypoxic tumor cells reveals a ROS-resistant phenotype that promotes metastasis. *Nat. Commun.* **2019**, *10*, 4862. [CrossRef] [PubMed]

22. Godet, I.; Mamo, M.; Thurnheer, A.; Rosen, D.M.; Gilkes, D.M. Post-Hypoxic Cells Promote Metastatic Recurrence after Chemotherapy Treatment in TNBC. *Cancers* **2021**, *13*, 5509. [CrossRef] [PubMed]
23. Stras, S.; Holleran, T.; Howe, A.; Sofou, S. Interstitial Release of Cisplatin from Triggerable Liposomes Enhances Efficacy against Triple Negative Breast Cancer Solid Tumor Analogues. *Mol. Pharm.* **2016**, *13*, 3224–3233. [CrossRef] [PubMed]
24. Stras, S.; Howe, A.; Prasad, A.; Salerno D.; Bhatavdekar, O.; Sofou, S. Growth of Metastatic Triple-Negative Breast Cancer Is Inhibited by Deep Tumor-Penetrating and Slow Tumor-Clearing Chemotherapy: The Case of Tumor-Adhering Liposomes with Interstitial Drug Release. *Mol. Pharm.* **2020**, *17*, 118–131. [CrossRef]
25. Bandekar, A.; Karve, S.; Chang, M.Y.; Mu, Q.; Rotolo, J.; Sofou, S. Antitumor efficacy following the intracellular and interstitial release of liposomal doxorubicin. *Biomaterials* **2012**, *33*, 4345–4352. [CrossRef]
26. Karve, S.; Bajagur Kempegowda, G.; Sofou, S. Heterogeneous domains and membrane permeability in phosphatidylcholine-phosphatidic acid rigid vesicles as a function of pH and lipid chain mismatch. *Langmuir* **2008**, *24*, 5679–5688. [CrossRef]
27. Bailey, A.L.; Cullis, P.R. Modulation of membrane fusion by asymmetric transbilayer distributions of amino lipids. *Biochemistry* **1994**, *33*, 12573–12580. [CrossRef]
28. Helmlinger, G.; Yuan, F.; Dellian, M.; Jain, R.K. Interstitial pH and pO2 gradients in solid tumors in vivo: High-resolution measurements reveal a lack of correlation. *Nat. Med.* **1997**, *3*, 177–182. [CrossRef]
29. Vaupel, P.; Kallinowski, F.; Okunieff, P. Blood flow, oxygen and nutrient supply, and metabolic microenvironment of human tumors: A review. *Cancer Res.* **1989**, *49*, 6449–6465.
30. Van Hennik, M.B.; van der Vijgh, W.J.; Klein, I.; Elferink, F.; Vermorken, J.B.; Winograd, B.; Pinedo, H.M. Comparative pharmacokinetics of cisplatin and three analogues in mice and humans. *Cancer Res.* **1987**, *47*, 6297–6301.
31. Newman, M.S.; Colbern, G.T.; Working, P.K.; Engbers, C.; Amantea, M.A. Comparative pharmacokinetics, tissue distribution, and therapeutic effectiveness of cisplatin encapsulated in long-circulating, pegylated liposomes (SPI-077) in tumor-bearing mice. *Cancer Chemother. Pharmacol.* **1999**, *43*, 1–7. [CrossRef] [PubMed]
32. Valencia, A.M.J.; Wu, P.H.; Yogurtcu, O.N.; Rao, P.; DiGiacomo, J.; Godet, I.; He, L.; Lee, M.H.; Gilkes, D.; Sun, S.X.; et al. Collective cancer cell invasion induced by coordinated contractile stresses. *Oncotarget* **2015**, *6*, 43438–43451. [CrossRef] [PubMed]
33. Prasad, A.; Nair, R.; Bhatavdekar, O.; Howe, A.; Salerno, D.; Sempkowski, M.; Josefsson, A.; Pacheco-Torres, J.; Bhujwalla, Z.M.; Gabrielson, K.L.; et al. Transport-driven engineering of liposomes for delivery of alpha-particle radiotherapy to solid tumors: Effect on inhibition of tumor progression and onset delay of spontaneous metastases. *Eur. J. Nucl. Med. Mol. Imaging* **2021**, *48*, 4246–4258. [CrossRef]
34. Li, J.Q.; Wu, X.; Gan, L.; Yang, X.L.; Miao, Z.H. Hypoxia induces universal but differential drug resistance and impairs anticancer mechanisms of 5-fluorouracil in hepatoma cells. *Acta Pharmacol. Sin.* **2017**, *38*, 1642–1654. [CrossRef] [PubMed]
35. Leite, E.A.; Lana, A.M.; Junior, A.D.; Coelho, L.G.; De Oliveira, M.C. Acute toxicity study of cisplatin loaded long-circulating and pH-sensitive liposomes administered in mice. *J. Biomed. Nanotechnol.* **2012**, *8*, 229–239. [CrossRef]
36. Rocha, H.L.; Godet, I.; Kurtoglu, F.; Metzcar, J.; Konstantinopoulos, K.; Bhoyar, S.; Gilkes, D.M.; Macklin, P. A persistent invasive phenotype in post-hypoxic tumor cells is revealed by fate mapping and computational modeling. *iScience* **2021**, *24*, 102935. [CrossRef]
37. Kelland, L. The resurgence of platinum-based cancer chemotherapy. *Nat. Rev. Cancer* **2007**, *7*, 573–584. [CrossRef]
38. Pandy, J.G.P.; Balolong-Garcia, J.C.; Cruz-Ordinario, M.V.B.; Que, F.V.F. Triple negative breast cancer and platinum-based systemic treatment: A meta-analysis and systematic review. *BMC Cancer* **2019**, *19*, 1065. [CrossRef]
39. Berry, D.A.; Ueno, N.T.; Johnson, M.M.; Lei, X.; Caputo, J.; Smith, D.A.; Yancey, L.J.; Crump, M.; Stadtmauer, E.A.; Biron, P.; et al. High-dose chemotherapy with autologous hematopoietic stem-cell transplantation in metastatic breast cancer: Overview of six randomized trials. *J. Clin. Oncol.* **2011**, *29*, 3224–3231. [CrossRef]
40. Stathopoulos, G.P.; Boulikas, T. Lipoplatin formulation review article. *J. Drug Deliv.* **2012**, *2012*, 581363. [CrossRef]
41. Boulikas, T. Clinical overview on Lipoplatin: A successful liposomal formulation of cisplatin. *Expert Opin. Investig. Drugs* **2009**, *18*, 1197–1218. [CrossRef] [PubMed]
42. Duan, X.; He, C.; Kron, S.J.; Lin, W. Nanoparticle formulations of cisplatin for cancer therapy. *Wiley Interdiscip. Rev. Nanomed. Nanobiotechnol.* **2016**, *8*, 776–791. [CrossRef]
43. De Luca, A.; Parker, L.J.; Ang, W.H.; Rodolfo, C.; Gabbarini, V.; Hancock, N.C.; Palone, F.; Mazzetti, A.P.; Menin, L.; Morton, C.J.; et al. A structure-based mechanism of cisplatin resistance mediated by glutathione transferase P1-1. *Proc. Natl. Acad. Sci. USA* **2019**, *116*, 13943–13951. [CrossRef] [PubMed]
44. Szturz, P.; Wouters, K.; Kiyota, N.; Tahara, M.; Prabhash, K.; Noronha, V.; Adelstein, D.; Van Gestel, D.; Vermorken, J.B. Low-Dose vs. High-Dose Cisplatin: Lessons Learned From 59 Chemoradiotherapy Trials in Head and Neck Cancer. *Front. Oncol.* **2019**, *9*, 86. [CrossRef] [PubMed]

pharmaceutics

Article

Co-Encapsulation of Simvastatin and Doxorubicin into pH-Sensitive Liposomes Enhances Antitumoral Activity in Breast Cancer Cell Lines

Jaqueline Aparecida Duarte [1], Eliza Rocha Gomes [1], André Luis Branco De Barros [2] and Elaine Amaral Leite [1,*]

[1] Department of Pharmaceutical Products, Faculty of Pharmacy, Federal University of Minas Gerais, Av. Antônio Carlos, 6627, Belo Horizonte 31270-901, Brazil
[2] Department of Clinical and Toxicological Analyses, Faculty of Pharmacy, Federal University of Minas Gerais, Av. Antônio Carlos, 6627, Belo Horizonte 31270-901, Brazil
* Correspondence: elaineleite@ufmg.br or leite_elaine@hotmail.com; Tel.: +55-3134096944; Fax: +55-3134096935

Abstract: Doxorubicin (DOX) is a potent chemotherapeutic drug used as the first line in breast cancer treatment; however, cardiotoxicity is the main drawback of the therapy. Preclinical studies evidenced that the association of simvastatin (SIM) with DOX leads to a better prognosis with reduced side effects and deaths. In this work, a novel pH-sensitive liposomal formulation capable of co-encapsulating DOX and SIM at different molar ratios was investigated for its potential in breast tumor treatment. Studies on physicochemical characterization of the liposomal formulations were carried out. The cytotoxic effects of DOX, SIM, and their combinations at different molar ratios (1:1; 1:2 and 2:1), free or co-encapsulated into pH-sensitive liposomes, were evaluated against three human breast cancer cell lines (MDA-MB-231, MCF-7, and SK-BR-3). Experimental protocols included cell viability, combination index, nuclear morphological changes, and migration capacity. The formulations showed a mean diameter of less than 200 nm, with a polydispersity index lower than 0.3. The encapsulation content was ~100% and ~70% for DOX and SIM, respectively. A more pronounced inhibitory effect on breast cancer cell lines was observed at a DOX:SIM molar ratio of 2:1 in both free and encapsulated drugs. Furthermore, the 2:1 ratio showed synergistic combination rates for all concentrations of cell inhibition analyzed (50, 75, and 90%). The results demonstrated the promising potential of the co-encapsulated liposome for breast tumor treatment.

Keywords: breast cancer; pH-sensitive liposomes; coencapsulation; doxorubicin; simvastatin

Citation: Duarte, J.A.; Gomes, E.R.; De Barros, A.L.B.; Leite, E.A. Co-Encapsulation of Simvastatin and Doxorubicin into pH-Sensitive Liposomes Enhances Antitumoral Activity in Breast Cancer Cell Lines. *Pharmaceutics* **2023**, *15*, 369. https://doi.org/10.3390/pharmaceutics15020369

Academic Editors: Ana Isabel Fraguas-Sánchez, Raquel Fernández García and Francisco Bolás-Fernández

Received: 15 December 2022
Revised: 9 January 2023
Accepted: 17 January 2023
Published: 21 January 2023

1. Introduction

Breast cancer was the most common cancer in the world in 2021, and more than 2.2 million cases were diagnosed [1]. Among chemotherapy regimens for treatment of this tumor, anthracyclines, especially doxorubicin (DOX), are the most often used. Despite the expressive clinical response rate, DOX induces serious adverse effects, mainly cardiotoxicity [2]. Furthermore, DOX can induce chemotherapeutic resistance, resulting in poor prognosis and survival of patients. The search for new strategies capable of overcoming these problems has become essential.

Nanomedicine has brought a favorable therapeutic option for DOX; it was the first approved DOX-liposomal formulation. Doxil® (Janssen Biotech, Inc., Johnson & Johnson, Horsham, PA, USA) showed antitumor efficacy comparable to free DOX, and also reduced heart damage [3].

Currently, other DOX-loaded nanoformulations are either approved or in advanced clinical studies for cancer treatment [4,5]. Although many of these products have been proven to be beneficial, with comparable efficacy to free DOX, side effects have still been reported with their use [6,7]. The association of DOX with other antitumor drugs has also been proposed as an alternative to improve therapeutic efficacy; however, this strategy has increased the side effects [8,9].

It has already been pointed out that the SIM increases the cytotoxic effect of DOX in breast cancer cell lines through negative regulation of the cell cycle or induction of apoptosis [10]. Nowadays, studies have investigated combinatorial chemotherapy regimens with compounds from different classes, such as statins, to increase the cytotoxic effect of conventional chemotherapeutic drugs [11]. Preclinical evidence suggests that simvastatin (SIM) has effects beyond its cholesterol-lowering properties, since it may have antitumor effects and decrease cardiac toxicity induced by DOX [12]. A meta-analysis of 1,111,407 cancer patients showed that the administration of SIM reduced cancer mortality by 40% [13]. In this context, the co-encapsulation of these drugs in liposomal formulation could be a promising strategy for improving efficacy and reducing toxicity. In addition, the association of both in the same nanosystem would allow simultaneous delivery to the target site [14]. Recently, a dual-drug liposomal encapsulation of daunorubicin and cytarabine (Vyxeos®) in a synergistic 1:5 molar ratio was approved by the Food and Drug Administration and European Medicines Agency for myeloid leukemia treatment [15].

Our group has developed pH-sensitive liposomes for carrying DOX, and the rationale behind the proposal is based on (i) the acidic pH of the tumor microenvironment and intracellular endosomes (around 6.5 and 5.0–6.0, respectively) compared to normal tissues (pH 7.4); (ii) presence of a polymorphic lipid capable of forming a lamellar bilayer at physiological pH as well as undergoing destabilization and change to a hexagonal phase, releasing the vesicle content at acidic pH; and (iii) drug circulation time prolonged by using a PEGylated liposome [16].

Herein, the aim was to develop and characterize a pH-sensitive liposomal formulation for co-delivery of DOX and SIM, as well as to evaluate the effect of different ratios of free or encapsulated drugs against human cancer cell lines to investigate their potential for breast cancer treatment.

2. Materials and Methods

2.1. Materials

1,2-Dioleoyl-sn-glycero-3-phosphoethanolamine (DOPE) and 1,2-distearoyl-sn-glycero-3-phosphoethanolamine-N-[amino(polyethylene glycol)-2000 (DSPE-PEG2000) were supplied by Lipoid GmbH (Ludwigshafen, Germany). Cholesterol hemisuccinate (CHEMS), phosphate-buffered saline (PBS), sodium hydroxide, 4-(2-hydroxyethyl)piperazine-1-ethane sulfonic acid (HEPES), ammonium sulfate, and sodium bicarbonate were obtained from Sigma-Aldrich (St. Louis, MI, USA). Polysorbate 80 (Tween™ 80) was provided by Croda Inc (Edison, NJ, USA). Chloroform and dimethylsulfoxide (DMSO) were provided from Synth (São Paulo, Brazil). Sodium chloride and HPLC-grade methanol were purchased from Merck (Frankfurt, Germany). Doxorubicin hydrochloride (DOX) was purchased from ACIC Chemicals (Brantford, ON, Canada). SIM was acquired from Fagron (São Paulo, Brazil) with a purity greater than 98.0%. The water used in the experiments was purified using the Milli-Q® distillation and deionization equipment (Millipore, MA, USA). The other substances used were of analytical grade.

Human breast tumor cell lines (MDA-MB-231, MCF-7, SK-BR-3) were purchased by American Type Culture Collection (Manassas, VA, USA). Culture media (Dulbecco's Modified Eagle's Medium, DMEM; Minimum Essential Medium, MEM and McCoy's, Fetal bovine serum (FBS), penicillin, and streptomycin were obtained from Gibco Life Technologies (Carlsbad, USA). Sulforhodamine B (SRB), tris(hydroxymethyl)aminomethane (Tris base), and trypsin were obtained from Sigma-Aldrich (St. Louis, MI, USA) and Hoechst 33258 (Thermo Fisher Scientific—Waltham, MA, USA).

2.2. Liposome Preparation

Blank liposomes (SpHL) and SIM-loaded liposomes (SpHL-S) were prepared by the lipid film hydration method. Chloroform aliquots of DOPE, CHEMS, DSPE-PEG2000 (molar ratio 5.8:3.7:0.5, respectively; total lipid concentration of 20 mM) were transferred to a round bottom flask. For SpHL-S, SIM chloroform solution (concentration 1 mg/mL) was added to lipids. The solvent was removed under reduced pressure using a Buchi Labortechnik AG Rotator CH-9233, model R-210, coupled to a V-700 vacuum pump (Flawil, Switzerland). After total solvent evaporation, a solution of NaOH in molar ratio NaOH:CHEMS, equal to 1, was added to the lipid films, followed by the addition of ammonium sulfate solution (300 mM), pH 7.4, under vigorous agitation. The unencapsulated SIM was then separated from the liposomes by centrifugation at 3000 rpm, 25 °C, for 10 min (Heraeus Multifuge X1R centrifuge, Thermo Fischer Scientific, Waltham, MA, USA).

The diameter of the vesicles was calibrated by the ultrasound (model CPX 500; 500 W, Cole-Parmer Instruments, Vernon Hills, IL, USA) using a Stepped microtip S&M 630-0418 nail with 21% amplitude for 5 min in an ice bath. The preparations were purified to eliminate external ammonium sulfate by ultracentrifugation (Ultracentrifuge Optima® L-80XP, Beckman Coulter, Brea, CA, USA) at 150,000× *g* and 4 °C for 120 min. The pellets were resuspended with 0.9% (*w*/*v*) NaCl solution, maintaining the initial lipid concentration.

For the preparation of liposomes containing DOX, freshly prepared liposomes (SpHL or SpHL-SIM) were incubated with DOX solution (1 or 2 mg/mL) for 2 h at 4 °C, and the encapsulation was performed by remote loading driven by a transmembrane sulfate gradient to obtain the final dispersion of SpHL-D and SpHL-D-S, respectively. Non-encapsulated DOX was removed by ultracentrifugation at the same conditions previously described (Ultracentrifuge Optima® L-80XP, Beckman Coulter, Brea, CA, USA). The purified pellet was resuspended with saline.

In order to guarantee the molar ratios in the liposomal form used in vitro studies, after quantifying SIM concentration, DOX was loaded, driven by the transmembrane ammonium sulfate gradient. As the DOX encapsulation efficiency is approximately 100%, DOX: SIM molar ratios 1:1, 1:2, or 2:1 were ensured.

2.3. *Physicochemical Characterization*

Mean Diameter, Polydispersity Index (PDI), and Zeta Potential

The mean diameter of the vesicles and the polydispersity index (PDI) were determined by dynamic light scattering (DLS) at 25 °C and a fixed angle of 90°. The zeta potential was determined by the electrophoretic mobility associated with DLS. All samples were diluted in 0.9% NaCl solution (*w*/*v*) at a ratio of 1:100 and measured, in triplicate, using Zetasizer NanoZS90 equipment (Malvern Instruments, Worcestershire, UK).

2.4. *Determination of DOX and SIM Content*

DOX and SIM quantification was carried out by high-performance liquid chromatography (HPLC). For DOX determination, the experimental conditions were the same as previously described [17].

SIM quantification was performed with the Agilent 1260 Infinity instrument (Santa Clara, CA, USA) using a mobile phase composed of methanol: 0.1% phosphoric acid solution (90:10 *v*/*v*) and a C18 reversed-phase column of 25 cm × 4.6 mm with a particle size of 5 µm (LichroCar, Merck, Frankfurt, Germany). An injection volume of 10 µL, a flow rate of 1.0 mL/min, and detection with a Diode Array detector G4212B (Santa Clara, CA, USA) at a wavelength of 238 nm and room temperature were used [18].

The liposome sample preparation consisted of the rupture of the lipid membrane with methanol 1:5 *v*/*v*, followed by dilution in the respective mobile phase. Liposomal formulations were quantified before (non-purified liposomes) and after (purified liposomes) purification, and the encapsulation percentage (EP) was calculated according to the following equation:

$$\text{Drug encapsulation percentage } (\%) = \frac{[\text{drug}] \text{ in purified liposomes}}{[\text{drug}] \text{ in non purified liposomes}} \times 100$$

2.5. Cryo-Transmission Electron Microscopy

SpHL-D-S images were obtained by cryo-transmission electron microscopy (cryo-TEM) using an FEI Tecnai Spirit G2-12 electron microscope (FEI, Hillsboro, OR, USA) operating at 120 kV. A 3 μL aliquot of the sample was deposited on the previously unloaded carbon grid. The grids were stained with filter paper for 5 s and vitrified by immersion in liquid ethane. The vitrified samples were stored under liquid nitrogen before being transferred to a TEM.

2.6. Drug Release Evaluation

The drug release study was carried out at pH 7.4 and 5.0 (corrected by adding 1 mol/L hydrochloric acid). Aliquots of 1 mL of SpHL-D-S (2:1) were transferred to a 10 KDa cut-off cellulose membrane (Sigma, St. Louis, MI, USA) with the ends sealed. The dialysis membrane was placed in an amber bottle containing 100 mL of HEPES buffer plus Tween 80 (0.1% *w/v*) to ensure sink condition for both drugs. The flasks were kept under agitation at 156 rpm and 37 °C in an IKA KS 4000i control incubator (Shanghai, China). At each time of investigation (0, 2, 4, 8, 12, and 24 h), a sample was taken and characterized as mean diameter and PDI. In addition, the drug release percentage over time was measured by quantifying DOX and SIM by HPLC, and data were plotted as cumulative percentages of drug release from three independent experiments.

2.7. Storage Stability

A freshly prepared liquid dispersion of SpHL-D-S at a molar ratio (DOX:SIM) of 2:1 was kept under a nitrogen atmosphere and protected from light at 4 °C. After 0, 7, 14, 30, 60, and 90 days of preparation, aliquots were collected and the physicochemical characteristics were measured as mentioned above. The mean values were compared with those obtained at day zero.

Storage stability was also evaluated in SpHL-D-S prepared after the reconstitution of lyophilized SpHL-S. In this case, liposomes were prepared as described above, except for the ammonium sulfate remotion step, in which dialysis against HEPES-buffered saline (HBS) pH 7.4 was performed. Then, the formulations were transferred to amber and cryo-resistant flasks containing glucose, as a cryoprotectant, in a sugar:lipid ratio of 2:1 (*w/w*). The vials were frozen in liquid nitrogen and lyophilized on a 24 h cycle using a Modulo lyophilizer (Thermo Electron Corporation, Waltham, MA, USA). After the lyophilization cycle, the amber vials were vacuum-sealed and stored at −20 °C. At 0, 7, 14, 30, 60, and 90 days after lyophilization, SpHL-S was reconstituted with ultrapure water and SIM concentration was determined by HPLC. Then, DOX was incubated, as described above, to obtain a DOX:SIM molar ratio of 2:1.

2.8. Cell Culture

Human breast adenocarcinoma cells MDA-MB-231 (ATCC HTB-26); MCF-7 (ATCC HTB-22) and SK-BR-3 (ATCC HTB-30) were cultured in DMEM, MEM supplemented with 0.01 mg/mL insulin, and McCoy media, respectively, and all media were supplemented with 10% FBS. Cell lines were cultivated in the presence of penicillin (100 IU/mL) and streptomycin (100 μg/mL) and maintained at 37 °C and 5% CO_2 in a humidified atmosphere. Prior to the experiments, all cell lines were screened for mycoplasma by polymerase chain reaction (PCR), with negative results.

2.9. Cytotoxicity Studies

Tumor cell viability was measured using the sulforhodamine B (SRB) assay. MDA-MB-231, MCF-7, or SK-BR-3 cells were seeded in 96-well plates (1×10^4 cells/well). After 24 h of incubation at 37 °C and 5 % CO_2, free DOX, free SIM, and free DOX:SIM at molar ratios of 1:1, 1:2, or 2:1, respectively; as well as SpHL-DOX, SpHL-SIM, or SpHL-DOX-SIM at molar ratios of 1:1, 1:2, or 2:1, respectively, were added to the wells (DOX concentration ranged from 0.0195 μM to 40 μM). Free SIM was dissolved in DMSO, and the DMSO concentration for all treatments was less than 1% *v*/*v*. After 48 h of incubation, 10% trichloroacetic acid (TCA) was added to each well in order to fix the cells for 1 h. The plates were then washed with water to remove TCA, followed by staining with SRB for 30 min. Then, the plates were washed with 1% *v*/*v* acetic acid to remove unbound dye. Finally, 10 mM Tris-Base solution (pH 10.5) was added to solubilize the protein-bound dye, and the optical density (OD) was read at 510 nm using a Spectra Max Plus 384 microplate spectrophotometer (Molecular Devices, Sunnyvale, CA, USA).

2.10. Determination of the Combination Index (CI)

For the different molar ratios of DOX:SIM, free or encapsulated, the percentage of viable cells was subjected to effect analysis and the combination index (CI) values were determined using CalcuSyn® (Biosoft, Ferguson, MO, USA). CalcuSyn® software allows for the simulation of synergism and antagonism at all dose and effect levels using the median effect algorithm. The values adopted to determine the effects were: synergistic effect, CI < 0.9; additive effect, CI between 0.9 and 1.45; and antagonistic effect, CI > 1.45 [19].

2.11. Nuclear Morphometric Analyzes (NMA)

To assess the nuclear morphological changes after treatment, the different cell lines were plated at a density of 2.0×10^5 cells/well in 6-well plates and incubated at 37 °C for 24 h. After incubation, cells were treated with 2 mL of different treatments (DOX, SpHL-D, SIM, SpHL-S, and the mixtures of free DOX:SIM and SpHL-D-S, at a 1:1; 1:2, or 2:1 molar ratio) at a total concentration of 80 nM. After incubation for 48 h, cells were fixed with 4% formaldehyde for 10 min and stained with a Hoescht 33342 (0.2 µg/mL) for another 10 min at room temperature in the dark. Fluorescent images of the nuclei were captured using an AxioVert 25 microscope with a Fluo HBO 50 fluorescence module connected to the Axio Cam MRC camera (Zeiss, Oberkochen, Germany). The analysis was made up of 300 nuclei per treatment using Image J 1.50i Software (National Institutes of Health, Bethesda, CA, USA) and the "NII_Plugin" plugin available at http://www.ufrgs.br/labsinal/NMA/ (accessed on 2 August 2022).

2.12. Migration Test

To study the two-dimensional migration, cells were plated at a density of 2.0×10^5 cells/well in 12-well plates and incubated at 37 °C for 24 h. Then, a straight wound was made into individual wells with a 10 µL pipette tip. This point was considered the "zero area" and was imaged using an AxioVert 25 microscope with an Axio Cam MRC camera attached (Zeiss, Oberkochen, Germany).

After obtaining the wounds, the control wells received 1 mL of medium with 1% FBS containing the different treatments (DOX, SIM, and the combination of DOX:SIM at ratios of 1:1; 1:2, or 2:1, respectively, in free or encapsulated form). The drug concentration used for treatment was 80 nM. This represents the total concentration of DOX or SIM alone or a combination of DOX: SIM at different molar ratios in the free or co-encapsulated forms. After 24 h of incubation at 37 °C, cells were fixed with 4% formaldehyde for 10 min. Images along the treated wounds were also obtained in phase contrast. The areas of all wounds were obtained using the MRI Wound Healing Tool plugin for the free version of the Image J 1.45 software (National Institutes of Health, Bethesda, CA, USA). The wound healing percentage was calculated according to the following equation:

$$\text{Wound healing}(\%) = 100 - \frac{\text{area of treated wound} \times 100}{\text{area of zero wound}}$$

2.13. Statistical Analyses

Statistical analyses were performed using GraphPad Software Prism (version 6.00, La Jolla, CA, USA). The normality and homoscedasticity of variance were tested by D'Agostino and Pearson and Brown–Forsythe, respectively. Variables without normal distribution were transformed [log(x + 1)]. The difference between the experimental groups was tested using a one-way analysis of variance (ANOVA), followed by the Tukey test. In vitro studies of nuclear morphology were evaluated two-way, followed by the Bonferroni test. Differences were considered significant when the *p*-value was less than 0.05 ($p < 0.05$). Results were expressed as mean ± SD of at least three independent experiments.

3. Results

In this study, we proposed that SIM and DOX be co-encapsulated into pH-sensitive liposomes, aiming to increase antitumor efficacy. Herein, we reported the development and physicochemical characterization of SpHL-D-S, as well as their effects against different human breast cancer cells (MDA-MB-231, MCF-7, and SK-BR-3).

3.1. Formulation Development and Physicochemical Characterization

The physicochemical characteristics of the liposomal formulations are summarized in Table 1. All formulations showed an average diameter ranging from 110 to 150 nm, which may allow for the efficient delivery of DOX and SIM to the tumor region due to the EPR effect [20]. In addition, a PDI lower than 0.3 and a zeta potential close to neutrality (−3.0 mV) indicate, respectively, adequate homogeneity and potential for reduced interaction with plasmatic proteins when injected by the intravenous route [21]. There were no significant differences between SpHL and SpHL-D for all parameters evaluated, and the values obtained were consistent with those previously reported [22,23]. Regarding SpHL-S, no significant difference was observed in PDI and zeta potential compared to SpHL and SpHL-D; however, mean vesicle diameter values were significantly higher. Furthermore, the vesicular size, PDI, and zeta potential were not affected for the formulations containing both drugs, when compared to SpHL-S.

Table 1. Physicochemical characteristics (mean diameter, PDI, zeta potential, encapsulation percentage—EP, and drug concentration) for the different liposomal formulations containing individual or co-encapsulated drugs.

Formulations	[Drug] Theoretical (mg/mL)		Mean Diameter (nm)	PDI	Zeta Potential (mV)	[Drug] Experimental (mg/mL)		EP (%)		Molar Ratio DOX:SIM
	DOX	SIM				DOX	SIM	DOX	SIM	
SpHL	0	0	113 ± 9.0	0.07 ± 0.03	−3.5 ± 0.80	-	-			
SpHL-D	0	1	123 ± 5.0	0.12 ± 0.03	−3.6 ± 0.90	0.99 ± 0.02	-	99 ± 0.1	-	-
SpHL-S	0	1	139 ± 2.6 [a]	0.22 ± 0.02	−3.72 ± 0.17	-	0.76 ± 0.06	-	76 ± 6	-
SpHL-D-S	1	1	145 ± 3.7 [a]	0.23 ± 0.03	−3.63 ± 0.14	0.98 ± 0.01	0.74 ± 0.05	98 ± 0.5	74 ± 0.5	1:1
	1	2	140 ± 1.1 [a]	0.12 ± 0.06	−3.39 ± 0.44	0.97 ± 0.01	1.26 ± 0.02	98 ± 0.5	63 ± 1.2	1:1.7
	2	2	147 ± 1.6 [a]	0.21 ± 0.02	−3.33 ± 0.32	1.97 ± 0.01	1.28 ± 0.02	99 ± 0.3	64 ± 0.7	1.2:1

[a] Represents a significant difference from the formulation containing SpHL and SpHL-D. Data are expressed as mean ± standard deviation (SD). $n = 3$.

Regarding encapsulation efficiency, values of almost 100% and above 60% were obtained for DOX and SIM, respectively. For SIM, data evidenced that an increase in concentration did not result in a proportional drug-encapsulated increase, suggesting a possible saturation of the bilayer. Encapsulation efficiency at the theoretical concentration of 2 mg/mL was around 16% lower compared to 1 mg/mL. On the other hand, no significant difference was observed after DOX encapsulation for any of the formulations, demonstrating that SIM co-encapsulation did not alter the ability of the liposomal system to carry DOX. The molar ratio values calculated for formulations containing both drugs were equal to 1:1, 1:1.7, and 1:1.2 when the liposomes were prepared with 1 mg/mL of each drug, 1 mg/mL of DOX and 2 mg/mL of SIM, and 2 mg/mL of both drugs, respectively.

Based on these results, we defined the initial SIM concentration at 1 mg/mL to prepare all formulations containing the co-encapsulated drugs at molar ratios (DOX:SIM) 1:1, 1:2, and 2:1, respectively. These liposomes were further used for in vitro assays. The same physicochemical investigations were carried out (data are provided in Supplementary Material, Table S1) and there was no significant difference in the parameters evaluated compared to those shown in Table 1.

3.2. Cell Viability and Synergism Analysis

The cytotoxicity was investigated by SRB assay, and we screened for synergistic, additive effects, or antagonism between DOX and SIM, free or co-encapsulated, against different subtypes of human breast cancer cells.

All three cell lines tested (MDA-MB-231, SK-BR-3, and MCF-7) were sensitive to treatment with DOX and SIM. However, DOX showed higher cytotoxicity than SIM, as can be observed by the values of half-maximum inhibitory concentration (IC_{50}) summarized in Table 2.

Table 2. IC_{50} values obtained for the breast cell lines exposed for 48 h to different proportions of DOX and SIM in free form or co-encapsulated into liposomes.

Treatments	IC_{50} (µM)		
	MDA-MB-231	**SK-BR-3**	**MCF-7**
DOX	0.80 ± 0.19	0.20 ± 0.07	0.71 ± 0.14
SIM	1.53 ± 0.37 [a]	0.85 ± 0.19 [a]	1.95 ± 0.63 [a]
DOX:SIM (1:1)	0.96 ± 0.27 [b,d]	0.33 ± 0.07 [b]	1.15 ± 0.33 [b]
DOX:SIM (1:2)	0.71 ± 0.17 [b]	0.19 ± 0.05 [b]	0.91± 0.23 [b]
DOX:SIM (2:1)	0.44 ± 0.07 [a,b]	0.19 ± 0.05 [b]	0.99 ± 0.35 [b]
SpHL-DOX	0.73 ± 0.14	0.32 ± 0.09	1.03 ± 0.32
SpHL-SIM	0.86 ± 0.23	0.83 ± 0.19 [c]	4.28 ± 0.99 [c]
SpHL-D-S (1:1)	0.47 ± 0.24	0.35 ± 0.06	3.98 ± 0.87 [c,e]
SpHL-D-S (1:2)	0.35 ± 0.12 [c]	0.35 ± 0.05	2.39 ± 1.07 [c,e]
SpHL-D-S (2:1)	0.31 ± 0.08 [c]	0.23 ± 0.07	0.87 ± 0.34

Data are expressed as mean ± DP. Letters represent significant differences compared to: [a] free DOX, [b] free SIM, [c] SpHL-D, [d] free DOX:SIM (2:1), [e] free form at the same molar ratio. $p < 0.05$ was considered a significant difference (Tukey's test).

For the MDA-MB-231 strain, it was possible to observe that the combination of free DOX:SIM at the molar ratio of 2:1, respectively, was twice as cytotoxic as the DOX in monotherapy or combination therapy at an equimolar ratio. Furthermore, the drug association led to a significantly greater inhibitory effect than SIM monotherapy at all proposed ratios (1:1, 1:2, and 2:1). Encapsulation of DOX into pH-sensitive liposomes did not significantly alter its cytotoxicity against MDA-MB-231 compared to the free drug. Analysis of SpHL-D-S at molar ratios of 1:2 and 2:1 demonstrated more pronounced cytotoxic effects (about 2.1 and 2.4-fold, respectively) than SpHL-D.

The SK-BR-3 cell line was the most sensitive to treatment with DOX and SIM, as demonstrated by IC_{50} values lower than those obtained for MDA-MB-231. The combination of drugs did not increase the cytotoxic activity compared to DOX, either in the free or the co-encapsulated form for the SK-BR-3 cell line.

For the MCF-7 strain, lower sensitivity was detected compared to others, especially after treatments with liposomal formulations. In this cell line, there was no significant difference between the free DOX and the DOX:SIM combination in the free form for any of the molar ratios evaluated. However, co-encapsulation of DOX and SIM at 1:1 and 1:2, respectively, significantly reduced cytotoxic activity compared to SpHL-D. It is noteworthy that the control group (SpHL) had no effects on cell viability and was similar to untreated cells, indicating no significant toxicity of the formulation excipients [17] (data not shown).

Taken together, the cell viability data suggest that the combination of DOX and SIM at a molar ratio of 2:1, respectively, either in the free form or co-encapsulated into liposomes, presented better results against the MDA-MB-231 cell line. However, no gains were observed against other cell lines.

Figure 1 shows the combination indices (CI) for the different treatments against MDA-MB-231, SK-BR-3, and MCF-7 cell lines, in three inhibition concentrations (50, 75, and 90% of the cells). For MDA-MB-231, the combination of DOX:SIM at a ratio of 2:1, respectively, showed a potential synergistic effect for free and co-encapsulated forms (Figure 1A). The CI values for DOX:SIM 2:1 and SpHL-D-S 2:1 were, respectively, approximately 0.7 and 0.5 for all cellular inhibition concentrations analyzed. Furthermore, the treatment with SpHL-D-S 1:2 was partially synergistic, showing a CI close to 0.9 for the higher inhibition fractions (75 and 90%), while free DOX:SIM 1:2 treatment showed an additive effect.

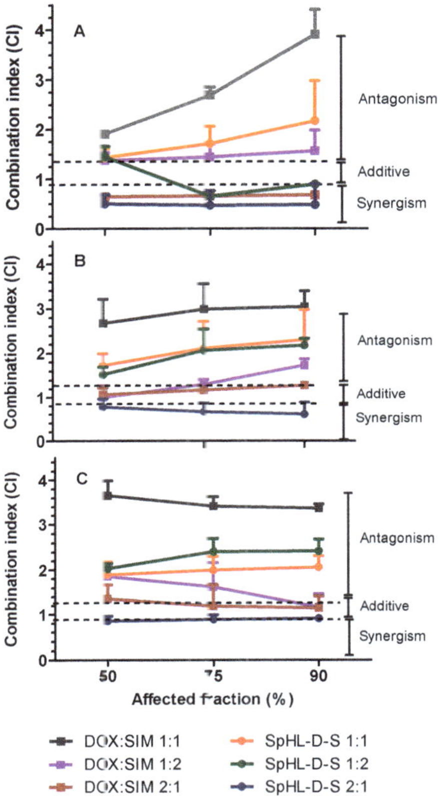

Figure 1. Fraction-affected X CI graph for free combinations and SpHL-D-S formulations in MDA-MB-231 (**A**), SK-BR-3 (**B**), and MCF-7 (**C**) cell lines. Note: All data are represented as mean ± SD (n = 3).

A synergistic effect was also observed for SK-BR-3 after treatment with SpHL-D-S 2:1, showing CI between 0.6 and 0.8. On the other hand, the same molar ratio of free drugs resulted in an additive effect, with CI ranging from 1.0 to 1.3 (Figure 1B). Similar results were obtained for the MCF-7 cell line (Figure 1C). The association of drugs at 1:1, either free or encapsulated, led to antagonism (CI close to 2) for all cell lines investigated.

3.3. Nuclear Morphometric Analyses

Evaluation of NMA was based on an analytical tool developed by Filippi-Chiela and collaborators that allows for the extraction of morphometric data to classify nuclei into populations: normal (N), irregular (I), small and regular (SR), and large and regular (LR). The change in nuclear morphology can occur in processes associated with cell death. These modifications include the nuclear condensation and fragmentation observed in apoptosis, the nuclear size increase observed in senescence, and increases in nuclear irregularity under chemical or physical stresses [24].

The NMA data obtained after different treatments are shown in Figure 2. There was no significant number of irregular nuclei after different treatments for any of the cell lines. Furthermore, apoptosis events (SR nuclei) showed a similar extent for the three cell lines

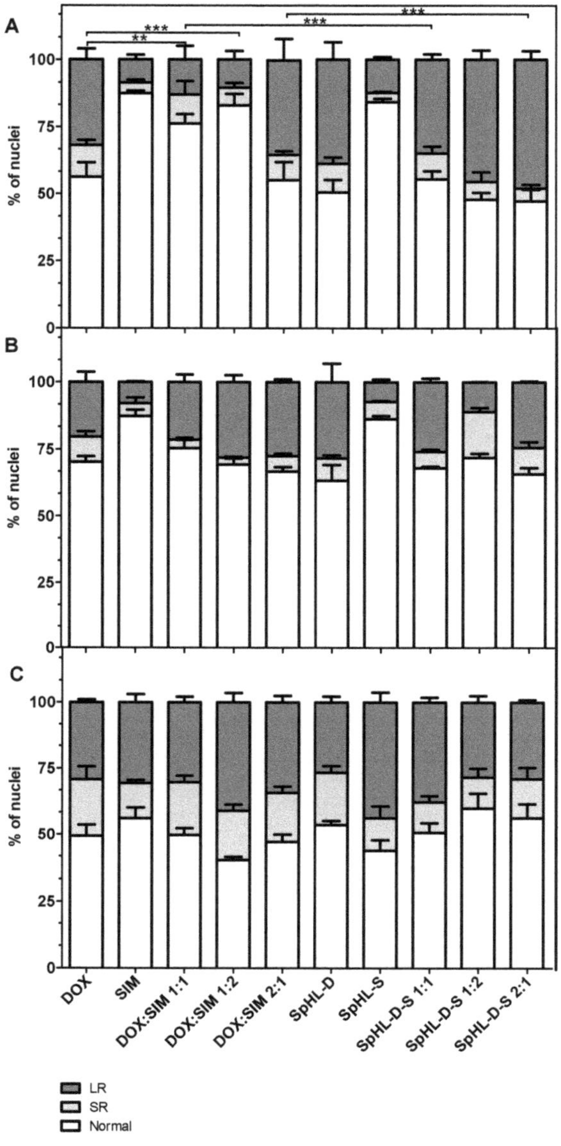

Figure 2. Nuclear morphometric distribution of cell lines (**A**) MDA-MB-231; (**B**) SK-BR-3, and (**C**) MCF-7, exposed to 80 nM of different treatments for 48 h. The bars represent normal (white bars), small and regular (light gray), and large and regular (dark gray) nuclei. Note: The data represent the mean ± SD of three independent experiments.; ** ($p < 0.01$) and *** ($p < 0.001$) represent a significant difference in relation to normal and LR nuclei (Bonferroni's test).

After DOX treatment, either in the free form or SpHL-D, MDA-MB-231 data analysis showed N nuclei ranging from 55 to 65%, SR equal to 10%, and LR varying from 25 to 35%. The values obtained after SIM treatment in both forms were 85%, 3%, and 12% for N, SR, and LR, respectively. These findings are in agreement with viability cell studies and reinforce the lower cytotoxic activity of SIM for this cell line. A significant reduction in LR nuclei was also verified, followed by increased N nuclei, after treatment with free DOX:SIM 1:1 or 1:2 compared to free DOX. In contrast, a significant increase in LR nuclei was detected after SpHL-D-S 1:2 and SpHL-D-S 2:1 treatments. It was also observed that the encapsulation of DOX:SIM 1:1 and 1:2 resulted in a significant increase ($p < 0.001$) in LR nuclei compared to free-form DOX at the same ratio. The increase in the levels of LR nuclei demonstrated an increase in senescence induction.

For SK-BR-3 cells, the percentage of distribution of nuclei was similar to MDA-MB-231 after SIM and DOX treatment. Furthermore, SIM treatment had a less pronounced cytotoxic effect compared to DOX treatments. No significant difference was observed between free or liposomal DOX, either alone or associated with SIM, for any of the molar ratios evaluated.

Concerning the MCF-7 cell line, no significant difference was detected between free DOX and other free forms or liposomal treatments. Similar to SK-BR-3, encapsulation of DOX:SIM at different molar ratios did not change the distribution of nuclei.

Figure 3 shows fluorescence photomicrographs of MDA-MB-231 nuclei stained with Hoescht 33342. An enlargement for cells exposed to the different treatments is evident compared to untreated cells. These characteristics correspond with the typical phenotypic morphology of senescence. It is also possible to observe the different distributions of LR and SR nuclei in relation to the control N that did not receive drug treatment. SK-BR-3 and MCF-7 cells had similar profiles to MDA-MB-231; thus, those images were not presented and are available in the Supplementary Materials (Figure S1).

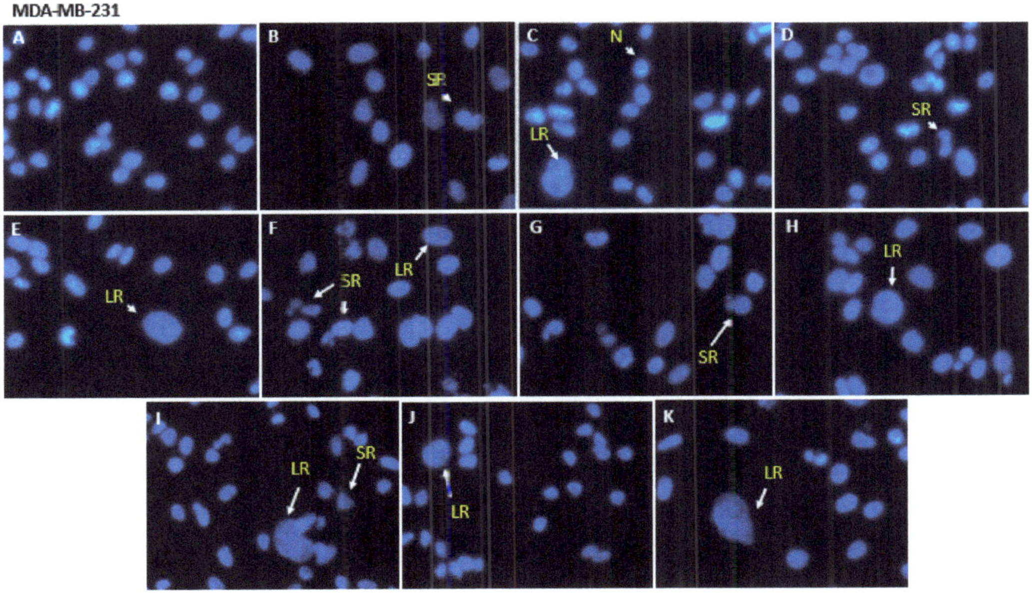

Figure 3. Representative fluorescence photomicrographs of breast cancer cell nuclei stained with Hoechst 33342 after treatments at a concentration of 80 nM, for 48 h: SpHL (**A**); free DOX (**B**); SIM free (**C**); DOX:SIM 1:1 (**D**); DOX:SIM 1:2 (**E**); DOX:SIM 2:1 (**F**) SpHL-D (**G**); SpHL-S (**H**); SpHL-D-S 1:1 (**I**); SpH-D-S 1:2 (**J**); or SpHL-D-S 2:1 (**K**). Note: Some of the different morphometric phenotypes of nuclei observed are indicated. N, normal; SR, apoptotic; LR, senescent. Images are representative of three independent experiments. Enhancement, 40×.

3.4. Migration Assay

Cell migration was evaluated by a wound-healing assay that allowed the observation of two-dimensional cell migration in confluent monolayer cell cultures. SK-BR-3 human breast cancer is non-metastatic; in attempted invasive assays, this cell line did not show invasiveness, so it was not used at this stage of the study [25,26].

Representative phase contrast photomicrographs of the scratches after 24 h of exposure to treatments are shown in Figure 4.

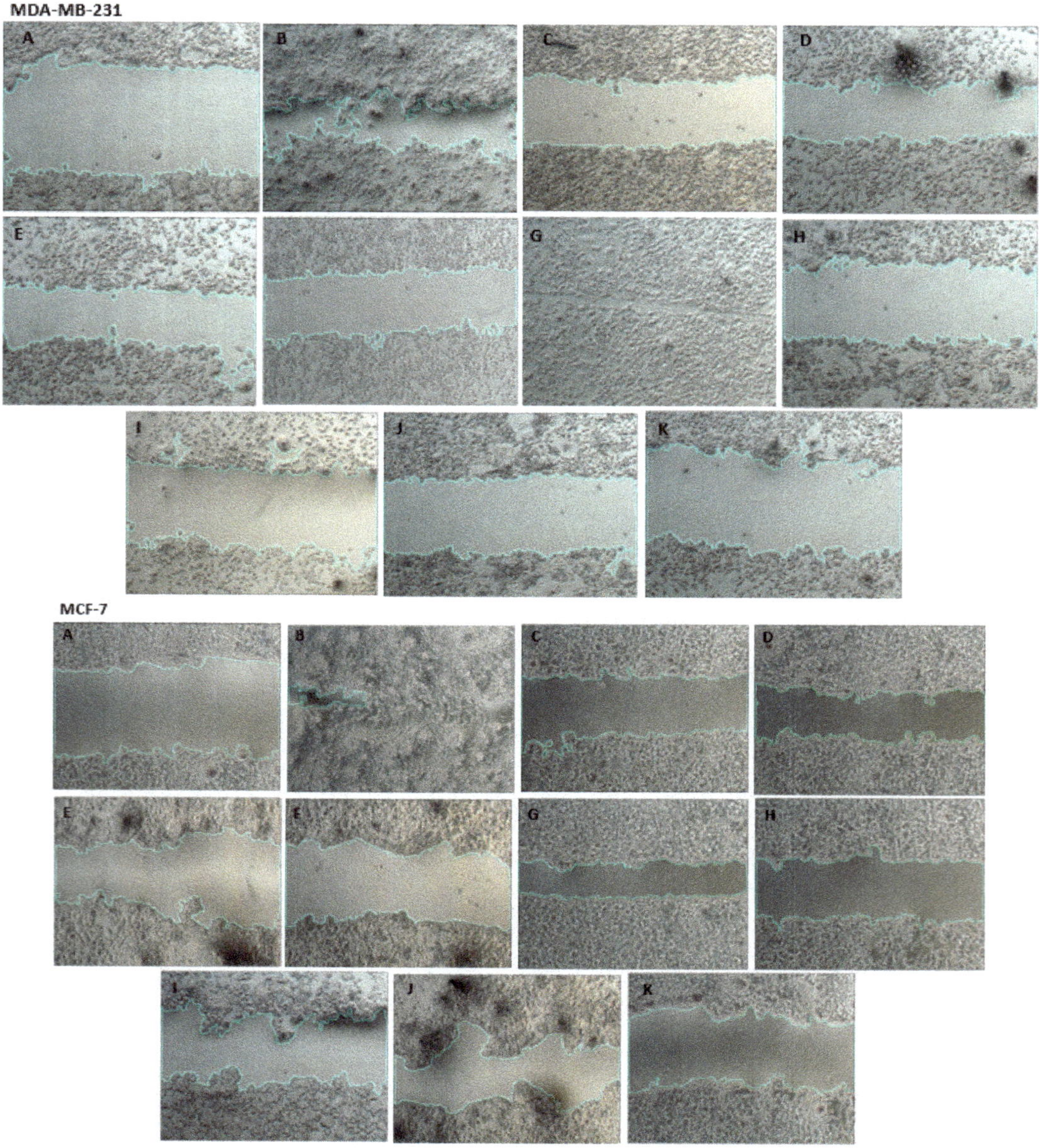

Figure 4. Representative phase contrast photomicrographs of MDA-MB-231 and MCF-7 cell lines exposed for 24 h at 80 nM to liposome treatments. Treatments: wound zero (control) (**A**); free DOX (**B**); SIM free (**C**); DOX:SIM 1:1 (**D**); DOX:SIM 1:2 (**E**); DOX:SIM 2:1 (**F**); SpHL-D (**G**); SpHL-S (**H**); SpHL-D-S 1:1 (**I**); SpH-D-S 1:2 (**J**); or SpHL-D-S 2:1 (**K**). 5× magnification.

As can be seen in Table 3, free DOX or SpHL-D did not inhibit MDA-MB-231 or MCF-7 cell migration. However, all treatments containing SIM significantly reduced the percentage of cell migration compared to treatments containing only DOX for both cell lines, except the DOX:SIM 1:1 treatment. For the MDA-MB-231 strain, it was observed that the combined treatments DOX:SIM 1:2 and 2:1 in the free form inhibited, respectively, two- and three-fold more cell migration compared to free DOX. On the other hand, SpHL-D-S therapy at a 1:2 molar ratio was about three-fold more inhibitory, and at a 2:1 ratio, about six-fold more inhibitory, when compared to SpHL-D. A similar profile was obtained for MCF-7. The combined treatments DOX:SIM 1:2 and 2:1 were, respectively, four and three times more inhibitory to migration compared to free DOX, while SpHL-D-S 1:2 and 2:1 inhibited two and three times more than SpHL-D.

Table 3. Percentage of cell migration in relation to control for MDA-MB-231 and MCF-7 cell lines evaluated after exposure to the free or encapsulated drugs at different molar ratios.

Treatments	MDA-MB-231	MCF-7
DOX	89.8 ± 6.0	90.1 ± 6.0
SIM	39.7 ± 5.0 [a]	37.9 ± 4.3 [a]
DOX:SIM (1:1)	47.9 ± 10.5 [c]	49.2 ± 3.7
DOX:SIM (1:2)	42.1 ± 6.7 [a]	22.0 ± 7.8 [a]
DOX:SIM (2:1)	27.8 ± 4.2 [a]	28.3 ± 8.1 [a]
SpHL-DOX	90.6 ± 5.8	87.9 ± 3.0
SpHL-SIM	24.5 ± 2.4 [b]	32.6 ± 8.8 [b]
SpHL-D-S (1:1)	25.2 ± 2.2 [b]	41.9 ± 5.4 [b]
SpHL-D-S (1:2)	24.8 ± 4.6 [b]	42.9 ± 1.3 [b]
SpHL-D-S (2:1)	15.5 ± 5.7 [b]	24.7 ± 2.2 [b]

[a] significant difference compared to treatment with free DOX; [b] significantly different from SpHL-D treatment; [c] significant difference compared to treatment with DOX:SIM 2:1. Data for cell lines MDA-MB-231 and MCF-7 were transformed as $y = \log(\text{value} + 1)$. A significant difference was considered for p-values < 0.05 (Tukey's test).

The in vitro studies clearly showed the difference in the response of cell lines to treatments. Furthermore, they were important as a screening to select the best molar ratio for DOX and SIM in order to proceed with formulation characterizations and guide future investigations. As previously reported, treatment with SpHL-D-S 2:1 showed a synergistic effect in all fractions and against all human breast tumor cell lines evaluated, so this ratio was used for a more detailed characterization of stability and morphological evaluation.

3.5. Drug Release Study

The DOX and SIM release profile from SpHL-D-S (2:1) was evaluated using a dialysis method at two different pH levels (7.4 and 5.0). Before the release study, various release conditions were tested to determine the sink conditions for both active substances (data not presented), and the HEPES buffer plus Tween 80 (0.1% w/v) was used. As shown in Figure 5, drug release was pH- and time-dependent. SpHL-D-S incubated at pH 5.0 showed higher DOX and SIM release than at pH 7.4. After 24 h of incubation, the DOX release was around 90% and 70% at pH 5.0 and 7.4, respectively. SIM release was more controlled, and near 65% and 56% was released after 24 h of incubation at pH 5.0 and 7.4.

At pH 7.4, the vesicle size was not changed for 24 h. In contrast, significant changes in the vesicle diameter were noted at pH 5.0 from 1 h of evaluation (Figure 5C), since the diameter of the vesicles increased by around 23% (142.6 ± 1.9 nm versus 176.7 ± 3.1 nm). The increase in vesicle size is also indicative that the SpHL-D-S responds to pH variation, since the low pH leads to vesicle aggregation and/or membrane fusion [16].

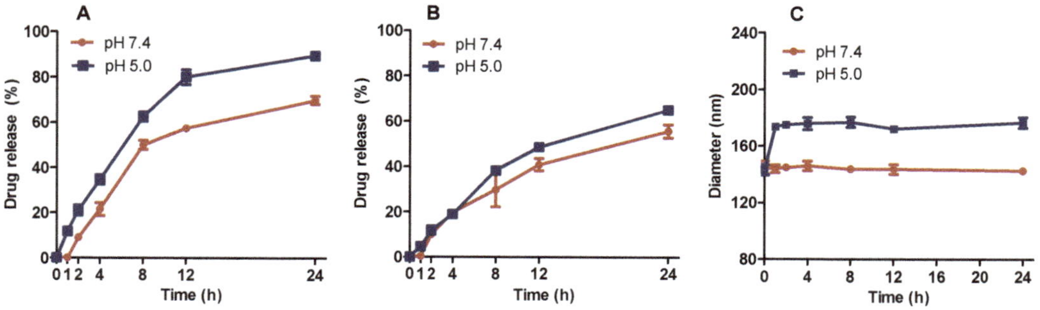

Figure 5. DOX (**A**) and SIM (**B**) release profiles from SpHL-D-S at pH 7.4 (red) and 5.0 (blue) and evaluation of vesicle diameter (**C**) at different times.

3.6. *Cryo-TEM*

Morphological analysis of SpHL-D-S at a molar ratio of 2:1 was also performed by cryo-TEM (Figure 6). Images showed the presence of vesicles which were spherical and non-spherical, unilamellar, and reasonably uniform in diameter. The non-spherical form can be attributed to the presence of DOX crystals that force a change in the shape of the vesicles from spherical to non-spherical [27].

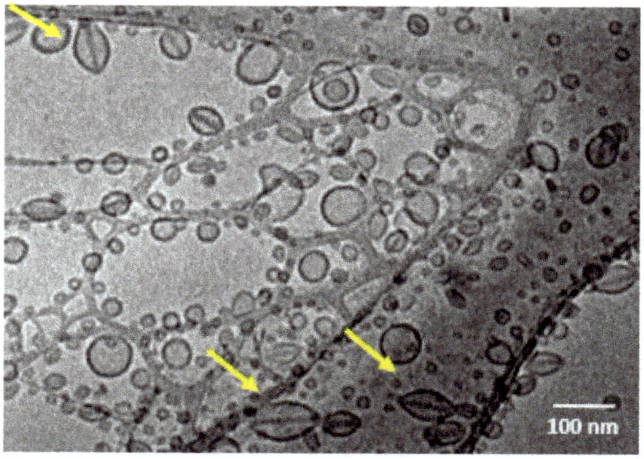

Figure 6. Cryo-TEM photomicrograph of SpHL-D-L 2:1. Note: Yellow arrows indicate DOX sulfate crystals within the liposomes.

3.7. *Storage Stability*

The physicochemical stability of SpHL-D-S 2:1 was studied over 90 days. No notable changes were observed in vesicle size and PDI (Figure 7A) for at least 90 days at 4 °C. Regarding the DOX and SIM retention into liposomes, both drugs were stable during the first 15 days. However, from the 15th day onwards, a gradual and significant reduction in the SIM-encapsulated level was observed, reaching about 50% in 90 days. The DOX concentration was maintained over time.

The reduction in the content of SIM may be due to its sensitivity to the aqueous solution. As SIM contains a lactone ring labile to hydrolysis, in an aqueous medium, hydrolysis may take place, resulting in a compound with lower lipophilicity. To avoid hydrolysis, SpHL-S was lyophilized and stored in its freeze-dried form for reconstitution with DOX at the moment of use. The results are presented in Figure 7B,D. Larger diameters (around 280 nm) with PDI near 0.25 were obtained after the lyophilization process using glucose as a lyoprotectant, and these values also remained unchanged for at least 90 days.

Furthermore, the SIM content and the DOX encapsulation capacity remained close to 100% for at least 90 days (Figure 7D).

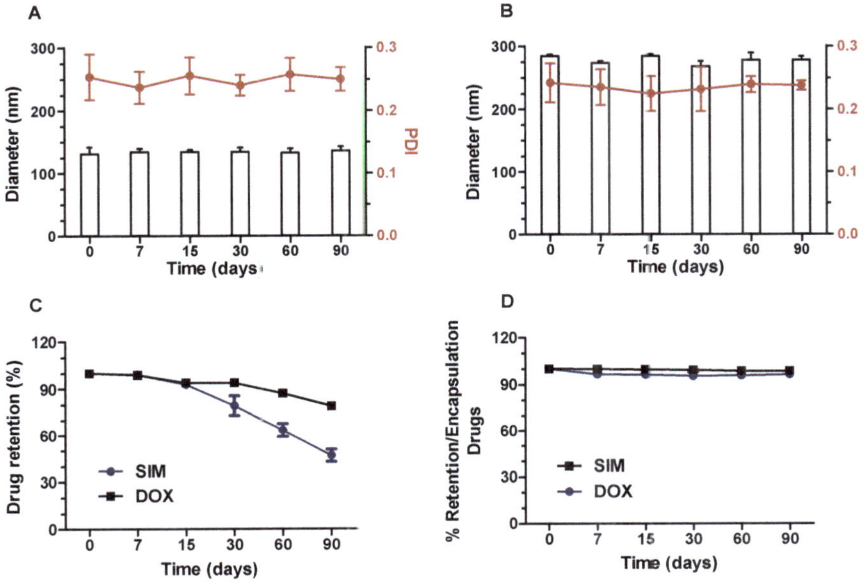

Figure 7. Average size, PDI, and % retention of drugs of SpHL-D-S 2:1, kept at 4 °C in liquid form (**A**,**C**) or prepared by reconstitution of lyophilized SpHL-S (**B**,**D**) and evaluated over 90 days.

4. Discussion

Although chemotherapy has played a central role in breast cancer treatment, the ability of drugs to kill cancer cells with minimal damage to healthy tissue is still a challenge, being one of the main requirements for the success of cancer therapy. It is well-described that most chemotherapeutic agents, such as DOX, may cause adverse effects that are potentially fatal to the patients. The most relevant, and sometimes irreversible, toxic effect of DOX is cardiomyopathy. To improve the safety profile of this antineoplastic drug, encapsulation into liposomes has been considered a promising alternative since it can promote an increase in drug selectivity, as it preferentially accumulates in the target tissue, reducing damage to healthy areas. Doxil®, the first liposomal formulation approved for breast cancer treatment, presented reduced cardiotoxicity and myelosuppression induced by DOX. Despite these advantages, there are still reports of cardiac toxicity in 11% of patients treated with this medication. Our research group has shown that pH-sensitive liposomes composed of DOPE, CHEMS, and DSPE-PEG carrying DOX and associated with other substances with antitumor potential are beneficial compared to liposomal formulations similar to Doxil® [28,29]. Recent studies have also reported that SIM exhibits anticancer activity since it can influence proliferation, migration, and cancer cell survival, and there are indications of protective factors during cancer chemotherapy in patients using SIM [30]. Therefore, we proposed that the potential of SIM to increase the DOX antitumor activity after short-term exposure of the breast cancer cell lines to treatment be investigated.

The first step of the study consisted of formulation development with suitable physicochemical properties for biological evaluation. All formulations showed homogeneity and small size (lower than 150 nm), despite the size having been increased by SIM presence (Table 1). This fact might be due to the hydrophobic nature of SIM, which favors its interaction with the lipid bilayer and increases the size of the vesicles [21,31]. It has been reported that small particle size and narrow size distribution are quality attributes of liposome drug products, especially for an injectable formulation, besides allowing the efficient delivery of antitumor agents to a tumor by passive targeting. These parameters did not change over time, as can be seen in Figure 7A. Furthermore, zeta potential values near the neutral range were obtained for all formulations, and can be attributed to the low electrophoretic mobility caused by the hydrodynamic resistance of the PEG molecules coupled to the DSPE-PEG2000 [21]. Previous studies have demonstrated that nanoparticle surfaces with no charge bind less protein than those that are negatively or positively charged, increasing blood circulation time [32].

As regards encapsulation efficiency, higher values were observed for SIM (>60%) and DOX (almost 100%). The high encapsulation obtained by the DOX active loading is often explained by the formation of insoluble DOX-sulfate crystals inside the aqueous core of liposomes [33]. These crystals, previously named "coffee bean," could be clearly observed by cryo-TEM (Figure 6). Regarding SIM, we suggest that the unsaturated phospholipid (DOPE) present in the formulation favored the "pockets" formation in the bilayer, in which the hydrophobic molecule as SIM was embedded. However, the SIM retention efficiency decreased over time (Figure 7C), likely due to the SIM hydrolysis in a more hydrophilic compound with less affinity by bilayer. To overcome this drawback, the formulation was lyophilized. The dry product was able to be stored for a long time and hydrated immediately before use [34]. After that, the concentration of both drugs was kept near 100% for 90 days. The mean diameter increased by around two-fold compared to liquid form. It has been reported that the lyophilization process, even with the use of cryoprotectants, can cause stress to the liposomal vesicles. In addition, at the time of reconstitution, the particles can aggregate, generating a larger diameter, as seen in Figure 5B [35].

It is well-known that the antitumor efficacy of pH-sensitive liposomes depends on their ability to release the drug into the tumor region. In an acidic environment, these formulations, composed of DOPE (a fusogenic lipid), can fuse or destabilize, releasing the encapsulated content [36,37]. Herein, the release study was carried out at pH 5.0 and 7.4. The release profile showed that the released total percentage of both drugs was higher at pH 5.0 than 7.4 (Figure 5). In addition, there was a significant change in the diameter of vesicles at pH 5.0. These data suggest the pH sensitivity property of the system, even with the addition of SIM to the lipid bilayer. Furthermore, assuming that the pH in the non-tumor environment were 7.4, most of the drugs would remain circulating retained into the liposomes for a longer time and, thus, could lead to less toxicity in normal tissues [22,38].

As breast cancer shows multiple subtypes with histopathological and biological differences that can lead to different treatment responses, we have chosen to evaluate the behavior of the formulations in two luminal subtype cell lines, namely MCF-7 and SK-BR-3, and one basal subtype cell line, MDA-MB-231. The first one is positive for estrogen receptors (ER) and progesterone receptors (PR) and negative for human epidermal growth factor receptor 2 (HER2). The second is ER-/PR-/HER2+, and the last is triple-negative breast cancer (ER−/PR−/HER2) [39].

The cytotoxicity assessment showed more pronounced sensitivity for SK-BR-3, followed by MDA-MB-231 and MCF-7, especially after DOX: SIM 2:1 treatment in free or co-encapsulated form. In addition, SpHL-D-S at the molar ratio of 2:1 presented a synergistic effect for all lines tested. Considering that the potential cytotoxic activity of SIM is related to its ability to modulate some effects on reactive oxygen species (ROS), deregulate caspase cascades, and inhibit 3-hydroxy-3methyl-glutaryl-coenzyme A reductase (overexpressed in cancer cells) [40–44], while the DOX mechanism of action refers to intercalation in DNA and interruption of DNA repair mediated by topoisomerase II [8], we may suggest that these different mechanisms favor the possibilities of synergism and increase the sensitivity of cells, thus minimizing the development of resistance [45]. This hypothesis is supported by previous studies that have reported that combined DOX and SIM therapy significantly stopped the growth of prostate cancer cells through multiple mechanisms such as increased levels of intracellular ROS, induced apoptosis, promoted cellular autophagy, and anti-angiogenesis [46]. Buranrat et al. reported that the combination of DOX and

SIM increased cytochrome c protein expression and caspase-3 activity compared to each drug alone, suggesting that SIM sensitizes MCF-7 breast tumor cells, potentiating the action of DOX [47]. Furthermore, Machado and coworkers suggested that MCF-7 cells are more resistant to oxidative damage caused by ROS compared to MDA-MB-231 cells, thus suffering less apoptosis [48]. This fact could explain the results obtained herein, in which IC50 values for MCF-7 were higher than MDA-MB-231 cells, especially after treatment with liposomal formulations.

5. Conclusions

In this study, we developed a novel formulation of pH-sensitive liposomes containing DOX and SIM. Our results show that this system is pH-responsive and stable in the lyophilized form for at least 90 days. The viability, CI, and NMA data pointed out that the 2:1 molar ratio can act synergistically, improving the inhibitory results of proliferation and induction of death of breast cancer cells. Furthermore, the migration results reinforce the notion that the combination of DOX and SIM significantly improves the inhibition of cell proliferation. However, further studies are needed to understand the molecular mechanisms involved

In summary, the present study identified a new strategy for a potential combination therapy. SpHL-D-L 2:1 showed suitable physicochemical properties, release behaviors, and cytotoxicity responses to be considered a promising alternative for further in vivo breast cancer therapy.

Supplementary Materials: The following supporting information can be downloaded at: https://www.mdpi.com/article/10.3390/pharmaceutics15020369/s1, Figure S1: Representative fluorescence photomicrographs of breast cancer cell nuclei stained with Hoechst 33342 after treatments at a concentration of 80 nM, for 48 h: SpHL (A); free DOX (B); SIM free (C); DOX:SIM 1:1 (D); DOX:SIM 1:2 (E); DOX:SIM 2:1 (F) SpHL-D (G); SpHL-S (H); SpHL-D-S 1:1 (I); SpH-D-S 1:2 (J) or SpHL-D-S 2:1 (L); Table S1: Physicochemical characteristics for the different formulations.

Author Contributions: Conceptualization, J.A.D., A.L.B.D.B. and E.A.L.; methodology, J.A.D. and E.R.G.; software, J.A.D. E.R.G.; A.L.B.D.B. and E.A.L. resources, E.A.L.; data curation, J.A.D., A.L.B.D.B. and E.A.L.; writing—original draft preparation, J.A.D.; writing—review and editing, J.A.D., A.L.B.D.B. and E.A.L.; visualization, J.A.D., A.L.B.D.B. and E.A.L.; supervision, A.L.B.D.B. and E.A.L.; project administration, E.A.L.; funding acquisition, A.L.B.D.B. and E.A.L. All authors have read and agreed to the published version of the manuscript.

Funding: This research was funded by Fundação de Amparo à Pesquisa do Estado de Minas Gerais (APQ-01764-17 and PPM-00387-17).

Institutional Review Board Statement: Not applicable.

Informed Consent Statement: Not applicable.

Data Availability Statement: Not applicable.

Acknowledgments: The authors thank Conselho Nacional de Desenvolvimento Científico e Tecnológico (CNPq, Brazil), Fundação de Amparo à Pesquisa do Estado de Minas Gerais (FAPEMIG, Brazil), and Coordenação de Aperfeiçoamento de Pessoal de Nível Superior (CAPES, Brazil) for their financial support and fellowships.

Conflicts of Interest: The authors declare no conflict of interest.

References

1. Sung, H.; Ferlay, J.; Siegel, R.L.; Laversanne, M.; Soerjomataram, I.; Jemal, A.; Bray, F. Global Cancer Statistics 2020: GLOBOCAN Estimates of Incidence and Mortality Worldwide for 36 Cancers in 185 Countries. *CA Cancer J. Clin.* **2021**, *71*, 209–249. [CrossRef] [PubMed]
2. Tan, Q.-W.; Luo, T.; Zheng, H.; Tian, T.-L. He, P.; Chen, J.; Zeng, H.-L.; Lv, Q. Weekly taxane–anthracycline combination regimen versus tri-weekly anthracycline-based regimen for the treatment of locally advanced breast cancer: A randomized controlled trial. *Chin. J. Cancer* **2017**, *36*, 27. [CrossRef] [PubMed]

3. Soundararajan, A.; Bao, A.; Phillips, W.T.; McManus, L.M.; Goins, B.A. Chemoradionuclide Therapy with ^{186}Re-Labeled Liposomal Doxorubicin: Toxicity, Dosimetry, and Therapeutic Response. *Cancer Biotherapy Radiopharm.* **2011**, *26*, 603–614. [CrossRef] [PubMed]
4. Zhao, N.; Woodle, M.C.; Mixson, A.J. Advances in Delivery Systems for Doxorubicin. *J. Nanomed. Nanotechnol.* **2018**, *9*, 519. [CrossRef]
5. Cagel, M.; Grotz, E.; Bernabeu, E.; Moretton, M.A.; Chiappetta, D.A. Doxorubicin: Nanotechnological overviews from bench to bedside. *Drug Discov. Today* **2017**, *22*, 270–281. [CrossRef]
6. Lao, J.; Madani, J.; Puértolas, T.; Álvarez, M.; Hernández, A.; Pazo-Cid, R.; Artal, Á.; Torres, A.A. Liposomal Doxorubicin in the Treatment of Breast Cancer Patients: A Review. *J. Drug Deliv.* **2013**, *2013*, 4564091. [CrossRef]
7. Gabizon, A.; Tzemach, D.; Mak, L.; Bronstein, M.; Horowitz, A.T. Dose Dependency of Pharmacokinetics and Therapeutic Efficacy of Pegylated Liposomal Doxorubicin (DOXIL) in Murine Models. *J. Drug Target.* **2002**, *10*, 539–548. [CrossRef]
8. Thorn, C.F.; Oshiro, C.; Marsh, S.; Hernandez-Boussard, T.; McLeod, H.; Klein, T.E.; Altman, R.B. Doxorubicin Pathways. *Pharm. Genom.* **2011**, *21*, 440–446. [CrossRef]
9. Gadisa, D.A.; Assefa, M.; Wang, S.-H.; Yimer, G. Toxicity profile of Doxorubicin-Cyclophosphamide and Doxorubicin-Cyclophosphamide followed by Paclitaxel regimen and its associated factors among women with breast cancer in Ethiopia: A prospective cohort study. *J. Oncol. Pharm. Pract.* **2020**, *26*, 1912–1920. [CrossRef]
10. Buranrat, B.; Senggunprai, L.; Prawan, A.; Kukongviriyapan, V. Effects of Simvastatin in Combination with Anticancer Drugs on Proliferation and Migration in Cholangiocarcinoma Cells. *Indian J. Pharm. Sci.* **2022**, *84*, 72–79. [CrossRef]
11. Li, N.; Xie, X.; Hu, Y.; He, H.; Fu, X.; Fang, T.; Li, C. Herceptin-conjugated liposomes co-loaded with doxorubicin and simvastatin in targeted prostate cancer therapy. *Am. J. Transl. Res.* **2019**, *11*, 1255–1269. [PubMed]
12. Duarte, J.A.; de Barros, A.L.B.; Leite, E.A. The potential use of simvastatin for cancer treatment: A review. *Biomed. Pharmacother.* **2021**, *141*, 111858. [CrossRef] [PubMed]
13. Jiang, W.; Hu, J.-W.; He, X.-R.; Jin, W.-L.; He, X.-Y. Statins: A repurposed drug to fight cancer. *J. Exp. Clin. Cancer Res.* **2021**, *40*, 241. [CrossRef] [PubMed]
14. Franco, M.S.; Roque, M.C.; Oliveira, M.C. Short and Long-Term Effects of the Exposure of Breast Cancer Cell Lines to Different Ratios of Free or Co-Encapsulated Liposomal Paclitaxel and Doxorubicin. *Pharmaceutics* **2019**, *11*, 178. [CrossRef]
15. Cortes, J.E.; Lin, T.L.; Uy, G.L.; Ryan, R.J.; Faderl, S.; Lancet, J.E. Quality-adjusted Time Without Symptoms of disease or Toxicity (Q-TWiST) analysis of CPX-351 versus 7 + 3 in older adults with newly diagnosed high-risk/secondary AML. *J. Hematol. Oncol.* **2021**, *14*, 110. [CrossRef]
16. Paliwal, S.R.; Paliwal, R.; Pal, H.C.; Saxena, A.K.; Sharma, P.R.; Gupta, P.N.; Agrawal, G.P.; Vyas, S.P. Estrogen-Anchored pH-Sensitive Liposomes as Nanomodule Designed for Site-Specific Delivery of Doxorubicin in Breast Cancer Therapy. *Mol. Pharm.* **2012**, *9*, 176–186. [CrossRef]
17. Ferreira, D.D.S.; Faria, S.D.; Lopes, S.C.d.A.; Teixeira, C.S.; Malachias, A.; Magalhães-Paniago, R.; Filho, J.D.d.S.; Oliveira, B.L.d.J.P.; Guimarães, A.R.; Caravan, P.; et al. Development of a bone-targeted pH-sensitive liposomal formulation containing doxorubicin: Physicochemical characterization, cytotoxicity, and biodistribution evaluation in a mouse model of bone metastasis. *Int. J. Nanomed.* **2016**, *11*, 3737–3751. [CrossRef]
18. Marques-Marinho, F.D.; Freitas, B.D.; Zanon, J.C.D.C.; Reis, I.A.; Lima, A.A.; Vianna-Soares, C.D. Development and Validation of a RP-HPLC Method for Simvastatin Capsules. *Curr. Pharm. Anal.* **2013**, *9*, 2–12. [CrossRef]
19. Chou, T.-C. Theoretical Basis, Experimental Design, and Computerized Simulation of Synergism and Antagonism in Drug Combination Studies. *Pharmacol. Rev.* **2006**, *58*, 621–681. [CrossRef]
20. Franco, M.S.; Gomes, E.R.; Roque, M.C.; Oliveira, M.C. Triggered Drug Release from Liposomes: Exploiting the Outer and Inner Tumor Environment. *Front. Oncol.* **2021**, *11*, 623760. [CrossRef]
21. Sariisik, E.; Koçak, M.; Baloglu, F.K.; Severcan, F. Interaction of the cholesterol reducing agent simvastatin with zwitterionic DPPC and charged DPPG phospholipid membranes. *Biochim. et Biophys. Acta (BBA)—Biomembr.* **2019**, *1861*, 810–818. [CrossRef] [PubMed]
22. Roque, M.C.; Franco, M.S.; Vilela, J.M.C.; Andrade, M.S.; de Barros, A.L.; Leite, E.A.; Oliveira, M.C. Development of Long-Circulating and Fusogenic Liposomes Co-encapsulating Paclitaxel and Doxorubicin in Synergistic Ratio for the Treatment of Breast Cancer. *Curr. Drug Deliv.* **2019**, *16*, 829–838. [CrossRef] [PubMed]
23. Silva, J.D.O.; Fernandes, R.; Oda, C.M.R.; Ferreira, T.H.; Botelho, A.F.M.; Melo, M.M.; Miranda, M.; Gomes, D.; Cassali, G.D.; Townsend, D.M.; et al. Folate-coated, long-circulating and pH-sensitive liposomes enhance doxorubicin antitumor effect in a breast cancer animal model. *Biomed. Pharmacother.* **2019**, *118*, 109323. [CrossRef] [PubMed]
24. Filippi-Chiela, E.C.; Oliveira, M.M.; Jurkovski, B.; Jacques, S.M.C.; da Silva, V.D.; Lenz, G. Nuclear Morphometric Analysis (NMA): Screening of Senescence, Apoptosis and Nuclear Irregularities. *PLoS ONE* **2012**, *7*, e42522. [CrossRef]
25. Liu, C.-L.; Chen, M.-J.; Lin, J.-C.; Lin, C.-H.; Huang, W.-C.; Cheng, S.-P.; Chen, S.-N.; Chang, Y.-C. Doxorubicin Promotes Migration and Invasion of Breast Cancer Cells through the Upregulation of the RhoA/MLC Pathway. *J. Breast Cancer* **2019**, *22*, 185–195. [CrossRef]
26. Miskey, C.; Botezatu, L.; Temiz, N.A.; Gogol-Döring, A.; Bartha, A.; Győrffy, B.; Largaespada, D.A.; Ivics, Z.; Sebe, A. *In Vitro* Insertional Mutagenesis Screen Identifies Novel Genes Driving Breast Cancer Metastasis. *Mol. Cancer Res.* **2022**, *20*, 1502–1515. [CrossRef]

27. Barenholz, Y. (Chezy) Doxil®—The first FDA-approved nano-drug: Lessons learned. *J. Control. Release* **2012**, *160*, 117–134. [CrossRef]
28. Boratto, F.; Franco, M.; Barros, A.; Cassali, G.; Malachias, A.; Ferreira, L.; Leite, E. Alpha-tocopheryl succinate improves encapsulation, pH-sensitivity, antitumor activity and reduces toxicity of doxorubicin-loaded liposomes. *Eur. J. Pharm. Sci.* **2020**, *144*, 105205. [CrossRef]
29. Silva, J.D.O.; Miranda, S.E.M.; Leite, E.A.; Sabino, A.D.P.; Borges, K.B.G.; Cardoso, V.N.; Cassali, G.D.; Guimarães, A.G.; Oliveira, M.C.; de Barros, A.L.B. Toxicological study of a new doxorubicin-loaded pH-sensitive liposome: A preclinical approach. *Toxicol. Appl. Pharmacol.* **2018**, *352*, 162–169. [CrossRef]
30. Di Bello, E.; Zwergel, C.; Mai, A.; Valente, S. The Innovative Potential of Statins in Cancer: New Targets for New Therapies. *Front. Chem.* **2020**, *8*, 516. [CrossRef]
31. Chen, Y.; Du, Q.; Guo, Q.; Huang, J.; Liu, L.; Shen, X.; Peng, J. A W/O emulsion mediated film dispersion method for curcumin encapsulated pH-sensitive liposomes in the colon tumor treatment. *Drug Dev. Ind. Pharm.* **2019**, *45*, 282–291. [CrossRef] [PubMed]
32. Aggarwal, P.; Hall, J.B.; McLeland, C.B.; Dobrovolskaia, M.A.; McNeil, S.E. Nanoparticle interaction with plasma proteins as it relates to particle biodistribution, biocompatibility and therapeutic efficacy. *Adv. Drug Deliv. Rev.* **2009**, *61*, 428–437. [CrossRef] [PubMed]
33. Lasic, D.; Frederik, P.; Stuart, M.; Barenholz, Y.; McIntosh, T. Gelation of liposome interior A novel method for drug encapsulation. *FEBS Lett.* **1992**, *312*, 255–258. [CrossRef] [PubMed]
34. Lee, M.-K. Liposomes for enhanced bioavailability of water-insoluble drugs: In vivo evidence and recent approaches. *Pharmaceutics* **2020**, *12*, 264. [CrossRef]
35. Mura, P.; Maestrelli, F.; Cirri, M.; Nerli, G.; Di Cesare Mannelli, L.; Ghelardini, C.; Mennini, N. Improvement of Butamben Anesthetic Efficacy by the Development of Deformable Liposomes Bearing the Drug as Cyclodextrin Complex. *Pharmaceutics* **2021**, *13*, 872. [CrossRef]
36. Gomes, E.R.; Carvalho, A.T.; Barbosa, T.C.; Ferreira, L.L.; Calado, H.D.R.; Sabino, A.P.; Oliveira, M.C. Fusion of Tumor-Derived Exosomes with Long-Circulating and pH-Sensitive Liposomes Loaded with Doxorubicin for the Treatment of Breast Cancer. *AAPS PharmSciTech* **2022**, *23*, 255. [CrossRef]
37. Kang, M.; Lee, K.-H.; Lee, H.S.; Jeong, C.W.; Ku, J.H.; Kim, H.H.; Kwak, C. Concurrent treatment with simvastatin and NF-κB inhibitor in human castration-resistant prostate cancer cells exerts synergistic anti-cancer effects via control of the NF-κB/LIN28/let-7 miRNA signaling pathway. *PLoS ONE* **2017**, *12*, e0184644. [CrossRef]
38. Galiullina, L.F.; Scheidt, H.A.; Huster, D.; Aganov, A.; Klochkov, V. Interaction of statins with phospholipid bilayers studied by solid-state NMR spectroscopy. *Biochim. Biophys. Acta (BBA)—Biomembr.* **2019**, *1861*, 584–593. [CrossRef]
39. Yousefnia, S.; Ghaedi, K.; Forootan, F.S.; Esfahani, M.H.N. Characterization of the stemness potency of *mammospheres* isolated from the breast cancer cell lines. *Tumor Biol.* **2019**, *41*, 1010428319869101. [CrossRef]
40. Rezano, A.; Ridhayanti, F.; Rangkuti, A.R.; Gunawan, T.; Winarno, G.N.A.; Wijaya, I. Cytotoxicity of Simvastatin in Human Breast Cancer MCF-7 and MDA-MB-231 Cell Lines. *Asian Pac. J. Cancer Prev.* **2021**, *22*, 33–42. [CrossRef]
41. O'grady, S.; Crown, J.; Duffy, M.J. Statins inhibit proliferation and induce apoptosis in triple-negative breast cancer cells. *Med Oncol.* **2022**, *39*, 142. [CrossRef] [PubMed]
42. Barbălată, C.I.; Porfire, A.S.; Sesarman, A.; Rauca, V.-F.; Banciu, M.; Muntean, D.; Ştiufiuc, R.; Moldovan, A.; Moldovan, C.; Tomuță, I. A Screening Study for the Development of Simvastatin-Doxorubicin Liposomes, a Co-Formulation with Future Perspectives in Colon Cancer Therapy. *Pharmaceutics* **2021**, *13*, 1526. [CrossRef] [PubMed]
43. Xie, L.; Zhu, G.; Shang, J.; Chen, X.; Zhang, C.; Ji, X; Zhang, Q.; Wei, Y. An overview on the biological activity and anti-cancer mechanism of lovastatin. *Cell. Signal.* **2021**, *87*, 110122. [CrossRef] [PubMed]
44. Bai, F.; Yu, Z.; Gao, X.; Gong, J.; Fan, L.; Liu, F. Simvastatin induces breast cancer cell death through oxidative stress up-regulating miR-140-5p. *Aging* **2019**, *11*, 3198–3219. [CrossRef]
45. Franco, M.S.; Oliveira, M.C. Ratiometric drug delivery using non-liposomal nanocarriers as an approach to increase efficacy and safety of combination chemotherapy. *Biomed. Pharmacother.* **2017**, *96*, 584–595. [CrossRef]
46. Li, Y.; Zhai, Y.; Liu, W.; Zhang, K.; Liu, J.; Shi, J.; Zhang, Z. Ultrasmall nanostructured drug based pH-sensitive liposome for effective treatment of drug-resistant tumor. *J. Nanobiotechnology* **2019**, *17*, 117. [CrossRef]
47. Mondal, L.; Mukherjee, B.; Das, K.; Bhattacharya, S.; Dutta, D.; Chakraborty, S.; Pal, M.M.; Gaonkar, R.H.; Debnath, M.C. CD-340 functionalized doxorubicin-loaded nanoparticle induces apoptosis and reduces tumor volume along with drug-related cardiotoxicity in mice. *Int. J. Nanomed.* **2019**, *14*, 8073–8094. [CrossRef]
48. Machado, K.L.; Marinello, P.C.; Silva, T.N.X.; Silva, C.F.N.; Luiz, R.C.; Cecchini, R.; Cecchini, A.L. Oxidative Stress in Caffeine Action on the Proliferation and Death of Human Breast Cancer Cells MCF-7 and MDA-MB-231. *Nutr. Cancer* **2021**, *73*, 1378–1388. [CrossRef]

pharmaceutics

Article

Delicate Hybrid Laponite–Cyclic Poly(ethylene glycol) Nanoparticles as a Potential Drug Delivery System

Shengzhuang Tang [1], Jesse Chen [1], Jayme Cannon [1], Mona Chekuri [1], Mohammad Farazuddin [1,2], James R. Baker, Jr. [1,2] and Su He Wang [1,2,*]

1 Michigan Nanotechnology Institute for Medicine and Biological Sciences and Department of Internal Medicine, University of Michigan, Ann Arbor, MI 48109, USA
2 Division of Allergy, Department of Internal Medicine, University of Michigan, Ann Arbor, MI 48109, USA
* Correspondence: shidasui@umich.edu

Abstract: The objective of the study was to explore the feasibility of a new drug delivery system using laponite (LAP) and cyclic poly(ethylene glycol) (cPEG). Variously shaped and flexible hybrid nanocrystals were made by both the covalent and physical attachment of chemically homogeneous cyclized PEG to laponite nanodisc plates. The size of the resulting, nearly spherical particles ranged from 1 to 1.5 μm, while PEGylation with linear methoxy poly (ethylene glycol) (mPEG) resulted in fragile sheets of different shapes and sizes. When infused with 10% doxorubicin (DOX), a drug commonly used in the treatment of various cancers, the LAP-cPEG/DOX formulation was transparent and maintained liquid-like homogeneity without delamination, and the drug loading efficiency of the LAP-cPEG nano system was found to be higher than that of the laponite-poly(ethylene glycol) LAP-mPEG system. Furthermore, the LAP-cPEG/DOX formulation showed relative stability in phosphate-buffered saline (PBS) with only 15% of the drug released. However, in the presence of human plasma, about 90% of the drug was released continuously over a period of 24 h for the LAP-cPEG/DOX, while the LAP-mPEG/DOX formulation released 90% of DOX in a 6 h burst. The results of the cell viability assay indicated that the LAP-cPEG/DOX formulation could effectively inhibit the proliferation of A549 lung carcinoma epithelial cells. With the DOX concentration in the range of 1–2 μM in the LAP-cPEG/DOX formulation, enhanced drug effects in both A549 lung carcinoma epithelial cells and primary lung epithelial cells were observed compared to LAP-mPEG/DOX. The unique properties and effects of cPEG nanoparticles provide a potentially better drug delivery system and generate interest for further targeting studies and applications.

Keywords: functional cyclized polyethylene glycol; PEGylation of laponite; hybrid nanoparticles; drug delivery

Citation: Tang, S.; Chen, J.; Cannon, J.; Chekuri, M.; Farazuddin, M.; Baker, J.R., Jr.; Wang, S.H. Delicate Hybrid Laponite–Cyclic Poly(ethylene glycol) Nanoparticles as a Potential Drug Delivery System. *Pharmaceutics* **2023**, *15*, 1998. https://doi.org/10.3390/pharmaceutics15071998

Academic Editors: Raquel Fernández García, Francisco Bolás-Fernández, Ana Isabel Fraguas-Sánchez and Inge S. Zuhorn

Received: 27 March 2023
Revised: 13 June 2023
Accepted: 20 June 2023
Published: 21 July 2023

1. Introduction

Following recent advancements in biomaterials and nanotechnology, drug delivery has undergone enormous developments [1–3]. With their flexibility and durability, hybrid organic–inorganic nanomaterials are considered a potential platform with applications in chemistry, physics, life sciences, medicine, and technology [4]. Hybrid nanomaterials based on silicate present an interesting group of materials due to their natural and widely used properties. In the last two decades, laponite (LAP), a synthetic magnesium silicate clay, has emerged as a novel drug delivery nanoplatform [5–7]. The dimension of this disc-shaped particle is 25 nm in diameter and 1 nm in thickness with a relatively stable chemical formula of $Na^{+0.7}[(Mg_{5.5}Li_{0.3})Si_8O_{20}(OH)_4]^{-0.7}$ [8]. The LAP nanoparticle has a net negatively charged plane and an unstable positively charged edge due to the release of sodium ions on its surface and the protonation of its hydroxyl groups on its edge. Electrostatic interactions amongst the surfaces and edges of the nano discs allows LAP to present as a homogenous dispersion, suspension, or gel, independent of the aqueous system [9,10]. The most basic application of the LAP nanoparticle is a drug–clay hybrid formula that uses the direct mixing of a drug with a LAP aqueous system, and then centrifugation to sediment the composite from solution. The resulting complex may also be further coated with polymer materials for a better release profile.

Chen et al. investigated the absorption of LAP nanoparticles with the enterohemorrhagic E. coli (EHEC) protein and found that the LAP nano-adjuvant was able to induce efficient humoral and cellular immune responses against the EHEC antigen [11]. Kalwar et al. centrifuged an LAP/ciprofloxacin complex, which was then disseminated into polycaprolactone to make nanofibers for more sustained drug release [12]. The silanol group, SiOH, on the edge of the clay sheet creates the potential to chemically modify clay for better solubility and organophilicity. Modifying the edge of the LAP clay using alkoxy silanes possessing additional primary amine groups has been reported by Wheeler et al. [13], allowing more complex polymers to be covalently grafted to the LAP nanoplate, creating a stable hybrid nanomaterial with an inorganic core. For example, a second generation of poly(amidoamine) dendrimer has been conjugated to the LAP nanoplate as a dendrimer-functionalized LAP hybrid nanomaterial [14]. After accreting doxorubicin (DOX), the dispersed composites demonstrated a pH-dependent sustained release profile and more potent inhibitory activities against KB human epithelial cancer cells than free DOX [14].

The excessive accumulation of LAP nano discs might lead to precipitation, so improving the dispersion stability of LAP particles would be a key to enhancing their performance. Polymers are one of the most commonly used stabilizers of inorganic particles such as silicate particles and gold nanoparticles (AuNPs). For example, Ling et al. illustrated different degrees of stability of poly(ethylene glycol) (PEG)-coated AuNPs based on the molecular weight of the linear PEGs used [15]. By adding sodium chloride, the coated AuNPs present visual color changes. Furthermore, the treatment of LAP silicate clay with poly(ethyleneoxide)alkyl ether enhanced stability and resulted in a nanocomposite suspension with spherical particles ranging from 70 nm to 1 μm [16]. Additionally, Gaharwar et al. cross-linked LAP with PEG to make a PEG-silicate nanocomposite hydrogel with flexible interconnective pores, which proved to be mechanically strong and structurally stable while maintaining a high water content [17]. In comparison with linear polymers, cyclized polymers exhibit distinct properties: higher density, higher glass transition temperature, smaller hydrodynamic volume, and lower viscosity [18,19]. By mixing cyclic poly(ethylene glycol) (c-PEG) with AuNPs, Wang et al. proved that physiosorbed c-PEG drastically enhanced the dispersion stability of AuNPs against an external environment and physiological conditions when compared with its linear counterpart [20].

To improve the drug delivery performance, we designed novel hybrid nanoparticles using LAP and cyclic PEG. We first synthesized cyclic PEG with an extra active OH group (cPEG-OH) by which the cyclic PEG was covalently attached to the LAP nanoplate. The chemical homogeneity of synthesized cPEG-OH was confirmed by NMR spectroscopy, specifically ^{13}C NMR, mass spectrometry (MS), and gel permeation chromatography (GPC). Moreover, the cPEGylation of LAP to construct the hybrid LAP-cPEG system was characterized by Fourier-transform infrared (FTIR) spectroscopy, ^{1}H NMR spectroscopy, dynamic light scattering (DLS), and scanning electron microscopy (SEM). Furthermore, the anticancer drug DOX was captured in the LAP-cPEG system, and the release profile of the LAP-cPEG/DOX formulation was determined in the presence of human plasma. Additionally, the in vitro cytotoxic effect of the LAP-cPEG/DOX formulation was measured by XTT and flow cytometric assays after incubation with A549 lung cancer cells or primary lung epithelial cells.

2. Materials and Methods

2.1. Materials

LAP (laponite-FN) was provided by BYK Netherlands B.V. (Deventer, Netherlands). Poly (ethylene glycol) 2000 (PEG); methoxy poly (ethylene glycol) 2000 (mPEG); DOX·HCl were obtained from AvaChem Scientific (San Antonio, TX, USA). 4-Nitrophenyl chloroformate;

1,3-diamino-2-propanol (Dimethylamino) pyridine (DMAP); N,N-diisopropylethylamine (DiPEA); 3-aminopropyldimethylethoxysilane (APMES); sodium hydroxide; hydrochloric acid and XTT reagents were all purchased from Sigma-Aldrich (St. Louis, MO, USA). A549 cells were purchased from Japanese Collection of Research Bioresources (JRCB) Cell Bank (Tokyo, Japan). Trypsin-EDTA 0.25%, 7-aminoactinomycin (7-AAD), Fixable Viability Dye eFluor™ 450 were obtained from Thermo Fisher Scientific (Waltham, MA, USA). Alexa Fluor® 647 anti-mouse CD326 (EpCAM) was purchased from BioLegend (San Diego, CA, USA). All solvents were purchased from Sigma-Aldrich and used as received. Deionized (DI) water was used in all the experiments. Dialysis membranes were purchased from Spectrum Laboratories (Rancho Dominquez, CA, USA).

2.2. Synthesis of LAP-cPEG Nanoparticles

The fundamental reaction was achieved by preparing the functional cyclic PEG (cPEG-OH). In the current study, cyclized PEG chains were synthesized by a practical and reliable method. First, to make LAP more active, the LAP nano discs were modified with amino groups via a condensation reaction of the LAP's silanol groups with 3-aminopropyldimethylethoxysilane (APMES) to form LAP-NH_2 (Scheme 1), as described in previous publications [13,14].

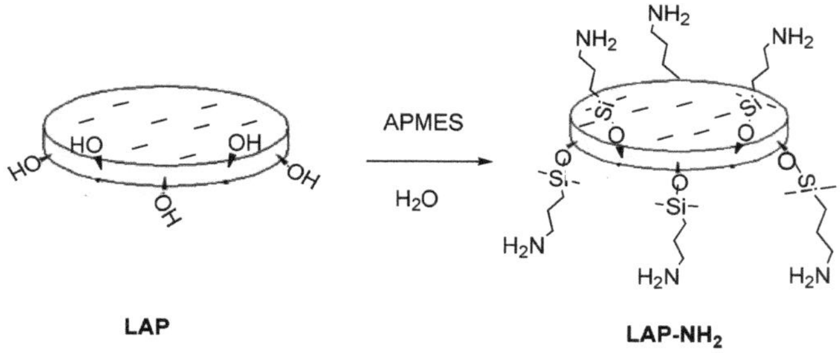

Scheme 1. Representation of a sheet of laponite (LAP) changed to LAP-NH_2.

Meanwhile, as shown in Scheme 2, medium-sized PEG2000 was activated with 4-nitrophenyl chloroformate in the presence of DMAP to form polyethylene glycol dinitrophenyl carbonate (PEG-NP). Purified PEG-NP was treated with equivalent 1,3-diamino-2-propanol to "lock" the terminals of PEG under dilute dichloromethane (DCM) solution in the presence of DiPEA. Thus, a cyclic PEG with a bare hydroxy group was constructed.

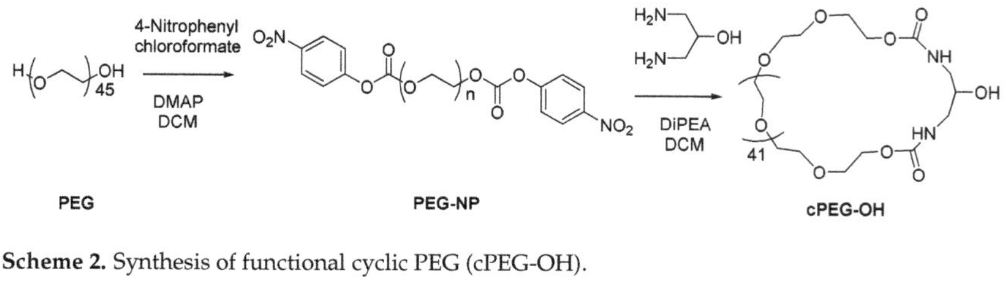

Scheme 2. Synthesis of functional cyclic PEG (cPEG-OH).

Using the same method for the activation of PEG, the desired product (cPEG-OH) was also activated to form cPEG-NP and was then ready for coupling. The active cPEG-NP was treated with LAP-NH_2 to construct hybrid LAP-cPEG particles (Scheme 3).

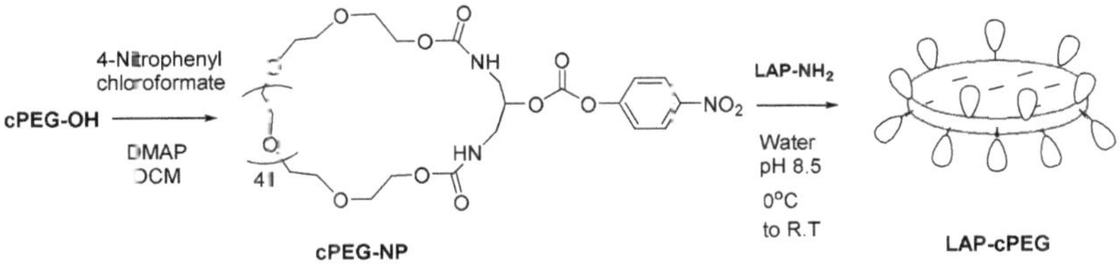

Scheme 3. Representation of covalent attachment of cyclic PEG to LAP.

To be used for comparison, linear mPEG with the same molecular weight as PEG was activated and then coupled to LAP nanoplates using the same procedure as above, forming the LAP-mPEG system (Scheme 4).

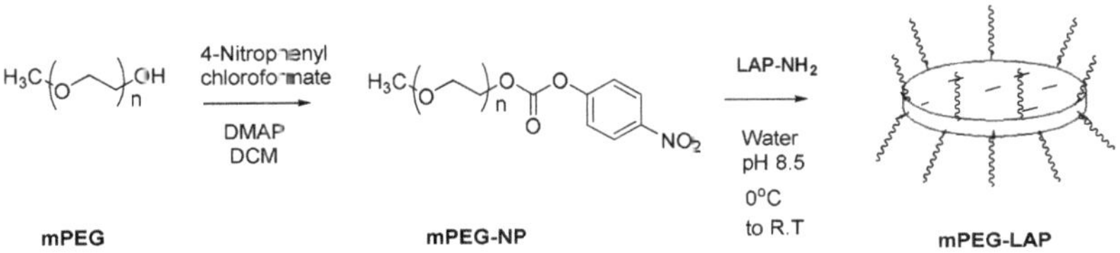

Scheme 4. Representation of covalent attachment of linear mPEG to LAP.

2.2.1. Procedure for Activation of PEG, mPEG, and cPEG

A single-step method for activation of PEG using 4-nitrophenyl chloroformate (4-NPCl) can produce a series of reactive PEG-phenylcarbonate derivatives. The PEG intermediates are stable for storage, and reaction with amino groups proceeds rapidly at near-neutral pH [21,22].

4-Nitrophenyl chloroformate (3 equiv) in DCM (100 mg/mL) and DMAP (3 equiv) in DCM (100 mg/mL) were added into separate solutions of PEG, mPEG, and cPEG (1 equiv) in DCM (50 mg/mL). The mixtures, now containing PEG-NP, mPEG-NP, and cPEG-NP, were stirred for 16 h at room temperature. After DCM was removed by rotatory evaporation, the residues were triturated from diethyl ether (50 mg/mL, 4 times), re-dissolved in DCM (50 mg/mL), washed with 1 M HCl (50 mg/mL, 2 times), and then with water (50 mg/mL). The resulting solutions were slowly added to an excess volume of diethyl ether (DCM:ether in a 1:10 ratio). The precipitates were filtered and washed with ether and then dried under vacuum.

For production of PEG-NP: activation of PEG (2.0 g, 1.0 mmol) yielded PEG-NP as a white solid (1.4 g, 60%). ^{1}H NMR (500 MHz, $CDCl_3$): δ 8.28–8.26 (d, J = 10 Hz, 4H, 4ArH-NP), 7.40–7.38 (d, J = 10 Hz, 4H, 4ArH-NP), 4.44–4.42 (t, J = 5 Hz, 4H, $2CH_2O$-(C=O)), 3.82–3.80 (t, J = 5 Hz, 4H, $2CH_2O$-(PEG)), 3.69–3.64 (m, PEG backbone) ppm.

For production of mPEG-NP: activation of mPEG (2.0 g, 1.0 mmol) yielded mPEG-NP as a white solid (1.9 g, 88%). ^{1}H NMR (500 MHz, $CDCl_3$): δ 8.29–8.27 (d, J = 10 Hz, 2H, 2ArH-NP), 7.40–7.38 (d, J = 10 Hz, 2H, 2ArH-NP), 4.44–4.42 (t, J = 5 Hz, 2H, CH_2O-(C=O)), 3.82–3.80 (t, J = 5 Hz, 2H, CH_2O-(PEG)), 3.69–3.54 (m, PEG backbone), 3.37 (s, 3H, CH_3O) ppm.

For production of cPEG-NP: activation of cPEG (212 mg, 0.1 mmol) yielded PEG-NP as a white solid (186 mg, 81%). ^{1}H NMR (500 MHz, $CDCl_3$): δ 8.28–8.26 (d, J = 10 Hz, 2H, 2ArH-NP), 7.44–7.42 (d, J = 10 Hz,2H, 2ArH-NP), 5.69 (br s, 2H, 2NH), 4.79 (m, 1H, CHO-(C=O)), 4.23–4.21 (t, J = 5 Hz, 4H, $2CH_2O$-(C=O)), 3.78–3.58 (m, PEG backbone) 3.50–3.39 (m, 4H, $2CH_2N$) ppm. ^{13}C (500 MHz, $CDCl_3$): δ 156.98 (NC=O), 155.45 (OC=O), 151.70 (ArC-NP), 145.40 (ArC-NP), 125.23 (ArC-NP), 121.96 (ArC-NP), 70.50 (PEG backbone), 69.39 (CH_2O-(C=O)), 64.25 (CH_2O-(PEG)), 40.04 (CH_2N) ppm.

2.2.2. Cyclization of PEG-NP to Form cPEG-OH

PEG-NP (300 mg, 0.13 mmol) was dissolved in DCM (300 mL) and cooled in an ice-water bath. A solution of 1,3-diamino-2-propanol (13 mg, 0.14 mmol) in DCM (13 mL) was added dropwise, followed by the addition of DiPEA (136 μL, 0.78 mmol). After being stirred for 24 h at 3–5 °C, the reaction mixture was allowed to warm up to room temperature and was then stirred for another 24 h. The resulting solution was concentrated by rotatory evaporation to 3 mL and slowly added to 30 mL of diethyl ether. The precipitate was filtered and washed with ether, and then further purified by flash column chromatography by eluting with 10% methanol in DCM. The eluted product was triturated from ether, filtered, and dried under vacuum to yield an off-white solid (177 mg, 64%). ^{1}H NMR (500 MHz, $CDCl_3$): δ 5.66 (br s, 2H, 2NH), 4.22–4.20 (t, J = 5 Hz, 4H, $2CH_2O$-(C=O)), 3.79–3.64 (m, PEG backbone), 3.51–3.49 (m, 1H, CHO), 3.28–3.27 (m, 2H, CH_2N), 3.19–3.16 (m, 2H, CH_2N). ^{13}C NMR (500 MHz, $CDCl_3$): δ 157.29 (C=O), 70.52 (PEG backbone), 70.00 (CHO), 69.48 (CH_2O-(PEG)), 64.02 (CH_2O-(C=O), 40.01 (CH_2N) ppm.

2.2.3. Modification of LAP to Form LAP-NH_2

LAP powder (100 mg) was suspended in water (80 mL) and stirred while heating at 50 °C overnight for an aqueous dispersion. Then, 32 mL of APMES aqueous solution (2% *w*/*w*, i.e., 1 mL of APMES was combined with 40 mL of water) was added dropwise under vigorous stirring. After stirring at 50 °C for 36 h, the reaction mixture was dialyzed against water (12 times over 3 days) using a dialysis membrane with a molecular weight cut-off (MWCO) of 15,000. The obtained aqueous solution was lyophilized to give a colorless solid LAP-NH_2 (74 mg).

2.2.4. PEGylation of LAP with mPEG or cPEG to Form LAP-mPEG or LAP-cPEG

First, 60 mg of activated mPEG-NP or cPEG-NP dissolved in acetonitrile (2 mL) was added to 20 mL of an LAP-NH_2 suspension (1 mg/mL) cooled in an ice-water bath. After stirring for 24 h at 3–5 °C, 1 drop of 1N NaOH was added to maintain the reaction mixture at a pH of 8–9. The mixture was stirred for another 24 h at 3–5 °C and then moved to room temperature and stirred overnight. The clear yellow solution was dialyzed against water (pH 8, 2 times), and water (pH 7.4, 10 times) using a dialysis membrane with an MWCO of 15,000. The final solution was lyophilized to give white solid LAP-mPEG (36 mg) or LAP-cPEG (31 mg).

2.3. LAP-PEG/DOX Formulation

LAP-PEG/DOX was formulated by mixing 10% (*w*/*w*) DOX·HCl with LAP-PEG (LAP-mPEG or LAP-cPEG) in water. First, 0.16 mL of DOX·HCl aqueous solution (5 mg/mL) was added to 8 mL of LAP-PEG solution (1 mg/mL). The mixture was stirred for 24 h at room temperature in the dark. The resulting solution was dialyzed against water (150 mL, 4 times) over 36 h in the dark using a membrane with a MWCO of 15,000. The LAP-PEG/DOX (LAP-mPEG/DOX or LAP-cPEG/DOX) formulation in the membrane bag was collected and stored at 3–5 °C in the dark for further application. Meanwhile, the combined dialysis medium was concentrated by rotatory evaporation in reduced pressure and analyzed by UV–Vis with a lambda 25 UV–Vis spectrophotometer (PerkinElmer, Waltham, MA, USA) at 480 nm. The amount of unencapsulated free DOX was determined using a DOX calibration curve. The DOX loading efficiency was determined using the following equation:

$$\text{DOX loading efficiency} = \frac{\text{Mass of feeding DOX} - \text{Mass free DOX}}{\text{Mass of feeding DOX}} \times 100\%$$

2.4. In Vitro DOX Release Kinetics from LAP-cPEG/DOX Formulation

The drug release kinetics of the LAP-cPEG/DOX formulation was determined in the presence of PBS or human plasma. Briefly, 1.8 mL of the formulation was mixed well with 0.2 mL of either PBS or human plasma and transferred to a dialysis bag with an MWCO of 15,000. The dialysis bag was then placed in 18 mL of PBS while stirring. At each time interval (0, 0.33, 1, 3, 6, 12, 24 and 48 h), 0.6 mL of PBS buffer was taken for UV analysis and replaced with an equal volume of fresh PBS solution. The concentration of DOX in the dialysis medium was measured using a Lambda 25 UV–Vis spectrophotometer at 480 nm. For comparison, DOX released from the LAP-mPEG/DOX formulation in the presence of plasma was conduct in the same manner.

2.5. Antitumor Efficacy of LAP-cPEG/DOX Formulation

2.5.1. XTT Assay

Cell viability was performed via the XTT assay for A549 cells. Cells were planted (15,000 cells/well) in a 96-well tissue culture plate with medium composed of RPMI, 10% FBS, and 1% Pen–Strep, and incubated at 37 °C with 5% CO_2 overnight. The cells were then fed with DOX, LAP-mPEG/DOX, and LAP-cPEG/DOX to reach the applied DOX concentrations. After 48 h, the supernatants were removed, PBS and XTT reagents were added, and the plate was again incubated for two hours. Using the Synergy HT plate reader (BioTek Instruments; Winooski, VT, USA), the absorbance could be measured as an indication of cell viability, determined from the optical density differences at 690 nm and 492 nm.

2.5.2. Flow Cytometric Assay

A549 cell death was analyzed by 7-AAD staining assay. Primary lung cell death was analyzed by staining with EpCAM (CD326) and Fixable Viability Dye. Briefly, A549 cells (2×10^5) or lung primary cells (1×10^6 cells) were seeded in 48-well plates and incubated at 37 °C with 5% CO_2 overnight. Concentrated DOX, LAP-mPEG/DOX, or LAP-cPEG/DOX was added to the wells to reach the DOX therapeutic concentration of 0.75 and 1.25 μM for A549 cells or 2 μM for primary lung cells. After 24 h of treatment, cells were trypsinized, washed twice with FBS, stained, and analyzed on the flow cytometer (Novocyte, Agilent, Santa Clara, CA, USA). Flow cytometric data were analyzed using Flow-Jo V10.9 software.

3. Results and Discussion

3.1. Synthesis of Functional Cyclic PEG

Various approaches to the cyclization of PEG have been attempted [23–25]. One of these studies prepared an early version of the fully closed cyclic PEGs as large crown ethers, based on the Williamson reaction in the presence of powdered KOH, a harsh reaction condition [23]. Another common approach uses "click" chemistry, regarded as a mild way to cyclize polymers. A no outlet PEG copolymer was cyclized by click reaction chemistry in the presence of copper cations based on traditional click chemistry [24]. A tadpole-shaped functional copolymer was made by coupling azido-terminated PEG with a dialkyne-terminated polymer [25]. As a result, heavy metals were ultimately introduced to the system due to the formation of stable PEG (Cu^+) complexes [26,27]. This study provided a gentle approach to synthesize chemically homogeneous cyclic PEG with extra functional groups.

^{13}C and ^{1}H NMR spectroscopy were used to analyze the cyclic PEG product. As shown in the comparison of the ^{13}C spectra of PEG, cPEG-OH, and cPEG-NP (Figure 1a), the signals of neighboring methylene carbons ($HO-CH_2-CH_2-PEG-CH_2-CH_2-OH$) of hydroxyl groups at the end of PEG appeared at 72.41 and 61.54 ppm, respectively. After cyclization, the signals moved to 69.48 ppm and 64.02 ppm, respectively. Meanwhile, new single signals appeared at 157.29, 70.00, and 40.01 ppm, belonging to a formed carbonyl carbon and the methylidyne and methylene carbons of 1,3-diamino-2-propanol on cyclized PEG rings, respectively. After activation of cPEG with 4-nitrophenyl chloroformate (4-NPCl) to form cPEG-NP, signals for a new carbamate bond and nitrophenyl group appeared clearly, while the resonance peak of the methylidyne carbon on the cPEG ring shifted downfield due to carbamation. Correspondingly, in the ^{1}H spectrum (Figure 1b), after cyclization to form cPEG, the resonance peaks at 3.51–3.49 and 3.28–3.16 ppm representing methylidyne and methylene protons on diamino-propanol were observed, while the resonance peaks of the methylene protons on the terminal PEG backbone shifted downfield due to the formation of the carbamate bond. Nitrophenyl chloroformate activation of cPEG led to a significant downfield shift for the methylidyne proton on the cPEG ring while new resonance peaks of nitrophenyl protons were present after carbamation.

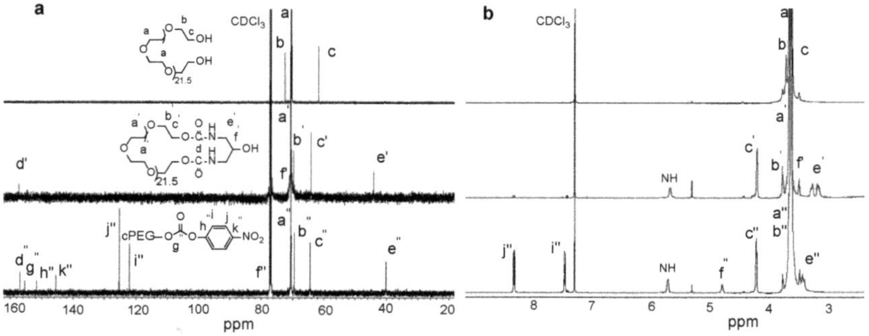

Figure 1. ^{13}C NMR spectra (**a**), and ^{1}H NMR spectra (**b**) of PEG, cPEG-OH, and cPEG-NP in deuterated chloroform $CDCl_3$.

Mass spectrometry (MS) was used to analyze the molecular weight changes in the reaction products. The mass spectra showed an overall increase in molecular weight, centering at 1940.1 for cPEG-OH and 1797.0 for PEG (Figure 2a), in which each peak distribution in cyclic PEG matched well with the precursor by an increase of ca. 142, which corresponds to the molar mass of the monomer lock unit. Incidentally, a regular *m/z* interval of ca. 44 was observed between neighboring peaks in each distribution for both linear and cyclic PEG, which corresponds to the molar mass of the PEG backbone units.

Gel permeation chromatography (GPC) was used to monitor the changes in linear PEG and cyclic PEG after the reaction. The observed GPC chromatogram of cPEG-OH was unimodal with Mw/Mn = 1.11, compared to mPEG and PEG with Mw/Mn = 1.11 and 1.12, respectively, by the same PEG analytic approach (Figure 2b). While the linear mPEG and PEG had similar retention times, cPEG-OH exhibited a distinctly longer retention time, indicating that the cyclic topology changes the hydrodynamic properties of PEG significantly.

^{13}C and ^{1}H NMR spectroscopy, mass spectrometry (MS), and gel permeation chromatography (GPC) results indicate cPEG-OH is a homogeneous product without linear PEG mixtures.

3.2. PEGylation of Laponite with cPEG and mPEG

The generic route for covalent modification of the LAP surface with additional activated amine groups was previously reported [8,9]. After modification, cPEG-OH or linear mPEG can be covalently attached to LAP nanoplates by the treatment of activated cPEG-NP or mPEG-NP with primary amine-functionalized LAP nanoplates (LAP-NH_2). As a result of PEGylation, cyclic PEG or linear mPEG molecules were both covalently and non-covalently attached to LAP, respectively. With the minimum loss of LAP during dialysis, there was a 55% weight increase with LAP-cPEG and an 80% weight increase with LAP-mPEG, indicating the composition ratio of LAP:cPEG was about 2:1 for LAP-cPEG, but 2:1.6 for LAP-mPEG.

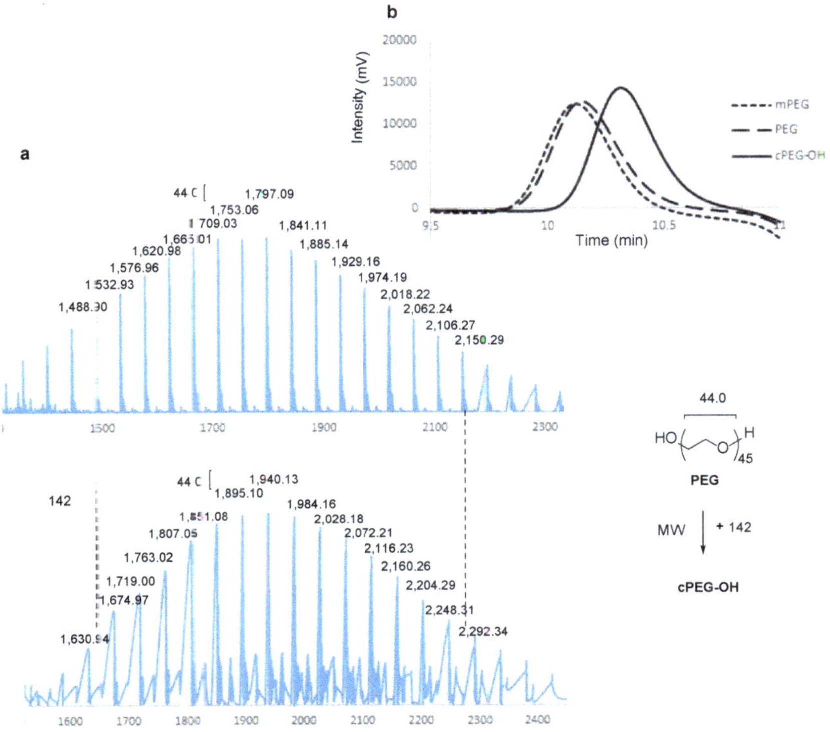

Figure 2. Representative mass spectra of PEG and cPEG-OH (**a**); gel permeation chromatography traces of mPEG, PEG, and cPEG-OH (**b**).

Fourier transform infrared (FTIR) and ^{1}H NMR spectra were used to verify the PEGylation of LAP. As shown in Figure 3a, all the FTIR signals of cPEG-OH were reflected on LAP-cPEG. The peak at 1648 cm^{-1} could be assigned to the carbamate bond formed between cPEG and LAP. In Figure 3b, the PEG backbone has a signal at 3.70 ppm that was observed after PEGylation, and the weaker signals at 3.30 to 3.10 ppm corresponded to the methylene groups of the lock molecule diamino-2-propanol in the LAP-cPEG system. Notably, the signal corresponding to the methylidyne proton in cPEG ring shifted from 3.55 to 4.42 ppm, confirming the formation of the carbamate bond between LAP and cPEG. Moreover, the corresponding integral of the signal ratio is 1:9, indicating that the ratio of covalently attached cPEG: non-covalently attached cPEG is about 1:2 (Supplementary Figure S2). Similarly, FTIR and NMR studies confirmed the successful coupling of linear mPEG to LAP. An FTIR signal at 1647 cm^{-1} was observed in LAP-mPEG, confirming the formation of the carbonyl bond between mPEG and LAP (Supplementary Figure S3a). In the NMR spectra (Supplementary Figure S3b), an expected peak at 4.65 observed in LAP-mPEG corresponded to the protons adjacent to the terminal hydroxy groups in mPEG while forming the carbamate, and the peak at 3.38 ppm corresponded to the terminal methyl group of mPEG.

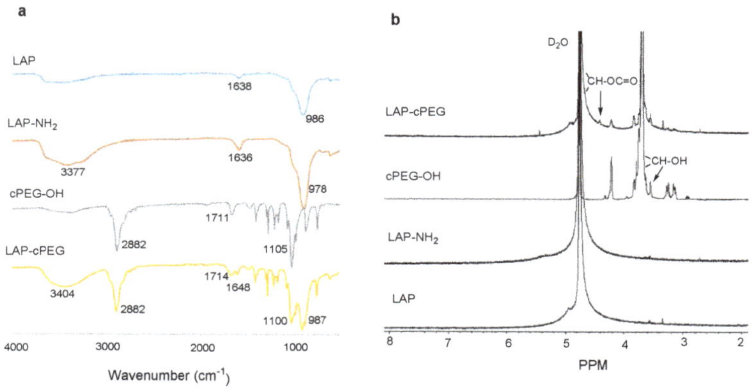

Figure 3. FTIR spectra (**a**) and ^1H NMR spectra (**b**) of LAP, LAP-NH_2, cPEG-OH, and LAP-cPEG.

3.3. Microstructure of PEG-cPEG Particle System

To investigate the size and shape of the synthesized LAP-PEG nano system, a scanning electron microscope (SEM) was used. While LAP particles physically absorbed PEG copolymer surfactant (Brij58) to form rough and stiff spheres ranging from 70 nm to 1000 nm [16] and while cross-linked by PEG copolymer chains led to a tough cellular fiber structure [17], LAP particles attached by cyclic PEG resulted in a distinguishable well-defined structure, a flexible and nearly spherical particle of about 1 μm (Figure 4(a-1,a-2)), in contrast to the attachment of linear PEG, which led to an irregular fiber sheet (Figure 4(b-1,b-2)). cPEGylation of LAP resulted in a stable LAP-PEG system as expected. Higher accumulation of LAP might lead to precipitation from the LAP suspension; however, owing to the specific properties of cPEG, LAP-cPEG remains a clear liquid without precipitate even when stored at lower temperature for longer times (Supplementary Figure S4). The cPEG endows inorganic LAP particles with greater hydrophilicity and organophilicity.

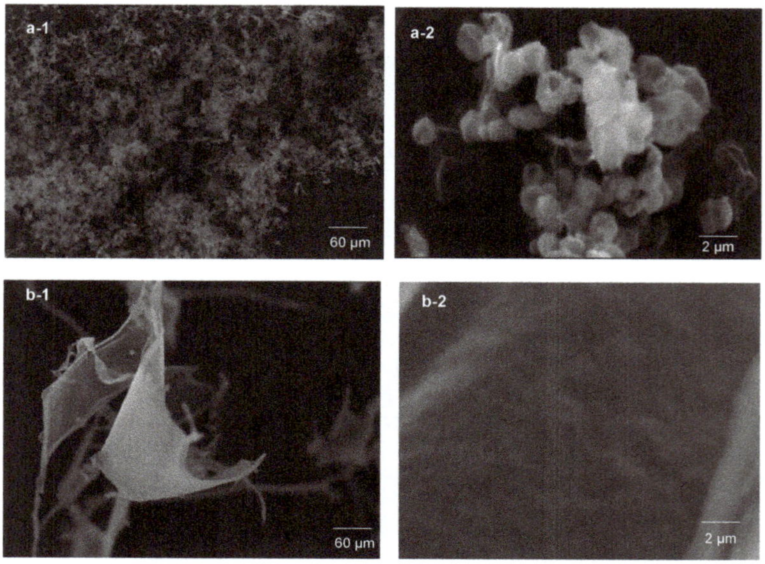

Figure 4. Scanning electron micrographs of LAP-cPEG and LAP-mPEG at magnifications of ×500 (**a-1**,**b-1**) and ×15,000 (**a-2**,**b-2**).

3.4. Dynamic Light Scattering (DLS) Characterization of PEG-cPEG Nanoparticles

The average hydrodynamic size of native LAP varies greatly from 100 nm to 300 nm depending on concentration, which is attributed to the stacking of LAP disc crystals in water [16]. Dynamic light scattering (DLS) was used to monitor the changes in hydrodynamic size and zeta potential of modified LAP (Figure 5). In the study, solid samples of LAP, LAP-NH_2, and synthesized LAP-PEG were dispersed in water at a concentration of 0.05 mg/mL for DLS analyses. As summarized in Table 1, from LAP to LAP-NH_2, a slight increase in average size and remarkable increase in average zeta potential were due to the modification of the LAP discs with amine groups, which are positively charged by protonation. The subsequent PEGylation of LAP discs with PEG leads to the expansion of average hydrodynamic size, and the recovery of average zeta potential due to the conversion of amine groups to carbamate groups after coupling. The hydrodynamic size for LAP-cPEG centered at 4661 nm is larger than the size of the mono LAP-cPEG nanoparticle, with an SEM measurement at roughly 1000 nm, indicating the higher order cluster behavior of LAP-cPEG nanoparticles.

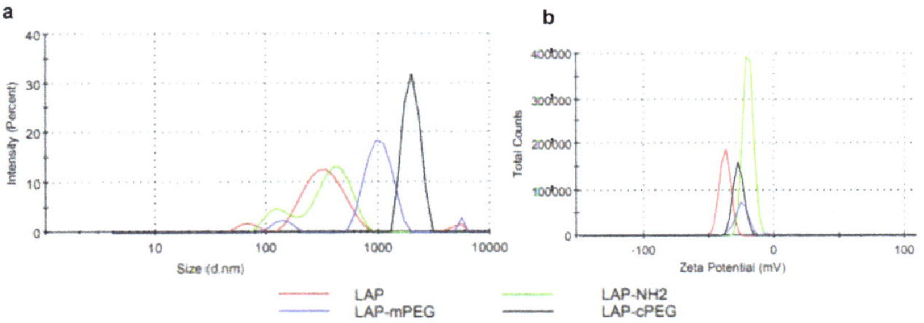

Figure 5. Dynamic light scattering for LAP, LAP–NH_2, LAP–mPEG, and LAP–cPEG at the same concentration of 0.05 mg/mL: hydrodynamic size (**a**) and zeta potential (**b**).

Table 1. Zeta potential, hydrodynamic size, and polydispersity of LAP, LAPNH_2, LAPm-PEG, and LAP-cPEG.

Nanoparticles	Hydrodynamic Size (nm)	Zeta Potential (mV)	Polydispersity (PDI)
LAP	284 ± 6	−37.5 ± 0.7	0.32
LAP-NH_2	360 ± 19	−18.8 ± 1.2	0.52
LAP-mPEG	2653 ± 42	−30.7 ± 5.5	0.85
LAP-cPEG	4661 ± 32	−27.2 ± 3.2	0.41

3.5. Primary Studies of LAP–cPEG/DOX Formulation

3.5.1. LAP–cPEG/DOX Formulation

In this study, 10% DOX was mixed well with LAP-cPEG (1 mg/mL) and then dialyzed against water using a membrane with an MWCO of 15,000 to remove any remaining DOX. The combined dialysates with free DOX were concentrated and quantified by UV–Vis using a standard curve as described in the Supplementary Materials. The drug loading efficiency of LAP-cPEG was found to be 64%, which was higher than that of mPEG (46%). In contrast, when 10% DOX was fed with LAP (1 mg/mL), the LAP/DOX complex precipitated from the solution during dialysis (Supplementary Figure S5).

The encapsulation of DOX in LAP-cPEG was confirmed by UV–Vis spectroscopy. The characteristic peak of DOX was observed in the absorption spectrum of the LAP-cPEG/DOX formulation with an absorption maximum at around 480 nm (Figure 6a). With its liquid-like properties, the LAP-cPEG/DOX formulation could be characterized by ultra-performance liquid chromatography (UPLC) chromatography. The retention time of the composite slightly lagged in contrast to DOX alone (Figure 6b).

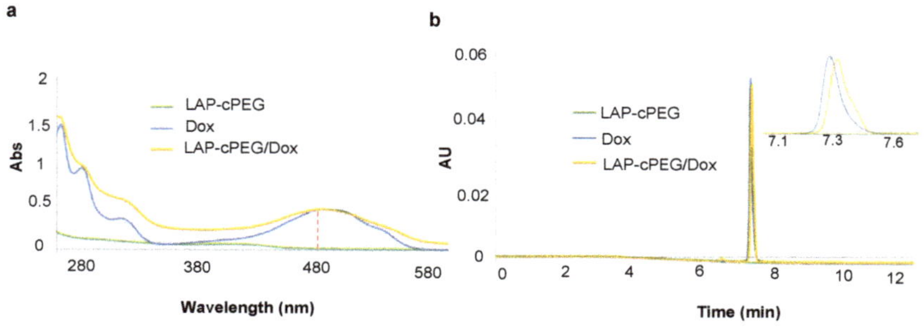

Figure 6. UV–Vis spectra (**a**) and UPLC chromatogram (UV traces at 480 nm) (**b**) representative of aqueous solutions of LAP-cPEG, DOX, and LAP-cPEG/DOX.

3.5.2. In Vitro Release Studies

The quantitative drug release profile in human plasma was determined by means of dialysis as described in the Supplementary materials. With the 15 kDa membrane, the free DOX was able to diffuse across the membrane and into the outer medium, which was measured by UV–Vis spectroscopy at predetermined time intervals. As shown in Figure 7a, in the presence of human plasma, compared to the LAP-mPEG/DOX formulation with a burst release of drug at 6 h, the LAP-cPEG/DOX formulation showed a prolonged release profile over 24 h. In the presence of PBS, while almost 100% of DOX was released from DOX solution in less than 3 h, only 15% of the drug was released from the LAP-cPEG/DOX system, indicating that the LAP-cPEG/DOX formulation remained stable in aqueous PBS. Free DOX would form a red precipitate in PBS due to the formation of covalently bonded DOX dimers [28]. Additionally, due to the degradation of free DOX in the presence of plasma [29], a reduction in the concentration of DOX in the measured solution was observed (Figure 7a).

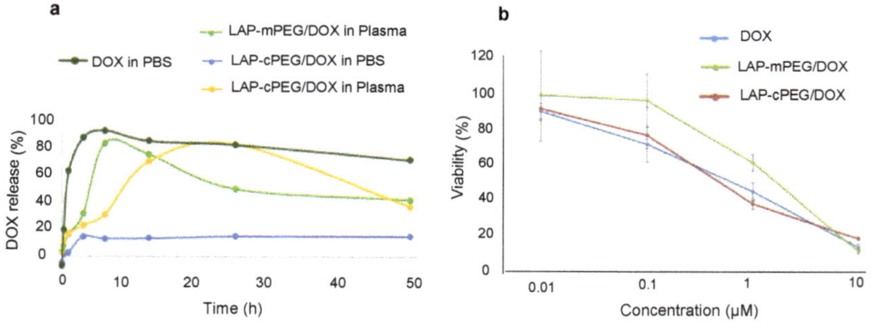

Figure 7. In vitro release profile from a dialysis bag of DOX in the free form, LAP-cPEG/Dox formulation in the presence of PBS or human plasma, and LAP-mPEG/DOX formation in human plasma (**a**); in vitro XTT cell viability assay of A549 cells treated with free DOX, LAP-mPEG/DOX, and LAP-cPEG/DOX at different DOX concentrations for 48 h (**b**).

3.5.3. Efficacy of LAP-cPEG/DOX Formulation on A549 Cell Growth Inhibition

After a 48-h incubation, A549 cells had similar levels of viability with DOX or LAP-cPEG/DOX (Figure 7b), suggesting that the DOX in the hybrid nanoparticles can still effectively inhibit cancer cell proliferation. While there was delayed and slow release of DOX from the delivery system, the A549 cell growth inhibition by LAP-cPEG/DOX was found to be similar to DOX in the free form. This indicates that the synthesized LAP-cPEG is functional and has potential as a novel drug delivery system. The OD value in each group was normalized against the OD value in cells cultured with only the appropriate medium.

3.5.4. Increased Drug Efficacy in LAP-cPEG/DOX in Comparison with LAP-mPEG/DOX

At lower DOX concentrations (<0.01 µM), DOX or its LAP-PEG formulations did not affect the survival of A549 cells, while at high DOX doses (e.g., 10 µM) , DOX or its LAP-PEG formulations demonstrated similar effects such that almost all A549 cells were killed indiscriminately. In this study, A549 cells were treated with either DOX alone or LAP-PEG/DOX formulations with a final DOX concentration, representing 0.75, 1, and 1.25 µM for 24 h. As summarized in Figure 8, a similar trend was seen in both DOX and LAP-cPEG/DOX treatments, in which cell survival decreased along with increased DOX concentration, whereas cells treated with LAP-mPEG/DOX maintained a consistently higher survival rate. At a DOX concentration of 1 µM or 1.25 µM, LAP-cPEG/DOX was twice as efficient as LAP-mPEG/DOX at inhibiting cancer cell proliferation. Toxicity analysis of these nanoparticles indicated that there was no remarkable interference from the agents (Supplementary Figure S6). The significant increase in the drug efficacy may be a result of the greater accumulation of LAP-cPEG, which enhanced permeability and retention (EPR) [30,31].

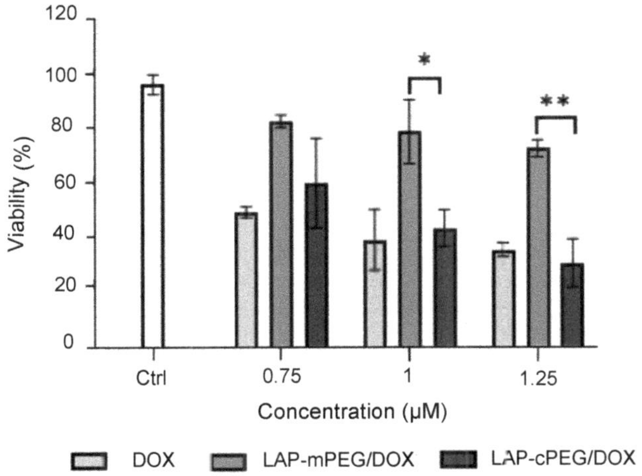

Figure 8. XTT assay results summary of A549 cells treated with DOX, LAP-mPEG/DOX, and LAP-cPEG/DOX at DOX concentrations of 0.75, 1, and 1.25 µM The viability of the cells treated with LAP-cPEG/DOX was significantly decreased compared to those treated with LAP-mPEG/DOX (* $p < 0.05$; ** $p < 0.01$).

Based on the series of XTT assays in A549 cells, the IC_{50} value for A549 cells was calculated as approximately 1 µM DOX, which corresponded to 9 µg/mL of the LAP-cPEG/DOX complex. This concentration is similar to the free DOX reported in this study. When using this complex to further target specific tumor biomarkers, the advantages of LAP-cPEG/DOX delivery system are enormous due to the lower toxicity.

Flow cytometry was also used to evaluate the effects of the formulations on A549 cells. As shown in Figure 9, LAP-cPEG/DOX kept pace with DOX, displaying rapidly increasing lethality with increasing DOX concentrations from 0.75 to 1.25 µM. In comparison, the effect of LAP-mPEG was much weaker. The 7-AAD staining results were in line with the data from the XTT assay.

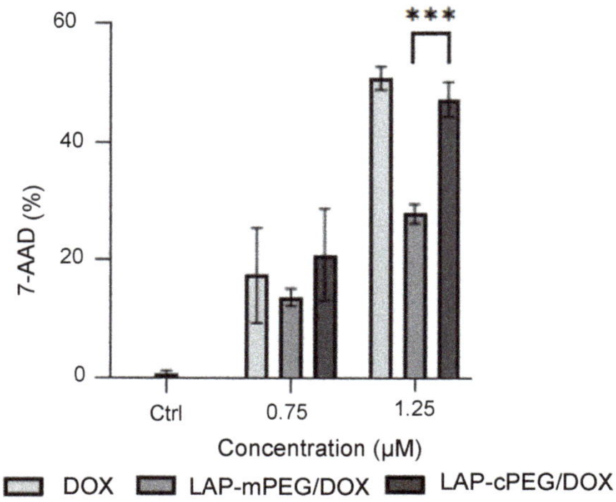

Figure 9. Evaluation of apoptosis in A549 cells by 7-AAD assay after 24 h of treatment with DOX, LAP-mPEG/DOX, and LAP-cPEG/DOX. As shown, there was a significant increase in the number of apoptotic cells treated with the LAP-cPEG/DOX formulation compared to the LAP-mPEG/DOX at a DOX concentration of 1.25 μM (*** $p < 0.001$).

3.5.5. Increased Drug Efficacy in LAP-cPEG/DOX in Primary Lung Epithelial Cells

The use of primary lung epithelial cells to evaluate the effects of LAP-cPEG/DOX has the clear advantage of a higher biological relevance compared to A549 cell data. After 24 h incubation, the cells were trypsinized and double-stained with epithelial and live–dead markers for the flow cytometry assay. The result showed that LAP-cPEG/DOX induced apoptosis in about 3% of lung primary epithelial cells, while LAP-mPEG/DOX induced apoptosis in about 1% (Figure 10). This suggests that conjugation of cyclized PEG, but not linear PEG, led to better accumulation and permeation of DOX. Free DOX had similar performance to LAP-cPEG/DOX, consistent with the previous XTT and flow cytometry assays in A549 cells.

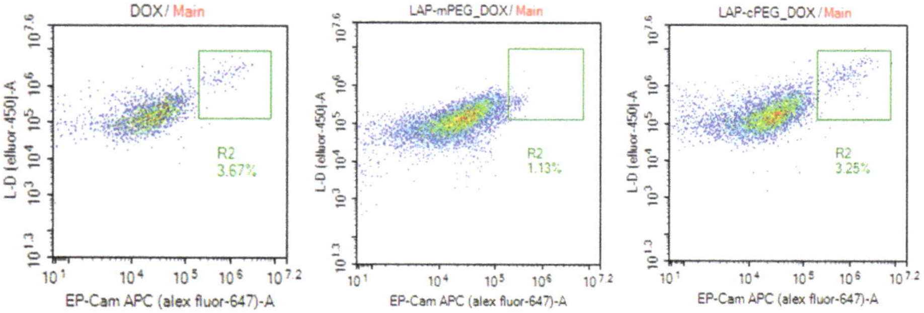

Figure 10. Evaluation of apoptosis in primary lung cells by EpCAM/L-D assay (flow cytometry) after 24 h of treatment with DOX, LAP-mPEG/DOX, and LAP-cPEG/DOX.

4. Conclusions

The goal of the current study was to design and assess the feasibility of a new drug delivery system using LAP and cPEG. Chemically homogeneous cyclic PEG with a bare functional hydroxy group was synthesized using gentle conditions. This synthetic approach produces the cPEG in a non-toxic manner and markedly enhances the biocompatibility. The cPEGylation leads to a variety of physical and covalent interactions between LAP nanoparticles and cPEG rings. The increase in surface area enhances the adsorption propensity for organic molecules. Moreover, the presence of cPEG molecules renders the system more hydrophilic and organophilic. LAP-cPEG nanoparticles have a greater solubility and are more biocompatible.

Our drug encapsulation studies indicate that DOX-loaded LAP-cPEG nanoparticles maintain their solubility after being fed with 10% of DOX and have a loading efficiency 1.5 times higher than that obtained with LAP-mPEG. The LAP-cPEG/DOX formulation increased stability over the LAP-mPEG formulation. Moreover, our results have demonstrated that the LAP-cPEG/DOX formulation displays efficient anticancer activity.

The unique properties, release profile, and enhanced cytotoxicity performance encourages further special affinity studies. Furthermore, uniform sizes and morphological factors of the LAP-cPEG nano system would be a priority for its advanced applications. This cPEGylation sets a precedent for constructing these unique organic–inorganic hybrid nanoparticles. Thus, this unique cPEGlyation has further potential in targeting approaches and biological applications.

Supplementary Materials: The following supporting information can be downloaded at: https://www.mdpi.com/article/10.3390/pharmaceutics15071998/s1, Figure S1: Calibration curve of DOX in water at 480 nm; Figure S2: Representative peak integration values of LAP-cPEG system; Figure S3: FTIR spectra (a), and ^{1}H NMR spectra (b) of LAP, LAP-NH_2, mPEG and LAP-mPEG; Figure S4: LAP and LAP-NH_2 suspensions (1 mg/mL) vs. LAP-mPEG and LAP-cPEG solutions (5 mg/mL); LAP/DOX, LAP-mPEG/DOX, and LAP-cPEG/DOX formulations are subjected in 15 K dialysis membranes after 6 h; Figure S6: In vitro cell cytotoxicity test of raw LAP, LAP-mPEG, and LAP-cPEG by means of XTT assay; Figure S7: ^{1}H NMR spectrum of PEG-NP (a) and mPEG-NP (b) in $CDCl_3$; ^{1}H NMR spectrum (a) and ^{13}C NMR spectrum (b) of cPEG-OH in $CDCl_3$; Figure S9: ^{1}H NMR spectrum of LAP-cPEG (a), and LAP-mPEG (b) in D_2O; Table S1: The summary of calculation of the DOX loading efficiency; Table S2: The absorbances of withdrawn dialysis medium at different time points; Table S3: The concentrations of DOX (mg/mL) in dialysis medium at different time points; Table S4: DOX release percentages from the formulations at different time points.

Author Contributions: Conceptualization, S.T. and S.H.W.; methodology, S.T., J.C. (Jesse Chen) and S.H.W.; Data curation, S.T. Formal analysis, S.T., J.C. (Jesse Chen) and J.C. (Jayme Cannon); Investigation, S.T., J.C. (Jesse Chen) and M.C. Writing—original draft, S.T. and J.C. (Jayme Cannon); Writing—review and editing, S.T., J.C. (Jayme Cannon), M.C., M.F., J.R.B.J. and S.H.W.; supervision, J.R.B.J. and S.H.W.; project administration, S.H.W.; Funding acquisition, J.R.B.J. All authors have read and agreed to the published version of the manuscript.

Funding: This research received no external funding.

Institutional Review Board Statement: Not applicable.

Informed Consent Statement: Not applicable.

Data Availability Statement: Data are contained within the article.

Acknowledgments: The authors are thankful to Biomedical Research Core Facilities (BRCF) for providing the SEM images. The authors are also thankful to University of Michigan Medical School for their support.

Conflicts of Interest: The authors declare no conflict of interest.

References

1. Liu, G.; Yang, L.; Chen, G.; Xu, F.; Yang, F.; Yu, H.; Li, L.; Dong, X.; Han, J.; Cao, C.; et al. A Review on Drug Delivery System for Tumor Therapy. *Front. Pharmacol.* **2021**, *12*, 735446. [CrossRef]
2. Mitchell, M.J.; Billingsley, M.M.; Haley, R.M.; Wechsler, M.E.; Peppas, N.A.; Langer, R. Engineering precision nanoparticles for drug delivery. *Nat. Rev. Drug Discov.* **2021**, *20*, 101–124. [CrossRef] [PubMed]
3. Mansour, A.; Romani, M.; Acharya, A.B. Rahman, B.; Verron, E.; Badran, Z. Drug Delivery Systems in Regenerative Medicine: An Updated Review. *Pharmaceutics* **2023**, *15*, 695. [CrossRef] [PubMed]
4. Ananikov, V.P. Organic–Inorganic Hybrid Nanomaterials. *Nanomaterials* **2019**, *9*, 1197. [CrossRef]

5. Wang, S.; Wu, Y.; Guo, R.; Huang, Y.; Wen, S.; Shen, M.; Wang, J.; Shi, X. Laponite Nanodisks as an Efficient Platform for Doxorubicin Delivery to Cancer Cells. *Langmuir* **2013**, *29*, 5030–5036. [CrossRef]
6. Das, S.S.; Neelam; Hussain, K.; Singh, S.; Hussain, A.; Faruk, A.; Tebyetekerwa, M. Laponite-based Nanomaterials for Biomedical Applications: A Review. *Curr. Pharm. Des.* **2019**, *25*, 424–443. [CrossRef]
7. Kiaee, K.; Dimitrakakis, N.; Sharifzadeh, S.; Kim, H.J.; Avery, R.K.; Moghaddam, K.M.; Haghniaz, R.; Yalcintas, E.P.; Barros, N.R.; Karamikamkar, S.; et al. Laponite-Based Nanomaterials for Drug Delivery. *Adv. Healthc. Mater.* **2022**, *11*, 2102054. [CrossRef]
8. BYK Additives & Instruments. *Laponite: Performance Additives*; Technical Information B-RI 21; BYK Additives & Instruments: Wesel, Germany, 2014.
9. Tawari, S.L.; Koch, D.L.; Cohen, C. Electrical Double-Layer Effects on the Brownian Diffusivity and Aggregation Rate of Laponite Clay Particles. *J. Colloid Interface Sci.* **2001**, *240*, 54–66. [CrossRef] [PubMed]
10. Tomas, H.; Alves, C.S.; Rodrigues, J. Laponite®: A key nanoplatform for biomedical applications? *Nanomed. Nanotechnol. Biol. Med.* **2018**, *14*, 2407–2420. [CrossRef]
11. Chen, W.; Zuo, H.; Mahony, T.J.; Zhang, B.; Rolfe, B.; Xu, Z.P. Efficient induction of comprehensive immune responses to control pathogenic E. coli by clay nano-adjuvant with the moderate size and surface charge. *Sci. Rep.* **2017**, *7*, 13367. [CrossRef]
12. Kalwar, K.; Zhang, X.; Bhutto, M.A.; Dali, L.; Shan, D. Incorporation of ciprofloxacin/laponite in polycaprolactone electrospun nanofibers: Drug release and antibacterial studies. *Mater. Res. Express* **2017**, *4*, 125401. [CrossRef]
13. Wheeler, P.A.; Wang, J.; Baker, J.; Mathias, L.J. Synthesis and Characterization of Covalently Functionalized Laponite Clay. *Chem. Mater.* **2005**, *17*, 3012–3018. [CrossRef]
14. Mustafa, R.; Luo, Y.; Wu, Y.; Guo, R.; Shi, X. Dendrimer-Functionalized Laponite Nanodisks as a Platform for Anticancer Drug Delivery. *Nanomaterials* **2015**, *5*, 1716–1731. [CrossRef]
15. Ling, K.; Jiang, H.; Zhang, Q. A colorimetric method for the molecular weight determination of polyethylene glycol using gold nanoparticles. *Nanoscale Res. Lett.* **2013**, *8*, 538. [CrossRef] [PubMed]
16. Bippus, L.; Jaber, M.; Lebeau, B. Laponite and hybrid surfactant/laponite particles processed as spheres by spray-drying. *New J. Chem.* **2009**, *33*, 1116–1126. [CrossRef]
17. Gaharwar, A.K.; Rivera, C.P.; Wu, C.-J.; Schmidt, G. Transparent, elastomeric and tough hydrogels from poly(ethylene glycol) and silicate nanoparticles. *Acta Biomater.* **2011**, *7*, 4139–4148. [CrossRef]
18. Kricheldorf, H.R.; Schwarz, G. Cyclic polymers by kinetically controlled step-growth polymerization. *Macromol. Rapid Commun.* **2003**, *24*, 359–381. [CrossRef]
19. Yamamoto, T.; Tezuka, Y. Cyclic polymers revealing topology effects upon self-assemblies, dynamics and responses. *Soft Matter* **2015**, *11*, 7458. [CrossRef] [PubMed]
20. Wang, Y.; Quinsaat, J.E.Q.; Ono, T.; Maeki, M.; Tokeshi, M.; Isono, T.; Tajima, K.; Satoh, T.; Sato, T.; Miura, Y.; et al. Enhanced dispersion stability of gold nanoparticles by the physisorption of cyclic poly(ethylene glycol). *Nat. Commun.* **2020**, *11*, 6089. [CrossRef]
21. Veronese, F.M.; Largajolli, R.; Boccu, E.; Benassi, C.A.; Schiavon, O. Surface modification of proteins. Activation of monomethoxy-polyethylene glycols by phenylchloroformates and modification of ribonuclease and superoxide dismutase. *Appl. Biochem. Biotechnol.* **1985**, *11*, 141–152. [CrossRef]
22. Kito, M.; Miron, T.; Wilchek, M.; Kojima, N.; Ohishi, N.; Yagi, K. A Simple and Efficient Method for Preparation of Monomethoxy-polyethylene Glycol Activated with p-Nitrophenylchloroformate and Its Application to Modification of L-Asparaginase. *J. Clin. Biochem. Nutr.* **1996**, *21*, 101–111. [CrossRef]
23. Sun, T.; Yu, G.-E.; Price, C.; Booth, C. Cyclic polyethers. *Polym. Commun.* **1995**, *36*, 3775–3778. [CrossRef]
24. Zhang, B.; Zhang, H.; Li, Y.; Hoskins, J.N.; Grayson, S.M. Exploring the Effect of Amphiphilic Polymer Architecture: Synthesis, Characterization, and Self-Assembly of Both Cyclic and Linear Poly(ethylene gylcol) b polycaprolactone. *ACS Macro Lett.* **2013**, *2*, 845–848. [CrossRef] [PubMed]
25. Tao, Y.; Zhao, H. Synthesis and self-assembly of amphiphilic tadpole-shaped block copolymer with disulfides at the junction points between cyclic PEG and linear PS. *Polymer* **2017**, *122*, 52–59. [CrossRef]
26. Stoychev, D. On the role of poly(ethylen glycol) in deposition of galvanic copper coatings. *Trans. IMF* **1998**, *76*, 73–80. [CrossRef]
27. Mroczka, R.; Słodkowska, A. The properties of the polyethylene glycol complex PEG(Na^+)(Cu^+) on the copper electrodeposited layer by Time-of-Flight Secondary-Ion Mass Spectrometry. The new insights. *Electrochim. Acta* **2020**, *339*, 135931. [CrossRef]
28. Yamada, Y. Dimerization of Doxorubicin Causes Its Precipitation. *ACS Omega* **2020**, *5*, 33235–33241. [CrossRef] [PubMed]
29. Laubrock, N.; Hempel, G.; Schulze-Westhoff, P.; Würthwein, G.; Flege, S.; Boos, J. The Stability of Doxorubicin and Idarubicin in Plasma and Whole Blood. *Chromatographia* **2000**, *52*, 9–13. [CrossRef]
30. Matsumura, Y.; Maeda, H. A new concept for macromolecular therapeutics in cancer chemotherapy: Mechanism of tumoritropic accumulation of proteins and the antitumor agent smancs. *Cancer Res.* **1986**, *46*, 6387–6392.
31. Maeda, H.; Tsukigawa, K.; Fang, J. A retrospective 30 years after discovery of the enhanced permeability and retention effect of solid tumors: Nextgeneration chemotherapeutics and photodynamic therapy—Problems, solutions, and prospects. *Microcirculation* **2016**, *23*, 173–182. [CrossRef]

pharmaceutics

MDPI

Article

Synthesis of Dipyridylaminoperylenediimide–Metal Complexes and Their Cytotoxicity Studies

José Garcés-Garcés [1], Marta Redrado [2], Ángela Sastre-Santos [1], María Concepción Gimeno [2,*] and Fernando Fernández-Lázaro [1,*]

1 Área de Química Orgánica, Instituto de Bioingeniería, Universidad Miguel Hernández de Elche, Avda. de la Universidad s/n, 03202 Elche (Alicante), Spain
2 Departamento de Química Inorgánica, Instituto de Síntesis Química y Catálisis Homogénea (ISQCH), CSIC-Universidad de Zaragoza, C/ Pedro Cerbuna 12, 50009 Zaragoza, Spain
* Correspondence: gimeno@unizar.es (M.C.G.); fdofdez@umh.es (F.F.-L.); Tel.: +34-(97)-6762291 (M.C.G.); +34-(96)-6658405 (F.F.-L.)

Abstract: A new family of perylenediimide (PDI) silver and copper complexes has been successfully synthesized by reacting *ortho*- and *bay*-substituted (dipyrid-2′,2″-ylamino)perylenediimide ligands with metal phosphine fragments. The coordination of the metal center did not reveal a significant effect on the photophysical properties, which are mainly due to the PDI ligands, and in some cases quenching of the luminescence was observed. The antiproliferative effect of the free perylenediimide ligands and the metallo-PDI complexes against the cervix cancer cell line HeLa was determined by MTT assay. The free perylenediimide ligands exhibited a moderate cytotoxic activity, but the coordination of silver or copper to the dypyridylamino fragment greatly enhanced the activity, suggesting a synergistic effect between the two fragments. In attempts to elucidate the cellular biodistribution of the PDIs and the complexes, a colocalization experiment using specific dyes for the lysosomes or mitochondria as internal standards revealed a major internalization inside the cell for the metal complexes, as well as a partial mitochondrial localization.

Keywords: perylenediimide; biological properties; cancer; cytotoxicity; metal complexes; silver; copper

Citation: Garcés-Garcés, J.; Redrado, M.; Sastre-Santos, Á.; Gimeno, M.C.; Fernández-Lázaro, F. Synthesis of Dipyridylaminoperylenediimide–Metal Complexes and Their Cytotoxicity Studies. *Pharmaceutics* **2022**, *14*, 2616. https://doi.org/10.3390/pharmaceutics14122616

Academic Editors: Raquel Fernández García, Francisco Bolás-Fernández and Ana Isabel Fraguas-Sánchez

Received: 3 November 2022
Accepted: 23 November 2022
Published: 27 November 2022

1. Introduction

Perylenediimides (PDIs) are one of the most important dyes known today due to their outstanding electrooptical properties, high fluorescence quantum yields, strong absorption of visible light and huge versatility in their chemistry [1]. The properties of PDIs can be modified by the functionalization of the aromatic core in their different positions, namely *bay* positions (1, 6, 7 and 12) and *ortho* positions (2, 5, 8, and 11). Depending on the nature of the substituents on the aromatic core, their absorption profile, as well as the electron accepting/donating character of PDIs, can be drastically modified [2]. For these reasons, the appropriate design of the PDIs plays a key role in modulating their properties and molecular organization, which will lead to the optimal performance of the material.

Although PDIs are mainly used in optoelectronic applications [3] and material science [4], the number of biological studies using PDIs has been growing in the last few years [5–7], becoming promising molecules for biological investigation. Water-soluble PDIs have been used in biological applications due to their biocompatibility, photostability and optical absorption and emission properties. Synthetic strategies to gain water solubility consist either of the functionalization of PDIs with carbohydrate or PEG moieties, or the formation of charged PDI salts. The latter allows the interaction with other charged molecules present in the organism, such as DNA or proteins contained in the cell membrane [6]. On the other hand, PDI–carbohydrate conjugates are excellent candidates to label protein–carbohydrate interactions as glycodendrimers, presenting the potential to recognize carbohydrate–protein (lectin) interactions involved in key biological processes [8].

There are some examples on the use of PDIs as biological labels, such as the PDI–estradiol conjugate used to monitor the estrogen receptor by confocal microscopy [9]. PDIs bearing biotin and maleimide moieties have been used to target specific receptors, such as maltoporin [10]. PDIs substituted with galactose, mannose and fucose [11] have been used as chemosensors. PDIs are also involved in nanomedicine [12]; an example of this is a glycosacharide–PDI attached to maghemite nanoparticles tested as a dual imaging agent in magnetic resonance imaging. PDIs are also used in photodynamic therapy [13].

A simple strategy to modulate the properties of PDI systems using metallic fragments is the functionalization of the perylene core with coordinating donor groups that can act as ligands for metal complex formation. Thus, PDI derivatives containing palladium [14] and gold [15] complexes have been synthesized for electrooptical applications and to prepare Langmuir films, respectively. A PDI self-assembly to construct silver nanohybrids with enhanced visible-light photocatalytic antibacterial effects has also been described [16]. Additionally, iridium-containing PDI complexes [17] have been used as organic light-emitting devices (OLEDs). Moreover, functionalization of PDIs with electron-donating groups to coordinate Cu^{+}, Cu^{2+} and Fe^{3+} allowed the development of photo-induced electron transfer systems with the aim to emulate the photosynthetic process [18]. On the other hand, the supramolecular chemistry of metallo-PDIs is an emerging research area; thus, metallo-cages based on PDIs [19] show high fluorescence quantum yields and the ability to host polycyclic aromatic hydrocarbon, such as pyrene or triphenylene. Biological properties of metal complex derivates of PDIs have been investigated too, as in the case of a PDI functionalized with phenanthroline moieties to coordinate ruthenium (II) [20], which was studied for photodynamic therapy. However, almost no studies have been published on PDI metallocomplexes as anticancer or theranostic agents.

One of the most promising metals that presents several biological properties is silver. For many years, silver complexes have been used for antiseptic, antibacterial or anti-inflammatory applications [21], taking advantage of their low cytotoxicity [22]. Silver organometallic complexes have also been studied as anticancer agents, as many silver (I) complexes have been found to exhibit a greater cytotoxic activity than cisplatin, with relatively low toxicity and greater selectivity toward cancer cells [23,24]. Cell death via apoptosis and depolarization of the mitochondrial membrane potential are the most accepted mechanisms of this anticancer activity [24–28]. On the other hand, copper salts have been less studied as drugs. Copper is an essential metal for organisms, playing a key role in numerous cellular processes. In particular, copper is the cofactor in important metalloenzymes for the mitochondrial metabolism and in detoxification of radical oxygen species (ROS). Copper complexes are potent topoisomerase inhibitors, the redox activity of [Cu(I)/Cu(II)] being one of the principal causes of cytotoxicity [29].

In this context, in order to study the synergistic influence of PDI ligands and their metal complexes as anticancer agents, we present here the synthesis and in vitro studies of a new family of silver and copper complexes derived from *ortho*- and *bay*-substituted (dipyrid-2′,2″-ylamino)perylenediimides, testing the free perylenediimide ligand and the metalloPDI complexes against HeLa cell line.

2. Materials and Methods

2.1. Synthetic Procedure

All chemicals were reagent grade, purchased from commercial sources, and were used as received unless otherwise specified. Column chromatography was performed on SiO_2 (40–63 lm) (Carlo Erba, Barcelona, Spain). TLC plates coated with SiO_2 60F254 were visualized under UV light (Macherey-Nagel, Düren, Germany).

^{1}H NMR and $^{31}P\{^{1}H\}$ NMR spectra were recorded at room temperature on a BRUKER AVANCE 400 spectrometer (Bruker, Billerica, MA, USA) (^{1}H, 400 MHz) or on a BRUKER AVANCE II 300 spectrometer (^{1}H, 300 MHz), with chemical shifts (ppm) reported relative to the solvent peaks in the ^{1}H spectra or external 85% H_3PO_4 in $^{31}P\{^{1}H\}$ of the deuterated solvent. CD_2Cl_2 and $CDCl_3$ were used as the deuterated solvents (Euroisotop, Saint-Aubin,

France). Chemical shifts were reported in the δ scale relative to residual CH_2Cl_2 (5.32 ppm) and TMS (0 ppms). NMR were recorded at ambient probe temperature. UV-vis spectra were recorded with a Perkin Elmer Lambda 365 spectrophotometer (Tres Cantos, Madrid, Spain) in $CHCl_3$ solutions in the range 250 to 800 nm. Fluorescence spectra were recorded with a HORIBA scientific SAS spectrophotometer (Palaiseau, France) in $CHCl_3$ solutions in the range 250 to 800 nm. High-resolution mass spectra were obtained from a Bruker Microflex LRF20 (Bruker, Boston, MA, USA) matrix-assisted laser desorption/ionization time of flight (MALDI-TOF), using dithranol as a matrix. IR spectra were recorded with a Nicolet Impact 400D spectrophotometer (ThermoFisher, Scienfic) in KBr in the range 4000–400 cm^{-1}.

The starting material [Ag(OTf)(PPh_3)] [30] was prepared according to published procedures. All other reagents and solvents were commercially available (Merk Life Science, Madrid, Spain).

2.1.1. Synthesis of *N,N′*-Diethylpropyl-1-(dipyrid-2′,2″-ylamine)perylene-3,4:9,10-tetracarboxydiimide (**PDI-2**)

N,N′-Diethylpropyl-1-bromoperylene-3,4:9,10-tetracarboxydiimide **PDI-1** (50 mg, 0.06 mmol), 2,2′-dipyridylamine (31 mg, 0.181 mmol), cesium carbonate (70 mg, 0.21 mmol) and 1,1′-bis[(diphenylphosphino)ferrocene]dichloropalladium (II) (4.4 mg, 0.0054 mmol) were added to a two-neck round-bottom flask and flushed with nitrogen for 30 min. Then, dry toluene (8 mL) was injected and stirred at 80 °C for 24 h under nitrogen atmosphere. The cooled mixture was extracted with dichloromethane and washed with water. The organic phase was dried over anhydrous sodium sulfate, filtered, and evaporated. Purification was carried out by silica gel column chromatography (toluene:acetone, 20:1), yielding 30 mg (70%) of **PD-2** as a purple solid. ^{1}H NMR (300 MHz, CD_2Cl_2) δ 9.24 (d, J = 8.3 Hz, 1H, H_g), 8.67-8.62 (m, 4H, H_{b-e}), 8.38 (bs, 1H, H_a,), 8.34 (d, J = 8.3 Hz, 1H, H_f) 8.22 (ddd, J = 4,93, 1.08, 0.89 Hz, 2H, H_k), 7.58 (dddd, J = 6.44, 5.32, 1.98, 1–95 Hz, 2H, H_m), 7.20 (d, J =7.36, 2H, H_n), 6.97 (ddd, J = 7.26, 4.91, 0.95 Hz, 2H, H_l), 5.04–4.92 (m, 2H, H_h), 2.28–2.10 (m, 4H, H_h), 1.96–1.80 (m, 4H, H_i), and 0.87 ppm (dt, J = 13.8, 7.5 Hz, 12 H, H_j). ^{13}C NMR (75 MHz, $CDCl_3$) δ 155.9, 149.1, 143.1, 138.1, 134.8, 134.4, 132.9, 129.3, 129.1, 129.0, 128.3, 128.2, 126.7, 126.5, 123.4, 123.6, 122.7, 119.5, 115.8, 57.8, 57.6, 25.1, 25.1, 11.4 and 11.41 ppm. FT-IR (KBr): 3457, 2962, 2872, 1704, 1650, 1593, 1458, 1426, 1401, 1332, 1242, 1193, 1144, 1086, 854, 813, 776, 743, and 694 cm^{-1}. UV-Vis ($CHCl_3$) λ_{max}/nm (log ε): 561 (4.48), 480 (4.55). HR-MALDI-TOF *m/z* [M^+] calc. for $C_{44}H_{37}N_5O_4$: 699.285, found: 699.280.

2.1.2. Synthesis of *N,N′*-Diethylpropyl-2,5,8,11-tetra(dipyrid-2′,2″-ylamine)perylene-3,4:9,10 tetracarboxydiimide (**PDI-6**)

N,N′-Diethylpropyl-2,5,8,11-tetrabromoperylene-3,4:9,10-tetracarboxydiimide **PDI-5** (50 mg, 0.06 mmol), 2,2′-dipyridylamine (123 mg, 0.72 mmol), cesium carbonate (273 mg, 0.84 mmol) and 1,1′-bis[(diphenylphosphino)ferrocene]dichloropalladium (II) (21 mg, 0.021 mmol) were added to a two-neck round-bottom flask and flushed with nitrogen for 30 min. Then, dry toluene (30 mL) was injected and stirred at 80 °C for 24 h under nitrogen atmosphere. The cooled mixture was extracted with dichloromethane and washed with water. The organic phase was dried over anhydrous sodium sulfate, filtered and evaporated. Purification was carried out by silica gel column chromatography (toluene:acetone, 20:1) yielding 30 mg (69%) of **PDI-6** as a purple solid. ^{1}H NMR (300 MHz, CD_2Cl_2) δ 8.15 (d, J = 3.7 Hz, 8H, H_e), 7.98 (s, 4H, H_a), 7.61–7.55 (m, 8H, H_g), 7.16 (d, J = 8.3 Hz, 8H, H_h), 6.93 (dd, J = 6.9, 5.2 Hz, 8H, H_f), 4.41–4.31 (m, 2H, H_b), 1.58–1.43 (m, 4 H, H_c), 1.36–1.22 (m, 4H, H_c) and 0.33 ppm (t, J = 7.4 Hz, 12H, H_d). ^{13}C NMR (75 MHz, $CDCl_3$) δ 162.3, 157.3, 148.5, 148.2, 138.0, 134.9, 133.3, 126.7, 123.6, 119.3, 119.1, 117.7, 57.7, 24.9 and 11.6 ppm. FT-IR (KBr): 3457, 2962, 2929, 2872, 1704, 1650, 1593, 1458, 1426, 1401, 1332, 1242, 1193, 1144, 1086, 854, 813, 776, 743, and 694 cm^{-1}.UV-Vis ($CHCl_3$) λ_{max}/nm (log ε): 536 (4.81), 496 (4.78). HR-MALDI-TOF *m/z* [M^+] calc. for $C_{74}H_{58}N_{14}O_4$: 1206.477, found: 1206.475.

2.1.3. Synthesis of Complex **PDI-3**

PDI-2 (10 mg, 0.014 mmol) was dissolved in DCM (2.5 mL) and then [Ag(OTf)PPh_3] (7.41 mg, 0.014 mmol) was added. The mixture was stirred at room temperature for 1 h and then the solvent was evaporated until dryness, yielding 14.97 mg (100%) of **PDI-3** as a purple solid. No purification step was needed. ^{1}H NMR (300 MHz, CD_2Cl_2) δ 9.20 (d, J = 8.3 Hz, 1 H, H_g), 8.74–8.61 (m, 4H_{b-e}),8.39 (s, 1H, H_a), 8.29 (d, J = 4.07 Hz, 2H, H_k), 8.24 (d, J =8.3 Hz, 2H, H_f), 7.67 (dddd, J = 8.38, 7.33, 1.89, 1.89 Hz, 2 H, H_m), 7.46–7.29 (m, 15 H, Ar-Ph), 7.24 (d, J = 8.36 Hz, 2H, H_n), 6.97 (dd, J = 6.69, 5.37 Hz, 2H, H_l), 5.07–4.91 (m, 2H, H_h), 2.26–2.10 (m, 4 H, H_i), 1.98–1.81 (m, 4 H, H_i), and 0.88 ppm (dt, J = 14.9, 7.5 Hz, 12 H, H_j). ^{31}P NMR (121 MHz, CD_2Cl_2) δ 16.7 and 12.2 ppm. FT-IR (KBr): 3473, 2962, 2365, 1699, 1654, 1593, 1434, 1328, 1242, 1021, 821, 756, 702, and 629 cm^{-1} UV-Vis ($CHCl_3$) λ_{max}/nm (log ε): 561 (4.91), 481 (4.75) and 274 (4.29). HR-MALDI-TOF *m/z* [M^+] calc. for $C_{62}H_{52}AgN_5O_4P$: 1069.288, found: 1069.282.

2.1.4. Synthesis of Complex **PDI-4**

PDI-2 (20 mg, 0.029 mmol) was dissolved in DCM (2.5 mL) and then [$Cu(NO_3)(PPh_3)_2$] (18.85 mg, 0.029 mmol) was added. The mixture was stirred at room temperature for 1 h and then the solvent was evaporated until dryness, yielding 37 mg (100%) of **PDI-4** as a purple solid. No purification step was needed. ^{1}H NMR (300 MHz, CD_2Cl_2) δ 9.28 (d, J = 8.3 Hz, 1H, H_g), 8.70–8.64 (m, 4H, H_{b-e}), 8.48 (s, 1H, H_a), 8.42 (d, J = 8.30 Hz, 1H, H_f) 8.31–(dd, J = 4.66, 1.1 Hz, 2 HH_k), 7.62–7.57 (m, 2H, H_m), 7.44–7.2 (m, 30 H, Ar-Ph), 7.19 (d, J = 8.3 Hz, 2H, H_n), 6.99 (dd, J = 6.8, 5.1 Hz, 2H, H_l), 5.12–5.0 (m, 2H, H_h), 2.38–2.16 (m, 4H, H_i), 2.03–1.86 (m, 4H, H_i), and 0.93 ppm (dt, J = 10.1, 7.5 Hz, 12 H, H_j). ^{31}P NMR (121 MHz, CD_2Cl_2) δ −0.47 ppm. FT-IR (KBr): 3052, 2958, 2925, 2872, 1691, 1654, 1597, 1458, 1433, 1405, 0380, 1331, 1249, 1192, 1090, 812, 738, 698, and 500 cm^{-1}. UV-Vis ($CHCl_3$) λ_{max}/nm (log ε). 561 (4.91), 481 (4.75) and 274 (4.29). MALDI-TOF *m/z* [M-PPh_3]$^+$ calc. for $C_{80}H_{67}CuN_5O_4P_2$_PPh_3: 1024.305, found for $C_{80}H_{67}CuN_5O_4P_2$–PPh_3: 1024.340.

2.1.5. Synthesis of Complex **PDI-7**

PDI-6 (10 mg, $8.28 \cdot 10^{-3}$ mmol) was dissolved in DCM (2.5 mL) and then [Ag(OTf)PPh_3] (17.20 mg, 0.033 mmol) was added. The mixture was stirred at room temperature for 1 h and then the solvent was evaporated until dryness, yielding 22 mg (99%) of **PDI-7** as a purple solid. No purification step was needed. ^{1}H NMR (300 MHz, CD_2Cl_2) δ 8.16 (bs, 12H, H_a, H_e), 7.58 (t, J = 7.1 Hz, 8H, H_g), 7.49–7.34 (m, 60H, Ar-Ph) 7.10 (d, J = 8.2 Hz, 8H, H_h), 6.93–6.89 (m, 8 H, H_f), 4.25–4.20 (m, 2H, H_b), 1.40–1.27 (m, 4H, H_c), 1.15–1.06 (m, 4H, H_c), and 0.16–0.09 ppm (m, 12H, H_d). ^{31}P NMR (121 MHz, CD_2Cl_2) δ 18.38 and 12.29 ppm. FT-IR (KBr): 3052, 2966, 2921, 2860, 1699, 1663, 1589, 1462, 1430, 1377, 1332, 1274, 1254, 1180, 1091, 1050, 776, 474, 694, 657, and 523 cm^{-1}. λ_{max}/nm (log ε): 536 (4.62), 271 (4.70).

2.1.6. Synthesis of Complex **PDI-8**

PDI-6 (10 mg, $8.28 \cdot 10^{-3}$ mmol) was dissolved in DCM (2.5 mL) and then [$Cu(NO_3)(PPh_3)_2$] (21.54 mg, 0.033 mmol) was added. The mixture was stirred at room temperature for 1 h and then the solvent was evaporated until dryness, yielding 29 mg (99%) of **PDI-8** as a purple solid. No purification step was needed. ^{1}H NMR (300 MHz, CD_2Cl_2) δ 8.13 (bs, 8H, H_e), 7.99 (bs, 4H, H_a), 7.60–7.55 (m, 8 H. H_g), 7.42–7.28 (m, 120H, Ar-Ph), 7.56 (bs, 8H, H_h), 6.91 (bs, 8H, H_f), 4.42–4.37 (m, 2H, H_b), 1.61–1.46 (m, 4H. H_c), 1.36–1.29 (m, 4H, H_c), and 0.35 ppm (t, J = 7.3 Hz, 12 H, H_d). ^{31}P NMR (121 MHz, CD_2Cl_2) δ −0.48 ppm. FT-IR (KBr): 3436, 3052, 3003, 2958, 2921, 2361, 1691, 1654, 1585, 1467, 1434, 1385, 1344, 1274, 1209, 1091, 1025, 988, 735, 694, 523, and 506 cm^{-1}. UV-Vis ($CHCl_3$) λ_{max}/nm (log ε): 536 (4.66), 274 (4.66).

2.2. Cell Culture

HeLa (cervical cancer) cell line (from ATCC, USA) was routinely cultured in high-glucose DMEM medium supplemented with 5% fetal bovine serum (FBS), L-glutamine and penicillin/streptomycin (hereafter, complete medium) at 37 °C in a humidified atmosphere of 95% air/5% CO_2.

2.3. Cell Viability Assays

The MTT-reduction assay was used to analyse cell metabolic activity as an indicator of cell sensitivity to compounds **PDI-2** to **PDI-4**, and **PDI-6** to **PDI-8** in the HeLa cell line. A total of 6000 cells/well were seeded in 96-well plates (100 μL/well) and allowed to attach for 24 h prior to addition of compounds. The complexes were dissolved in DMSO and added to cells in concentrations ranging from 0.2 to 50 μM in quadruplicate. Cells were incubated with our compounds for 24 h, then 10 μL of MTT (5 mg/mL in PBS) were added to each well and plates were incubated for 2 h at 37 °C. Finally, the culture medium was removed and DMSO (100 μL/well) was added to dissolve the formazan crystals. The optical density was measured at 550 nm using a 96-well multiscanner autoreader (ELISA) and IC_{50} was calculated. Each compound was analyzed at least in three independent experiments.

2.4. Cytotoxicity Assays

Apoptotic cell death was determined by measuring phosphatidyl-serine exposure on cell surface in HeLa cells. A total of 60,000 cells/well were seeded in 12-well plates (1 mL/well) and left overnight to be attached to the bottom. Cells were treated for 24 h with complexes **PDI-3** and **PDI-4** at IC_{50} and $2{\cdot}IC_{50}$ concentrations, respectively, in duplicate. After treatment, cells were trypsinised and resuspended in 50 μL of a mixture of Anexin-binding buffer (ABB; 140 mM NaCl, 2.5 mM $CaCl_2$, 10 mM HEPES/NaOH pH 7.4), FITC-conjugated Annexin V and incubated at room temperature in the dark for 15 min. Finally, cells were diluted to 250 μL with ABB and a total of 10,000 cells were acquired on a FACSCalibur flow cytometer (BD Biosciences, Franklin Lakes, NJ, USA). Cell death was analyzed using CellQuest Pro (BD Biosciences, Franklin Lakes, NJ, USA), FlowJo 7.6.1 (Becton Dickinson (BD), Franklin Lakes, NJ, USA) and GraphPad Prism 5 (GraphPad Software, San Diego, CA, USA) software.

2.5. Fluorescence Confocal Microscopy

A total of 10^4 HeLa cells/well were seeded in complete medium in μ-slide 8 well (ibiTreat) (300 μL/well) and left 24 h to be attached to the bottom. Then, 200 μL of culture medium were removed and 100 μL of a solution of species **PDI-2**, **-3**, **-4** and **-8** were added to a final concentration of 2 μM. The compounds were incubated with the cells for 2 h. Thereafter, MitoTracker Green (MTG) or LysoTracker Green (LTG) was added to a final concentration of 75 nM and 500 nM, respectively, and it was incubated with the cells for 30–45 min at room temperature. Eventually the medium was replaced with fresh medium without phenol red. Images were collected in a sequential mode in a FluoView FV10i (Olympus, Shinjuku, Japan) confocal microscope with a 40 oil immersion lens, a line average of 4, and a format of 1024 × 1024 pixels using excitation wavelength of either 488 or 561 nm. The confocal pinhole was 1 Airy unit. Images were analysed with FV10-ASW 3.1. Viewer software.

2.6. Cell Morphology Analysis

Alterations in cell morphology and behavior as a consequence of the exposure to complexes **PDI-3** and **PDI-4** were analyzed using an inverted microscope Olympus IX71 Inverted. A total of 10,000 cells/well were seeded in 12-well plates (1 mL/well) and left overnight to be attached to the bottom. Thereafter, cells were treated for 24 h with complexes at IC_{50} and $2{\cdot}IC_{50}$ concentrations, respectively, in duplicate.

3. Results and Discussion

3.1. Synthesis of PDIs and Metal Complexes

PDI-1 and **PDI-5** were synthesized as described in the literature [31–33]. **PDI-2** and **PDI-6** were synthesized for the first time using a Buchwald–Hartwig cross-coupling reaction [34,35]. Thus, bromo **PDI-1** and tetrabromo **PDI-5** were reacted with 2,2′-dipyridylamine in the presence of bis[(diphenylphosphino)ferrocene]dichloropalladium(II) in a basic media to obtain **PDI-2** and **PDI-6** with 70% and 69% yield, respectively (Scheme 1). Both PDIs were fully characterized by spectroscopic and spectrometric methods (see the Supporting Information).

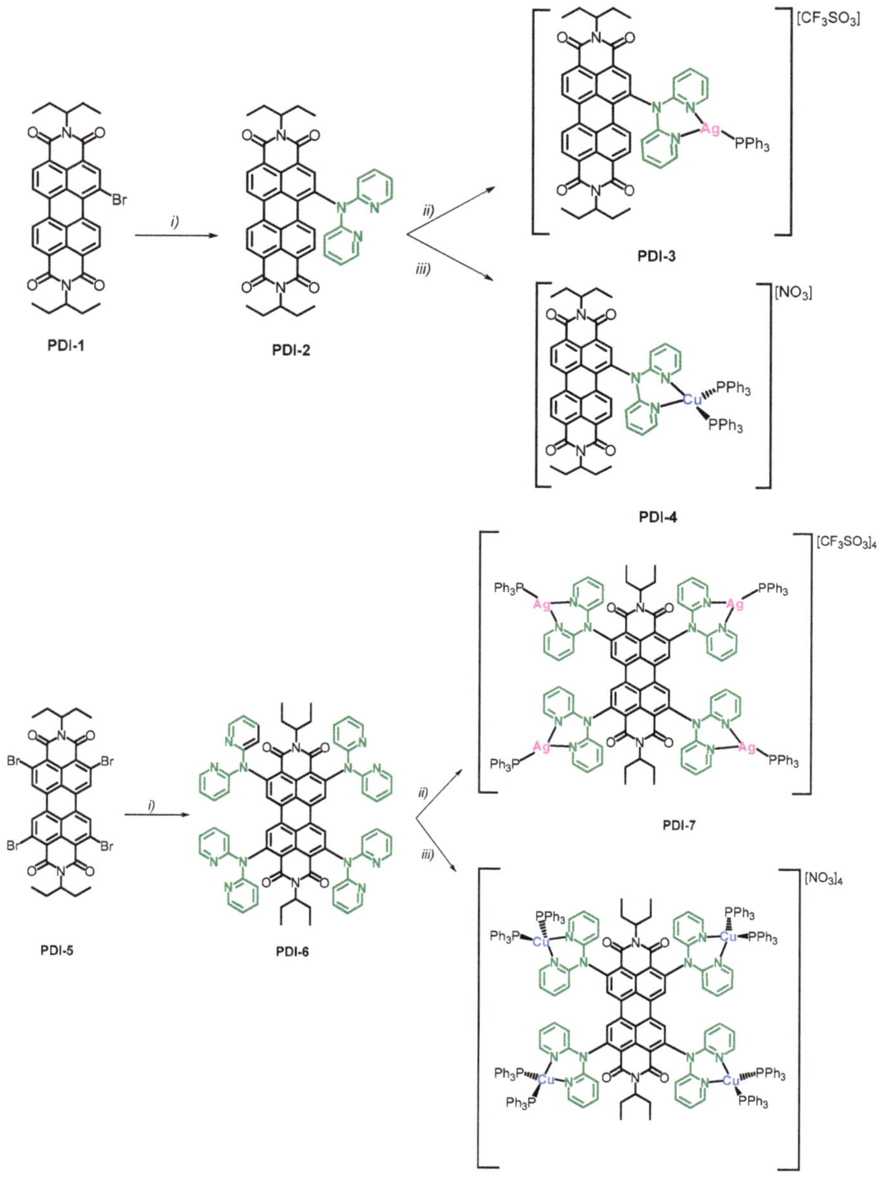

Scheme 1. Reagents and conditions: **(i)** 2,2′-dipyridylamine, $[Pd(dppf)_2Cl_2]$, DCM, Cs_2CO_3, toluene, 24 h, 80 °C, nitrogen; **(ii)** $[Ag(OTf)(PPh_3]$, DCM, 1 h, rt; **(iii)** $[CuNO_3(PPh_3)_2]$, DCM, 1 h, rt.

The addition of either [Ag(OTf)(PPh_3)] or [CuNO_3(PPh_3)$_2$] to a solution of **PDI-2** or **PDI-6** in a 1:1 or 4:1 molar ratio, respectively, led to the formation of the phosphine silver (I) complexes **PDI-3** and **PDI-7**, and the phosphine copper(I) complexes **PDI-4** and **PDI-8** (Scheme 1). In all cases, complexation reactions were quantitative, and no purification steps were required.

Figure 1 shows the comparison between **PDI-2** and the mono-copper complex **PDI-4**. We can observe that all aromatic protons of the pyridyl group were weakly deshielded in **PDI-4** in comparison with **PDI-2** due to copper complexation, Hk being the most affected. At 7.44–7.26 ppm we found the signal attributed to the phosphine groups integrating for 30 H corresponding to two phosphine groups. The mono-silver complex **PDI-3** followed the same pattern (see Supporting Information Figure S11).

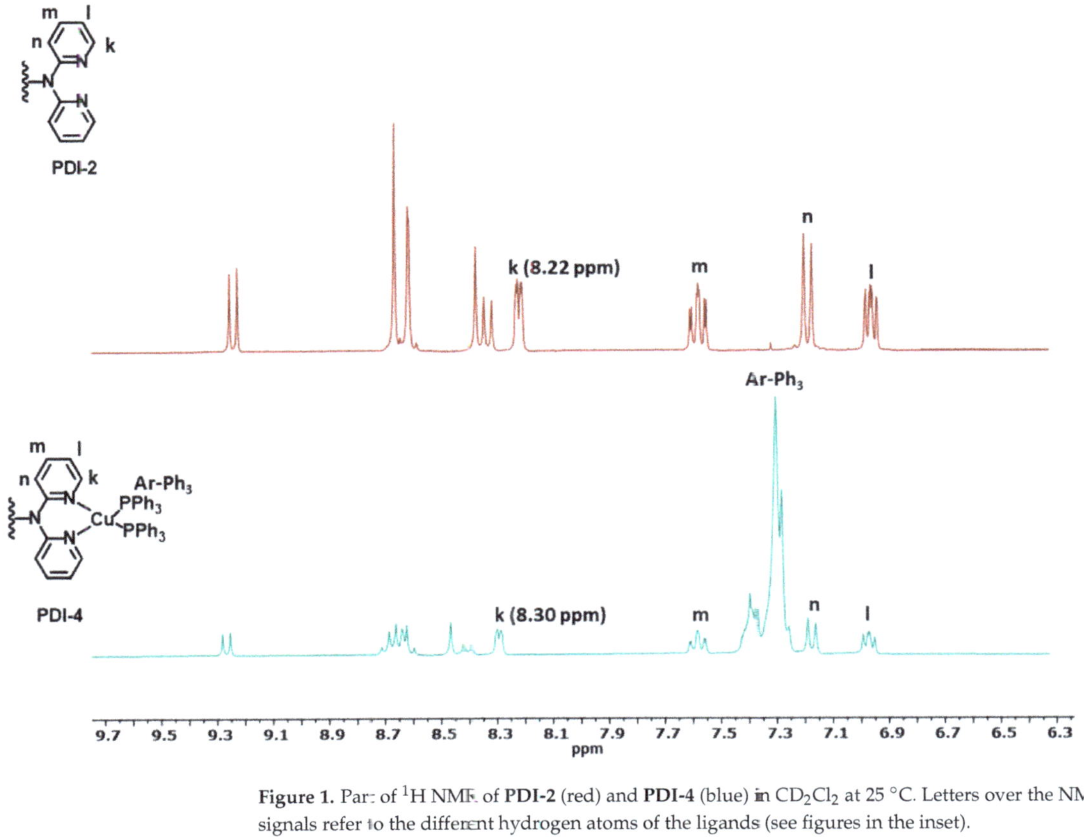

Figure 1. Part of ^{1}H NMR of **PDI-2** (red) and **PDI-4** (blue) in CD_2Cl_2 at 25 °C. Letters over the NMR signals refer to the different hydrogen atoms of the ligands (see figures in the inset).

Figure 2 shows the comparison between **PDI-6** and the tetra-copper complex **PDI-8**. In this case, all signals were broadened, possibly because of the rotation of the four substituted dipyridylamino metallo units in **PDI-6–8.** Additionally, we can observe the resonance corresponding to the aromatic protons of the phosphine groups between 7.28 and 7.45 ppm integrating for 120 H, indicating the presence of two phosphine groups for each copper unit. The same broadening effect was observed in the tetra-silver complex **PDI-7**. In this case, an integration of 60 H of the phosphine signals agrees with the existence of four triphenylphosphine units (see Supporting Information Figure S17).

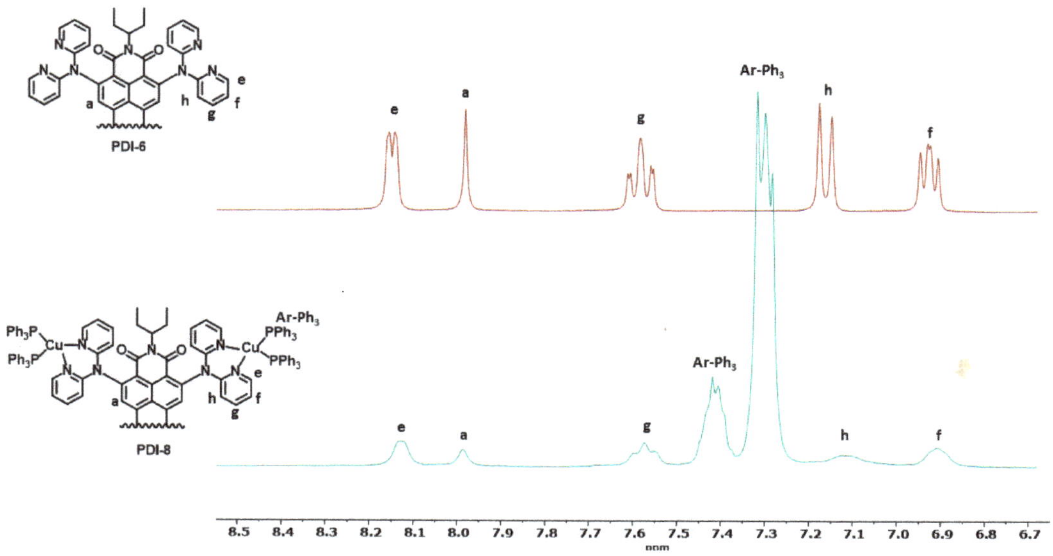

Figure 2. Part of ^{1}H NMR of **PDI-6** (red) and **PDI-8** (blue) in CD_2Cl_2 at 25 °C.

In the case of silver complexes, **PDI-3** and **PDI-7**, the $^{31}P\{^1H\}$ NMR spectrum showed a broad doublet at 12.02 and 17.12 ppm, respectively, due to the coupling of the phosphorus atom with the two silver isotopes ^{109}Ag and ^{107}Ag, corresponding to the average coupling. The copper complexes **PDI-4** and **PDI-8** showed a signal at −0.5 ppm in the $^{31}P\{^1H\}$ NMR spectrum in agreement with the presence of equivalent phosphorus atoms (Figure 3).

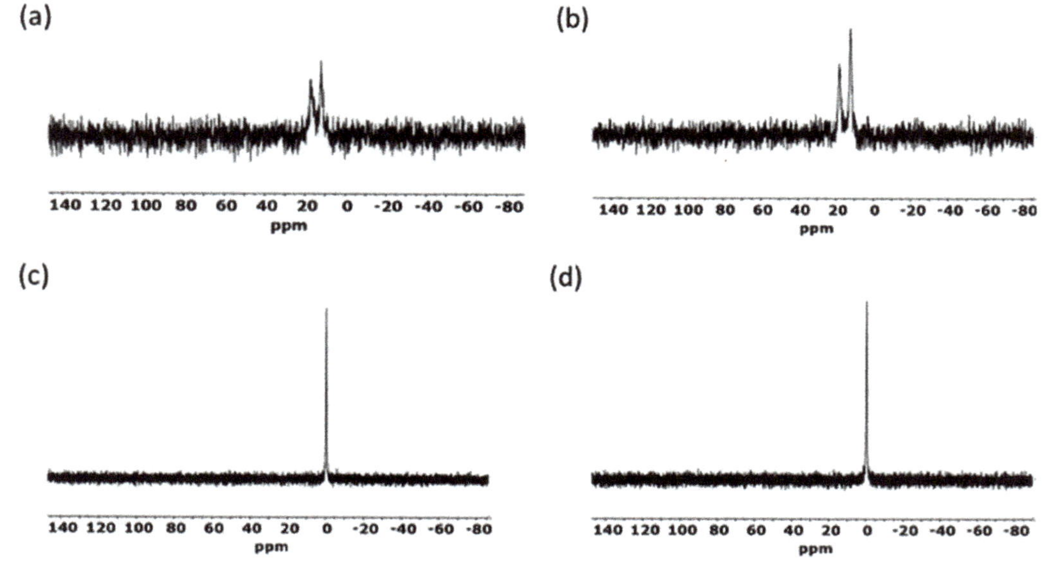

Figure 3. $^{31}P\{^1H\}$ NMR spectra of PDI metal complexes (**a**) **PDI-3**, (**b**) **PDI-7**, (**c**) **PDI-4**, (**d**) **PDI-8** in CD_2Cl_2 at 25 °C.

3.2. Absorption and Fluorescence Studies

The presence of N atoms in **PDI-2** and **PDI-6** quenches the fluorescence in these PDIs. Thus, while **PDI-1** has a fluorescence quantum yield of 91%, it drops to 35% in **PDI-2**. For **PDI-6**, fluorescence is completely quenched (see Supporting Information, Figure S9). In the case of the mono-substituted complexes **PDI-3** and **PDI-4**, the fluorescence quantum yields were 49 and 57%, respectively, being higher than in the precursor **PDI-2**.

The absorption spectrum of **PDI-2** in chloroform solution changed totally in respect to the precursor **PDI-1**, which located its maximum at 524 nm, typical for a *bay*-substituted PDI with electron withdrawing groups. **PDI-2** showed a broad band at 561 nm, which corresponds to the charge transfer from the dipyridylamine moieties to the perylene core (Figure 4a). On the other hand, functionalization of **PDI-5** in the *ortho* positions with dipyridylamine induced a dramatic bathochromic shift, changing the maximum of **PDI-5** located at 508 nm to 536 nm in **PDI-6** (Figure 4b).

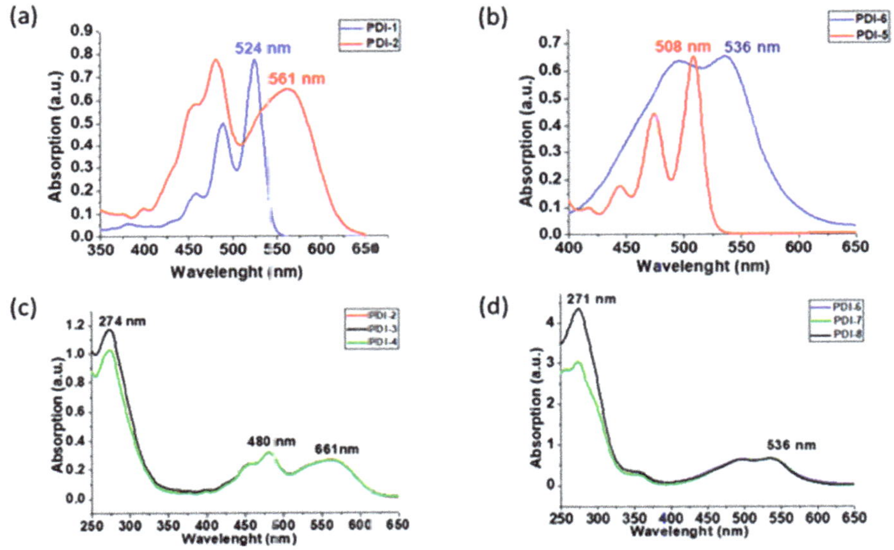

Figure 4. Normalized absorption in $CHCl_3$ as solvent at 25 °C of (**a**) **PDI-1** and **PDI-2**, (**b**) **PDI-5** and **PDI-6**, (**c**) **PDI-2**, **PDI-3** and **PDI-4**, and (**d**) **PDI-6**, **PDI-7** and **PDI-8**.

The UV-vis spectra in chloroform of the four metal complexes, **PDIs-3–4** and **PDIs-7–8**, show new absorption bands at 274 and 271 nm, attributed to the phenyl groups of the phosphine moieties, while the absorption band attributed to the perylene core remains unaffected after complexation reaction (Figure 4c,d).

3.3. Antiproliferative Studies

Antiproliferative studies were carried out for all compounds against human cervical carcinoma (HeLa) cancer cell line using the MTT assay [36], and the results are shown in Table 1. We tested the stability of all compounds in DMSO, the medium used in the in vitro assays, ^{1}H NMR, corroborating that they remained stable after a few days. In addition, the stability of the complexes in the biological media (Phosphate Buffer Solution PBS with 5% of DMSO) was measured using Uv-Vis spectra. The spectra measured at 0 and 24 h showed that the PDI and the corresponding silver complexes remained stable in solution (see Figure S23). However, some differences in the high energy absorptions appeared for the copper complex **PDI-8** and, consequently, we can not discard that this complex could dissociate some PPh_3 ligands in DMSO or biological solutions. The effect of this dissociation in the cytotoxic properties will be studied in due course.

Table 1. IC_{50} values of **PDI-2–PDI-4** and **PDI-6–PDI-8** incubated for 24 h in HeLa cells.

Compound	IC_{50} (μM)
PDI-2	11.51 ± 0.9
PDI-3	2.46 ± 0.1
PDI-4	3.08 ± 0.6
PDI-6	10.54 ± 0.8
PDI-7	2.05 ± 0.9
PDI-8	1.90 ± 0.1

The data show that the starting **PDI-2** and **PDI-6** ligands were moderately active, with half minimum inhibitory concentrations (IC_{50}) of 11.51 ± 0.86 and 10.54 ± 0.82 μM, respectively. Coordination of the silver or copper fragments greatly enhanced the cytotoxic activity, and the final complexes exhibited IC_{50} values in the low micromolar range. Analyzing the results as a function of the metal, a clear tendency was not observed because for **PDI-3** and **PDI-4**, the silver complex presented a slightly higher activity than the copper one, but the opposite result was obtained for **PDI-7** and **PDI-8**. However, these differences may not be significant, as the complexes in general exhibited excellent activity.

3.4. *Morphological Appearance and Cell Death Mechanism*

Cellular behavior and morphological alterations of HeLa cells after exposure to the complexes were analyzed under an inverted microscope. Untreated cells were healthy, grew exponentially and exhibited their characteristic morphology, whereas the cells treated with the silver and copper compounds at concentrations about and double the IC_{50} showed alterations in the morphology (Figure 5). It is noticeable that for copper compound **PDI-4**, the formation of apoptotic death cells was observed, whereas at higher concentration some of the cells were greatly disturbed and presented a necrotic morphology. For the silver compound **PDI-3**, an apoptotic cell death envisaged an even higher concentration.

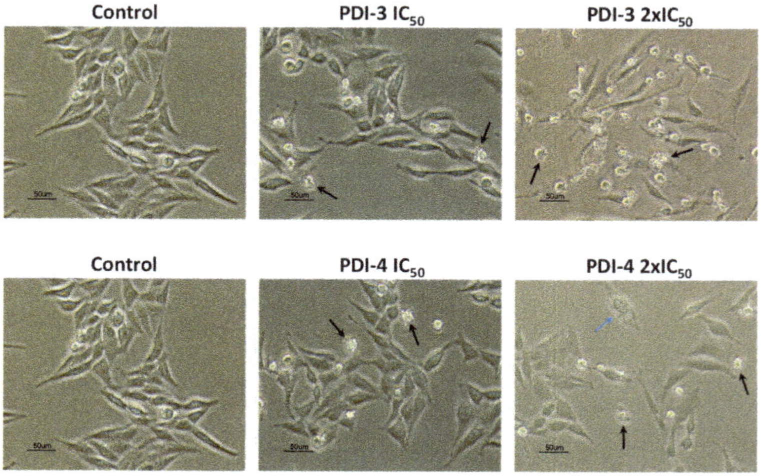

Figure 5. Phase contrast microscopy images of HeLa cells untreated (control) and treated with **PDI-3** and **PDI-4** at concentrations equal to the IC_{50} and 2 × IC_{50} μM for 24 h. Black arrows point to apoptotic cells and blue arrow to necrotic cells.

With the purpose of corroborating the mechanism of cellular death, flow cytometry studies were performed. Evaluation of their ability to promote cell death based on specific cell death markers, in particular, phosphatidylserine (PS) exposure on the outer face of the plasma membrane to detect apoptosis using Annexin V-DY634 as a marker, were conducted. As can be observed in Figure 6, both complexes induced apoptosis as cell death, and a more potent cytotoxic effect at higher concentrations was observed, especially for the compound silver species **PDI-3**.

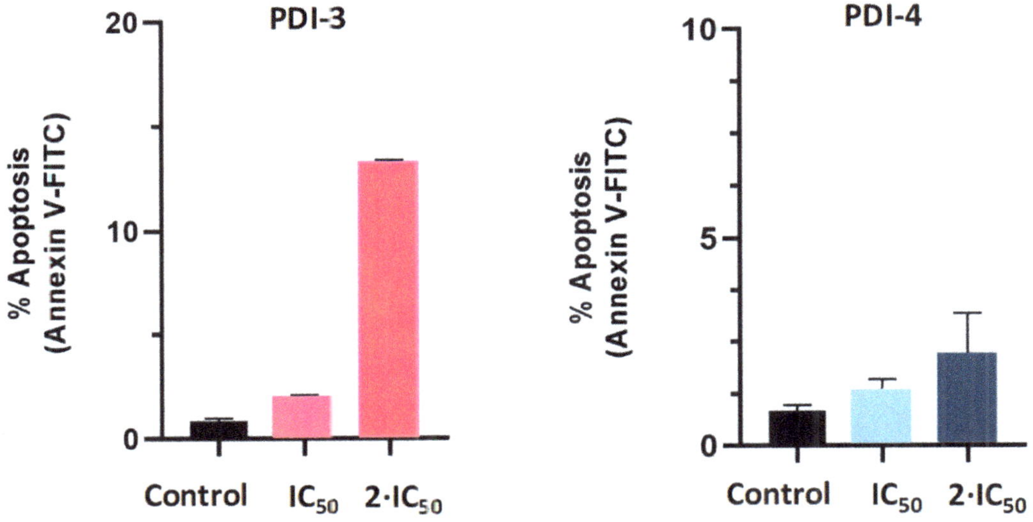

Figure 6. Cytotoxicity assays of compounds **PDI-3** and **PDI-4** incubated in HeLa cells for 24 h, in concentrations of IC_{50} and 2 IC_{50} values.

3.5. Confocal Fluorescence Microscopy

Cell biodistribution of the ligand **PDI-2** and the metal complexes **PDI-3** and **PDI-4** was studied in HeLa cells. Quenching of the luminescent properties in the tetra-metallic complexes precluded the analysis of the biodistribution in cancer cells. A colocalization assay was performed where the ligand **PDI-2** and the copper complex **PDI-4** were incubated with HeLa cells together with a commercially available selective dye for a specific organelle as internal standard. The superimposition of the images obtained from the internal standard with those of the study compounds provides the cellular internalization of the compounds.

As many of these small molecules enter the cell with a passive transport and localize in the lysosomes, the colocalization experiment was performed using the LysoTracker Green with a different emission energy from the compounds. Figure 7 shows the emission inside the cells of the ligand and copper complexes in red, and in green the emission of the LysoTracker and the superimposition images, observing a slightly different emission pattern for each compound.

The **PDI-2** ligand presents a lower internalization inside the cells than the corresponding metal complexes, and all of them spread through the cytoplasm of the cell, non-entering in the nucleus. It can be observed in the superimposition images that neither the ligand or the complexes colocalized with the signal emitted by LysoTracker, indicating the absence of a lysosomal localization.

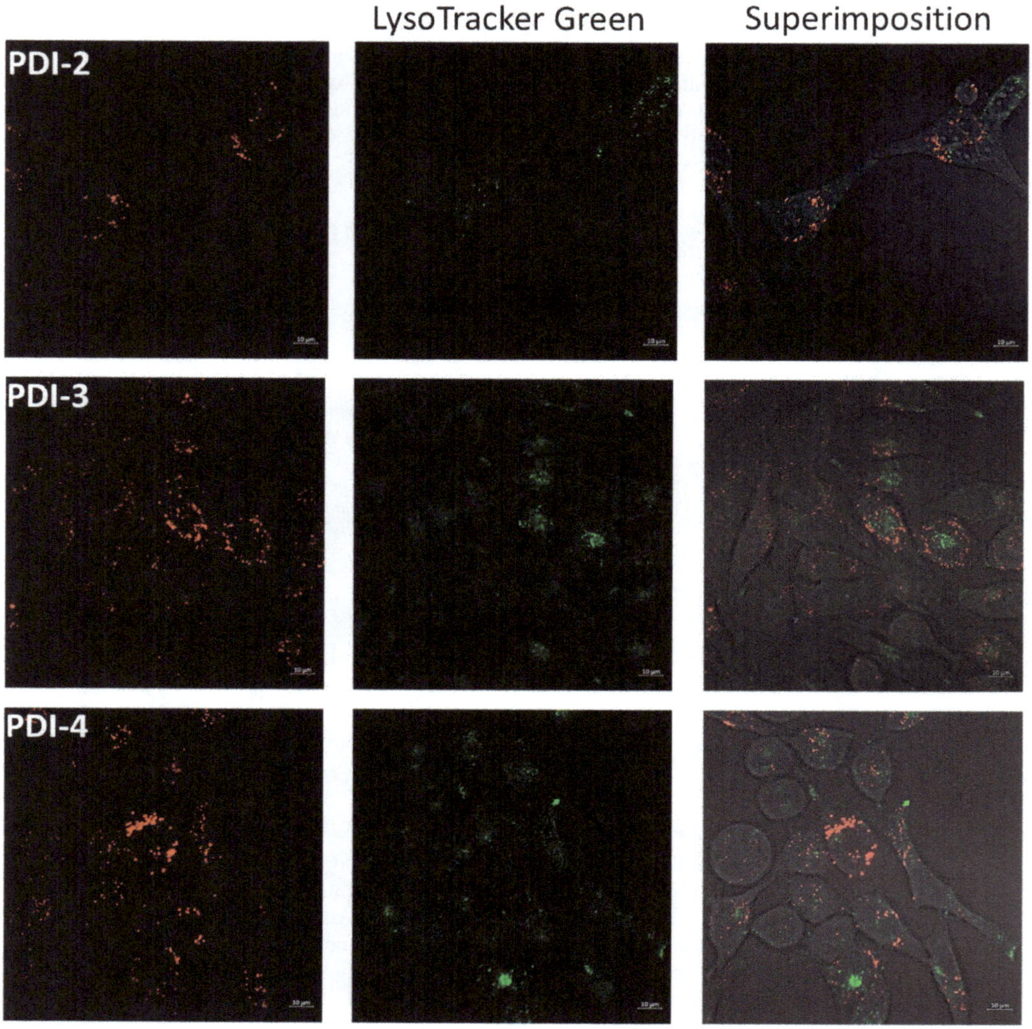

Figure 7. Fluorescence confocal microscopy images in HeLa cells incubated with the ligand **PDI-2** and the **PDI-3** and **PDI-4** complexes at 2 h (red, irradiated at 561 nm) and stained with LysoTracker Green (green, irradiation at 488 nm).

In an attempt to elucidate the biodistribution and considering the previous experiment, compounds were incubated in HeLa cells for 2 h and MitoTracker Green, a mitochondrial selective dye, was added as internal standard. Mitochondria is an important biological target and several metal complexes targeting mitochondria have been encountered. Superimposition of the images reveals a partial mitochondrial localization for the ligand **PDI-2** and the copper complex **PDI-4** (Figure 8). Additionally, small spots near the nuclear region that do not match with the mitochondrial biodistribution can be observed. This accumulation may point to a localization in the Golgi apparatus, although further experiments with this specific dye as internal standard should be performed.

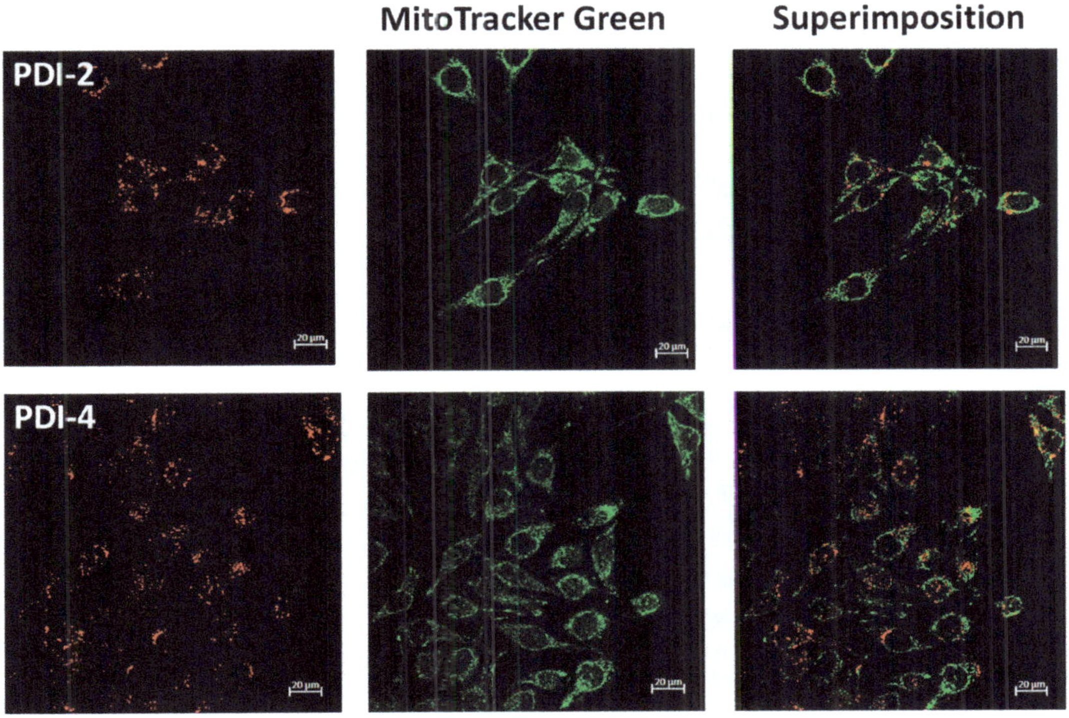

Figure 8. Fluorescence confocal microscopy images in HeLa cells incubated with the ligand **PDI-2** and the copper complex **PDI-4** at 2 h (red, irradiated at 561 nm) and stained with MitoTracker Green (green, irradiation at 488 nm).

4. Conclusions

We report the synthesis of perylenediimide (PDI) derivatives bearing one or four dipyridylamino fragments with the purpose of studying the coordination properties to silver and copper phosphine complexes. These ligands coordinate to the metal fragments in a chelate fashion and mononuclear or tetranuclear complexes have been achieved. As perylenediimides are very interesting chromophore groups, the photophysical properties of the ligands and complexes have been studied. The coordination of the metal center did not reveal a significant effect on the emission energy in the complexes, which are mainly based on the PDI ligands, although a higher quantum yield was observed upon coordination of the metal complexes. For the tetranuclear silver or copper derivatives, quenching of the luminescence was observed.

The antiproliferative effect of the free perylenediimide ligand and the metal complexes against the cervix cancer cell line HeLa was determined by the MTT assay. The free perylenediimide ligands exhibit a moderate cytotoxic activity, but the coordination of silver or copper to the dypyridylamino fragment greatly enhanced the activity, suggesting a synergistic effect between the two fragments. Flow cytometry experiments showed that the metal complexes induce an apoptotic cell death. To assert the cellular biodistribution of the PDIs and the complexes, a colocalization experiment using specific dyes for the lysosomes or mitochondria as internal standards revealed a major internalization inside the cell for the metal complexes as well as a partial mitochondrial localization.

Supplementary Materials: The following supporting information can be downloaded at: https://www.mdpi.com/article/10.3390/pharmaceutics14122616/s1. Figure S1: ^{1}H NMR spectrum of PDI-2. Figure S2: ^{13}C NMR spectrum of PDI-2. Figure S3: MALDI-TOF spectrum of PDI-2. Figure S4: UV-Vis and fluorescence spectra of PDI-2. Figure S5: IR spectrum (KBr) of PDI-2. Figure S6: ^{1}H NMR spectrum of PDI-6. Figure S7: 1^3C NMR spectrum of PDI-6. Figure S8: MALDI-TOF spectrum of PDI-6. Figure S9: UV-Vis and fluorescence spectra of PDI-6. Figure S10: IR spectrum (KBr) of PDI-6. Figure S11: ^{1}H NMR spectrum of PDI-3. Figure S12: MALDI-TOF spectrum of PDI-3. Figure S13: IR spectrum (KBr) of PDI-3. Figure S14: ^{1}H NMR spectrum of PDI-4. Figure S15: MALDI-TOF spectrum of PDI-4. Figure S16: IR spectrum (KBr) of PDI-4. Figure S17: ^{1}H NMR spectrum of PDI-7. Figure S18: IR spectrum (KBr) of PDI-7. Figure S19: ^{1}H NMR spectrum of PDI-8. Figure S20: IR spectrum (KBr) of PDI-8. Figure S21: UV-Vis spectra of PDI-complexes. Figure S22: Fluorescence spectra of PDI-3 and PDI-4. Figure S23: UV-Vis spectra of PDI-2, -3, -7, -8 in PBS solution + 5% DMSO at 37.5 °C, at 0 and 24 h. Figure S24: Dose–response curves of HeLa cells after incubation with cationic PDI-2, -3, -4, and PDI-6, -7, -8 for 24 h.

Author Contributions: Conceptualization, M.C.G. and F.F.-L.; methodology, J.G.-G. and M.R.; formal analysis, M.C.G., Á.S.-S. and F.F.-L.; writing—original draft preparation, M.C.G., Á.S.-S. and F.F.-L.; writing—review and editing, M.C.G., Á.S.-S., F.F.-L., J.G.-G. and M.R.; funding acquisition, M.C.G., Á.S.-S. and F.F.-L. All authors have read and agreed to the published version of the manuscript.

Funding: This research was funded by Agencia Estatal de Investigación (AEI), projects PID2019-109200GB-I00, PID2019-104379RB-C21/AEI/10.13039/501100011033, RED2018-102471-T (MCIN/AEI/10.13039/501100011033) and Gobierno de Aragón-Fondo Social Europeo (Research Group E07_20R).

Institutional Review Board Statement: Not applicable.

Informed Consent Statement: Not applicable.

Data Availability Statement: Not applicable.

Conflicts of Interest: The authors declare no conflict of interest.

References

1. Nowak-Król, A.; Würthner, F. Progress in the synthesis of perylene bisimide dyes. *Org. Chem. Front.* **2019**, *6*, 1272–1318. [CrossRef]
2. Gutiérrez-Moreno, D.; Sastre-Santos, Á.; Fernández-Lázaro, F. Direct amination and N-heteroarylation of perylenediimides. *Org. Chem. Front.* **2019**, *6*, 2488–2499. [CrossRef]
3. Seetharaman, S.; Zink-Lorre, N.; Gutierrez-Moreno, D.; Karr, P.A.; Fernández-Lázaro, F.; D´Souza, F. Quadrupolar Ultrafast Charge Transfer in Diaminoazobenzene-Bridged Perylenediimide Triads. *Chem. Eur. J.* **2022**, *28*, e202104574. [CrossRef] [PubMed]
4. Sideri, I.K.; Jang, J.; Garcés-Garcés, J.; Sastre-Santos, Á.; Canton-Vitoria, R.; Kitaura, R.; Fernández-Lázaro, F.; D´Souza, F.; Tagmatarchis, N. Unveiling the Photoinduced Electron-Donating Character of MoS_2 in Covalently Linked Hybrids Featuring Perylenediimide. *Angew. Chem. In. Ed.* **2021**, *60*, 9120–9126. [CrossRef]
5. Singh, P.; Hirsch, A.; Kumar, S. Perylene diimide-based chemosensors emerging in recent years: From design to sensing. *Trends Anal. Chem.* **2021**, *138*, 116–327. [CrossRef]
6. Sun, M.; Müllen, K.; Yin, M. Water-soluble perylenediimides: Design concepts and biological applications. *Chem. Soc. Rev.* **2016**, *45*, 1513–1528. [CrossRef]
7. Lu, L.; Sun, H.-J.; Zeng, Y.-T.; Shao, Y.; Bermeshev, M.V.; Zhao, Y.; Sun, B.; Chen, Z.-J.; Ren, X.-K.; Zhu, M. Perylene diimide derivative *via* ionic self-assembly: Helical supramolecular structure and selective detection of ATP. *J. Mater. Chem. C* **2020**, *8*, 10422–10430. [CrossRef]
8. Wang, K.; An, H.; Qian, F.; Wang, Y.; Zhang, J.; Li, X. Synthesis, optical properties and binding interactions of a multivalent glycocluster based on a fluorescent perylene bisimide derivative. *RSC Adv.* **2013**, *3*, 23190–23196. [CrossRef]
9. Céspedes-Guirao, F.J.; Ropero, A.B.; Font-Sanchis, E.; Nadal, Á.; Fernández-Lázaro, F.; Sastre-Santos, Á. A water-soluble perylenedye functionalised with a 17β-estradiol: A new fluorescent tool for steroid hormones. *Chem. Commun.* **2011**, *47*, 8307–8309. [CrossRef]
10. Yang, S.K.; Shi, X.; Park, S.; Doganay, S.; Ha, T.; Zimmerman, S.C. Monovalent, Clickable, Uncharged, Water-Soluble Perylenediimide-Cored Dendrimers for Target-Specific Fluorescent Biolabeling. *J. Am. Chem. Soc.* **2011**, *133*, 9964–9967. [CrossRef]
11. Donnier-Marechal, M.; Galanos, N.; Grandjean, T.; Pascal, Y.; Ji, D.K.; Dong, L.; Gillon, E.; He, X.P.; Imberty, A.; Kipnis, E.; et al. Perylenediimide-based glycoclusters as high affinity ligands of bacterial lectins: Synthesis, binding studies and anti-adhesive properties. *Org. Biomol. Chem.* **2017**, *15*, 10037–10043. [CrossRef] [PubMed]
12. Gálvez, N.; Kedracka, E.J.; Carmona, F.; Céspedes-Guirano, F.J.; Font-Sanchis, E.; Fernández-Lázaro, F.; Sastre-Santos, Á.; Domínguez-Vera, J.M. Water soluble fluorescent-magnetic perylenediimide-containing maghemite-nanoparticles for bimodal MRI/OI imaging. *J. Inorg. Biochem.* **2012**, *117*, 205–211. [CrossRef] [PubMed]

13. Li, H.; Yue, L.; Li, L.; Liu, G.; Zhang, J.; Luo, X.; Wu, F. Triphenylamine-perylene diimide conjugate-based organic nanoparticles for photoacoustic imaging and cancer phototherapy. *Colloids Surf. B Biointerfaces* **2021**, *205*, 111841. [CrossRef] [PubMed]
14. Büyükekçi, S.I.; Orman, E.B.; Sangül, A.; Altindal, A.; Özkaya, A.R. Electrochemical and photovoltaic studies on water soluble triads: Metallosupramolecular self-assembly of ditopic bis(imidazole)perylene diimide with platinum(II)-, and palladium(II)-2,2′:6′,2″-terpyridyl complex ions. *Dyes Pigm.* **2017**, *144*, 190–202. [CrossRef]
15. Dominguez, C.; Baena, M.J.; Coco, S.; Espinet, P. Perylenecarboxydiimide-gold(I) organometallic dyes. Optical properties and Langmuir films. *Dyes Pigm.* **2017**, *140*, 375–383. [CrossRef]
16. Cai, Y.; Cheng, W.; Ji, C.; Su, Z.; Yin, M. Perylenediimide/silver nanohybrids with visible-light photocatalysis enhanced antibacterial effect. *Dyes Pigm.* **2021**, *195*, 109698. [CrossRef]
17. Costa, R.D.; Céspedes-Guirao, F.J.; Ortí, E.; Bolink, H.J.; Gierschner, J.; Fernández-Lázaro, F. Sastre-Santos, Á. Efficient deep-red light-emitting electrochemical cells based on a perylenediimide-iridium-complex dyad. *Chem. Commun.* **2009**, *26*, 3886–3888. [CrossRef]
18. Qvortrup, K.; Bond, A.D.; Nielsen, A.; McKenize, C.J.; Kilså, K.; Nielsen, M.B. Perylenediimide—Metal ion dyads for photo-induced electron transfer. *Chem. Commun.* **2008**, 1986–1988. [CrossRef]
19. Hou, Y.; Zhang, Z.; Lu, S.; Yuan, J.; Zhu, Q.; Chen, W.P.; Ling, S.; Li, X.; Zheng, Y.Z.; Zhu, K.; et al. Highly Emissive Perylene Diimide-Based Metallacages and Their Host–Guest Chemistry for Information Encryption. *J. Am. Chem. Soc.* **2020**, *142*, 18763–18768. [CrossRef]
20. Aksakal, N.E.; Kazan, H.H.; Ecik, E.T.; Yuksel, F. Novel photosensitizer based on a ruthenium(ii) phenanthroline bis(perylenediimide) dyad: Synthesis, generation of singlet oxygen and in vitro photodynamic therapy. *New J. Chem.* **2018**, *42*, 17538–17545. [CrossRef]
21. Zhang, S.; Du, C.; Wang, Z.; Han, X.; Zhang, K.; Liu, L. Carboplatin resistant human laryngeal carcinoma cells are cross resistant to curcumin due to reduced curcumin accumulation. *Toxicol. Vitr.* **2013**, *27*, 739–744. [CrossRef] [PubMed]
22. Eloy, L.; Jarrousse, A.S.; Teyssot, M.L.; Gautier, A.; Morel, L.; Jolivalt, C.; Cresteil, T.; Roland, S. Anticancer Activity of Silver–*N*-Heterocyclic Carbene Complexes: Caspase-Independent Induction of Apoptosis via Mitochondrial Apoptosis-Inducing Factor (AIF). *ChemMedChem* **2012**, *7*, 805–814. [CrossRef]
23. Kumar Raju, S.; Karunakaran, A.; Kumar, S.; Sekar, P.; Murugesan, M.; Karthikeyan, M. Silver Complexes as Anticancer Agents: A Perspective Review. *German J. Pharm. Biomater.* **2022**, *1*, 6–28. [CrossRef]
24. Santini, C.; Pellei, M.; Gandin, V.; Porchia, M.; Tisato, F.; Marzano, C. Advances in Copper Complexes as Anticancer Agents. *Chem. Rev.* **2014**, *114*, 815–862. [CrossRef] [PubMed]
25. Canudo-Barreras, G.; Ortego, L.; Izaga, A.; Marzo, I.; Herrera, R.P.; Gimeno, M.C. Synthesis of New Thiourea-Metal Complexes with Promising Anticancer Properties. *Molecules* **2021**, *26*, 6891. [CrossRef]
26. Mármol, I.; Montanel-Perez, S.; Royo, J.C.; Gimeno, M.C.; Villacampa, M.D.; Rodríguez-Yoldi, M.J.; Cerrada, E. Gold(I) and Silver(I) Complexes with 2-Anilinopyridine-Based Heterocycles as Multitarget Drugs against Colon Cancer. *Inorg. Chem.* **2020**, *59*, 17732–17745. [CrossRef]
27. Johnson, A.; Marzo, I.; Gimeno, M.C. Heterobimetallic propargyl gold complexes with π-bound copper or silver with enhanced anticancer activity. *Dalton Trans.* **2020**, *49*, 11736–11742. [CrossRef]
28. Salvador-Gil, D.; Ortego, L.; Herrera, R.P.; Marzo, I.; Gimeno, M.C. Highly active group 11 metal complexes with α-hydrazidophosphonate ligands. *Dalton Trans.* **2017**, *46*, 13745–13755. [CrossRef]
29. Molinaro, C.; Martoriati, A.; Pelinski, L.; Cailliau, K. Copper Complexes as Anticancer Agents Targeting Topoisomerases I and II. *Cancers* **2020**, *12*, 2863. [CrossRef]
30. Bardají, M.; Crespo, O.; Laguna, A.; Fischer, A.K. Structural characterization of silver(I) complexes [Ag(O_3SCF_3)(L)] (L=PPh_3, PPh_2Me, SC_4H_8) and [AgL_n](CF_3SO_3) (n=2–4), (L=PPh_3, PPh_2Me). *Inorg. Chim. Acta* **2000**, *304*, 7–16. [CrossRef]
31. Rajasingh, P.; Cohen, R.; Shirman, E.; Shimon, L.J.W.; Rybtchiski, B. Selective Bromination of Perylene Diimides under Mild Conditions. *J. Org. Chem.* **2007**, *72*, 5973–5979. [CrossRef] [PubMed]
32. Battagliarin, G.; Li, C.; Enkelmann, V.; Müllen, K. 2,5,8,11-Tetraboronic Ester Perylenediimides: A Next Generation Building Block for Dye-Stuff Synthesis. *Org. Lett.* **2011**, *13*, 3012–3015. [CrossRef] [PubMed]
33. Teraoka, T.; Hiroto, S.; Shinokubo, H. Iridium-Catalyzed Direct Tetraborylation of Perylene Bisimides. *Org. Lett.* **2011**, *13*, 2532–2535. [CrossRef]
34. Guram, A.S.; Rennels, R.A.; Buchwald, S.L. A Simple Catalytic Method for the Conversion of Aryl Bromides to Arylamines. *Angew Chem. Int. Ed. Engl.* **1995**, *34*, 1348–1350. [CrossRef]
35. Louie, L.; Hartwig, J.F. Palladium-catalyzed synthesis of arylamines from aryl halides. Mechanistic studies lead to coupling in the absence of tin reagents. *Tetrahedron Lett.* **1995**, *36*, 3609–3612. [CrossRef]
36. Van Meerloo, J.; Kaspers, G.J.; Cloos, J. Cell sensitivity assays: The MTT assay. *Methods Mol. Biol.* **2011**, *731*, 237–245.

pharmaceutics

MDPI

Article

A Pseudovirus Nanoparticle-Based Trivalent Rotavirus Vaccine Candidate Elicits High and Cross P Type Immune Response

Ming Xia [1,†], Pengwei Huang [1,†] and Ming Tan [1,2,*]

[1] Division of Infectious Diseases, Cincinnati Children's Hospital Medical Center, Cincinnati, OH 45229, USA; ming.xia@cchmc.org (M.X.); pengwei.huang@cchmc.org (P.H.)
[2] Department of Pediatrics, University of Cincinnati College of Medicine, Cincinnati, OH 45229, USA
* Correspondence: ming.tan@cchmc.org
† These authors contributed equally to this work.

Abstract: Rotavirus infection continues to cause significant morbidity and mortality globally. In this study, we further developed the S_{60}-VP8* pseudovirus nanoparticles (PVNPs) displaying the glycan receptor binding VP8* domains of rotavirus spike proteins as a parenteral vaccine candidate. First, we established a scalable method for the large production of tag-free S_{60}-VP8* PVNPs representing four rotavirus P types, P[8], P[4], P[6], and P[11]. The approach consists of two major steps: selective precipitation of the S-VP8* proteins from bacterial lysates using ammonium sulfate, followed by anion exchange chromatography to further purify the target proteins to a high purity. The purified soluble proteins self-assembled into S_{60}-VP8* PVNPs. Importantly, after intramuscular injections, the trivalent vaccine consisting of three PVNPs covering VP8* antigens of P[8], P[4], and P[6] rotaviruses elicited high and broad immunogenicity in mice toward the three predominant P-type rotaviruses. Specifically, the trivalent vaccine-immunized mouse sera showed (1) high and balanced IgG and IgA antibody titers toward all three VP8* types, (2) high blocking titer against the VP8*-glycan receptor interaction, and (3) high and broad neutralizing titers against replications of all P[8], P[4], and P[6] rotaviruses. Therefore, trivalent S_{60}-VP8* PVNPs are a promising non-replicating, parenteral vaccine candidate against the most prevalent rotaviruses worldwide.

Keywords: rotavirus; S_{60}-VP8* pseudovirus nanoparticle; rotavirus vaccine; rotavirus VP8*; non-replicating rotavirus vaccine; norovirus S_{60} nanoparticle

Citation: Xia, M.; Huang, P.; Tan, M. A Pseudovirus Nanoparticle-Based Trivalent Rotavirus Vaccine Candidate Elicits High and Cross P Type Immune Response. *Pharmaceutics* **2022**, *14*, 1597. https://doi.org/10.3390/pharmaceutics14081597

Academic Editors: Ana Isabel Fraguas-Sánchez, Raquel Fernández García and Francisco Bolás-Fernández

Received: 5 July 2022
Accepted: 27 July 2022
Published: 30 July 2022

1. Introduction

Rotaviruses, a group of double-stranded RNA viruses in the family Reoviridae, are causative agents of contagious gastroenteritis in infants and young children with typical symptoms of severe watery diarrhea, vomiting, abdominal pain, and/or fever, often leading to dehydration, and occasional death. Before a vaccine was available, nearly every child was infected with rotavirus at least once by the age of five, with the first infection usually occurring before three years of age [1]. Through the implementation of live attenuated vaccines since 2006, the rotavirus disease burden around the globe has significantly decreased, particularly in developed countries [2,3]. Nevertheless, the effectiveness of oral vaccines has been found to be diminished in source-deprived, low-income nations [4,5]. Consequently, rotavirus-associated diseases continue to cause about 24 million outpatient visits, 2.3 million hospitalizations, and 200,000 deaths worldwide each year [6,7]. Therefore, rotavirus-associated diarrhea remains a global public health threat, and a new generation of rotavirus vaccine tactics with improved efficacy is urgently needed, especially for children in developing countries where rotavirus infection occurs the most.

The reasons underlying the reduced effectiveness of current live rotavirus vaccines in low-income nations are not fully understood [8,9]. The growing literature points to multiple factors that affect the intestinal environment of children in developing countries [9]. These include microbiota dysbiosis [10], malnutrition [11], enterovirus infection [12], and the simultaneous immunization of poliovirus and other oral vaccines [9,13]. These factors may play a role in altering the intestinal conditions necessary for optimal replication of the live rotavirus vaccines, thus negatively impacting the immune responses and the efficacy of the oral vaccines, which are also common to other live, oral vaccines [9].

In summary of related literature, a recent study [14] quantified rotavirus vaccine impact, investigated the reduced vaccine effectiveness using sophisticated mathematical models, and proposed a parenteral vaccine tactic to circumvent the negative impact of the above-mentioned intestine-associated factors. Therefore, a non-replicating subunit vaccine administrated via a parenteral route could enhance rotavirus vaccine efficacy for children in developing nations. In addition, the known risk of intussusception associated with the live rotavirus vaccine [15–21] may result from the replication of oral vaccines within the intestine. Thus, a non-replicating parenteral vaccine may also avoid intussusception risk offering an improved safety feature.

Our development of a non-replicating subunit rotavirus vaccine started with the P_{24}-VP8* nanoparticle [22–24] that consists of a 24 valent P_{24} nanoparticle core made by 24 norovirus protruding (P) domains [25,26] and 24 surface displayed VP8* antigens The VP8* antigens form the distal heads of rotavirus spikes, which are composed of rotavirus VP4s. Since VP8* interacts with glycan receptors to initiate a viral infection, it is a major neutralizing antigen and thus an important vaccine target of a rotavirus subunit vaccine [23,27–34]. The P_{24}-VP8* nanoparticles were shown to elicit high immune responses in mice [23] and pigs [35] towards the displayed VP8* antigens after intramuscular immunization and protected immunized mice and gnotobiotic pigs from rotavirus challenge [23,35]. In this regard, rotavirus-like particles consisting of VP2, VP6, and/or VP7 [36,37], P2-VP8-P[8] fusion proteins composed of a tandem of two VP8* with a T cell epitope in between [38,39], and truncated VP4 trimers [40] have been generated and studied as non-replicating rotavirus vaccine candidates by others.

The rotavirus virion is a triple-layered particle about 85 nm in diameter. It consists of a core shell constituted by VP2, a middle layer formed by VP6, and an outer layer consists of two surface proteins, VP7 and VP4. Rotaviruses are categorized into G and P genotypes based on the gene sequences encoding the surface proteins VP7 and VP4/VP8*, respectively. P[8] and P[4] are the two most prevalent P genotypes [41], contributing to up to 95% of circulated rotaviruses around the world. It has also been noted that P[6] rotaviruses are frequently detected in Africa, accounting for up to 30% of the detected rotaviruses [42,43]. These data indicate that a potent rotavirus vaccine should be able to protect vaccinees against P[8], P[4], and P[6] rotaviruses, particularly for use in developing countries. In addition, although less prevalent than P[8], P[4], and P[6] rotaviruses, the P[11] genotype is often found in India [44–47]. In fact, India has developed and licensed a live Rotavac® vaccine (Bharat Biotech) that contains a single P[11] rotavirus strain.

In an attempt to create a new non-replicating subunit rotavirus vaccine, we took advantage of our recently developed S_{60} nanoparticle that consists of 60 norovirus shell (S) domains, to generate an S_{60}-VP8* pseudovirus nanoparticle (PVNP) that displays 60 copies of VP8* antigen of a P[8] rotavirus on the surface [48]. This polyvalent S_{60}-VP8* PVNP preserves the pathogen-associated molecular patterns (PAMPs) of both norovirus and rotavirus and thus induces high immune responses toward the VP8* antigens and protects mice from the rotavirus challenge [33,48,49]. The S_{60}-VP8* PVNP was purified using a His tag that appears to reduce the solubility and thus the production yield of the PVNP, which may impose a negative factor in the downstream development of the vaccine candidate. In this study, we designed tag-free S_{60}-VP8* PVNPs displaying VP8* antigens representing the four predominant rotavirus P types and developed an efficient, scalable production approach to generate tag-free PVNPs in a large amount. A trivalent vaccine consisting of S_{60}-VP8* PVNPs covering VP8* antigens of P[8], P[4], and P[6] rotaviruses elicited high and broad immune responses to all three VP8* types, offering a promising vaccine candidate against predominant rotaviruses circulating globally.

2. Materials and Methods

2.1. Plasmids for Expression of Four Tag-Free S-VP8 Fusion Proteins*

Three DNA fragments that encode the major functional sections of the VP8* domains, spanning from L65 to L223 of rotavirus VP4 proteins of a P[8] (strain 13851), a P[4] (strain BM5256), and a P[6] (strain 11597) virus, respectively, were amplified by PCR from our lab stock plasmids [22,30,50]. The DNA fragments were then cloned into the previously made pET-24b (Novagen)-based vector that was generated for production of the C-terminally His-tagged S_{60}-VP8* P[8] PVNP [48] by replacing its VP8* encoding sequences. The S domain-encoding region in the plasmids contains an R69A mutation to remove the exposed protease recognition site [48]. In addition, a DNA fragment encoding the same VP8* region of a P[11] rotavirus (GenBank Code: EU200796) was codon-optimized to *Escherichia coli* (*E. coli*) and synthesized by GenScript (Piscataway, NJ, USA). The synthesized DNA fragment was subcloned into the above-mentioned plasmid using the same approach. A stop codon was added in front of the His tag-encoding sequences of pET 24b to remove the His tag.

2.2. Expression and Purification of Tag-Free S-VP8 Fusion Proteins*

Tag-free S-VP8* proteins were expressed using the *E. coli* (strain BL21, DE3) system through an induction with 0.25 mM isopropyl-β-D-thiogalactopyranoside (IPTG) at ~22 °C overnight as described elsewhere [25,51]. For protein purification, bacteria were lysed by sonication, and the bacterial lysates were clarified by centrifugation at 10,000 rpm for 30 min using an Avanti J26XP centrifuge (Beckman Coulter Life Sciences, Indianapolis, IN, USA) and a JA-17 rotor. Clarified supernatants were treated with ammonium sulfate [$(NH_4)_2SO_4$] at 1.2 M end concentrations for 30 min to selectively precipitate the target proteins. The protein precipitations were collected by centrifugation at 5000 rpm for 20 min using the same centrifuge and rotor (see above), washed twice using 1.2 M $(NH_4)_2SO_4$ solution in 20 mM Tris buffer (pH 8.0), and then dissolved in 20 mM Tris buffer (pH 8.0), as described previously [22].

2.3. Anion Exchange Chromatography

Anion exchange chromatography was conducted to further purify the $(NH_4)_2SO_4$-precipitated S-VP8* proteins using an AKTA Fast Performance Liquid Chromatography System (AKTA Pure 25L, GE Healthcare Life Sciences, Piscataway, NJ, USA) with a HiPrep Q HP 16/10 column (20 mL bed volume, GE Healthcare Life Sciences, Piscataway, NJ, USA), as described previously [22]. Briefly, the column was equilibrated with 5 column volumes (CV) of 20 mM Tris-HCl buffer (pH 8.0, referred to as buffer A). After loading the protein samples (~5 mL), the column was washed using 7 CVs of buffer A. The bound proteins were eluted using 7 CVs 1 M NaCl in buffer A (referred to as buffer B) through a linear gradient (0 to 100% buffer B). The column was washed with 7 CVs of buffer B, followed by a final equilibration with 7 CVs of Buffer A. Relative protein amounts in the effluent were shown by A280 absorbance.

2.4. Sodium Dodecyl Sulfate Polyacrylamide Gel Electrophoresis (SDS-PAGE)

SDS-PAGE was performed to analyze the protein quality using 10% separating gels. Protein concentrations were determined by SDS-PAGE using serially diluted bovine serum albumin (BSA, Bio-Rad, Hercules, CA, USA), with known concentrations as standards on the same gels [23].

2.5. Transmission Electron Microscopy (TEM)

TEM was performed to inspect the morphology of the S_{60}-VP8* PVNPs. PVNP samples from gel filtration chromatography or a CsCl density gradient in 6.0 µL volume were absorbed to a grid (FCF200-CV-50, Electron Microscopy Sciences, Hatfield, PA, USA) for 20 min in a humid chamber and were negatively stained with 1% ammonium molybdate After washing and air drying, the grids were observed using a Hitachi microscope (model H-7650) at 80 kV for a magnification between 15,000× and 60,000× as described elsewhere [48]

2.6. Cesium Chloride (CsCl) Density Gradient Ultracentrifugation

This method was utilized to analyze the density of the S_{60}-VP8* PVNPs as described previously [48]. Briefly, 0.5 mL of the purified PVNPs were mixed with CsCl solution to a volume of 10 mL with a density of 1.3630 and centrifuged at 41,000 rpm (288,000× *g*) for 45 h using the Optima L-90K ultracentrifuge (Beckman Coulter Life Sciences, Indianapolis, IN USA). By bottom puncture of the centrifugation tubes, the CsCl gradients were fractionated into 22 fractions, with about 0.5 mL each. The S-VP8* PVNPs in the fractions were detected by EIA assays after 100-fold dilution in phosphate buffer saline (PBS, pH 7.4) and coated on 96-well microtiter plates (Thermo Scientific, Waltham, MA, USA) using our in-house-made hyperimmune guinea pig serum against norovirus VLPs [52]. The CsCl densities of the fractions were determined using the refractive index.

2.7. Mouse Immunization with the S_{60}-VP8 PVNPs and Controls

Rotavirus-free BALB/c mice at age about six weeks with body weight ranging from 19 to 23 g were randomly divided into five groups with 6 to 8 mice each (N = 6–8) that were immunized with following immunogens, respectively: (1) the trivalent PVNP vaccine consisting of three S_{60}-VP8* PVNPs that display the VP8* antigens of P[8], P[4], and P[6] rotaviruses, respectively, in equal molar ratio at 30 µg/mouse/dose (10 µg of each PVNP type); (2) the S_{60}-VP8* PVNPs of P[8] rotavirus at 10 µg/mouse/dose; (3) the S_{60}-VP8* PVNPs of P[4] rotavirus at 10 µg/mouse/dose; (4) the S_{60}-VP8* PVNPs of P[6] rotavirus at 10 µg/mouse/dose; and (5) the S_{60} nanoparticles without the VP8* antigens [25,26] at 10 µg/mouse/dose as a negative control. All immunogens were treated with endotoxin removal resin (Pierce, Waltham, MA, USA) to remove endotoxin contamination. The immunogens were delivered with an Alum adjuvant (Thermo Scientific aluminum hydroxide, 40 mg/mL) at 25 µL/dose through 1:1 mixing with immunogens at 20 µg/mouse/dose, as described elsewhere [22]. This resulted in an end aluminum hydroxide dose of 1.0 mg/dose/mouse. Immunogens in 50 µL volumes were injected intramuscularly into the thigh muscle. Immunizations were performed three times at 2-week intervals. Blood samples were taken before the first immunization, as well as two weeks after the second and the third immunization, through tail veins (before the first immunization and after the second immunization) and the heart puncture approach (after the third immunization) for serum sample preparations [23].

2.8. Enzyme Immunoassays (EIAs)

EIAs were performed to detect the S-VP8* proteins in the fractions of the CsCl gradients (see above) and to determine the VP8*-specific antibody titers [48]. For antibody determination, gel filtration purified GST-VP8* fusion proteins of P[8], P[4], and P[6] rotaviruses from our lab stock [30,50] were coated on microtiter plates at 1 µg/mL overnight. After blocking with nonfat milk, the plates were incubated with mouse sera at serial 2x dilutions. Bound antibodies were measured with goat-anti-mouse IgG-horse radish peroxidase (HRP) conjugate (1:5000, MP Biomedicals, Santa Ana, CA, USA) for VP8*-specific IgG or goat-anti-mouse IgA-horse radish peroxidase (HRP) conjugate (1:2000, Invitrogen, Waltham, MA, USA) for VP8*-specific IgA. Antibody titers were defined as the maximum dilutions of sera that exhibited at least cut-off signals of OD_{450} = 0.15, as described previously [48].

2.9. 50% Blocking Titer (BT_{50}) of Sera against Rotavirus VP8*-Glycan Receptor Attachment

This was determined as described previously [53]. Briefly, well-characterized human saliva samples with Lewis b (Le^b) antigens from our lab stock [52] were boiled and coated on microtiter plates at 1:1000 dilution. The P_{24}-VP8* nanoparticle at 0.625 μg/mL was pre-incubated with the PVNP-immunized mouse sera at different dilutions before the P_{24}-VP8* nanoparticles were added to the coated saliva samples. The BT_{50} was defined as the serum dilutions that caused at least 50% blocking effects compared with the unblocked positive controls.

2.10. Rotavirus Neutralization Assays

This fluorescence-based plaque reduction assay was performed as described previously [22,49]. Briefly, rotaviruses of the P[8] (Wa strain, G1P8), P[6] (ST-3 strain, G4P6), and P[4] (DS-1 strain, G2P4) types were treated with trypsin and incubated with serially diluted mouse sera after various PVNP immunizations. The treated rotaviruses were then added to the MA104 cells on 96-well plates, and the cells were continually cultured for 16 h. The cells on the plates were then fixed with pre-cooled 80% (v/v) acetone, followed by blocking with nonfat milk. The rotavirus-infected cells were stained with guinea pig antiserum (1:800) against rotaviruses. The bound antibodies were shown by fluorescein DyLight 594-labeled goat anti-guinea pig IgG (H +L) antibodies (Jackson Immuno Research Labs, West Grove, PA, USA). Fluorescence-formation plaques on plates were photographed using a Cytation 5 imaging reader, and fluorescence plaques (rotavirus-infected cells) were counted. Neutralization titers were described as the maximum dilutions of the mouse sera, showing at least a 50% reduction in fluorescence-formation plaques compared with the positive control with mouse serum.

2.11. Statistical Analyses

Statistical differences between data groups were analyzed using software GraphPad Prism version 9.3.1 (471) (GraphPad Software, Inc., San Diego, CA, USA) via unpaired *t* tests. Differences were classified as follows: (1) non-significant (labeled as ns), when a p value is >0.05, (2) significant (labeled as *), when a p value is <0.05, (3) highly significant (labeled as **), when a p value is <0.01, and (4) extremely significant, when a p value is <0.001 (labeled as ***), or <0.0001 (labeled as ****).

3. Results

3.1. Expression and Selective Precipitation of the S-VP8* Proteins

Four S-VP8* fusion proteins (Figure 1A), each containing the VP8* domain of a P[4], a P[6], a P[8], or a P[11] rotavirus, were expressed using the *E. coli* system. After IPTG induction, bacterial cultures were collected and sonicated to release soluble S-VP8* proteins. The clarified bacterial lysates were treated with 1.2 M $(NH_4)_2SO_4$ to selectively precipitate the target proteins, which were then dissolved in 20 mM Tris buffer (pH 8.0). The S-VP8* proteins at about 43 kDa were shown on an SDS-PAGE gel (Figure 1B), revealing the S-VP8* proteins as the major precipitated proteins, with a number of co-precipitated bacterial proteins.

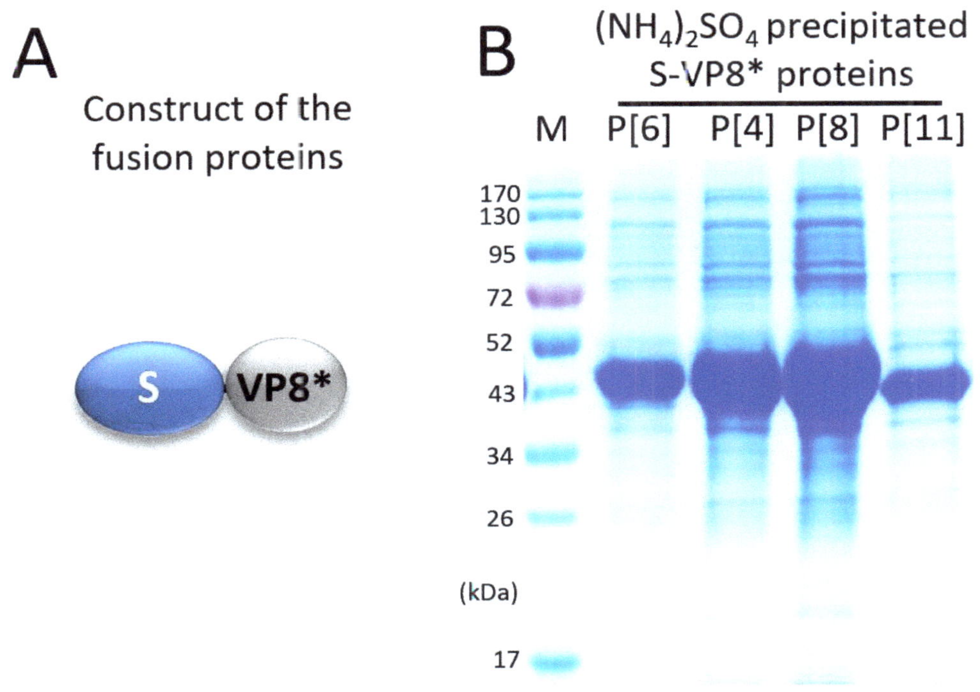

Figure 1. Expression and selective precipitation of the S-VP8* fusion proteins. (**A**) Schematic diagram of the S-VP8* fusion proteins. S, modified norovirus shell (S) domain; VP8*, rotavirus VP8* domain. (**B**) SDS-PAGE of the ammonium sulfate [$(NH_4)_2SO_4$] precipitated S-VP8* fusion proteins at about 43 kDa, which contain the VP8* domains of P[6], P[4], P[8], and P[11], respectively. Lane M is a pre-stained protein standards with indicated molecular weights in kDa.

3.2. Purification of S-VP8* Proteins by Ion Exchange Chromatography

The $(NH_4)_2SO_4$ precipitated S-VP8* proteins of the four rotavirus P types were further purified using anion exchange chromatography, with their elusion curves shown in Figure 2A (P[4]), Figure S1A (P[6]), Figure S2A (P[8]), and Figure S3A (P[11]), respectively. The major elution peaks of the corresponding chromatography were analyzed by SDS-PAGE (Figures 2B, S1B, S2B and S3B), showing three common features among these four ion exchanges. First, the vast majority of the co-precipitated bacterial proteins did not bind or did not bind well to the HiPrep Q HP 16/10 column. As a result, they either flowed directly through the column or were washed away during the washing step afterwards. Second, all four target proteins were eluted in single narrow peaks with relatively low salt concentrations, corresponding to 34.7% to 38.7% of buffer B, equivalent to 347 mM to 387 mM NaCl. Third, the S-VP8* proteins were separated well from the co-precipitated bacterial proteins, reaching to high yields of the proteins at >30 mg/liter of bacterial culture and a high purity of >95% (Figures 2B, S1B, S2B and S3B). Thus, this production method serves as a simple but effective and scalable approach for low-cost production of tag-free PVNPs (see below).

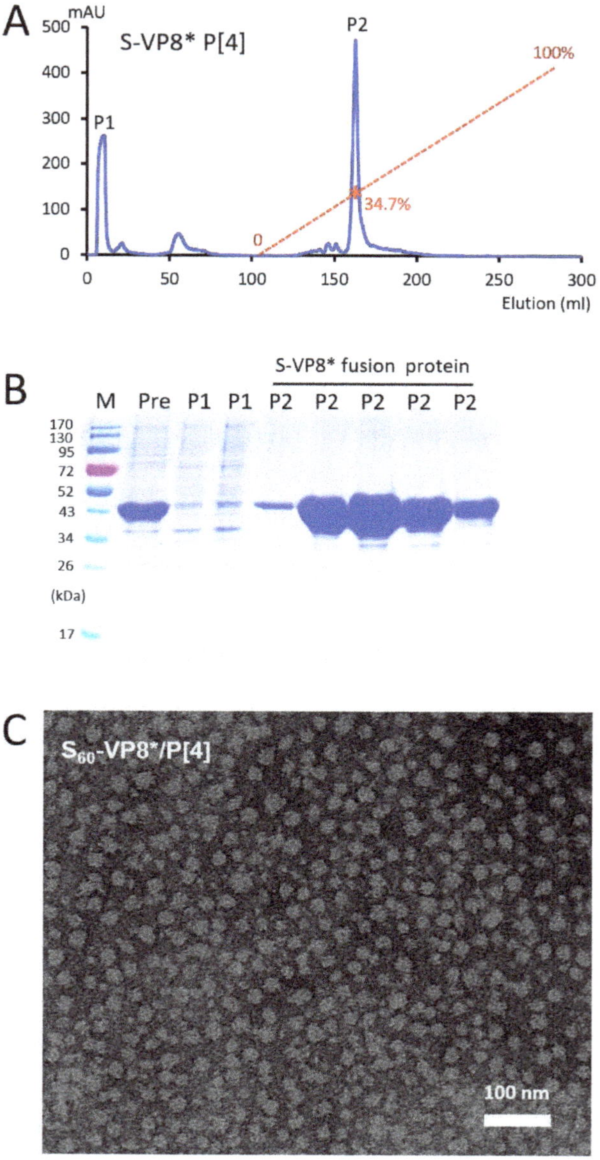

Figure 2. Purification of tag-free S-VP8* P[4] protein and its self-assembly into pseudovirus nanoparticles (PVNPs). (**A**) An anion exchange elution curve of the ammonium sulfate [$(NH_4)_2SO_4$] precipitated S-VP8* P[4] protein. The *X*-axis indicates elution volume (mL), whereas the *Y*-axis shows UV (A_{280}) absorbances (mAU). The red dashed line indicates the linear increase of elution buffer B (0–100%), with a red star symbol indicating the percentage of buffer B at the elution peak of the S-VP8* P[4] protein (34.7%). Two major peaks that were analyzed by SDS-PAGE are indicated as P1 and P2. (**B**) SDS-PAGE of the pre-loaded protein (Pre), as well as proteins from peak 1 (P1) and peak 2 (P2) from the anion exchange chromatography. Pre is the $(NH_4)_2SO_4$ precipitated protein samples before loading to the column; M is the pre-stained protein standards with indicated molecular weights in kDa. The S-VP8* P[4] protein was eluted in P2. (**C**) A micrograph of negative-staining transmission electron microscopy (TEM) of the protein from P2 shows spheric-shaped PVNPs.

3.3. Self-Formation of Purified S-VP8* Proteins into PVNPs

The ion exchange chromatography purified S-VP8* fusion proteins were inspected by negative strain TEM, revealing large numbers of nanoparticles at about 25 nm in diameter, with some size variations (Figures 2C, S1C, S2C and S3C). Since the previously solved 3-dimensional structure of the His tagged S_{60}-VP8 P[8] PVNPs exhibited about 25 nm in diameters [48], these micrographs indicated that the four tag-free S-VP8* fusion proteins self-assembled into S_{60}-VP8* PVNPs. The size variations disappeared after the PVNPs were further analyzed by CsCl gradient ultracentrifugation (see below).

3.4. CsCl Gradient Ultracentrifugation of the PVNPs

The four S-VP8* fusion proteins were analyzed by CsCl gradient ultracentrifugation, which revealed a major and minor peak for each S-VP8* fusion protein (Figure 3A,C,E,G left panel). The major peaks were located at or near fraction 17, whereas the minor peaks were at fraction 11 of the gradients, equivalent to densities of 1.305 and 1.311 mg/cm^3, respectively. TEM inspection of the protein samples from the major peaks (fractions 17 or 18) showed uniform, ring shaped S_{60}-VP8* PVNPS (Figure 3B,D,F,H right panel). Inspection of the proteins from the minor peaks (fraction 11) also showed similar ring-shaped PVNPs, but the PVNP numbers were apparently less abundant (data not shown) than those of the major peaks. It remains unclear why similar PVNPs are distributed in two distinct peaks with different densities.

3.5. Trivalent PVNP Vaccine and Its IgG Responses in Mice

Surveillance data showed that P[8], P[4], and P[6] rotaviruses are the predominant rotavirus P types [41–43], thus three S_{60}-VP8* PVNP types, displaying the VP8* antigens of P[8], P[4], and P[6] rotaviruses, respectively, were mixed at equal molar ratios as a trivalent vaccine. Mice were immunized intramuscularly with the trivalent vaccine, using aluminum hydroxide as an adjuvant. The three individual PVNPs were used as single-valent PVNP vaccine controls, and the S_{60} nanoparticle without the VP8* antigen was used as a platform control for comparisons (see Materials and methods). Serum samples were collected after two and three immunizations to determine the VP8*-specific antibody responses by EIA assays using recombinant VP8* proteins of P[8], P[4], and P[6] rotaviruses, respectively, as capture antigens.

The results (Figure 4) showed that, after three immunizations, the trivalent vaccine induced high and balanced IgG titers (341,333 to 614,533) to all P[8], P[4], and P[6] VP8*s to levels similar to those elicited by the single-valent PVNPs against their homologous VP8* antigens (*Ps* > 0.05, Figure 4B). It was noted that the sera after immunization with the individual single-valent PVNPs showed significantly lower IgG titers against the two heterologous VP8* antigens (*Ps* < 0.05, Figure 4B). Similar scenarios of immune responses of the trivalent vaccine and individual PVNP and S_{60} controls were also observed after two immunizations (Figure 4A), but the resulting IgG titers were significantly lower compared with those after three immunizations (*Ps* < 0.05), which was expected. We also noted that the sera after immunizations with the single-valent P[8] or P[4] PVNP revealed higher cross-reactivity against each other of the two VP8* antigens compared with that against the P[6] VP8* antigen. These observations reflect their evolutionary distances, as P[8] and P[4] rotaviruses are members of the same genetic lineage in the P[II] genogroup; in contrast, P[6] rotavirus belongs to another lineage of the same P[II] genogroup [54]. The S_{60} nanoparticle without VP8* an antigen did not elicit detectable VP8*-specific IgG (<25).

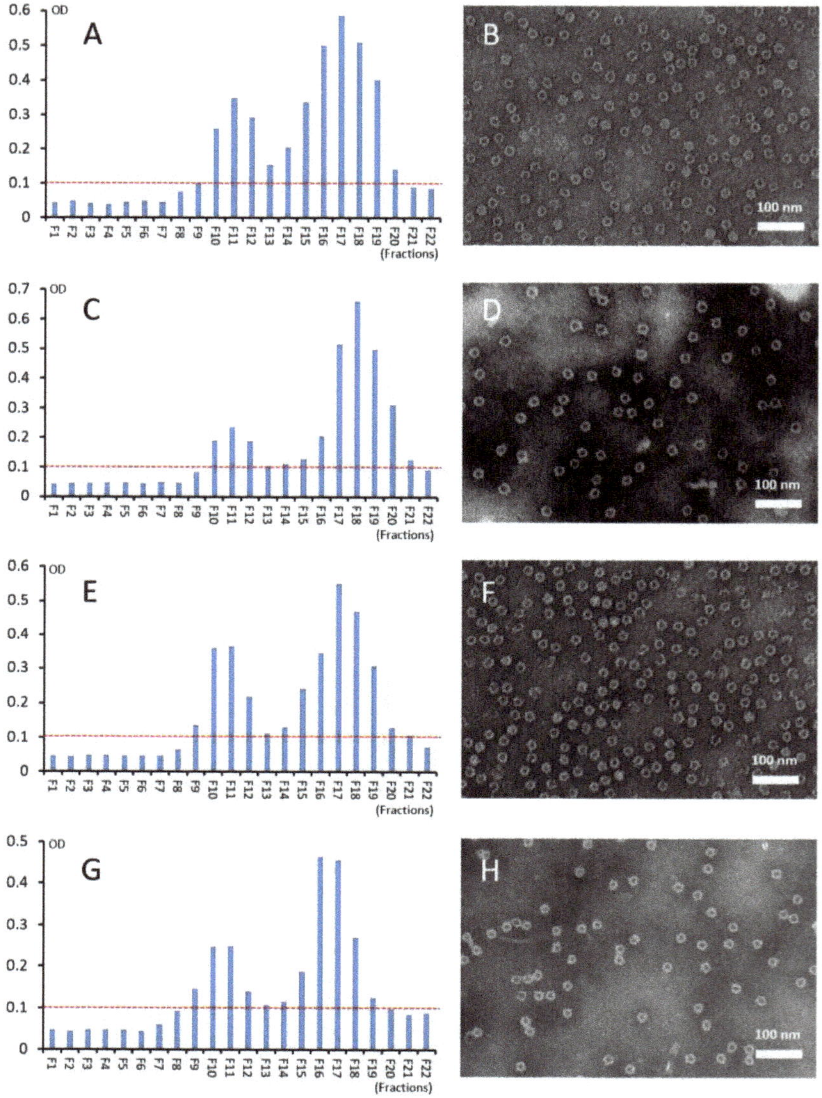

Figure 3. Analyses of the four S_{60}-VP8* PVNPs using cesium chloride (CsCl) density gradient centrifugation and transmission electron microscopy (TEM). (**A**,**C**,**E**,**G**) Following centrifugation, the CsCl density gradients containing the S_{60}-VP8* PVNPs of P[4] (**A**), P[6] (**C**), P[8] (**E**), and P[11] (**G**) rotaviruses, respectively, were fractionated into 22 portions. The relative S_{60}-VP8* protein amounts in the fractions were measured by EIA assays using a hyperimmune antibody against norovirus VLP [52]. Y-axes show signal intensities in optical density (OD), with red dashed lines showing the cut-off signal at OD = 0.1, while X-axes indicate the fraction numbers. (**B**,**D**,**F**,**H**) Negative stain TEM micrographs of the S_{60}-VP8* PVNPs from fractions 17 (**B**,**F**,**H**), or 18 (D), showing uniform, ring-shaped PVNPs containing VP8* antigens of the P[4] (**B**), P[6] (**D**), P[8] (**F**) rotaviruses, and P[11] (**H**) rotaviruses, respectively.

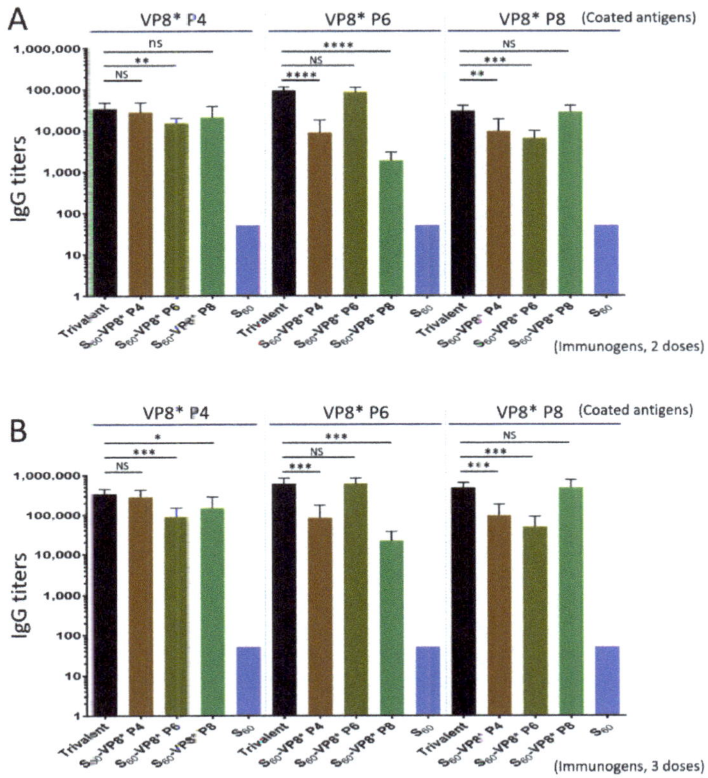

Figure 4. The trivalent S_{60}-VP8* PVNP vaccine (trivalent) induced higher and broader IgG responses in mice toward the three homologous VP8* antigens (black columns) compared with those elicited by the three single-valent S_{60}-VP8* PVNPs (brawn/cyan/green columns) after two (**A**) and three (**B**) immunizations. The *Y*-axis shows the VP8*-specific IgG titers, while the *X*-axis shows different vaccines or immunogens, as indicated. Statistical differences between data groups with corresponding *p*-values are calculated and shown in the Supplementary Materials. "NS", non-significant for *p*-values > 0.05; "*", significant for *p*-values < 0.05; "**", highly significant for *p*-values < 0.01; "***", extremely significant for *p*-values < 0.001; "****", extremely significant for *p*-values < 0.0001.

3.6. *Serum IgA Responses of the Trivalent PVNP Vaccine*

The mouse serum IgA titers after three immunizations of the trivalent PVNP vaccine, as well as the three single-valent PVNP vaccines, were also determined by EIAs (Figure 5). The outcomes showed that the trivalent vaccine elicited broad IgA titers (1600 to 2933) toward all P[8], P[4], and P[6] VP8* antigens, resembling those induced by the individual single-valent PVNP vaccines against their homologous VP8* antigens (*Ps* > 0.05, Figure 5). Like the IgG responses (Figure 4), the sera after immunization with each single-valent PVNP vaccine showed substantially lower IgA titers against the two heterologous VP8* antigens (*Ps* < 0.05, Figure 5). As expected, the S_{60} nanoparticle without VP8* antigens did not induce detectable VP8*-specific IgA (<12.5). The serum IgA titers after two immunizations of the trivalent PVNP vaccine were not determined due to a lack of sufficient serum samples after they were used for IgG titer determinations.

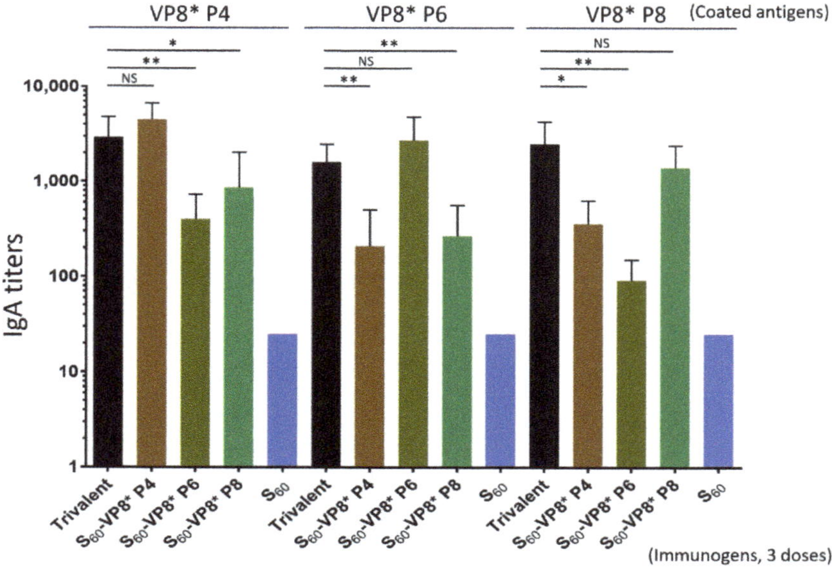

Figure 5. The trivalent S_{60}-VP8* PVNP vaccine (trivalent) induced higher and broader serum IgA responses in mice toward the three homologous VP8* antigens (black columns) compared with those elicited by the three single-valent S_{60}-VP8* PVNPs (brawn/cyan/green columns) after three immunizations. The *Y*-axis shows the VP8*-specific serum IgA titers, while the *X*-axis shows different vaccines or immunogens, as indicated. Statistical differences between data groups with corresponding *p*-values are calculated and shown in the Supplementary Materials. "NS", non-significant for *p*-values > 0.05; "*", significant for *p*-values < 0.05; "**", highly significant for *p*-values < 0.01.

3.7. BT_{50} of the Trivalent Vaccine-Immunized Mouse Sera against VP8-Glycan Receptor Attachment*

The VP8* domain of P[8] rotavirus binds Le^b glycans for viral infection [30,50,55] and a blocking assay using the P_{24}-VP8* nanoparticle as rotavirus VP8* surrogates and Le^b positive saliva samples as Le^b glycan source have been developed and used as a surrogate neutralization assay [48,53]. Here, we determined the BT_{50} of the trivalent vaccine-immunized mouse sera against P_{24}-VP8* P[8]-glycan receptor attachment using the three individual single-valent PVNP-immunized sera as controls for comparisons. The results (Figure 6A) showed that the trivalent vaccine-immunized mouse sera exhibited a high BT_{50} titer (3733) against the P_{24}-VP8* P[8]-Le^b interaction, which was similar to that (3200) of the sera after immunization with the single-valent S_{60}-VP8* P[8] PVNP ($P > 0.05$). Corresponding to their IgG and IgA titers, the sera after immunization with the single-valent S_{60}-VP8* P[4] or S_{60}-VP8* P[6] PVNP revealed significantly lower BT_{50} (1000 or 208, $Ps < 0.05$) compared with that of the sera after immunization with the trivalent PVNP vaccine. The sera after immunization with the S_{60} nanoparticle without VP8* antigens did not show detectable blocking activity (<12.5).

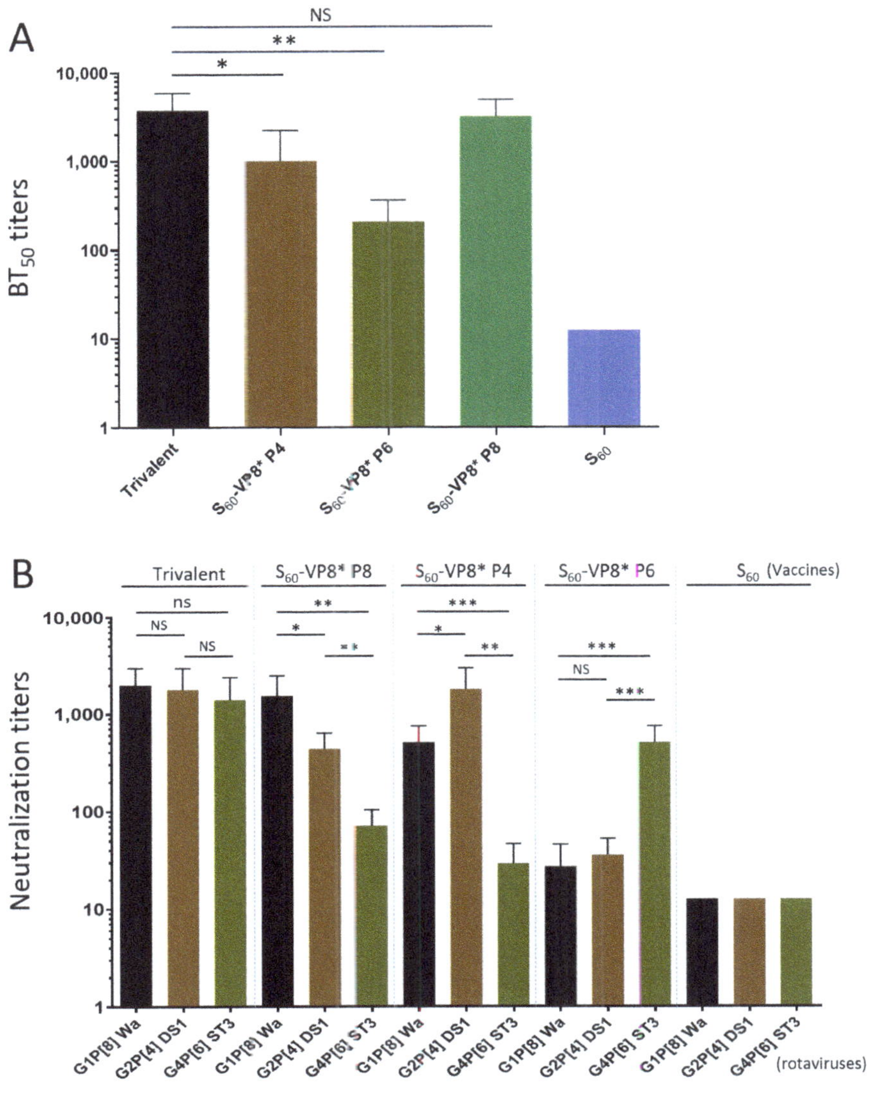

Figure 6. Blocking (**A**) and neutralization (**B**) titers of the mouse sera after immunization with the trivalent PVNP vaccine and controls against predominant rotavirus P types. (**A**) 50% blocking titers (BT_{50}, *Y*-axis) of the mouse sera after immunization with the trivalent PVNP vaccine (trivalent) and the three single-valent PVNPs (*X*-axis) against attachment of the P_{24} nanoparticle displaying P[8] VP8* to glycan receptors in a Le^b positive saliva sample. (B) 50% neutralization titers (*Y*-axis) of mouse sera after administration with the trivalent vaccine (trivalent) against replication of a P[8] (Wa strain, G1P8, black columns), a P[4] (DS-1 strain, G2P4, brown columns), and a P[6] (ST-3, G4P6, green columns) rotavirus, respectively, in cell culture, using the mouse sera after immunization with the three single-valent PVNPs and the S_{60} nanoparticle without VP8* antigens (S_{60}) as controls (indicated on the top). Statistical differences between data groups with corresponding *p*-values are calculated and shown in the Supplementary Materials. "NS", non-significant for *p*-values > 0.05; "*", significant for *p*-values < 0.05; "**", highly significant for *p*-values < 0.01; "***", extremely significant for *p*-values < 0.001.

3.8. Neutralization of the Trivalent Vaccine-Immunized Mouse Sera

The mouse sera after immunization with the trivalent PVNP vaccine were determined for their 50% neutralization titers through fluorescence plaque reduction assays. This revealed high neutralization titers against all three homologous rotavirus strains representing the predominant P[8] (Wa strain, G1P8), P[4] (DS-1, G2P4), and P[6] (ST-3, G4P6) types, reaching titers of 2000, 1800, and 1400, respectively (Figure 6B, $Ps > 0.05$ among the three titers). It was noted that the two titers against P[8] and P[4] rotaviruses were similar to that of sera after immunization with the individual P[8] or P[4] PVNPs against their homologous rotaviruses ($Ps > 0.05$), but the titer against P[6] rotavirus appeared significantly higher than that of sera after immunization with the single-valent P[6] PVNP against the homologous P[6] rotavirus ($Ps < 0.05$), suggesting a potential antigen sparing effect of the trivalent vaccine against P[6] rotavirus.

Unlike the trivalent vaccine that elicited high and balanced neutralization titers against all three P type rotaviruses, which were consistent with their high and broad IgG and IgA responses, the sera after immunization with the individual single-valent PVNPs showed significantly lower neutralization titers against the two heterologous rotaviruses (Figure 6B, $Ps < 0.05$). In addition, corresponding to their evolutionary distances among P[8], P[4], and P[6] rotaviruses (see above), the sera after immunizations with the single-valent P[8] or P[4] PVNP vaccines exhibited higher cross-neutralization titers against each other of the two rotaviruses compared with that against the P[6] rotavirus. These data provide strong evidence that trivalent S_{60}-VP8* PVNPs are a promising candidate vaccine against major rotavirus P types circulating around the world.

4. Discussion

This report represents a new advancement of our long-term efforts to develop a non-replicating subunit rotavirus vaccine for parenteral administration to circumvent the intestinally related issues associated with the current live, oral rotavirus vaccines. We were able to generate His-tagged S_{60}-VP8* PVNPs displaying the VP8* antigens of a P[8] rotavirus previously [33,48]. In this study, based on the success of generating tag-free P_{24}-VP8* nanoparticles [22], we developed a scalable approach for large productions of four tag-free S_{60}-VP8* PVNPs covering the VP8* antigens of the three predominant rotavirus P types, P[8], P[4], and P[6], as well as a minor P[11] rotavirus, respectively. This was a major improvement because it provides a low-cost production method for our vaccine candidates. Importantly, after intramuscular immunizations, the trivalent vaccine consisting of the three PVNPs displaying the P[8], P[4], and P[6] VP8* antigens induced a high and balanced immune response in mice against all three VP8* antigens. The resulting mouse sera exhibited high and broad neutralization titers against replications of all P[8], P[4], and P[6] rotaviruses. By contrast, the single-valent PVNPs elicited higher titers of IgG, IgA, and neutralization antibodies against the homologous VP8* but significantly lower titers against the two heterologous VP8* antigens and rotaviruses. Therefore, trivalent PVNPs represent a promising non-replicating rotavirus vaccine candidate for parenteral immunization.

The method developed in this study for S_{60}-VP8* PVNP production is relatively simple and scalable for the future manufacturing of the vaccine product on an industrial scale. The procedure consists of two major steps: a selective chemical precipitation of the S-VP8* fusion protein from the bacterial lysates, followed by an ion exchange chromatography to further purify the target proteins. Compared with the method that we developed previously to produce the tag-free P_{24}-VP8* nanoparticle [22], the one established in this study was apparently more efficient, reaching higher PVNP yields at higher purity. The main reason for this improvement was that the vast majority of the co-precipitated bacterial proteins by ammonium sulfate did not bind or bound only weakly to the ion exchange column. Consequently, the vast majority of the co-precipitated bacterial proteins flow through the column directly or were washed out by the washing step afterwards. This feature led to a scenario in which nearly no contaminated proteins were found in the elution peaks of the target proteins. This method worked well in producing all four tested PVNPs, providing a low-cost approach for the large production of our trivalent rotavirus vaccine candidate. In addition, our data strongly suggest that the method can be applied to generate S_{60}-VP8* PVNPs of other P-type rotaviruses.

Due to the propensity of the norovirus shell (S) protein to self-assemble into the S_{60} nanoparticles, the His-tagged S-VP8* fusion protein spontaneously forms the S_{60}-VP8* PVNPs spontaneously [48]. The tag-free S-VP8* protein apparently retained this feature and thus assembled into PVNPs automatically, as shown by the negative stain TEM inspections. It was noted that the PVNPs from different steps of the purification procedure exhibited variable morphologies under TEM. Those from an anion exchange column appeared to be in spheric shapes with variations in sizes. However, they showed uniform ring shapes after CsCl density gradient ultracentrifugation. It is not clear whether the specific buffer conditions with presence of CsCl play a role in these morphological differences under TEM. Future studies may be necessary to clarify this phenomenon. In addition, after CsCl density gradient ultracentrifugation, the S-VP8* proteins formed two peaks differing in their densities, but similar PVNPs were seen in both peaks. Thus, it remains elusive for reasons behind the formation of the two peaks in the CsCl density gradient ultracentrifugation.

Literature has shown that anti-rotavirus serum IgA [56,57] and IgG [58] titers, as well as serum neutralizing antibody titers [57] are correlated with rotavirus vaccine efficacy or protection against rotavirus infection. Another study [59] showed that anti-rotavirus serum IgA titers were correlated with IgA titers in the intestines. In a previous study [22] to investigate the immunogenicity of the trivalent P_{24}-VP8* nanoparticle vaccine candidate, the same dosage of antigens with the same adjuvant, as well as the same intramuscular immunization routes as those in this study, were used. These similar conditions allowed us to compare the immune responses elicited by the P_{24}-VP8* nanoparticles and the S_{60}-VP8* PVNPs. We noted that the IgG titers elicited by the trivalent S_{60}-VP8* PVNP vaccine (341,333 to 614,533) in this study were at least 3.5-fold higher than those (95,600 to 128,000) induced by the trivalent P_{24}-VP8* nanoparticle vaccine in the earlier study [22], after a three-dose immunization ($Ps < 0.05$). Accordingly, the neutralization titers of the sera after immunization with the trivalent S_{60}-VP8* PVNP vaccine (1400 to 2000) in this study were over 4.0-fold higher than those (346 to 362) induced by the trivalent P_{24}-VP8* nanoparticle vaccine in the previous study [22] ($Ps < 0.05$). Similar higher IgG titers elicited by the individual single-valent S_{60}-VP8* PVNPs than those induced by the individual single-valent P_{24}-VP8* nanoparticles were also observed ($Ps < 0.05$). The significantly higher immune responses induced by the trivalent S_{60}-VP8* PVNP vaccine than those elicited by the trivalent P_{24}-VP8* nanoparticle vaccine were most likely due to the greater valences of the S_{60}-VP8* PVNPs than those of the P_{24}-VP8* nanoparticle (60 vs. 24 valences). In addition, the S_{60} nanoparticle resembling the inner shell of the norovirus capsid may retain better pathogen-specific molecular patterns (PSMPs) than those of the artificially made P_{24} nanoparticles [25,26]. Finally, the adjuvant effects of the S_{60} shell may be stronger than those of the P_{24} nanoparticle. All three factors may contribute more or less to the higher immunogenicity of the trivalent S_{60}-VP8* PVNP vaccine than that of the trivalent P_{24}-VP8* nanoparticle vaccine.

Unlike their high effectiveness in developed countries, current live rotavirus vaccines show reduced efficacy in low-income nations [4,5], where rotavirus infection occurs the most. As a result, rotavirus infection continues to cause significant morbidity and mortality in developing countries [6,7], even with the implementation of the live virus. The literature shows that intestine-related factors contribute to reduced vaccine efficacy [9–13], because these factors may change intestinal conditions needed for optimal replication of live rotavirus vaccines, leading to reduced vaccine immune responses and efficacies [9,14]. In addition, the risk of intussusception associated with live vaccines [15–21] may also result from vaccine rotavirus replication in the intestine. Thus, a non-replicating, parenteral vaccine may help circumvent the intestine-related issues of the live vaccines for improved vaccine efficacy in developing nations [14] and our nanoparticle-based subunit vaccine may serve as an excellent choice in this direction. In particular, our trivalent S_{60}-VP8* PVNP vaccine containing VP8* antigens of P[8], P[4], and P[6] rotaviruses elicited high and broad immune responses to the predominant rotavirus P types, offering broad immunity against the most prevalent rotaviruses worldwide.

5. Conclusions

Our results in this investigation showed that the trivalent S_{60}-VP8* PVNP vaccine covering P[8], P[4], and P[6] rotavirus antigens is a promising non-replicating subunit rotavirus vaccine candidate for parenteral administration for broad immunity against predominant rotaviruses around the world.

Supplementary Materials: The following supporting information can be downloaded at: https://www.mdpi.com/article/10.3390/pharmaceutics14081597/s1, Figure S1: Purification of tag-free S-VP8* P[6] protein and its self- assembly into pseudovirus nanoparticles (PVNPs); Figure S2: Purification of tag-free S-VP8* P[8] protein and its self-assembly into pseudovirus nanoparticles (PVNPs); Figure S3: Purification of tag-free S-VP8* P[11] protein and its self-assembly into pseudovirus nanoparticles (PVNPs); Statistical analyses for Figure 4; Statistical analyses for Figure 5; and Statistical analyses for Figure 6.

Author Contributions: Conceptualization, M.T.; methodology, M.T., M.X. and P.H.; validation, M.T., M.X. and P.H.; formal analysis, M.T., M.X. and P.H.; investigation, M.X., P.H. and M.T.; data curation, M.T.; writing—original draft preparation, M.T.; writing—review and editing, M.T., M.X. and P.H.; visualization, M.T. and M.X.; supervision, M.T.; project administration, M.T.; funding acquisition, M.T. All authors have read and agreed to the published version of the manuscript.

Funding: The research in this article was supported by the National Institute of Health, the National Institute of Allergy and Infectious Diseases (1 R56 AI148426-01A1 to M.T.), two institutional Innovation Fund awards (Innovation Fund 2019, and Innovation Fund 2020, to M.T.) of Cincinnati Children's Hospital Medical Center (CCHMC), a CCHMC GAP Fund award (GAP Fund 2020 to M.T.) and a pilot grant from the Center for Clinical & Translational Science & Training (CCTST, to M.T.). The project described was also supported by the National Center for Advancing Translational Sciences of the National Institutes of Health, under Award Number UL1TR001425.

Institutional Review Board Statement: All animal experiments were performed in compliance with the recommendations in the Guide for the Care and Use of Laboratory Animals (23a) of the National Institute of Health (NIH). The protocols were approved by the Institutional Animal Care and Use Committee (IACUC) of the Cincinnati Children's Hospital Research Foundation (Animal Welfare Assurance No. A3108-01). This study was not involved in a human subject; thus it did not need an Institutional Review Board approval.

Informed Consent Statement: Not applicable.

Data Availability Statement: Not applicable.

Conflicts of Interest: The authors declare no conflict of interest. The funders of this research had no role in the design of the study; in the collection, analyses, or interpretation of data; in the writing of the manuscript, or in the decision to publish the results.

References

1. Crawford, S.E.; Ramani, S.; Tate, J.E.; Parashar, U.D.; Svensson, L.; Hagbom, M.; Franco, M.A.; Greenberg, H.B.; O'Ryan, M.; Kang, G.; et al. Rotavirus infection. *Nat. Rev. Dis. Primers* **2017**, *3*, 17083. [CrossRef] [PubMed]
2. Yen, C.; Tate, J.E.; Patel, M.M.; Cortese, M.M.; Lopman, B.; Fleming, J.; Lewis, K.; Jiang, B.; Gentsch, J.; Steele, D.; et al. Rotavirus vaccines: Update on global impact and future priorities. *Hum. Vaccines* **2011**, *7*, 1282–1290. [CrossRef] [PubMed]
3. Vesikari, T.; Karvonen, A.; Prymula, R.; Schuster, V.; Tejedor, J.C.; Cohen, R.; Meurice, F.; Han, H.H.; Damaso, S.; Bouckenooghe, A. Efficacy of human rotavirus vaccine against rotavirus gastroenteritis during the first 2 years of life in European infants: Randomised, double-blind controlled study. *Lancet* **2007**, *370*, 1757–1763. [CrossRef]
4. Madhi, S.A.; Cunliffe, N.A.; Steele, D.; Witte, D.; Kirsten, M.; Louw, C.; Ngwira, B.; Victor, J.C.; Gillard, P.H.; Cheuvart, B.B.; et al. Effect of human rotavirus vaccine on severe diarrhea in African infants. *N. Engl. J. Med.* **2010**, *362*, 289–298. [CrossRef] [PubMed]
5. Armah, G.E.; Sow, S.O.; Breiman, R.F.; Dallas, M.J.; Tapia, M.D.; Feikin, D.R.; Binka, F.N.; Steele, A.D.; Laserson, K.F.; Ansah, N.A.; et al. Efficacy of pentavalent rotavirus vaccine against severe rotavirus gastroenteritis in infants in developing countries in sub-Saharan Africa: A randomised, double-blind, placebo-controlled trial. *Lancet* **2010**, *376*, 606–614. [CrossRef]

6. Tate, J.E.; Burton, A.H.; Boschi-Pinto, C.; Steele, A.D.; Duque, J.; Parashar, U.D.; Network, W.H. 2008 estimate of worldwide rotavirus-associated mortality in children younger than 5 years before the introduction of universal rotavirus vaccination programmes: A systematic review and meta-analysis. *Lancet Infect. Dis.* **2012**, *12*, 136–141. [CrossRef]
7. Parashar, U.D.; Gibson, C.J.; Bresse, J.S.; Glass, R.I. Rotavirus and severe childhood diarrhea. *Emerg. Infect. Dis.* **2006**, *12*, 304–306 [CrossRef]
8. Desselberger, U. Differences of Rotavirus Vaccine Effectiveness by Country: Likely Causes and Contributing Factors. *Pathogens* **2017**, *6*, 65. [CrossRef]
9. Parker, E.P.; Ramani, S.; Lopman, B.A.; Church, J.A.; Iturriza-Gomara, M.; Prendergast, A.J.; Grassly, N.C. Causes of impaired oral vaccine efficacy in developing countries. *Future Microbiol.* **2018**, *13*, 97–118. [CrossRef] [PubMed]
10. Harris, V.C.; Haak, B.W.; Handley, S.A. Jiang, B.; Velasquez, D.E.; Hykes, B.L., Jr.; Droit, L.; Berbers, G.A.M.; Kemper, E.M.; van Leeuwen, E.M.M.; et al. Effect of Antibiotic-Mediated Microbiome Modulation on Rotavirus Vaccine Immunogenicity: A Human, Randomized-Control Proof-of-Concept Trial. *Cell Host Microbe* **2018**, *24*, 197–207 e194. [CrossRef] [PubMed]
11. Rytter, M.J.; Kolte, L.; Briend, A.; Friis, H.; Christensen, V.B. The immune system in children with malnutrition–a systematic review. *PLoS ONE* **2014**, *9*, e105017. [CrossRef] [PubMed]
12. Taniuchi, M.; Platts-Mills, J.A.; Begum, S.; Uddin, M.J.; Sobuz, S.U.; Liu, J.; Kirkpatrick, B.D.; Colgate, E.R.; Carmolli, M.P.; Dickson, D.M.; et al. Impact of enterovirus and other enteric pathogens on oral polio and rotavirus vaccine performance in Bangladeshi infants. *Vaccine* **2016**, *34*, 3068–3075. [CrossRef] [PubMed]
13. Ramani, S.; Mamani, N.; Villena, R.; Bandyopadhyay, A.S.; Gast, C.; Sato, A.; Laucirica, D.; Clemens, R.; Estes, M.K.; O'Ryan, M.L. Rotavirus Serum IgA Immune Response in Children Receiving Rotarix Coadministered With bOPV or IPV. *Pediatric Infect. Dis. J.* **2016**, *35*, 1137–1139. [CrossRef]
14. Pitzer, V.E.; Bennett, A.; Bar-Zeev, N.; Jere, K.C.; Lopman, B.A.; Lewnard, J.A.; Parashar, U.D.; Cunliffe, N.A. Evaluating strategies to improve rotavirus vaccine impact during the second year of life in Malawi. *Sci. Transl. Med.* **2019**, *11*, eaav6419. [CrossRef] [PubMed]
15. Desai, R.; Cortese, M.M.; Meltzer, M.I.; Shankar, M.; Tate, J.E.; Yen, C.; Patel, M.M.; Parashar, U.D. Potential intussusception risk versus benefits of rotavirus vaccination in the United States. *Pediatric Infect. Dis. J.* **2013**, *32*, 1–7. [CrossRef] [PubMed]
16. Bauchau, V.; Van Holle, L.; Mahaux, O.; Holl, K.; Sugiyama, K.; Buyse, H. Post-marketing monitoring of intussusception after rotavirus vaccination in Japan. *Pharmacoepidemiol. Drug Saf.* **2015**, *24*, 765–770. [CrossRef] [PubMed]
17. Yung, C.-F.; Chan, S.P.; Soh, S.; Tan, A.; Thoon, K.C. Intussusception and Monovalent Rotavirus Vaccination in Singapore: Self-Controlled Case Series and Risk-Benefit Study. *J. Pediatrics* **2015**, *167*, 163–168.e161. [CrossRef] [PubMed]
18. Rosillon, D.; Buyse, H.; Friedland, L.R.; Ng, S.-P.; Velazquez, F.R.; Breuer, T. Risk of Intussusception After Rotavirus Vaccination: Meta-analysis of Postlicensure Studies. *Pediatric Infect. Dis. J.* **2015**, *34*, 763–768. [CrossRef] [PubMed]
19. Yih, W.K.; Lieu, T.A.; Kulldorff, M.; Martin, D.; McMahill-Walraven, C.N.; Platt, R.; Selvam, N.; Selvan, M.; Lee, G.M.; Nguyen, M. Intussusception risk after rotavirus vaccination in U.S. infants. *N. Engl. J. Med.* **2014**, *370*, 503–512. [CrossRef]
20. Weintraub, E.S.; Baggs, J.; Duffy, J.; Vellozzi, C.; Belongia, E.A.; Irving, S.; Klein, N.P.; Glanz, J.M.; Jacobsen, S.J.; Naleway, A.; et al. Risk of intussusception after monovalent rotavirus vaccination. *N. Engl. J. Med.* **2014**, *370*, 513–519. [CrossRef]
21. Glass, R.I.; Parashar, U.D. Rotavirus vaccines–balancing intussusception risks and health benefits. *N. Engl. J. Med.* **2014**, *370*, 568–570. [CrossRef] [PubMed]
22. Xia, M.; Huang, P.; Jiang, X.; Tan, M. A Nanoparticle-Based Trivalent Vaccine Targeting the Glycan Binding VP8* Domains of Rotaviruses. *Viruses* **2021**, *13*, 72. [CrossRef] [PubMed]
23. Tan, M.; Huang, P.; Xia, M.; Fang, P.A.; Zhong, W.; McNeal, M.; Wei, C.; Jiang, W.; Jiang, X. Norovirus P particle, a novel platform for vaccine development and antibody production. *J. Virol.* **2011**, *85*, 753–764. [CrossRef]
24. Tan, M.; Jiang, X. Norovirus Capsid Protein-Derived Nanoparticles and Polymers as Versatile Platforms for Antigen Presentation and Vaccine Development. *Pharmaceutics* **2019**, *11*, 472. [CrossRef] [PubMed]
25. Tan, M.; Jiang, X. The p domain of norovirus capsid protein forms a subviral particle that binds to histo-blood group antigen receptors. *J. Virol.* **2005**, *79*, 14017–14030. [CrossRef] [PubMed]
26. Tan, M.; Fang, P.; Chachiyo, T.; Xia, M.; Huang, P.; Fang, Z.; Jiang, W.; Jiang, X. Noroviral P particle: Structure, function and applications in virus-host interaction. *Virology* **2008**, *382*, 115–123. [CrossRef] [PubMed]
27. Desselberger, U. Rotaviruses. *Virus Res.* **2014**, *190*, 75–96. [CrossRef] [PubMed]
28. Dormitzer, P.R.; Sun, Z.Y.; Blixt, O.; Paulson, J.C.; Wagner, G.; Harrison, S.C. Specificity and affinity of sialic acid binding by the rhesus rotavirus VP8* core. *J. Virol.* **2002**, *76*, 10512–10517. [CrossRef]
29. Hu, L.; Crawford, S.E.; Czako, R.; Cortes-Penfield, N.W.; Smith, D.F.; Le Pendu, J.; Estes, M.K.; Prasad, B.V. Cell attachment protein VP8* of a human rotavirus specifically interacts with A-type histo-blood group antigen. *Nature* **2012**, *485*, 256–259. [CrossRef] [PubMed]
30. Huang, P.; Xia, M.; Tan, M.; Zhong, W.; Wei, C.; Wang, L.; Morrow, A.; Jiang, X. Spike protein VP8* of human rotavirus recognizes histo-blood group antigens in a type-specific manner. *J. Virol.* **2012**, *86*, 4833–4843. [CrossRef] [PubMed]
31. Ramani, S.; Cortes-Penfield, N.W.; Hu, L.; Crawford, S.E.; Czako, R.; Smith, D.F.; Kang, G.; Ramig, R.F.; Le Pendu, J.; Prasad, B.V.; et al. The VP8* Domain of Neonatal Rotavirus Strain G10P[11] Binds to Type II Precursor Glycans. *J. Virol.* **2013**, *87*, 7255–7264. [CrossRef] [PubMed]

32. Liu, Y.; Huang, P.; Tan, M.; Liu, Y.; Biesiada, J.; Meller, J.; Castello, A.A.; Jiang, B.; Jiang, X. Rotavirus VP8*: Phylogeny, host range, and interaction with histo-blood group antigens. *J. Virol.* **2012**, *86*, 9899–9910. [CrossRef] [PubMed]
33. Xia, M.; Huang, P.; Jiang, X.; Tan, M. Immune response and protective efficacy of the S particle presented rotavirus VP8* vaccine in mice. *Vaccine* **2019**, *37*, 4103–4110. [CrossRef] [PubMed]
34. Xue, M.; Yu, L.; Jia, L.; Li, Y.; Zeng, Y.; Li, T.; Ge, S.; Xia, N. Immunogenicity and protective efficacy of rotavirus VP8* fused to cholera toxin B subunit in a mouse model. *Hum. Vaccines Immunother.* **2016**, *12*, 2959–2968. [CrossRef]
35. Ramesh, A.; Mao, J.; Lei, S.; Twitchell, E.; Shiraz, A.; Jiang, X.; Tan, M.; Yuan, A.L. Parenterally Administered P24-VP8* Nanoparticle Vaccine Conferred Strong Protection against Rotavirus Diarrhea and Virus Shedding in Gnotobiotic Pigs. *Vaccines* **2019**, *7*, 177. [CrossRef] [PubMed]
36. Azevedo, M.P.; Vlasova, A.N.; Saif, L.J. Human rotavirus virus-like particle vaccines evaluated in a neonatal gnotobiotic pig model of human rotavirus disease. *Expert Rev. Vaccines* **2013**, *12*, 169–181. [CrossRef] [PubMed]
37. Li, Z.; Cui, K.; Wang, H.; Liu, F.; Huang, K.; Duan, Z.; Wang, F.; Shi, D.; Liu, Q. A milk-based self-assemble rotavirus VP6-ferritin nanoparticle vaccine elicited protection against the viral infection. *J. Nanobiotech.* **2019**, *17*, 13. [CrossRef] [PubMed]
38. Groome, M.J.; Fairlie, L.; Morrison, J.; Fix, A.; Koen, A.; Masenya, M.; Jose, L.; Madhi, S.A.; Page, N.; McNeal, M.; et al. Safety and immunogenicity of a parenteral trivalent P2-VP8 subunit rotavirus vaccine: A multisite, randomised, double-blind, placebo-controlled trial. *Lancet Infect. Dis.* **2020**, *20*, 851–863. [CrossRef]
39. Groome, M.J.; Koen, A.; Fix, A.; Page, N.; Jose, L.; Madhi, S.A.; McNeal, M.; Dally, L.; Cho, I.; Power, M.; et al. Safety and immunogenicity of a parenteral P2-VP8-P[8] subunit rotavirus vaccine in toddlers and infants in South Africa: A randomised, double-blind, placebo-controlled trial. *Lancet Infect. Dis.* **2017**, *17*, 843–853. [CrossRef]
40. Li, Y.; Xue, M.; Yu, L.; Luo, G.; Yang, H.; Jia, L.; Zeng, Y.; Li, T.; Ge, S.; Xia, N. Expression and characterization of a novel truncated rotavirus VP4 for the development of a recombinant rotavirus vaccine. *Vaccine* **2018**, *36*, 2086–2092. [CrossRef] [PubMed]
41. Todd, S.; Page, N.A.; Steele, A.D.; Peenze, I.; Cunliffe, N.A. Rotavirus Strain Types Circulating in Africa: Review of Studies Published during 1997-2006. *J. Infect. Dis.* **2010**, *202*, S34–S42. [CrossRef] [PubMed]
42. Santos, N.; Hoshino, Y. Global distribution of rotavirus serotypes/genotypes and its implication for the development and implementation of an effective rotavirus vaccine. *Rev. Med. Virol.* **2005**, *15*, 29–56. [CrossRef] [PubMed]
43. Ouermi, D.; Soubeiga, D.; Nadembega, W.M.C.; Sawadogo, P.M.; Zohoncon, T.M.; Obiri-Yeboah, D.; Djigma, F.W.; Nordgren, J.; Simpore, J. Molecular Epidemiology of Rotavirus in Children under Five in Africa (2006–2016): A Systematic Review. *Pak. J. Biol. Sci.* **2017**, *20*, 59–69. [CrossRef]
44. Jain, V.; Parashar, U.D.; Glass, R.I.; Bhan, M.K. Epidemiology of rotavirus in India. *Indian J. Pediatr.* **2001**, *68*, 855–862. [CrossRef] [PubMed]
45. Iturriza Gomara, M.; Kang, G.; Mammen, A.; Jana, A.K.; Abraham, M.; Desselberger, U.; Brown, D.; Gray, J. Characterization of G10P[11] rotaviruses causing acute gastroenteritis in neonates and infants in Vellore, India. *J. Clin. Microbiol.* **2004**, *42*, 2541–2547. [CrossRef] [PubMed]
46. Libonati, M.H.; Dennis, A.F.; Ramani, S.; McDonald, S.M.; Akopov, A.; Kirkness, E.F.; Kang, G.; Patton, J.T. Absence of Genetic Differences among G10P[11] Rotaviruses Associated with Asymptomatic and Symptomatic Neonatal Infections in Vellore, India. *J. Virol.* **2014**, *88*, 9060–9071. [CrossRef]
47. Gazal, S.; Taku, A.K.; Kumar, B. Predominance of rotavirus genotype G6P[11] in diarrhoeic lambs. *Vet. J.* **2012**, *193*, 299–300. [CrossRef] [PubMed]
48. Xia, M.; Huang, P.; Sun, C.; Han, L.; Vago, F.S.; Li, K.; Zhong, W.; Jiang, W.; Klassen, J.S.; Jiang, X.; et al. Bioengineered Norovirus S60 Nanoparticles as a Multifunctional Vaccine Platform. *ACS Nano.* **2018**, *12*, 10665–10682. [CrossRef] [PubMed]
49. Liu, C.; Huang, P.; Zhao, D.; Xia, M.; Zhong, W.; Jiang, X.; Tan, M. Effects of rotavirus NSP4 protein on the immune response and protection of the SR69A-VP8* nanoparticle rotavirus vaccine. *Vaccine* **2020**, *39*, 263–271. [CrossRef] [PubMed]
50. Xu, S.; Ahmed, L.U.; Stuckert, M.R.; McGinnis, K.R.; Liu, Y.; Tan, M.; Huang, P.; Zhong, W.; Zhao, D.; Jiang, X.; et al. Molecular basis of P[II] major human rotavirus VP8* domain recognition of histo-blood group antigens. *PLoS Pathog.* **2020**, *16*, e1008386. [CrossRef]
51. Tan, M.; Hegde, R.S.; Jiang, X. The P domain of norovirus capsid protein forms dimer and binds to histo-blood group antigen receptors. *J. Virol.* **2004**, *78*, 6233–6242. [CrossRef] [PubMed]
52. Huang, P.; Farkas, T.; Zhong, W.; Tan, M.; Thornton, S.; Morrow, A.L.; Jiang, X. Norovirus and histo-blood group antigens: Demonstration of a wide spectrum of strain specificities and classification of two major binding groups among multiple binding patterns. *J. Virol.* **2005**, *79*, 6714–6722. [CrossRef] [PubMed]
53. Xia, M.; Wei, C.; Wang, L.; Cao, D.; Meng, X.J.; Jiang, X.; Tan, M. Development and evaluation of two subunit vaccine candidates containing antigens of hepatitis E virus, rotavirus, and astrovirus. *Sci. Rep.* **2016**, *6*, 25735. [CrossRef] [PubMed]
54. Jiang, X.; Liu, Y.; Tan, M. Histo-blood group antigens as receptors for rotavirus, new understanding on rotavirus epidemiology and vaccine strategy. *Emerg. Microbes Infect.* **2017**, *6*, e22. [CrossRef]
55. Xu, S.; McGinnis, K.R.; Liu, Y.; Huang, P.; Tan, M.; Stuckert, M.R.; Burnside, R.E.; Jacob, E.G.; Ni, S.; Jiang, X.; et al. Structural basis of P[II] rotavirus evolution and host ranges under selection of histo-blood group antigens. *Proc. Natl. Acad. Sci. USA* **2021**, *118*, e2107963118. [CrossRef]
56. Patel, M.; Glass, R.I.; Jiang, B.; Santosham, M.; Lopman, B.; Parashar, U. A systematic review of anti-rotavirus serum IgA antibody titer as a potential correlate of rotavirus vaccine efficacy. *J. Infect. Dis.* **2013**, *208*, 284–294. [CrossRef]

57. Clarke, E.; Desselberger, U. Correlates of protection against human rotavirus disease and the factors influencing protection in low-income settings. *Mucosal. Immunol.* **2015**, *8*, 1–17. [CrossRef]
58. Ward, R.L.; Bernstein, D.I.; Shukla, R.; Young, E.C.; Sherwood, J.R.; McNeal, M.M.; Walker, M.C.; Schiff, G.M. Effects of antibody to rotavirus on protection of adults challenged with a human rotavirus. *J. Infect. Dis.* **1989**, *159*, 79–88. [CrossRef]
59. Azevedo, M.S.; Yuan, L.; Iosef, C.; Chang, K.O.; Kim, Y.; Nguyen, T.V.; Saif, L.J. Magnitude of serum and intestinal antibody responses induced by sequential replicating and nonreplicating rotavirus vaccines in gnotobiotic pigs and correlation with protection. *Clin. Diagn. Lab. Immunol.* **2004**, *11*, 12–20. [CrossRef]

pharmaceutics

MDPI

Article

Native Study of the Behaviour of Magnetite Nanoparticles for Hyperthermia Treatment during the Initial Moments of Intravenous Administration

Valentina Marassi [1,2,*], Ilaria Zanoni [3], Simona Ortelli [3], Stefano Giordani [1], Pierluigi Reschiglian [1,2], Barbara Roda [1,2], Andrea Zattoni [1,2], Costanza Ravagli [4], Laura Cappiello [4], Giovanni Baldi [4], Anna L. Costa [3] and Magda Blosi [3]

1 Department of Chemistry G. Ciamician, University of Bologna, Via Selmi 2, 40126 Bologna, Italy
2 Stem Sel srl, University of Bologna, 40129 Bologna, Italy
3 CNR-ISSMC, Institute of Science, Technology and Sustainability for Ceramics (Former ISTEC), Via Granarolo 64, 48018 Faenza, Italy
4 Ce.Ri.Col, Colorobbia Consulting S.R.L., 50059 Sovigliana Vinci, Italy
* Correspondence: valentina.marassi@unibo.it

Abstract: Magnetic nanoparticles (MNPs) present outstanding properties making them suitable as therapeutic agents for hyperthermia treatments. Since the main safety concerns of MNPs are represented by their inherent instability in a biological medium, strategies to both achieve long-term stability and monitor hazardous MNP degradation are needed. We combined a dynamic approach relying on flow field flow fractionation (FFF)-multidetection with conventional techniques to explore frame-by-frame changes of MNPs injected in simulated biological medium, hypothesize the interaction mechanism they are subject to when surrounded by a saline, protein-rich environment, and understand their behaviour at the most critical point of intravenous administration. In the first moments of MNPs administration in the patient, MNPs change their surrounding from a favorable to an unfavorable medium, i.e., a complex biological fluid such as blood; the particles evolve from a synthetic identity to a biological identity, a transition that needs to be carefully monitored. The dynamic approach presented herein represents an optimal alternative to conventional batch techniques that can monitor only size, shape, surface charge, and aggregation phenomena as an averaged information, given that they cannot resolve different populations present in the sample and cannot give accurate information about the evolution or temporary instability of MNPs. The designed FFF method equipped with a multidetection system enabled the separation of the particle populations providing selective information on their morphological evolution and on nanoparticle–proteins interaction in the very first steps of infusion. Results showed that in a dynamic biological setting and following interaction with serum albumin, PP-MNPs retain their colloidal properties, supporting their safety profile for intravenous administration.

Keywords: biological identity; biological fluids; flow field flow fractionation (FFF)-multidetection; hyperthermia treatment; intravenous administration; magnetic nanoparticles; native characterization; protein corona

Citation: Marassi, V.; Zanoni, I.; Ortelli, S.; Giordani, S.; Reschiglian, P.; Roda, B.; Zattoni, A.; Ravagli, C.; Cappiello, L.; Baldi, G.; et al. Native Study of the Behaviour of Magnetite Nanoparticles for Hyperthermia Treatment during the Initial Moments of Intravenous Administration. *Pharmaceutics* **2022**, *14*, 2810. https://doi.org/10.3390/pharmaceutics14122810

Academic Editors: Raquel Fernández García, Francisco Bolás-Fernández and Ana Isabel Fraguas-Sánchez

Received: 18 November 2022
Accepted: 13 December 2022
Published: 15 December 2022

1. Introduction

Nanoparticles (NPs) and nanomaterials (NMs) have been a focus of the biomedical sciences and engineering for over a century because of their enormous potential in nanotechnologies. Magnetic nanoparticles represent one of the most investigated class of nanomaterials for biomedical application due to their unique physicochemical properties that make them suitable for many applications in biotechnology, magnetic separation, targeted drug delivery, diagnostics (MRI, CT, PET, ultrasound, SERS), optical imaging, and as cytotoxic agents [1]. Furthermore, magnetic nanoparticles can be synthetized and modified with various chemical functional groups, which enables their conjugation with antibodies, ligands, and drugs of interest, thus opening their application for theragnostic purposes in cancer treatment, combining diagnosis with therapy [2–4]. Iron oxides particles, such as magnetite (Fe_3O_4) and its oxidized form (α-Fe_2O_4), are some of the most used magnetic carriers in biomedical applications. They have good biocompatibility, low toxicity [5], and are protagonists of one of the most promising cancer therapies: magneto fluid hyperthermia (MFH), which uses magnetic NPs to heat biological tissues and destroy cancer cells. In fact, cancer cells are more sensitive to high temperatures than healthy cells and die of apoptosis above a temperature of 43–46 °C [6]. The treatment can be used both alone or paired with other treatments such as chemotherapy and radiotherapy to optimize its efficiency. Fe_3O_4 magnetic nanoparticles (MNPs) should have a narrow size distribution and good dispersibility in aqueous media to be relevant for the human body. The narrow size distribution of the iron oxide core ensures high heating capabilities in a low concentration under biocompatible alternating magnetic field (AMF) conditions [7].

The main issues of these particles are represented by their loss of magnetism under oxidation and long-term inherent instability due to the high surface energy and the strong magnetic attraction between particles. High salt concentrations typical of biological matrixes further affect the colloidal stability of MNPs [8]. These two main instability routes can be handled by surface functionalization. Several classes of biocompatible chelating agents (lipids, gelatin, dextran, chitosan, polyvinyl alcohol, etc.) are nowadays used to form a polymeric layer on the surface of magnetic NPs to improve their stabilization considering their biological application [9,10]. Among various coatings, PEG—polyethylene glycol—stands out because of its hydrophilicity, biocompatibility, non-antigenicity, and antifouling properties [11]. In fact, PEG-coated iron oxide NPs have shown good results which remarkably extend NPs circulation in the blood [12]. Another interesting coating used on iron oxide NPs is the biodegradable copolymer PLGA, widely used for the preparation of biodegradable carriers and offering the possibility of tuning the drug release properties and the biological behaviour of Fe_3O_4 NPs [13–15].

Properly-coated MNPs, exploited for their biomedical applications, are typically dispersed in a biocompatible fluid and injected either directly into the tumor or in the blood system [16]. After entering the blood stream, they encounter serum proteins (i.e., human serum albumin, HSA, which makes up 60% protein content). As the infusion progresses, particles and proteins mix with an increasing imbalance towards the latter, generating a protein corona which likely allows MNPs to reach a new biological identity determined by this new biochemical surrounding. Corona effects are crucial for clinical applications since NPs properties and bioavailability are altered (in a positive or negative way) by their formation [17,18]. The process is a complex self-evolving scenario [19]; once MNPs in contact with the medium given the change in the medium MNPs encounter, an initial destabilization/precipitation/aggregation of MNPs, even with a subsequent restabilization, could occur and determine adverse reactions and potentially be very toxic for the patient.

Evaluating this transition proves challenging, since the interacting parts are numerous, and different parameters are needed to paint a full scenario. Studies focusing on the stability on MNPs in biological matrixes [20] and describing the formation and evolution of the protein corona [21] are typically performed with batch sizing and imaging tools [22]. These methodologies clarify whether NPs are subjected to modification but cannot give any answer other than an averaged one, without being able to identify the evolution of single populations [23]. Overall, this represents a major limitation, since the matrices involved are complex and the NPs samples are not always as monodispersed as presumed. A way to improve upon the limitations of these widespread methodologies is represented by the exploitation of Field Flow Fractionation (FFF) techniques. These techniques are a single phase-based platform which allow the separation of a wide range of different analytes (1 nm to tens of µm in size, corresponding to 15 orders of magnitude in molar mass) in native conditions based on their interactions with an external field [24,25]. A series of detectors coupled with the separation systems then provide a characterization of the separated analytes by the means of spectroscopy, laser scattering, and MS analysis. Different FFF subvariants can be described based on the external field exploited, and the Asymmetrical Flow FFF (AF4) variant represents by far the most exploited and successful of these [26]. AF4 has been widely used to separate and characterize systems of biomedical interest [27–29], biological matrices of high complexity [30,31], and to evaluate the binding interaction between different species [32,33]. Hollow Fiber Asymmetrical Flow FFF (HF5) represent the miniaturized version of AF4. Compared to AF4 and other typical particle-separation techniques, this variant typically has comparable or greater efficiency and higher sensitivity [34]. The separative channel is also disposable upon the need to avoid the risk of cross contamination. HF5 has recently been shown to characterize the behaviour of serum components in hemolysis conditions, allowing the discrimination of how each component separately interacts with heme in a competitive environment [35]. Moreover, its application on the characterization of metal NPs [36–38] and on their conjugation studies [39] is widely documented.

This paper reports the results collected in the framework of the EU project BIORIMA (H2020-760928_ BIOmaterial RIsk MAnagement), on Fe_3O_4 NPs coated by PEG/PLGA (PP-MNPs) intended for drug delivery application. PP-MNO were analysed by an HF5 platform at increasing amounts of HSA to simulate the first stages of intravenous administration and investigate their stability and behaviour in simulated use conditions. HF5 represents the best technique to monitor the morphological evolution of coated magnetic NPs applied by injection for therapy and subjected to a laminar flow. After characterizing PP-MNPs, we first monitored the size and zeta potential changes by a titration with HSA at four different points. Then, the same experiment was translated to a dynamic mode by exploiting a specifically designed HF5 multidetection method to observe the behaviour of PP-MNPs at a growing concentration of HSA, mimicking the first instants of administration. This platform provided a separation of the NPs-HSA conjugates from the leftover components and the simultaneous characterization of each separated species by the means of spectroscopy and laser scattering (MW and gyration radius). Moreover, the determination of the corresponding morphologies through the calculation of their v-values [40] provided us with outstanding information concerning the shape of the PP-MNPs and conjugates, the mechanisms with which HSA binds PP-MNPs, and helped address crucial gave us outstanding information concerning the shape of the PP-MNPs and conjugates, the mechanisms with which HSA binds PP-MNPs, and helped addressing address safety concerns.

2. Materials and Methods

2.1. Materials

Fe_3O_4 PEG-PLGA NPs (PP-MNP) were provided by Colorobbia Consulting S. r. l. (Sovigliana Vinci (FI), Italy) in the form of a suspension at a an Fe_3O_4 concentration of 2000 mg L^{-1} and prepared according to the patented procedure [41,42]. Briefly, MNPMNPs suspended in diethylene glycol were superficially functionalized with [N-(3,4-dihydroxyphenethyl) dodecanamide (DDA)] and dispersed in tetrahydrofuran (THF). Then, a THF solution of PLGA-b-PEG-COOH block copolymer was added to the magnetite-DDA NPs suspension. The formation of hybrid Fe_3O_4 PEG-PLGA was achieved by the nanoprecipitation method: two streams of fluid ((1) organic dispersion of functionalized magnetite and PLGA-b-PEG-COOH and (2) phosphate-buffered solution in a volumetric ratio of 1/10) were mixed and recovered. The formed dispersion was then dialyzed (Cogent M system, Pellicon membrane 2 Mini, cut-off 100 kDa) to remove the organic phase using a pure phosphate-buffered aqueous solution. The system was then concentrated to the final concentration and filtered through a polyethersulfone membrane syringe filter (0.22 mm). The overall process was carried out in sterile conditions. Human serum albumin (HSA) was purchased from Sigma-Aldrich (Milan, Italy).

2.2. Preparation of PP-MNP Stock Suspensions

The PP-MNP suspension, as provided, was diluted to 256 ppm in an aqueous solution containing 0.05%wt of filtered human serum albumin (HSA) by vortex treatment (30 s).

2.3. Characterization

2.3.1. X-ray Diffraction (XRD)

XRD analysis was carried out on powder obtained by drying PP-MNP suspensions. The measurement was performed at room temperature with a Bragg/Brentano diffractometer (X'pertPro PANalytical) equipped with a fast X'Celerator detector, using a Cu anode as the X-ray source (Kα, λ = 1.5418 Å). Diffractogram was recorded in the range of 20–70° 2θ counting for 0.2 s every 0.05° 2θ step.

2.3.2. Colloidal Characterization

The colloidal behaviour of PP-MNPMNPs was evaluated on stock and diluted stock suspensions in MilliQ water at 256 and 50 mg L^{-1} to determine the hydrodynamic size distribution and Zeta Potential (ZP), by means of dynamic light scattering (DLS) and electrophoresis light scattering (ELS) techniques, respectively. The measurements were performed using a Zetasizer Nanoseries (Malvern Instruments, Malvern, UK). Each sample was prepared and analysed in triplicate. Particle size diameter (d_{DLS}) and zeta potential ($Zpot_{ELS}$) values were obtained by averaging three measurements.

2.3.3. HSA Titration

PP-MNP stock (2000 mg L^{-1}) was diluted to 200 mg L^{-1}. Four different batches of HSA were prepared in phosphate buffer to be mixed with magnetite to obtain an Fe_3O_4/HSA weight ratio of 2:1, 1:1, 1:2, and 1:4 as described in Table 1. The samples were prepared by mixing and homogenizing by vortex (30 s) the same volume of the two compounds (1 mL + 1 mL) at different concentrations.

Table 1. Experimental concentration setup for the DLS/ELS measurements.

PP-MNP HSA Weight Ratio	PP-MNP		HSA	
	Volume (mL)	Concentration (mg L^{-1})	Volume (mL)	Concentration (mg L^{-1})
2:1	1	200	1	100
1:1		200		200
1:2		200		400
1:4		200		800

The hydrodynamic diameter and Zeta Potential measurements were carried out in Phosphate Buffer (Sodium Phosphate 1 mM, pH 7.4) by the DLS/ELS technique.

2.3.4. Transmission Electron Microscopy

PP-MNPs were observed by using an FEI TECNAI F20 microscope operating at 200 keV. The suspension was applied on a holey carbon-coated grid. The specimen was then dried at 60 °C. The images were collected in phase-contrast mode and high-angle annular dark-field scanning transmission mode (HAAD-FSTEM). High-resolution (HREM) and Selected Area Electron Diffraction (SAED) analyses were performed to investigate the crystalline phase structure and composition. The mean particle diameter was calculated on more than 100 particles.

2.3.5. FFF UV FLD MALS

HF5 analyses were performed using an Agilent 1200 HPLC system (Agilent Technologies, Santa Clara, CA, USA) consisting of a degasser, an isocratic pump with an Agilent 1100 DAD UV/Vis spectrophotometer and an Agilent 1200 Fluorimeter combined with an

Eclipse® DUALTEC separation system (Wyatt Technology Europe, Dernbach, Germany), followed by an 18-angle multiangle light scattering detector model DAWN HELEOS (Wyatt Technology Corporation, Santa Barbara, CA, USA). The HF5 cartridge (Wyatt Technology, Europe) is commercially available and has a 10 kDa cutoff. The scheme of the HF5 cartridge, its assembly, and the modes of operation of the Eclipse® DUALTEC system have already been described [43,44]. The ChemStation version B.04.02 (Agilent Technologies) data system for Agilent instrumentation was used to set and control the instrumentation and for the computation of various separation parameters, complete with the Wyatt Eclipse @ ChemStation version 3.5.02 (Wyatt Technology Europe). ASTRA® software version 6.1.7 (Wyatt Technology Corporation) was used to handle signals from the detectors (MALS and UV) and to compute the sample Rg (radius of gyration), also named the RMS (root mean square radius) values. The HF5 method is composed of four steps: focus, focus–injection, elution, and elution–injection, allowing for flow equilibration, sample injection, sample separation and system cleaning. Longitudinal (transport) and transversal (focus/cross) flow settings are adjusted to customize the method. Longitudinal flow was kept constant at 0.35 mL/min, while cross/focus flow expressed as Vx are shown in Table 2. In normal fractionation mode, particle retention is a function of its apparent diffusion coefficient, relating retention time to hydrodynamic radius (*R*h). The Rh is approximated as a radius of a sphere having similar hydrodynamic behaviour in terms of diffusion and friction of the eluted particle [45]. Multi-angle laser light scattering (MALLS) was used to determine colloidal size. This technique allows for the determination of particle root mean square radius of gyration (Rg, or RMS) by measuring the net intensity of light scattered by such particles at a range of fixed angles. The particle Rg is determined by the mass distribution within the particle. The single mass increments are weighed by the square of the radius distance from the center of mass. Consequently, two particles with same hydrodynamic radius (Rh), but with different Rg values, may have a different mass distribution, and thus, different shapes [46].

Table 2. Flow conditions for the HF5 analyses.

Focus (mL min^{-1})	Focus-Injection (mL min^{-1})	Elution (mL min^{-1})			Elution-Inject (mL min^{-1})
Vx = 0.8 T = 1 min	Vx = 0.8 T = 5 min	Vx = 0.55 to 0.04 T = 6 min	Vx = 0.04 T = 18 min	Vx = 0.00 T = 3 min	Vx = 0.00 T = 2 min

The radius of gyration and molar mass distributions determined by FFF-MALS provide information on the scaling behaviours in the solution. The scaling exponent ν is defined by the slope in a double logarithmic logMW–logRg plot and gives information about the conformation of the molecules in the solution. It is theoretically defined for spheres ν = 0.33, random-coil ν = 0.5–0.6, and rod-like structures ν~1 [47,48].

3. Results and Discussion

3.1. Batch and Static Characterization

The first steps of the characterization of the evolution involved building a data set with the most common characterization techniques, which involved imaging, X-ray diffraction, and batch measurement of size (DLS) and zeta potential.

3.1.1. X-ray Diffraction of MNP

PP-MNPs were characterized through XRD. The main peaks identified on target NPs are consistent with the magnetite phase (JCPDS card n. 19-0629) with XRD reflections at 2Theta = 30.1°; 35.4°; 43.0°; 56.9°; and 62.5°, as shown by Figure 1.

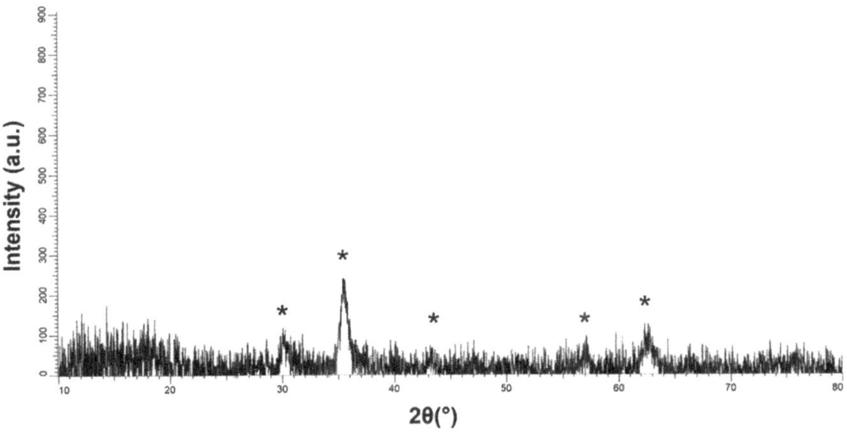

Figure 1. XRD diffractogram of MNPs (Fe_3O_4-PEG/PLGA). * = magnetite (JCPDS card n. 19-0629).

The collected peaks were typically broad in agreement with the particle nanosized dimensions.

3.1.2. Size and Zeta Potential Measurements

PP-MNPs were observed by TEM. The images acquired in phase-contrast (Figure 2a) and HAADF-STEM (Figure 2b) modes revealed a regular spheroidal morphology of the particles with a mean diameter of 12 ± 4 nm. The higher magnification HREM image (Figure 2c) showed a cubic crystal structure consistent with the magnetite lattice; crystalline magnetite was the unique phase composition resulting from the SAED analysis of the collected polycrystalline pattern rings (inset of figure-c).

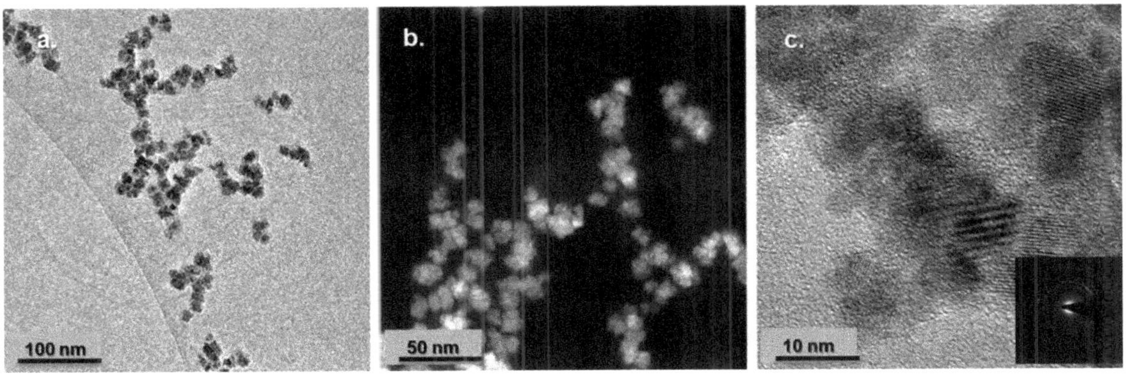

Figure 2. Transmission electron microscopy images of PP-MNPs (**a**) TEM phase-contrast image; (**b**) HAADF-STEM image; (**c**) HREM image and in the inset SAED polycrystalline pattern rings. Scale bars: (**a**) 100 nm; (**b**) 50 nm; (**c**) 10 nm.

PP-MNPs dispersed in phosphate buffer and evaluated at two concentrations showed a neutral pH, a hydrodynamic diameter of about 70 nm, and a negative Z potential (~50 mV) as reported in Table 3. Results were consistent with previously-published works on PEG-PLGA coating [49,50].

Table 3. Colloidal properties (hydrodynamic diameter, d_{DLS} and Z potential, $Zpot_{ELS}$) of PP-MNPs and HSA.

Sample	Concentration (ppm)	dDLS (nm)	PDI	Z_{pot} (mV)	pH
PP-MNP	50	74 ± 1	0.1	−49.5 ± 3.3	7.3
	256	76 ± 2	0.2	−49.0 ± 2.4	7.4
HSA	800	9.8 ± 2.4	0.7	−31.5 ± 9.6	7.3
	100	10.4 ± 2.2	0.7	−33.5 ± 4.7	7.3

As expected, the hydrodynamic diameter, comprehensive of the grafted polymers, was larger than the size assessed by TEM.

We also evaluated the colloidal properties of HSA at the highest and lowest concentrations used in dynamic-flow conditions, which as expected is present as predominantly a monomer in phosphate buffer with a size around 10 nm and a negative charge for both concentrations. It is interesting to note that for PP-MNPs, we obtained similar data at both concentrations, pointing out that the main colloidal properties were not affected by dilution and the change of stability, and the aggregation state is therefore due to the medium change following interactions in the biological setting.

3.1.3. Titration with HSA in Static Conditions

By means of DLS/ELS measurements, we monitored the colloidal evolution of magnetite nanoparticles titrated by HSA according to the mass ratios reported in Table 2. In our previous work [51], we reported that the addition of albumin increased the DLS diameters registered for the suspended nanoparticles. However, by titrating PP-MNPs with HSA in phosphate buffer, we observed a decrease in the hydrodynamic diameter for higher HSA amounts (Figure 3), consistent with a dispersion action or a size rearrangement promoted by the protein adsorption on nanoparticles.

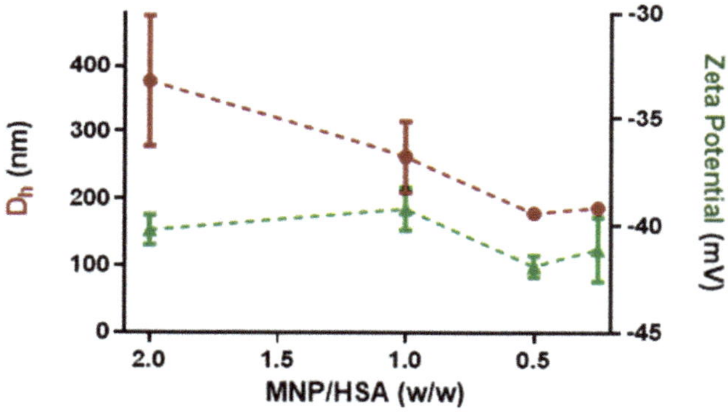

Figure 3. Titration of PP-MNPs with HSA in water. Red points: hydrodynamic diameter. Green triangles: zeta potential.

From the DLS results, it is reasonable to infer that the increasing presence of HSA provides shielding and favors colloidal stability. For PP-MNPs with HSA ratios < 1, i.e., at predominant concentrations of HSA, the hydrodynamic diameter reached a plateau value around 180 nm (Table 4).

Table 4. DLS/ELS data for the titration of PP-MNPs with HSA.

PP-MNP/HSA	pH	Size d_{DLS} (nm)	Deviation (nm)	PDI	ζ-pot (mV)	Deviation (mV)
2	6.4	377	99	0.500	−40.2	0.7
1	6.7	263	53	0.450	−39.2	1.0
0.5	6.7	179	9	0.370	−41.9	0.5
0.25	6.6	187	4	0.400	−41.1	1.5

The PP-MNP-HSA suspensions showed Z potentials leveling off at around −40 mV, close to the MNPs value and slightly reduced for the presence of HSA, characterized by a lower Z potential.

Most importantly, the size deviation obtained for lower ratios (0.5 and 0.25, i.e., where HSA is more concentrated) is much lower, indicating that the structures obtained are more stable and defined.

3.2. *Native and Dynamic Characterization with FFF-Multidetection*

To simulate the intravenous injection administration, the titration experiment was translated from static conditions to an in-flow approach, using HF5 as separation device to isolate different populations, followed by online detection to monitor the profile changes in UV-Vis absorption, fluorescence, and measured size. PP-MNPs were characterized alone and in the presence of an increasing amount of HSA to understand their stability and behaviour once injected into a simulated biological medium. The points chosen, which were the same as those for the batch characterization, aimed to ideally photograph what occurs in the first moments of administration, when PP-MNPs shift from a scenario where they are the main species to one where the biological medium surrounds them. The analyses were carried out in phosphate buffer (Sodium Phosphate 1 mM, pH 7.4). The amount of PP-MNPs injected was the same for all analyses, and as shown in Table 2. All mixes were 1:1 in volume as to avoid changes due to different medium proportions.

The separation method was designed and optimized to elute HSA and PP-MNPs at different retention times. Method precision was assessed in triplicate on retention times and on signal intensity, which both exhibited deviations < 1%. The limit of quantification (LOQ) expressed as 10× the baseline noise resulted in 8.4 ng (0.42 pmol) and 48 ng for HSA and PP-MNPs, respectively. The final method envisioned a combination of gradient and isocratic crossflow which allowed for their baseline separation and elution in 30 min.

In this way, for the mixed suspensions, the insurgence of new bands or the coexistence of typical signals for the two species directly indicates an interaction between the two.

To obtain information about the composition of combined species, it was necessary to attribute a peak to one species, the other, or both, and "diagnostic" signals were selected. First, HSA displays intrinsic fluorescence (excitation at 280, emission at 340 nm), typical for proteins [48], while PP-MNPs only have a faint emission at 550 nm. Second, PP-MNPs absorb at 480 nm, while HSA does not. Thus, 480 nm was chosen to monitor the presence of PP-MNPs. The results are shown in Figure 4.

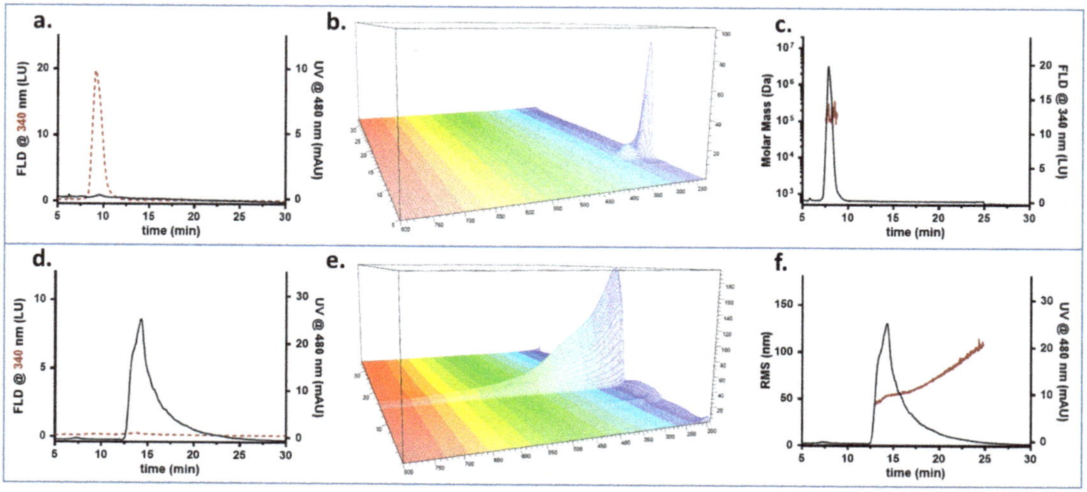

Figure 4. FFF fractogram (red dashed line: fluorescence signal; grey line: absorption signal), UV-Vis absorption spectrum, and Molar Mass/RMS radius (red) and fluorescence/UV profile (grey) obtained for HSA (**a–c**) and MNPs (**d–f**).

Figure 4a,d show the fractogram profiles recorded as absorption at 480 nm and fluorescence at 340 nm for the optimized method. As observed from the different profiles for the two signals and samples, the method developed ensured that HSA and PP-MNPs were potentially baseline-separated, and that both had a characteristic signal which could be followed individually.

HSA is eluted at 9 min as a single peak (Figure 4a) highlighting an absorption spectrum (Figure 4b) typical for a protein, with a local maximum at 280 nm and no absorption past the UV range. The molar mass averaged about 100 kDa (Figure 4c), indicating that HSA is present as a mix of monomer (66.7 kDa, prevalent) and oligomers as already observed in similar conditions with a native separation [serum heme].

PP-MNPs were eluted as a single band of a broad size distribution (red distribution, Figure 4f) peaking at 15 min (Figure 4d). The UV-Vis spectrum (Figure 4e) was broad and intense, with scattering at higher wavelengths. The population of NPs was found to be monomodal (Figure 4f)—the majority of PP-MNPs (min 14.0 to 17.5, 75% of peak area) had an Rg of 51 ± 5 nm while the peak tail reached 110 nm. This agrees with the DLS data measuring an Rh of 75 nm, since the shape factor obtained [52], expressed as the Rg/Rh ratio, would be equal to 0.7, corresponding to a solid sphere.

It is possible to see that the peak tailing contains aggregated forms of a higher radius, formed following contact with the saline environment.

We then monitored the system evolution after mixing PP-MNPs with an increasing amount of has. Results referred to PP-MNP:HSA mixes at 2:1 and 1:1 mass ratios are shown in Figure 5. MALS measurements show the overlay of the RMS radius calculation on the signal at 480 nm used to visualize when NPs are eluted and their size/aggregation state. This signal allows the monitoring of the evolution in all mixtures. For each mix of PP-MNPs and HSA, the fractogram overlaying the HSA fluorescence and PP-MNPs absorption, the UV-Vis absorption spectrum, and the radius distribution are displayed.

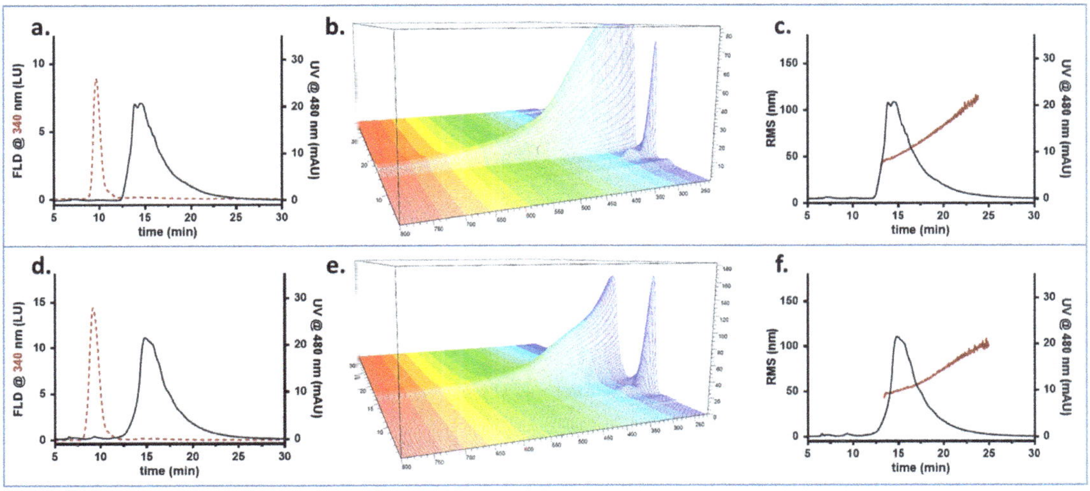

Figure 5. FFF fractogram (red dashed line: fluorescence signal; grey line: absorption signal), UV-Vis absorption spectrum, and Molar Mass/RMS radius (red) and fluorescence/UV profile (grey) obtained for suspensions at PP-MNP:HSA 2:1 (**a–c**) and 1:1 (**d–f**) mass ratios.

In a 2:1 proportion, PP-MNPs and HSA are eluted at different times (Figure 5a, red dotted for HSA and grey line for MNP) and do not exhibit interactions apart from a slight absorption at 480 found at the HSA retention time, consisting of about 0.2% of the 480 signal-integrated area. The two different absorption spectra are shown by the 3D output (Figure 5b).

PP-MNPs are present as a single band of a broad size distribution similar to what is observed for PP-MNPs alone (Figure 5c). The largest part of the PP-MNPs is eluted from minute 14 to 17.5, corresponding to an average radius of 50 nm, while the peak tail reached a dimension of 110 nm (red distribution). For PP-MNPs and HSA mixed at a 1:1 ratio, we detected at 9 min a small peak at 480 nm (Figure 5d), meaning that some NPs are eluted earlier following conformational/surface modification. The absorption spectrum shows that the HSA profile is slightly different (absorbs at higher wavelengths as well, similar to the broad absorption of PP-MNPs), suggesting that some interactions take place between the two phases. In Figure 5d PP-MNPs are identified as a small band (more visible than the previous mixture) at 9 min (the intensity is however too low for a reliable RMS calculation) and a main monomodal band at 15 min with a broad size distribution as visible from the MALS radius calculation (Figure 5f). The majority of PP-MNPs (min 14.0 to 17.5) average 50 nm while the peak tail reaches 100 nm.

Data collected on the 1:2 PP-MNPs: HSA ratio, corresponding to a doubled HSA content, revealed a completely different situation, showing a clear interaction between the compounds (Figure 6).

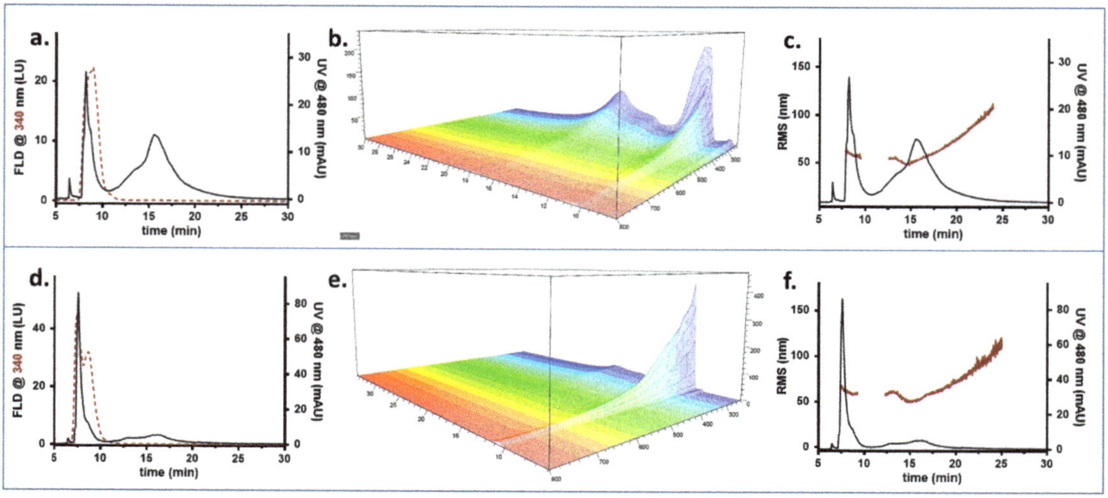

Figure 6. FFF fractogram (red dashed line: fluorescence signal; grey line: absorption signal), UV-Vis absorption spectrum, and Molar Mass/RMS radius (red) and fluorescence/UV profile (grey) obtained for 1:2 PP-MNP:HSA (**a–c**) and 1:4 PP-MNP:HSA (**d–f**) suspensions.

The profile at 480 nm shows that nanoparticles from different species are eluted at different times. A new band absorbing at 8 min at 480 nm is clearly visible in Figure 6a, preceding the peak corresponding to HSA alone (Figure 6a), and the PP-MNP band at 14 min decreases the same amount since the total integrated area was verified to be constant for all analyses. Due to the fluorescence signal, we hypothesized that such new band also contains HSA, indicating that PP-MNPs and proteins interact to form a differently arranged system with a completely different retention behaviour and involving both species. The absorption spectrum appears as a combined band of HSA and PP-MNPs (Figure 6b). The MALS calculation pointed out that the newly-formed species had an RMS radius comparable to the previously characterized PP-MNPs (55 nm vs. 58 nm, Figure 6c). The early retention time for species with same RMS radius indicates a different shape and/or surface charge which impact the retentive behaviour in HF5. Since the DLS and Zeta potential results show a decreasing hydrodynamical radius, it is possible that HSA takes part in coating PP-MNPs competing with PEG/PLGA, the formal coating, and creates a hybrid coating less influenced by the polymer encaging. We hypothesize the formation of an HSA protein corona on PP-MNPs, with consequent formation of HSA-PP-MNPs composite. Last, the PP-MNPs: HSA 1:4 ratio showed a progression in the PP-MNPs shift to the earlier peak. The signal relative to HSA is split into a PP-MNP-containing fraction (eluted at 8 min) and its typical retention peak at 10 min, where the PP-MNPs also tailed (Figure 6d). The UV-Vis spectrum shows the migration of the absorption profile towards the earlier peak (Figure 6e); in terms of the RMS radius, the two species eluted at 8 and 15 min are measured at 60 nm and average at 59 nm, respectively (Figure 6f). A second shoulder of 60 nm at 12 min stems from the later band, suggesting a reconversion of the PP-MNPs towards the newly-formed band.

The fluorescence signal of HSA is split with a maximum at the same time of early-eluted PP-MNPs (whose peak increases compared to the 1:2 mix), and a second maximum at its characteristic retention time. The UV absorption shows that PP-MNPs are mainly present as an HSA-PP-MNPs composite (8 to 10 min) rather than particles alone (12 to 20 min). In the HSA excess condition (PP-MNPs: HSA $\geq$ 1:2), an HSA-PP-MNPs composite is formed. HSA gives rise to a protein corona on PP-MNPs, minimizing the agglomeration phenomena between PP-MNPs due to maximization of electrostatic and steric repulsion [53]. Thus, the HSA-PP-MNPs system was characterized by well-dispersed NPs and a net negative charge.

The FFF-multidetection data suggested that in the presence of a low amount of HSA, the two phases—HSA and PP-MNPs—coexist separately. As the HSA content increases, they begin to interact, and HSA becomes part of the existing PEG/PLGA coating, creating a protein corona on PP-MNPs, up to the encapsulation of most of the MNPs in the HSA matrix.

Evidence of this transition also comes from the conformational study of the peaks of the HSA-PP-MNPs (7.5–10 min interval) and PP-MNPs (14–18 min interval), namely, population 1 and population 2, obtained for all mixes and shown in Figure 7.

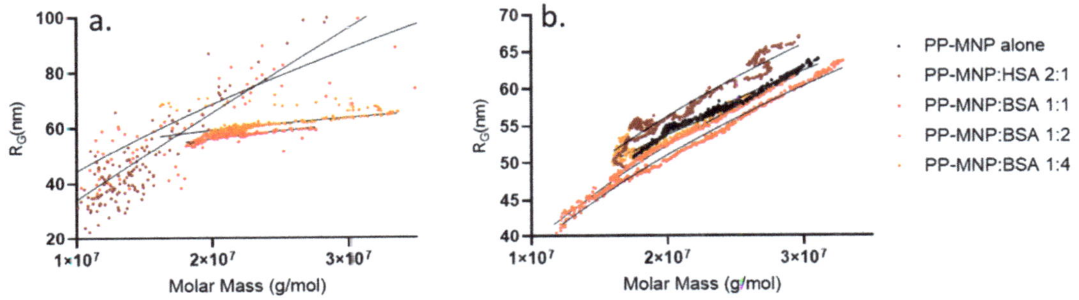

Figure 7. Conformation plots obtained for population 1 (**a**) and population 2 (**b**) expressed as double logarithmic molar mass/gyration radius regression lines.

A conformation plot considers the double logarithmic dependency between the mass and radius values calculated with MALS, where the slope "v" (v value) is an indication of the shape of the particles analysed. A solid sphere has a v value of about 0.33—higher values describe elongated or deformed structures (e.g., a rod has a v value of 1, whereas for a random coil v nears 0.7)—while lower values describe a denser core and a softer shell. In our case, population 2, i.e., free PP-MNPs still non-interacting with HSA, had a v value of 0.4 decreasing to 0.33 (0.40–0.41–0.40–0.36–0.33) at the highest ratio measured. These values indicate a spherical shape decreasing to a solid sphere at the lowering of the free PP-MNP amount, without evident conformational changes apart from what is expected from a lowering concentration. At the same time, when HSA increases, population 1 starts to form. In this case, the change in the conformation is very clear; it starts as a very elongated (and polydisperse) form (v value = 0.9 and 0.7 for 2:1 and 1:1 ratios), which can be attributed to HSA surrounding the PP-MNP system and solvating it. Then, the conformation plot evolves towards a core-shell form where dense PP-MNP particles are surrounded by a less-dense, stable coating of PEG/PLGA-HSA (v value = 0.21 and 0.19 for 1:2 and 1:4 ratios), which remained stable even when increasing the HSA:PP-MNP ratio.

This information is extremely relevant, since nanoparticle activity also depends on shape, surface, and conformation. Combined with the size results obtained from DLS, these data confirm that MNPs retain a spherical shape, and the change in retention time previously noted is not due to a new conformation, but rather to a different apparent radius. In fact, the retention time of the observed species is not compatible with the radius measured by MALS—the explanation for such little retention can be due to a reversed elution mode, meaning that the species is behaving as hydrodynamically very big while actually being smaller, which is only possible when species such as PEG surround it. Weak interactions between particles and free PEG/PLGA could contribute to creating a high apparent hydrodynamic radius which is eluted in inversed mode. The evidence for surface interactions occurring with the increase in HSA (as opposed to simple coelution) can be gathered also by observing a change in the emission spectra of the conjugate, similar to that of HSA (whereas PP-MNPs do not emit, see Figure 4d) but presenting additional peaks (not shown). The interaction can be due to electrostatic interactions between MNPs and the negative charge of HSA in a physiological pH (due to a pI of 4.7), but also on the chemisorption on the thiol groups from albumin onto the MNP surface. Moreover, the presence of a complex structure involving both PEG/PLGA and HSA over MNPs is confirmed by the absorption spectrum which is typical for PP-MNPs. As for PEG/PLGA behaviour, it is true that the protein-repellent properties of coatings such as PEG are reported to prevent nonspecific interactions of serum proteins with nanoparticles, reducing the interaction with the immune system and leading to longer circulation times in the bloodstream [54]. However, there are also some reports that BSA was able to rapidly couple to PEG-encapsulated nanoparticles to increase their stability and biocompatibility in the cell culture media and intracellularly by preventing aggregation [55,56], corroborating the mechanism hypothesized above.

Last, to summarize our findings, we evaluated the area of the signal at 480 nm for all mixtures. The total area values were identical (within a 3% deviation), showing that the increase in HSA did not modify PP-MNPs absorption at this wavelength, and recovery was constant in the FFF analyses. Then, we considered the area percentage of HSA-PP-MNPs eluted at 8 min, obtaining the curve in Figure 8. To evaluate the binding trend we also increased the ratio between PP-MNPs and HSA to 1.6, 1:8, and 1:10, where population 2 was no longer visible and the only species was the core-shell structure already observed in population 1.

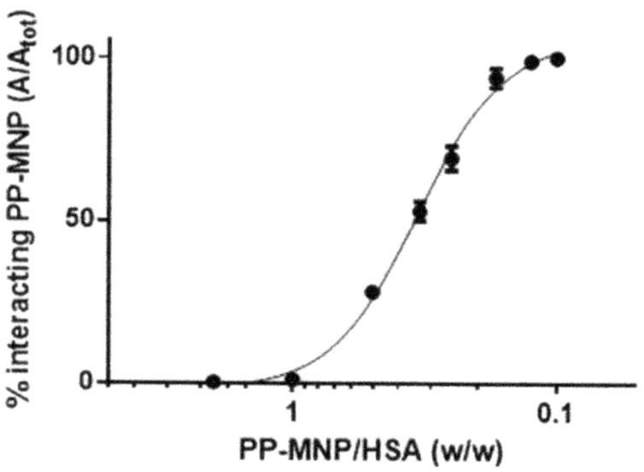

Figure 8. HSA/PP-MNP interaction vs. HSA increase expressed as the percentage of PP-MNPs interacting with HSA (black dots and error bars, n = 3) calculated from independent runs of supensions at 2:1, 1:1, 1:2, 1:4, 1:6, 1:8, 1:10 PP-MNPs:HSA mass ratio.

Until the HSA amount is double that of the PP-MNPs, there is very little interaction. This rapidly changes with a 1:2 ratio, indicating that only a higher amount of protein can interact with the PP-MNPs, with HSA encapsulation on PP-MNPs. When a 1:8 ratio is reached, all PP-MNPs are converted into HSA-PP-MNPs eluted as population 1.

Following a further HSA increase and PP-MNP dilution in the biological medium, until reaching the albumin range in healthy human blood (34–54 g/L), all PP-MNPs are coated with an HSA protein corona, acting as an HSA-PP-MNPs composite. The latter can be considered as biocompatible NPs due to the HSA shell, and suitable for potential therapeutic medical applications [57].

Some study limitations apply, such as the need for FFF method adjustment according to the type of sample, which requires a reoptimization if the methodology is applied to another system. The current FFF setup requires very little sample but is not indicated for particle collection and further study. If necessary, a scaling up to the flat, non-miniaturized channel can be performed. Limitations aside, combining these results with those obtained with batch techniques, it is evident how the information obtained is complementary and the approach is advantageous. Whereas DLS and Z potential evaluation allow an observation of the evolution of PP-MNPs when injected in a biological fluid, it is only through the selective size/conformation analysis obtained from FFF-multidetection that it is possible to visualize what species are present in a frame-by-frame approach, to observe the evolving PP-MNP surface, and to and understand the high excess of protein needed to achieve full conversion into their biological identity.

4. Conclusions

Understanding the evolution of MNP-based therapeutics upon injection into the patient is both necessary and challenging. It is crucial to identify possible particle instability that may raise safety concerns, but at the same time several parameters (size, conformation, coating, surface properties) need to be monitored in a dynamic way, which is difficult to achieve. While current techniques can monitor these parameters, their response is mediated upon all the possible populations present in the sample, since measurements are performed statically. A separation approach can instead provide selective information and identify particle evolution in the native state, monitoring the evolution of injected MNPs at increasing levels of protein and simulating their dispersion in a biological medium. In this work, a method based on miniaturized FFF-multidetection allowed us to confirm that the particles are relatively stable in the medium (though some aggregation can occur) and progressively interact with proteins to form a new biological identity, with a process that involves a very imbalanced mass ratio. By combining conformation studies to batch characterization results, it was also possible to confirm the unchanged morphology of particles which is strictly linked to their activity and cytotoxicity. With this approach and setup, it is possible to monitor nanoparticles–protein interactions in the very first steps of infusion and evaluate the effect of the concentration and ratio on the size, shape, and arrangement of PP-MNPs.

Author Contributions: Conceptualization, M.B. and V.M.; methodology, V.M., M.B. and A.L.C.; formal analysis, I.Z., S.G. and S.O.; investigation, I.Z., S.G. and S.O.; writing—original draft preparation, V.M., I.Z., S.O. and M.B.; writing—review and editing, V.M., I.Z., S.O., S.G., P.R., B.R., A.Z., C.R., L.C., G.B., A.L.C. and M.B.; funding acquisition, P.R. and M.B. All authors have read and agreed to the published version of the manuscript.

Funding: This work was supported by the European Union's Horizon 2020 Research and Innovation Programme under grant agreement No. 760928 (BIORIMA).

Institutional Review Board Statement: Not applicable.

Informed Consent Statement: Not applicable.

Data Availability Statement: The datasets generated for this study can be obtained from the corresponding author upon reasonable request.

Conflicts of Interest: The authors declare no conflict of interest. Valentina Marassi, Pierluigi Reschiglian, Barbara Roda, and Andrea Zattoni are associates of the spinoff company byFlow srl; the company mission includes know-how transfer, development, and application of novel technologies and methodologies for the analysis and characterization of samples of nano-biotechnological interest.

References

1. Maldonado-Camargo, L.; Unni, M.; Rinaldi, C. Magnetic Characterization of Iron Oxide Nanoparticles for Biomedical Applications. *Methods Mol. Biol.* **2017**, *1570*, 47–71. [CrossRef] [PubMed]
2. Shubayev, V.I.; Pisanic, T.R., 2nd; Jin, S. Magnetic nanoparticles for theragnostics. *Adv. Drug Deliv. Rev.* **2009**, *61*, 467–477. [CrossRef] [PubMed]
3. Wankhede, M.; Bouras, A.; Kaluzova, M.; Hadjipanayis, C.G. Magnetic nanoparticles: An emerging technology for malignant brain tumor imaging and therapy. *Expert Rev. Clin. Pharmacol.* **2012**, *5*, 173–186. [CrossRef] [PubMed]
4. Lin, Y.; Zhang, K.; Zhang, R.; She, Z.; Tan, R.; Fan, Y.; Li, X. Magnetic nanoparticles applied in targeted therapy and magnetic resonance imaging: Crucial preparation parameters, indispensable pre-treatments, updated research advancements and future perspectives. *J. Mater. Chem. B* **2020**, *8*, 5973–5991. [CrossRef] [PubMed]

5. Laurent, S.; Dutz, S.; Häfeli, U.O.; Mahmoudi, M. Magnetic fluid hyperthermia: Focus on superparamagnetic iron oxide nanoparticles. *Adv. Colloid Interface Sci.* **2011**, *166*, 8–23. [CrossRef]
6. Wong, R.S.Y. Apoptosis in cancer: From pathogenesis to treatment. *J. Exp. Clin. Cancer Res.* **2011**, *30*, 87. [CrossRef]
7. Samanta, B.; Yan, H.; Fischer, N.O.; Shi, J.; Jerry, D.J.; Rotello, V.M. Protein-passivated Fe_3O_4 nanoparticles: Low toxicity and rapid heating for thermal therapy. *J. Mater. Chem.* **2008**, *18*, 1204–1208. [CrossRef]
8. Park, J.Y.; Patel, D.; Choi, E.S.; Baek, M.J.; Chang, Y.; Kim, T.J.; Lee, G.H. Salt effects on the physical properties of magnetite nanoparticles synthesized at different NaCl concentrations. *Colloids Surf. A Physicochem. Eng. Asp.* **2010**, *367*, 41–46. [CrossRef]
9. Hayashi, K.; Tomonaga, H.; Matsuyama, T.; Ida, J. Facile synthesis, characterization of various polymer immobilized on magnetite nanoparticles applying the coprecipitation method. *J. Appl. Polym. Sci.* **2022**, *139*, 51581. [CrossRef]
10. Mylkie, K.; Nowak, P.; Rybczynski, P.; Ziegler-Borowska, M. Polymer-Coated Magnetite Nanoparticles for Protein Immobilization. *Materials* **2021**, *14*, 248. [CrossRef]
11. Anbarasu, M.; Anandan, M.; Chinnasamy, E.; Gopinath, V.; Balamurugan, K. Synthesis and characterization of polyethylene glycol (PEG) coated Fe_3O_4 nanoparticles by chemical co-precipitation method for biomedical applications. *Spectrochim. Acta Part A Mol. Biomol. Spectrosc.* **2015**, *135*, 536–539. [CrossRef]
12. Patsula, V.; Horák, D.; Kučka, J.; Macková, H.; Lobaz, V.; Francová, P.; Herynek, V.; Heizer, T.; Páral, P.; Šefc, L. Synthesis and modification of uniform PEG-neridronate-modified magnetic nanoparticles determines prolonged blood circulation and biodistribution in a mouse preclinical model. *Sci. Rep.* **2019**, *9*, 10765. [CrossRef]
13. Mosafer, J.; Teymouri, M. Comparative study of superparamagnetic iron oxide/doxorubicin co-loaded poly (lactic-co-glycolic acid) nanospheres prepared by different emulsion solvent evaporation methods. *Artif. Cells Nanomed. Biotechnol.* **2018**, *46*, 1146–1155. [CrossRef]
14. Sah, H.; Thoma, L.A.; Desu, H.R.; Sah, E.; Wood, G.C. Concepts and practices used to develop functional PLGA-based nanoparticulate systems. *Int. J. Nanomed.* **2013**, *8*, 747–765. [CrossRef]
15. Danhier, F.; Ansorena, E.; Silva, J.M.; Coco, R.; Le Breton, A.; Préat, V. PLGA-based nanoparticles: An overview of biomedical applications. *J. Control. Release* **2012**, *161*, 505–522. [CrossRef]
16. Tombácz, E.; Tóth, I.Y.; Nesztor, D.; Illés, E.; Hajdú, A.; Szekeres, M.; Vékás, L. Adsorption of organic acids on magnetite nanoparticles, pH-dependent colloidal stability and salt tolerance. *Colloids Surf. A Physicochem. Eng. Asp.* **2013**, *435*, 91–96. [CrossRef]
17. Han, M.; Li, Y.; Lu, S.; Yuan, B.; Cheng, S.; Cao, C. Amyloid Protein-Biofunctionalized Polydopamine Nanoparticles Demonstrate Minimal Plasma Protein Fouling and Efficient Photothermal Therapy. *ACS Appl. Mater. Interfaces* **2022**, *14*, 13743–13757. [CrossRef]
18. Wang, X.; Zhang, W. The Janus of Protein Corona on nanoparticles for tumor targeting, immunotherapy and diagnosis. *J. Control. Release* **2022**, *345*, 832–850. [CrossRef]
19. Cox, A.; Andreozzi, P.; Dal Magro, R.; Fiordaliso, F.; Corbelli, A.; Talamini, L.; Chinello, C.; Raimondo, F.; Magni, F.; Tringali, M.; et al. Evolution of Nanoparticle Protein Corona across the Blood–Brain Barrier. *ACS Nano* **2018**, *12*, 7292–7300. [CrossRef]
20. Bychkova, A.V.; Sorokina, O.N.; Kovarskii, A.L.; Leonova, V.B.; Rozenfel'd, M.A. Interaction between blood plasma proteins and magnetite nanoparticles. *Colloid J.* **2010**, *72*, 696–702. [CrossRef]
21. Dell'Orco, D.; Lundqvist, M.; Oslakovic, C.; Cedervall, T.; Linse, S. Modeling the Time Evolution of the Nanoparticle-Protein Corona in a Body Fluid. *PLoS ONE* **2010**, *5*, e10949. [CrossRef]
22. Xiao, Q.; Zoulikha, M.; Qiu, M.; Teng, C.; Lin, C.; Li, X.; Sallam, M.A.; Xu, Q.; He, W. The effects of protein corona on in vivo fate of nanocarriers. *Adv. Drug Deliv. Rev.* **2022**, *186*, 114356. [CrossRef] [PubMed]
23. Mourdikoudis, S.; Pallares, R.M.; Thanh, N.T.K. Characterization techniques for nanoparticles: Comparison and complementarity upon studying nanoparticle properties. *Nanoscale* **2018**, *10*, 12871–12934. [CrossRef] [PubMed]
24. Reschiglian, P.; Rambaldi, D.C.; Zattoni, A. Flow field-flow fractionation with multiangle light scattering detection for the analysis and characterization of functional nanoparticles. *Anal. Bioanal. Chem.* **2011**, *399*, 197–203. [CrossRef] [PubMed]
25. Ventouri, I.K.; Loeber, S.; Somsen, G.W.; Schoenmakers, P.J.; Astefanei, A. Field-flow fractionation for molecular-interaction studies of labile and complex systems: A critical review. *Anal. Chim. Acta* **2022**, *1193*, 339396. [CrossRef]
26. Zattoni, A.; Roda, B.; Borghi, F.; Marassi, V.; Reschiglian, P. Flow field-flow fractionation for the analysis of nanoparticles used in drug delivery. *J. Pharm. Biomed. Anal.* **2014**, *87*, 53–61. [CrossRef]
27. Zhang, X.; Li, Y.; Shen, S.; Lee, S.; Dou, H. Field-flow fractionation: A gentle separation and characterization technique in biomedicine. *TrAC Trends Anal. Chem.* **2018**, *108*, 231–238. [CrossRef]
28. Marassi, V.; Macis, M.; Giordani, S.; Ferrazzano, L.; Tolomelli, A.; Roda, B.; Zattoni, A.; Ricci, A.; Reschiglian, P.; Cabri, W. Application of Af4-Multidetection to Liraglutide in Its Formulation: Preserving and Representing Native Aggregation. *Molecules* **2022**, *27*, 5485. [CrossRef]
29. Wankar, J.; Bonvicini, F.; Benkovics, G.; Marassi, V.; Malanga, M.; Fenyvesi, E.; Gentilomi, G.A.; Reschiglian, P.; Roda, B.; Manet, I. Widening the Therapeutic Perspectives of Clofazimine by Its Loading in Sulfobutylether β-Cyclodextrin Nanocarriers: Nanomolar IC(50) Values against MDR S. epidermidis. *Mol. Pharm.* **2018**, *15*, 3823–3836. [CrossRef]
30. Leeman, M.; Choi, J.; Hansson, S.; Storm, M.U.; Nilsson, L. Proteins and antibodies in serum, plasma, and whole blood-size characterization using asymmetrical flow field-flow fractionation (AF4). *Anal. Bioanal. Chem.* **2018**, *410*, 4867–4873. [CrossRef]

31. Zappi, A.; Marassi, V.; Kassouf, N.; Giordani, S.; Pasqualucci, G.; Garbini, D.; Roda, B.; Zattoni, A.; Reschiglian, P.; Melucci, D. A Green Analytical Method Combined with Chemometrics for Traceability of Tomato Sauce Based on Colloidal and Volatile Fingerprinting. *Molecules* **2022**, *27*, 5507. [CrossRef]
32. Ashby, J.; Schachermeyer, S.; Duan, Y.; Jimenez, L.A.; Zhong, W. Probing and quantifying DNA-protein interactions with asymmetrical flow field-flow fractionation. *J. Chromatogr. A* **2014**, *1358*, 217–224. [CrossRef]
33. Marassi, V.; Mattarozzi, M.; Toma, L.; Giordani, S.; Ronda, L.; Roda, B.; Zattoni, A.; Reschiglian, P.; Careri, M. FFF-based high-throughput sequence shortlisting to support the development of aptamer-based analytical strategies. *Anal. Bioanal. Chem.* **2022**. [CrossRef]
34. Marassi, V.; Roda, B.; Zattoni, A.; Tanase, M.; Reschiglian, P. Hollow fiber flow field-flow fractionation and size-exclusion chromatography with MALS detection: A complementary approach in biopharmaceutical industry. *J. Chromatogr. A* **2014**, *1372*, 196–203. [CrossRef]
35. Marassi, V.; Giordani, S.; Reschiglian, P.; Roda, B.; Zattoni, A. Tracking Heme-Protein Interactions in Healthy and Pathological Human Serum in Native Conditions by Miniaturized FFF-Multidetection. *Appl. Sci.* **2022**, *12*, 6762. [CrossRef]
36. Tan, Z.Q.; Liu, J.F.; Guo, X.R.; Yin, Y.G.; Byeon, S.K.; Moon, M.H.; Jiang, G.B. Toward full spectrum speciation of silver nanoparticles and ionic silver by on-line coupling of hollow fiber flow field-flow fractionation and minicolumn concentration with multiple detectors. *Anal. Chem.* **2015**, *87*, 8441–8447. [CrossRef]
37. Marassi, V.; Casolari, S.; Panzavolta, S.; Bonvicini, F.; Gentilomi, G.A.; Giordani, S.; Zattoni, A.; Reschiglian, P.; Roda, B. Synthesis Monitoring, Characterization and Cleanup of Ag-Polydopamine Nanoparticles Used as Antibacterial Agents with Field-Flow Fractionation. *Antibiotics* **2022**, *11*, 358. [CrossRef]
38. Bai, Q.; Yin, Y.; Liu, Y.; Jiang, H.; Wu, M.; Wang, W.; Tan, Z.; Liu, J.; Moon, M.H.; Xing, B. Flow field-flow fractionation hyphenated with inductively coupled plasma mass spectrometry: A robust technique for characterization of engineered elemental metal nanoparticles in the environment. *Appl. Spectrosc. Rev.* **2021**, 1–22. [CrossRef]
39. Marassi, V.; Calabria, D.; Trozzi, I.; Zattoni, A.; Reschiglian, P.; Roda, B. Comprehensive characterization of gold nanoparticles and their protein conjugates used as a label by hollow fiber flow field flow fractionation with photodiode array and fluorescence detectors and multiangle light scattering. *J. Chromatogr. A* **2021**, *1636*, 461739. [CrossRef]
40. Thielking, H.; Kulicke, W.-M. Determination of the structural parameters of aqueous polymer solutions in the molecular, partially aggregated, and particulate states by means of FFFF/MALLS. *J. Microcolumn Sep.* **1998**, *10*, 51–56. [CrossRef]
41. Baldi, G.; Ravagli, C.; Comes Franchini, M.; D'Elios, M.M.; Benagiano, M.; Bitossi, M. Magnetic Nanoparticles Functionalized with Cathecol, Production and Use Thereof. WO 2015104664-A1, 16 July 2015.
42. D'Elios, M.M.; Aldinucci, A.; Amoriello, R.; Benagiano, M.; Bonechi, E.; Maggi, P.; Flori, A.; Ravagli, C.; Saer, D.; Cappiello, L.; et al. Myelin-specific T cells carry and release magnetite PGLA–PEG COOH nanoparticles in the mouse central nervous system. *RSC Adv.* **2018**, *8*, 904–913. [CrossRef] [PubMed]
43. Marassi, V.; Roda, B.; Casolari, S.; Ortelli, S.; Blosi, M.; Zattoni, A.; Costa, A.L.; Reschiglian, P. Hollow-fiber flow field-flow fractionation and multi-angle light scattering as a new analytical solution for quality control in pharmaceutical nanotechnology. *Microchem. J.* **2018**, *136*, 149–156. [CrossRef]
44. Roda, B.; Marassi, V.; Zattoni, A.; Borghi, F.; Anand, R.; Agostoni, V.; Gref, R.; Reschiglian, P.; Monti, S. Flow field-flow fractionation and multi-angle light scattering as a powerful tool for the characterization and stability evaluation of drug-loaded metal–organic framework nanoparticles. *Anal. Bioanal. Chem.* **2018**, *410*, 5245–5253. [CrossRef] [PubMed]
45. Baalousha, M.; Kammer, F.V.D.; Motelica-Heino, M.; Hilal, H.S.; Le Coustumer, P. Size fractionation and characterization of natural colloids by flow-field flow fractionation coupled to multi-angle laser light scattering. *J. Chromatogr. A* **2006**, *1104*, 272–281. [CrossRef] [PubMed]
46. Marassi, V.; Di Cristo, L.; Smith, S.G.J.; Ortelli, S.; Blosi, M.; Costa, A.L.; Reschiglian, P.; Volkov, Y.; Prina-Mello, A. Silver nanoparticles as a medical device in healthcare settings: A five-step approach for candidate screening of coating agents. *R. Soc. Open Sci.* **2018**, *5*, 171113. [CrossRef]
47. Marassi, V.; De Marchis, F.; Roda, B.; Bellucci, M.; Capecchi, A.; Reschiglian, P.; Pompa, A.; Zattoni, A. Perspectives on protein biopolymers: Miniaturized flow field-flow fractionation-assisted characterization of a single-cysteine mutated phaseolin expressed in transplastomic tobacco plants. *J. Chromatogr. A* **2021**, *1637*, 461806. [CrossRef]
48. Marassi, V.; Maggio, S.; Battistelli, M.; Stocchi, V.; Zattoni, A.; Reschiglian, P.; Guescini, M.; Roda, B. An ultracentrifugation—Hollow-fiber flow field-flow fractionation orthogonal approach for the purification and mapping of extracellular vesicle subtypes. *J. Chromatogr. A* **2021**, *1638*, 461861. [CrossRef]
49. Wassel, R.A.; Grady, B.; Kopke, R.D.; Dormer, K.J. Dispersion of super paramagnetic iron oxide nanoparticles in poly(d,l-lactide-co-glycolide) microparticles. *Colloids Surf. A Physicochem. Eng. Asp.* **2007**, *292*, 125–130. [CrossRef]
50. Liu, X.; Kaminski, M.D.; Chen, H.; Torno, M.; Taylor, L.; Rosengart, A.J. Synthesis and characterization of highly-magnetic biodegradable poly(d,l-lactide-co-glycolide) nanospheres. *J. Control. Release* **2007**, *119*, 52–58. [CrossRef]
51. Ortelli, S.; Costa, A.L.; Zanoni, I.; Blosi, M.; Geiss, O.; Bianchi, I.; Mehn, D.; Fumagalli, F.; Ceccone, G.; Guerrini, G.; et al. TiO_2@BSA nano-composites investigated through orthogonal multi-techniques characterization platform. *Colloids Surf. B Biointerfaces* **2021**, *207*, 112037. [CrossRef]

52. Marassi, V.; Casolari, S.; Roda, B.; Zattoni, A.; Reschiglian, P.; Panzavolta, S.; Tofail, S.A.M.; Ortelli, S.; Delpivo, C.; Blosi, M.; et al. Hollow-fiber flow field-flow fractionation and multi-angle light scattering investigation of the size, shape and metal-release of silver nanoparticles in aqueous medium for nano-risk assessment. *J. Pharm. Biomed. Anal.* **2015**, *106*, 92–99. [CrossRef]
53. Kennedy, D.C.; Qian, H.; Gies, V.; Yang, L. Human serum albumin stabilizes aqueous silver nanoparticle suspensions and inhibits particle uptake by cells. *Environ. Sci. Nano* **2018**, *5*, 863–867. [CrossRef]
54. Free, P.; Shaw, C.P.; Lévy, R. PEGylation modulates the interfacial kinetics of proteases on peptide-capped gold nanoparticles. *Chem. Commun.* **2009**, 5009–5011. [CrossRef]
55. Boulos, S.P.; Davis, T.A.; Yang, J.A.; Lohse, S.E.; Alkilany, A.M.; Holland, L.A.; Murphy, C.J. Nanoparticle–Protein Interactions: A Thermodynamic and Kinetic Study of the Adsorption of Bovine Serum Albumin to Gold Nanoparticle Surfaces. *Langmuir* **2013**, *29*, 14984–14996. [CrossRef]
56. Nicoară, R.; Ilieș, M.; Uifălean, A.; Iuga, C.A.; Loghin, F. Quantification of the PEGylated Gold Nanoparticles Protein Corona. Influence on Nanoparticle Size and Surface Chemistry. *Appl. Sci.* **2019**, *9*, 4789. [CrossRef]
57. Nosrati, H.; Sefidi, N.; Sharafi, A.; Danafar, H.; Kheiri Manjili, H. Bovine Serum Albumin (BSA) coated iron oxide magnetic nanoparticles as biocompatible carriers for curcumin-anticancer drug. *Bioorg. Chem.* **2018**, *76*, 501–509. [CrossRef]

pharmaceutics

MDPI

Article

Mitigating Cardiotoxicity of Dendrimers: Angiotensin-(1-7) via Its Mas Receptor Ameliorates PAMAM-Induced Cardiac Dysfunction in the Isolated Mammalian Heart

Saghir Akhtar [1,*], Fawzi Babiker [2,*], Usman A. Akhtar [3] and Ibrahim F. Benter [4]

1 College of Medicine, QU Health, Qatar University, Doha P.O. Box 2713, Qatar
2 Departments of Physiology, Faculty of Medicine, Health Science Center, Kuwait University, Safat P.C. Box 24923, Kuwait
3 Department of Mechanical and Chemical Engineering, College of Engineering, Qatar University, Doha P.O. Box 2713, Qatar
4 Faculty of Medicine, Eastern Mediterranean University, Famagusta 99628, North Cyprus, Turkey
* Correspondence: s.akhtar@qu.edu.qa (S.A.); fawzi.babiker@ku.edu.kw (F.B.)

Abstract: Aim: The influence of the physiochemical properties of dendrimer nanoparticles on cardiac contractility and hemodynamics are not known. Herein, we investigated (a) the effect of polyamidoamine (PAMAM) dendrimer generation (G7, G6, G5, G4 and G3) and surface chemistry (-NH_2, -COOH and -OH) on cardiac function in mammalian hearts following ischemia-reperfusion (I/R) injury, and (b) determined if any PAMAM-induced cardiotoxicity could be mitigated by Angiotensin-(1-7) (Ang-(1-7), a cardioprotective agent. Methods: Hearts isolated from male Wistar rats underwent regional I/R and/or treatment with different PAMAM dendrimers, Ang-(1-7) or its MAS receptors antagonists. Thirty minutes of regional ischemia through ligation of the left anterior descending coronary artery was followed by 30 min of reperfusion. All treatments were initiated 5 min prior to reperfusion and maintained during the first 10 min of reperfusion. Cardiac function parameters for left ventricular contractility, hemodynamics and vascular dynamics data were acquired digitally, whereas cardiac enzymes and infarct size were used as measures of cardiac injury. Results: Treatment of isolated hearts with increasing doses of G7 PAMAM dendrimer progressively exacerbated recovery of cardiac contractility and hemodynamic parameters post-I/R injury. Impairment of cardiac function was progressively less on decreasing dendrimer generation with G3 exhibiting little or no cardiotoxicity. Cationic PAMAMs (-NH_2) were more toxic than anionic (-COOH), with neutral PAMAMs (-OH) exhibiting the least cardiotoxicity. Cationic G7 PAMAM-induced cardiac dysfunction was significantly reversed by Ang-(1-7) administration. These cardioprotective effects of Ang-(1-7) were significantly revoked by administration of the MAS receptor antagonists, A779 and D-Pro^7-Ang-(1-7). Conclusions: PAMAM dendrimers can impair the recovery of hearts from I/R injury in a dose-, dendrimer-generation-(size) and surface-charge dependent manner. Importantly, PAMAM-induced cardiotoxicity could be mitigated by Ang-(1-7) acting through its MAS receptor. Thus, this study highlights the activation of Ang-(1-7)/Mas receptor axis as a novel strategy to overcome dendrimer-induced cardiotoxicity.

Keywords: PAMAM dendrimer; Ang-(1-7); cardiac ischemia/reperfusion; Mas receptor; surface chemistry; dendrimer generation; toxicity

Citation: Akhtar, S.; Babiker, F.; Akhtar, U.A.; Benter, I.F. Mitigating Cardiotoxicity of Dendrimers: Angiotensin-(1-7) via Its Mas Receptor Ameliorates PAMAM-Induced Cardiac Dysfunction in the Isolated Mammalian Heart. *Pharmaceutics* **2022**, *14*, 2673. https://doi.org/10.3390/pharmaceutics14122673

Academic Editors: Ana Isabel Fraguas-Sánchez, Raquel Fernández García and Francisco Bolás-Fernández

Received: 28 October 2022
Accepted: 27 November 2022
Published: 1 December 2022

1. Introduction

Polyamidoamine (PAMAM) dendrimers, or "starburst dendrimers", are nano-sized, spherical and highly-branched polymers that have important applications in nanomedicine, including as drug delivery carriers [1–5]. They can be synthesized by defined nanoparticle size, molecular architecture and surface charge or terminal functional group chemistry [2,3,5]. During PAMAM synthesis, sequential layers of radially repeating units are attached to a defined core (e.g., ethylenediamine), leading to progressive generations (G) of dendrimers with each consecutive generation having an increased molecular diameter and molecular weight due to the doubling of the number of surface functional groups compared to the previous generation [2,5]. Additionally, PAMAM dendrimers, can be produced with cationic amino-(-NH_2), anionic carboxyl-(-COOH) or neutral hydroxyl-(-OH) terminal groups, all of which have been widely studied, including as potential drug delivery vectors [2,5,6]. Thus, PAMAMs with defined physicochemical properties, which are commercially available as a homologous series of low polydispersity polymers with increasing molecular weight and defined surface charge, readily lend themselves to structure activity relationship studies.

There is now growing evidence to suggest that beyond their ability to enhance drug delivery, PAMAM dendrimers have innate biological and toxicological actions that are highly dependent on their physicochemical properties (for recent review see [3]). Previously, we have shown that naked PAMAM dendrimers (without any drug cargo) can modulate key cell signaling networks, including those involving the epidermal growth factor receptor (EGFR), in a generation- (molecular weight) and surface charge- (functional group) dependent manner both in vitro and in vivo [7–9]. Due to passive accumulation of dendrimers within organs of the reticuloendothelial system, including the heart (for review see [3]), PAMAMs have been successfully used to deliver both small molecular weight drugs and gene-based therapies to cardiac tissue (e.g., [10–13]). However, little is known of their toxicological profile in the mammalian heart.

We previously showed that systemically (intraperitoneally) administered PAMAM dendrimers could improve peripheral vascular function in vivo [8]. Thus, in a subsequent study, we hypothesized that PAMAMs might act similarly in the vasculature of the heart and thereby offer pharmacological benefit especially after cardiac ischemia-reperfusion injury (as would be required therapeutically after a "heart attack"). Contrary to our expectations, we recently reported that a G6 cationic PAMAM dendrimer actually impaired the ability of mammalian hearts to recover from ischemia-reperfusion injury ex vivo and in vivo [14]. Both systemic administration in vivo (daily i.p injections for 4 weeks) as well as acute, ex vivo administration directly to the isolated heart during reperfusion led to qualitatively similar effects on the heart with a cationic G6 PAMAM dendrimer [14]. However, the impact of other PAMAM dendrimer generations and surface chemical groups on cardiac function have not been studied. Thus, in the present study, we utilized the less time consuming and less costly approach of ex vivo (rather than in vivo) administration of dendrimers to isolated hearts during reperfusion to study the influence of PAMAMs of different generations and surface chemistries on cardiac recovery following ischemic injury, in the hope that lower generations or non-cationic PAMAMs might show some pharmacological benefit in acute cardiac ischemic injury. Another advantage of using the isolated perfused heart as a model is that perfusion with aqueous buffers largely avoids any potential blood complications, such as hemolysis or coagulation that might otherwise occur following direct, rapid intravenous administration of at least the cationic PAMAMs in vivo (for recent review see [3]).

Ischemic heart disease is one of the major health concerns globally [15–17]. Restriction of coronary blood supply (e.g., from atherosclerotic plaques) eventually leads to myocardial infarction (MI) and potentially death [18,19]. The extent of infarction and disease outcome can be mitigated to some extent by restoration of blood flow following ischemia [18,19]. However, reperfusion itself contributes to unavoidable damage in the myocardium, referred to as reperfusion or ischemia/reperfusion (I/R) injury [18,19]. Several pharmacological and mechanical cardioprotective procedures, including balloon-angioplasty, have been used to limit the devastating effects of I/R injury in the myocardium [20–24]. Pharmacologically, the use of thrombolytics such as streptokinase to degrade fibrin clots, or anticoagulation therapy with clopidogrel or aspirin, can also reduce thrombus size and restore coronary blood flow [25]. Several updated clinical and pre-clinical strategies for the pharmacological targeting of the underlying signaling pathways of MI have been reviewed recently [17].

Pharmacological conditioning of the heart (induced with drug(s)) can also provide protection akin to that of classical postconditioning [26–28]. However, we have been studying the cardioprotective effects of Angiotensin-(1-7), a member of the renin-angiotensin-aldosterone system (RAAS) that is crucial to the homeostasis of the cardiovascular system (for review see [29–31]).

Ang-(1-7) is a heptapeptide that generally acts via its Mas receptor to counter-regulate the functions of Angiotensin II (Ang II), the main peptide component of the RAAS. It can be synthesized by enzymatic cleavage of Ang II by Angiotensin converting enzyme 2 (ACE2)—which also doubles as the receptor for SARS-CoV2 in human cells [29,32]. The ACE2-Ang-(1-7)-Mas receptor axis of the RAAS promotes anti-oxidative stress, anti-inflammatory, anti-fibrotic and pro-vasodilatory effects that typically protect cardiovascular organs against various pathological injuries [29]. We have shown that Ang-(1-7)-mediated cardio-protection in animal models of diabetes and/or hypertension can occur via multiple mechanisms [33–37]. Thus, in this study, in addition to studying the impact of PAMAM dendrimer generation (G7, G6, G5, G4 and G3) and surface chemistry (-NH_2, -COOH and -OH) on cardiac function, we sought to investigate whether Ang-(1-7) could mitigate the cardiotoxicity of high-generation cationic PAMAM dendrimers in an isolated, perfused rat heart model of I/R injury.

2. Materials and Methods

2.1. Materials

All materials and chemicals were purchased from Sigma Aldrich (St. Louis, Missouri, USA) unless stated otherwise. PAMAM dendrimers with an ethylenediamine core were produced by Dendritech (USA) and purchased from the Sigma Chemical Company (St Louis, MO, USA). The properties of PAMAMs were characterized previously and we showed them to be mono-disperse structures [8]. The nominal physicochemical properties of PAMAM dendrimers and the doses used in this study are summarized in Table 1.

Table 1. List of PAMAM dendrimers, their nominal physicochemical properties and dosages used in this study.

Terminal Surface Chemistry $	Surface Charge	Generation $	Molecular Weight (Da) $	Diameter (nm) $	No. of Surface Groups $	Dose (s) Administered in Isolated Rat Heart
-NH_2	Cationic	3	6909	3.6	32	100 nM
-NH_2	Cationic	4	14,215	4.5	64	100 nM
-NH_2	Cationic	5	28,826	5.4	128	100 nM
-NH2	Cationic	6	58,048	6.7	256	100 nM
-NH_2	Cationic	7	116,493	8.1	512	100 nM and for dose-dependent studies: 1 µg, 5 µg, 7.5 µg, 10 µg or 20 µg/mL
-OH	Neutral	6	58,304	NA	256	100 nM
-COOH	Anionic	5.5	52,913	NA	256	100 nM

$ Manufacturer provided information. NA, Information not made available. Anionic PAMAM dendrimers are produced as half-generations. All dendrimers had an ethylenediamine core structure.

2.2. Animals and Procedures

Male Wistar rats with body weights in the range of 250–350 g were obtained from the Kuwait University Animal Resources Centre. The study was approved by the Health

Science Center, Kuwait University Animal Ethics Committee. The study was conducted as per the EU Directive 2010/63/EU for experiments in animals. All rats were kept under controlled conditions within a temperature range of 21–24 °C, a 12 h light/dark cycle (7 a.m.–7 p.m.) and a humidity of 50%. The rats were kept in plastic cages (2 rats/cage), with *ad libitum* access to food and water. The rats received anesthesia via an intraperitoneal (i.p) injection of a 60 mg/kg dose of sodium pentobarbital as well as an injection of the anticoagulant, heparin (1000 U/kg body weight). Animal sacrifice was performed via cervical dislocation under general anesthesia. Surgery to isolate hearts [38] as well as cannulation and perfusion of the heart has been described by us previously [39]. Hearts underwent 30 min of regional ischemia through occlusion of the left anterior descending (LAD) branch of the coronary artery. We maintained a constant preload of 6 mmHg under basal controlled conditions and a constant perfusion pressure (PP) of 50 mmHg throughout the experimental procedures detailed in Figure 1. PP was measured using a Statham pressure transducer (P23 Db) and regulated electronically in the perfusion assembly (Module PPCM type 671 (Hugo Sachs Elektronik-Harvard Apparatus GmbH, Germany)) similar to that described previously [39].

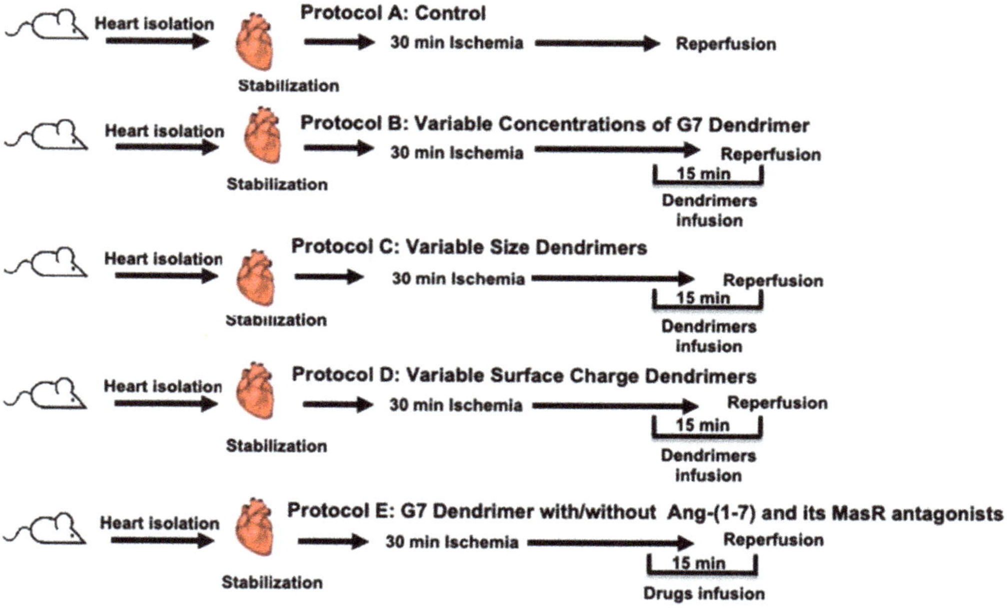

Figure 1. Schematic representation showing the experimental protocols used in the study (n = 8). A: Untreated ischemia-reperfusion control (C). B: Dose response relationship for the G7 PAMAM dendrimer. C: Effect of the dendrimer size (generation) on heart subjected to ischemia and reperfusion. D: Effect of the surface charge/chemistry of dendrimers on hearts subjected to ischemia and reperfusion. E: Effect of the G7 PAMAM dendrimer in the presence or absence of Ang-(1-7) and its Mas receptors antagonists on the effects of ischemia and reperfusion.

2.3. Experimental Study Protocols

Rats were randomly assigned to 5 groups addressing 5 experimental protocols labelled as A-E (see Figure 1). Isolated hearts from rats (n = 8) in the first group (Protocol A) underwent 30 min ischemia and 30 min of reperfusion with no other treatment and served as controls (Figure 1). In protocol B, rat hearts (n = 8 for each dose) were subjected to 5 different concentrations of cationic G7 PAMAM dendrimer (1 µg, 5 µg, 7.5 µg, 10 µg or 20 µg/mL) to evaluate the dose-dependent effect of this dendrimer (Figure 1). In protocol C, we studied the cardiac effects of different dendrimer generations (molecular size) ranging from the smallest, G3 to G4, G5, G6, to the largest, G7, PAMAM dendrimers at a fixed concentration of 100 nM in isolated rat hearts (n = 8 for each dendrimer generation) (Figure 1, Protocol C). Protocol D was used to investigate the cardiac effects of the different surface chemistries (or charge) of the dendrimers whereby isolated hearts (n = 8 for each surface chemistry) were treated with either cationic G6, anionic G5.5 or neutral G6 PAMAM dendrimers at a fixed concentration of 100 nM (Figure 1, Protocol D). In protocol E, we investigated the effects of Ang-(1-7) and its Mas receptor antagonists on reversing G7 dendrimer cardiotoxicity. In addition to having control hearts subjected to I/R with no other treatment, other isolated rat hearts (N = 8 for each subgroup) were treated with either Ang-(1-7), cationic G7 PAMAM dendrimer; (G7) G7+(Ang-(1-7), G7+Ang-(1-7)+A779 (i.e., D-Ala^7-Ang-(1-7) or G7+Ang-(1-7)+D-Pro (i.e., D-Pro^7-Ang-(1-7)) (Figure 1, protocol E). All treatments were administered to isolated hearts 5 min before reperfusion and were continued during the first 10 min of reperfusion post I/R. Hearts undergoing I/R injury alone (without any other treatment) served as controls.

2.4. Assessment of Heart Function

The various cardiac function parameters relating to hemodynamics and contractility were determined during the period of stabilization (baseline) and after I/R injury as previously described [38–40]. Left ventricular (LV) dynamics were assessed through measuring the left ventricular (LV) end-diastolic pressure (LVEDP)- a measure of ventricular compliance that is typically elevated following acute myocardial infarction; and also the maximum developed pressure (DPmax) and LV contractility (+dP/dt or -dP/dt) parameters. The coronary vascular dynamics were determined through measuring coronary vascular resistance (CVR) and coronary flow (CF) as previously described [38–40].

2.5. Assessment of Cardiac Damage through Infarct Size Measurement and Determination of Cardiac Enzyme Levels

The size of LV infarcts was determined after staining with triphenyltetrazolium chloride (TTC) as described previously [41]. Images of infarcts from a given tissue slice were obtained using a Nikon camera and subsequently analyzed using Leica ImageJ (Wayne Rasb and National Institute of Health, USA), manually indicated on the image for each slice. The infarcted area (expressed as a percentage) on the image was calculated relative to total LV area. The cardiac enzymes, creatine kinase (CK) and lactate dehydrogenase (LDH) that were released in the coronary effluent during reperfusion were measured as described by us previously [42] as markers for cardiomyocyte injury.

2.6. Data Analysis

A two-way analysis of variance (ANOVA) followed by the least significant difference (LSD) post-hoc analysis of the data was performed using SPSS software. Comparisons between the data means of the different experimental groups and the mean for their respective controls was undertaken. All experimental data were presented as the mean ± standard error of the mean and statistically significance ascertained when values for $p < 0.05$.

3. Results

3.1. The Effects of Increasing Doses of Cationic G7 PAMAM Dendrimers on Cardiac Function Recovery following I/R Injury in Isolated Rat Hearts

In this study, the animal body weights (mean 300 ± 50 g) and heart size (1.5 ± 0.3 g) were not significantly different among the experimental groups studied. Regional ischemia followed by reperfusion caused a significant deterioration in the LV hemodynamics, contractility and coronary vascular dynamics compared to baseline data ($p < 0.05$). For example, % recovery in Pmax was only around 50% (Figure 2). Infusion of increasing doses of cationic G7 PAMAM dendrimer (1 µg, 5 µg, 7.5 µg, 10 µg or 20 µg/mL) at reperfusion resulted in a gradual increase in the deterioration of the LV hemodynamic, contractility and coronary vascular dynamics. For example, % recovery of Pmax gradually decreased with a statistically significant decline noted at doses of 7.5 μg/mL and above ($p < 0.05$) (Figure 2a). A similar deterioration was observed in LVEDP ($p < 0.01$), a measure of ventricular compliance (Figure 2b) as well as the other LV contractility parameters (+dp/dt; dp/dt) (Figure 2c,d). Hemodynamic parameters of CF and CVR also deteriorated with a significant decrease being observed at the higher doses ($p < 0.05$) (Figure 2e,f). For almost all cardiac function parameters, G7 PAMAM cardiotoxicity appeared to plateau at doses of 10 μg/mL and above (see Figure 2). For example, %R values for DPmax, +dp/dt; dp/dt plateaued at around 14%, whereas for CF, this value was around 10%. Similarly, a plateau was also observed for G7 PAMAM at doses of 10 μg/mL and above with LVEDP and CVR.

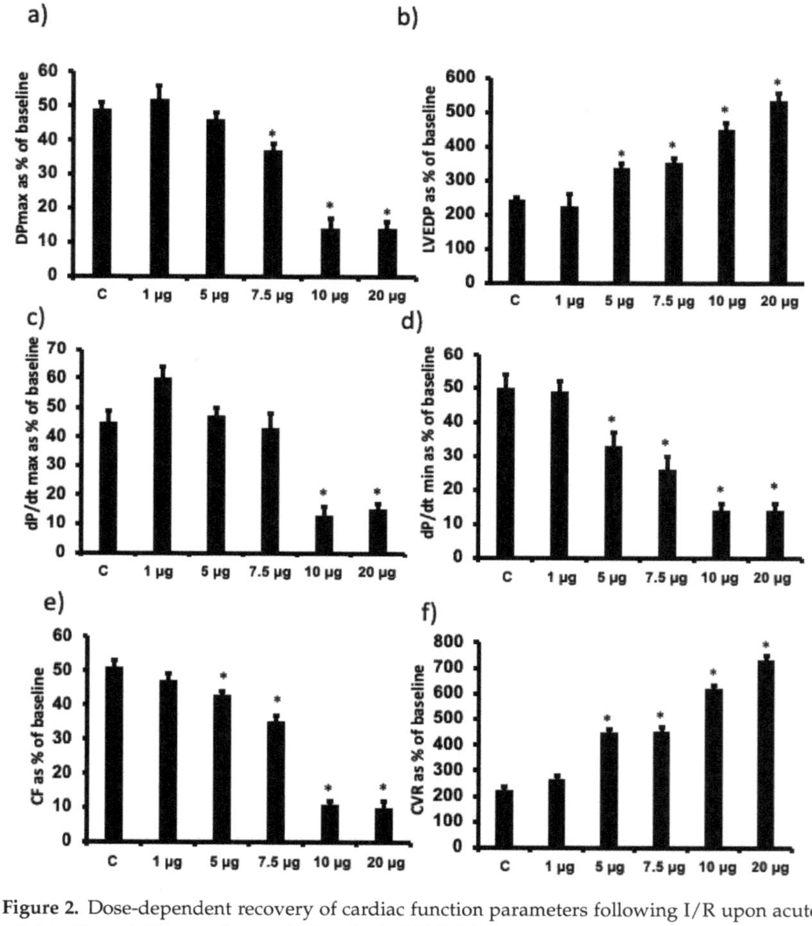

Figure 2. Dose-dependent recovery of cardiac function parameters following I/R upon acute administration of different doses of G7 cationic PAMAM (1.0 through 20 μg/mL). Percent recovery of cardiac function data (**a**–**f**) following I/R for left ventricle function (DPmax (**a**) and LVEDP (**b**)), contractility indices (+dP/dt (**c**) and −dP/dt (**d**) and coronary vascular dynamics (CF (**e**) and CVR (**f**)) are shown. The data were computed after 30 min reperfusion and expressed as the mean ± SEM. DPmax: maximum developed pressure; LVEDP: left ventricular end-diastolic pressure; CF: coronary flow; CVR: coronary vascular resistance. Control hearts, C = I/R alone. N = 8. Mean ± SEM. Asterix (*) indicates significant difference ($p < 0.05$) from controls.

3.2. The Influence of Cationic Dendrimer Generation on Cardiac Function Recovery following I/R Injury in Isolated Rat Hearts

To determine the influence of PAMAM dendrimer generation (i.e., molecular size/weight) on cardiac function recovery post-ischemic injury, we infused a fixed dose (100 nM) of each of G7, G6, G5, G4 and G3 cationic (-NH_2) PAMAM dendrimers. G3 generally exhibited little or no cardiac toxicity, whereas there was a gradual and significant decline in cardiac function recovery with progressively increasing dendrimer generation in terms of LV hemodynamics, contractility and coronary vascular dynamics (Figure 3). There was a 2-fold or greater decline in cardiac function from G4 to G7 cationic dendrimers as evidenced by the relative changes in %R values for Pmax, LVEDP, +dp/dt, dp/dt, CF and CVR parameters (see Figure 3).

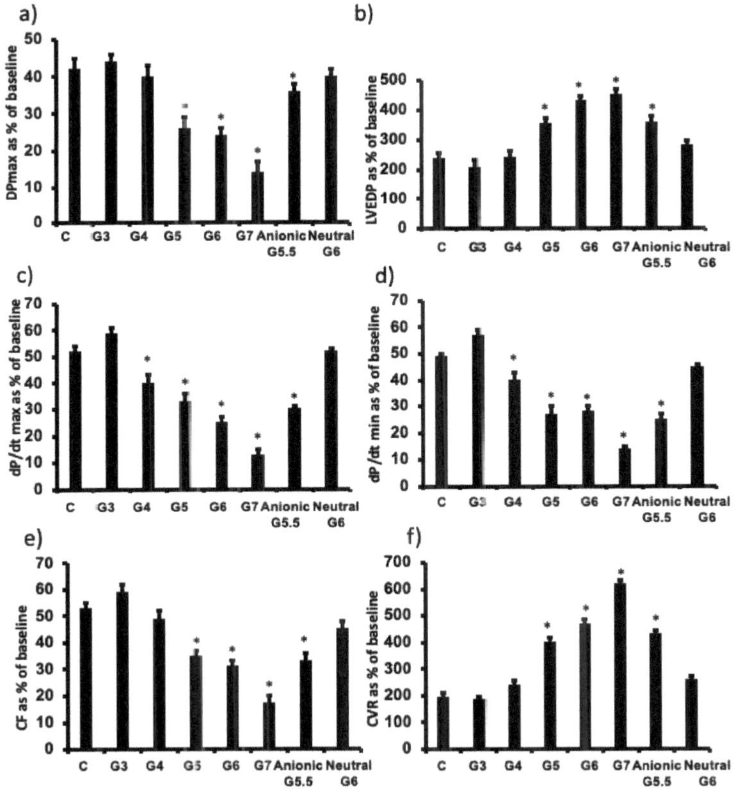

Figure 3. PAMAM-induced impairment in cardiac function is dependent on physicochemical properties of molecular size (generation) and surface charge of PAMAM dendrimers. Post I/R recovery in the left ventricle function (DPmax (**a**) and LVEDP (**b**)), contractility indices (+dP/dt (**c**) and –dP/dt (**d**)) and coronary vascular dynamics (CF (**e**) and CVR (**f**)) after treatment with various PAMAM dendrimer generations with variable molecular sizes (G3, G4, G5, G6, G7) or variable surface charge (cationic G6, anionic G5.5 or neutral G6). The data were computed after 30 min reperfusion and expressed as the mean ± SEM. DPmax: maximum developed pressure; LVEDP: left ventricular end-diastolic pressure; CF: coronary flow; CVR: coronary vascular resistance; G3: third generation PAMAM dendrimer; G4: fourth generation PAMAM; G5: fifth generation PAMAM; G6: sixth generation PAMAM; G7: seventh generation PAMAM G4. Control hearts, C = I/R alone. N = 8. Asterix (*) indicates significant difference ($p < 0.05$) from controls.

3.3. The influence of PAMAM Dendrimer Surface Chemistry on Cardiac Function Recovery after I/R Injury in Isolated Rat Hearts

To investigate the influence of dendrimer surface chemistry, we compared the cardiac effects of G6 neutral, G6 cationic and G5.5 anionic PAMAM dendrimers housing the following terminal chemical groups, respectively: hydroxyl- (-OH), amino- (–NH_2) and carboxyl- (-COOH). Note that anionic PAMAM are only produced in half generations, hence the use of G5.5 -COOH (anionic) PAMAM for comparative purposes as the nearest molecular size to G6 that was used for cationic and neutral PAMAMs. Neutral G6 PAMAM exhibited little or no cardiotoxicity compared to charged PAMAMs, whereby cationic G6 PAMAM was more cardiotoxic than anionic G5.5 PAMAM (Figure 3). For example, following cardiac I/R injury, G6 cationic PAMAM reduced % recovery in Pmax by over 50%, whereas anionic reduced the same parameter by only around 25% and neutral surface chemistry had no effect ($p < 0.05$). Similar trends were observed for all other cardiac function parameters measured (LVEDP, +dp/dt, CF and CVR) except that for the dp/dt (max and min) function where both cationic and anionic PAMAMs compromised recovery to a similar degree (approximately 40–50%) (Figure 3).

3.4. PAMAM-Induced Cardiac Dysfunction Can Be Rescued by Ang-(1-7) in a Mas Receptor-Dependent Mechanism of Action

To examine the potential beneficial effect of Ang-(1-7) in protecting the rat heart against the cardiotoxic effects of G7 PAMAM dendrimer, we administered this drug during reperfusion in the absence or presence of the G7 PAMAM dendrimer and/or its Mas receptor blockers, A-779 or D-Pro (see Section 2. The infusion of G7 PAMAM dendrimer (10 μg/mL) induced a significant deterioration in almost all cardiac function parameters compared to control (Figure 4). Ang-(1-7) treatment significantly improved ($p < 0.001$) recovery of DPmax, LVDP and LV contractility from I/R injury alone or upon treatment with the cationic G7 PAMAM dendrimer (Figure 4a–d). A similar cardioprotective effect was noticed on coronary vascular dynamics as the deterioration caused by I/R alone or following G7 PAMAM dendrimer treatment was rescued by adjunct administration of Ang-(1-7) ($p < 0.001$) (Figure 4e,f). The cardioprotection afforded by Ang-(1-7) was largely revoked in the presence of its Mas receptor antagonist, A-779 or D-Pro (Figure 4), implying that the beneficial effects of Ang-(1-7) in mitigating dendrimer-induced cardiotoxicity were mediated, at least in part, via its Mas receptor. These results from cardiac function recovery studies were confirmed by evaluation of the cardiac enzyme levels and the infarct size (see Table 2). Ang-(1-7) treatment largely neutralized both the I/R injury and cationic G7 PAMAM-induced cardiac damage as evidenced by decreased CK and LDH enzyme levels and myocardial infarct size ($p < 0.05$ and $p < 0.01$ respectively) (see Table 2 and Figure 5).

Table 2. Effects of Ang-(1-7) and its Mas receptor antagonists, ischemia/reperfusion (I/R) and cationic G7 PAMAM dendrimer on cardiac enzymes levels. CK = Creatinine kinase; LDH = lactate dehydrogenase. G7: seventh generation cationic PAMAM dendrimer; Ang-(1-7): angiotensin-1-7; D-Pro and A779 are Ang-(1-7) selective antagonists. Asterix * refers to significant difference ($p < 0.05$) compared to control I/R alone.

Treatment	CK (IU/L)	*p* Value	LDH (IU/L)	*p* Value
I/R	35.77 ± 0.46	-	28.27 ± 1.12	-
Ang-(1-7)	26.97 ± 1.43 *	0.001	20.24 ± 0.39 *	0.001
G7	46.26 ± 1.39 *	0.022	40.41 ± 0.99 *	0.01
G7 + Ang-(1-7)	28.34 ± 0.86 *	0.002	21.73 ± 0.73 *	0.001
G7 + Ang-(1-7) + DPro	35.22 ± 1.21	0.709	29.40 ± 0.76	0.294
G7 + Ang-(1-7) + A779	35.32 ± 0.96	0.633	29.33 ± 0.39	0.383

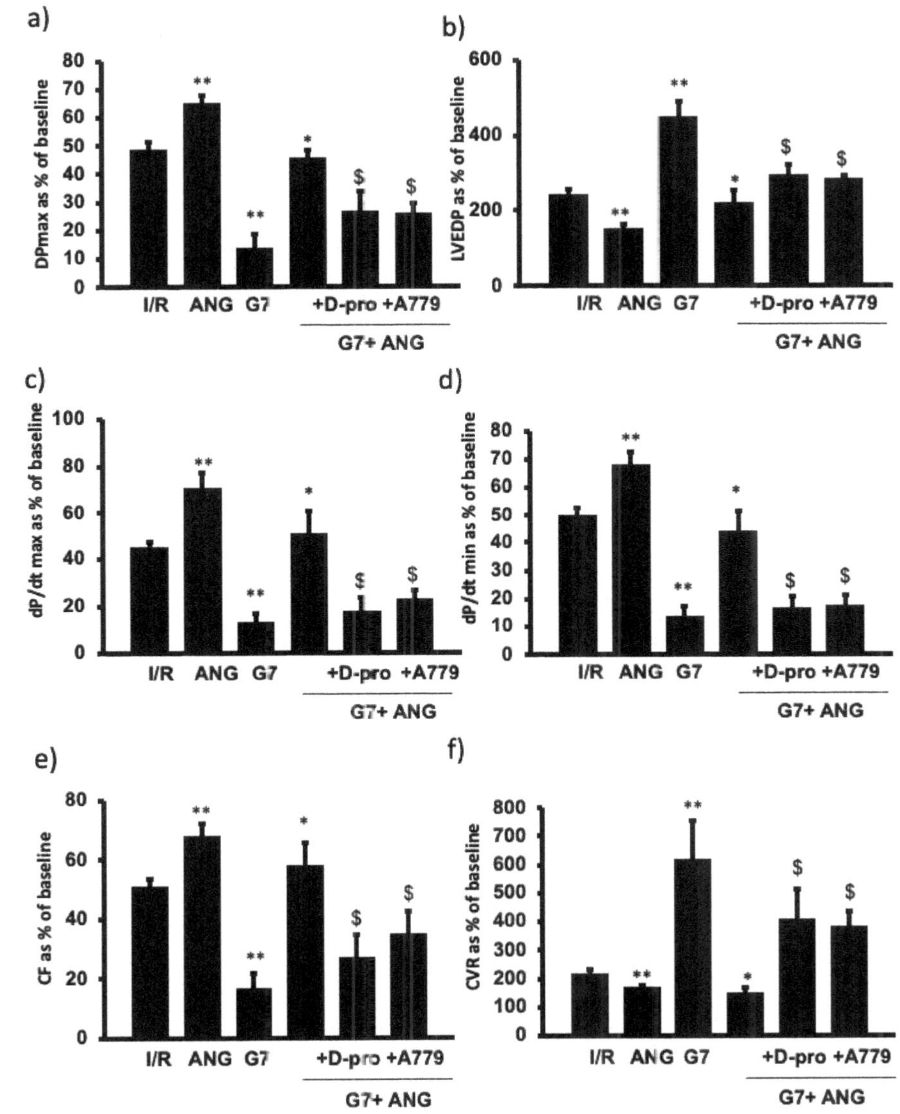

Figure 4. Ang-(1-7) via its Mas Receptor rescues cationic G7 PAMAM-induced impairment of cardiac function (**a**–**f**). Post I/R recovery in the left ventricle function (DPmax (**a**) and LVEDP (**b**)), contractility indices (+dP/dt (**c**) and −dP/dt (**d**)) and coronary vascular dynamics (CF (**e**) and CVR (**f**)) after treatment with G7 PAMAM in presence or absence of Ang-(1-7) and its Mas receptor blockers D-Pro and A779 The data were computed after 30 min reperfusion and expressed as the mean ± SEM. DPmax: maximum developed pressure; LVEDP: left ventricular end-diastolic pressure; CF: coronary flow; CVR: coronary vascular resistance; Ang-(1-7): angiotensin-91-7); D-Pro: Ang-(1-7) selective antagonist; A779: Ang-(1-7) selective antagonist (see Section 2). Double Asterix ** refers to significant difference ($p < 0.05$) compared to control I/R alone and single Asterix * refers to significant difference ($p < 0.05$) compared G7 values. Dollar sign ($) indicates significant difference ($p < 0.05$) compared to G7 + Ang-(1-7).

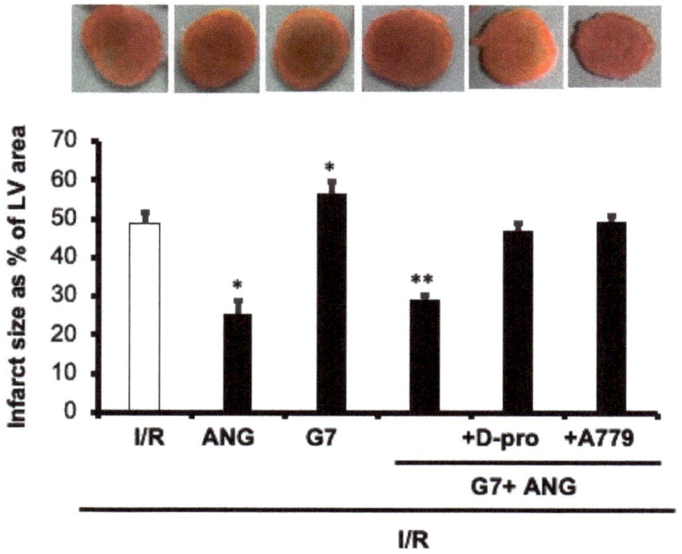

Figure 5. Ang-(1-7) via its Mas Receptor rescues cationic G7 PAMAM-induced myocardial infarction. Infarct size post-I/R injury was determined after treatment with G7 PAMAM in the presence or absence of Ang-(1-7) and its Mas receptor blockers D-Pro and A779 (n = 4). Top panel: representative 2,3,5-triphenyl-2H-tetrazolium chloride-stained heart slices for each treatment condition. Bottom Panel: measured infarct size, normalized to the LV area, in isolated rat hearts at the end of reperfusion. C: control; G7: seventh generation cationic PAMAM dendrimer; Ang-(1-7): angiotensin-1-7; D-Pro: Ang-(1-7) selective antagonist; A779: Ang-(1-7) selective antagonist. Single Asterix * refers to significant difference ($p < 0.05$) compared to control I/R alone and double Asterix ** to significant difference ($p < 0.05$) compared to G7 values.

4. Discussion

PAMAM dendrimers have been proposed to have multiple roles in clinical nanomedicine including as drug delivery vectors [3]. However, the toxicological profiles of these dendrimers in specific organs and tissues are not fully elucidated. Indeed, naked dendrimer nanoparticles (without any drug cargo) are known to exert biological and toxicological actions of their own in several biological systems [3] but their direct biological/toxicological impact on the mammalian heart is understudied. We previously showed that a cationic G6 dendrimer administered chronically over four weeks to healthy and diabetic rats could partially impair recovery of heart function following I/R injury [14]. However, the influence of the different PAMAM dendrimer physiochemical properties, such as generation (molecular size/number of surface groups) and surface charge, on cardiac contractility and hemodynamics functions are not known. Thus, we examined the effect of cationic PAMAM dendrimer generation (G7, G6, G5, G4 and G3) and surface chemistry (-NH_2 (cationic), -COOH (anionic) and -OH (neutral)) on recovery of cardiac function parameters in mammalian hearts after I/R injury. The key findings of this study are that cationic G7 PAMAM dendrimer dose-dependently impaired cardiac contractility and hemodynamics in the isolated, perfused rat heart and that impairment of cardiac function was generally dependent on the key physicochemical properties of dendrimer generation (G7 > G6 > G5 > G4 > G3 that had little or no effect) and surface chemistry (cationic > anionic > neutral that had little or no effect)). Importantly, we further showed that cardiotoxicity of cationic PAMAM dendrimer nanoparticles could be mitigated by co-administering the cardioprotective agent, Ang-(1-7). Mechanistically, the cardio-protection afforded by Ang-(1-7) in reversing PAMAM-induced cardiac injury occurred, at least in part, via its Mas receptor, as two different Mas receptor antagonists largely revoked the cardio-protection afforded by this heptapeptide (see also Figure 6). Thus, our studies show, for the first time, that the physiochemical properties of dendrimer generation (molecular size) and surface charge are important determinants of PAMAM cardiotoxicity, and critically, that administration of Ang-(1-7) may represent a novel strategy to mitigate cardiotoxicity of PAMAM dendrimers and possibly other nanoparticle drug delivery systems.

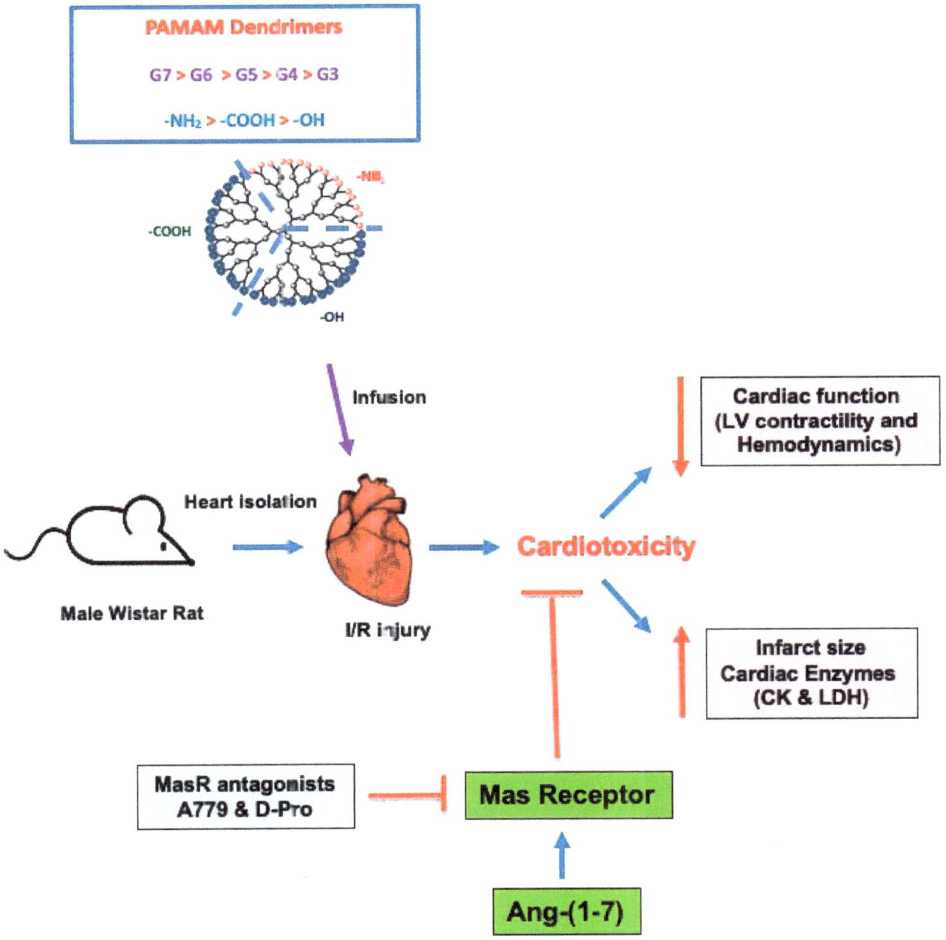

Figure 6. A schematic summary of the impact of different PAMAMs in the mammalian heart and the ability of Ang-(1-7) to mitigate their cardiotoxicity. In isolated rat hearts subjected to I/R injury, administration of PAMAM dendrimers exacerbated recovery of cardiac function in terms of LV contractility and hemodynamics parameters as well by increasing infarct size and cardiac enzyme levels (LDH and CK)—hallmarks of cardiac damage and toxicity. These effects of PAMAMs were dependent on dendrimer generation (G7 > G6 > G5 > G4 > G3) and surface charge ((-NH_2 (cationic) > -COOH (anionic) > -OH (neutral)). The adjunct administration of Ang-(1-7) rescued the cardiotoxicity caused by cationic PAMAM dendrimers. The beneficial effects of Ang-(1-7) were revoked by two Mas receptor (MasR) antagonists (A779 and D-Pro), confirming that Ang-(1-7) actions were, at least in part, mediated through MasR. Thus, Ang-(1-7) may represent a viable strategy to mitigate the cardiotoxicity of PAMAM dendrimers.

The fact that we found nanoparticle surface charge to be a key determinant of PAMAM-mediated cardiac dysfunction is consistent with our own studies on the biological and toxicological effects of PAMAMs in other systems [8,9]. Charged PAMAMs especially those bearing cationic surface chemistry generally exhibit a greater cellular toxicity than neutral PAMAMs [6]. The greater cardiotoxicity observed with cationic PAMAMs in this study is further supported by the discovery that cationic PAMAMs, compared to their neutral counterparts, reportedly exhibit greater biodistribution to the heart [43]. Concerning the heart, there is also evidence in the literature suggesting that PAMAMs preferentially accumulate in ischemic cardiac tissue following I/R injury compared to the normal non-diseased myocardium [44], implying that the ischemic heart may be more prone to the adverse toxicological effects of charged PAMAM dendrimers compared to healthy heart tissue, though this requires further study and validation experimentally. The impairment of cardiac function recovery was also dependent on dendrimer generation (see Figure 3). G7 dose-dependently compromised cardiac contractility and hemodynamics following I/R injury and the cardiotoxicity of cationic PAMAMs markedly decreased with progressively lower generations, with G3 having little or no effect on cardiac functional recovery post-I/R injury. These data implied that lower generation PAMAMs, even those bearing cationic surface charges, may be safer to use in vivo than the higher generation cationic PAMAMs that exhibited marked cardiotoxicity. The dependency of cardiac function on dendrimer generation may be suitably explained by the fact that higher generations have progressively greater positively charged surface groups that facilitate increased cellular accumulation and thus result in greater biological and toxicological actions (for reviews see [3,45]). This is additional to the general phenomenon of nanoparticles administered systemically, passively bio-distributing to organs of the reticulo-endothelial system that include the heart [3,45].

The mechanism by which PAMAMs result in impairment of cardiac function recovery from I/R injury was not studied here and is a potential limitation of our study. However, the outcomes of several biological and toxicological studies from our group, as well as others, do offer some insights [7–9,46–53]. Collectively, these studies suggest that beyond their role as drug delivery agents, PAMAM dendrimers house the potential to modulate important cellular genes and protein signaling networks in vitro and in vivo, which can lead to increased oxidative stress-induced injury and apoptosis. PAMAMs can also interfere with key receptor signaling networks such as those involving the epidermal growth factor receptor (EGFR) family of receptor tyrosine kinases (RTKs) (for review see [3]). EGFR RTKs have immense importance in physiological functions such as cell proliferation, growth, differentiation, motility, migration and apoptosis [54,55]. Dysregulated EGFR signaling has long been established to be associated with cancer [54,56] but our previous studies have also highlighted its importance in cardiovascular pathology (for review see [30]). For example, we previously showed that EGFR signaling mediates cardiac preconditioning [57] and is also critical for recovery of hearts post-I/R injury [58,59], implying that EGFR likely represents an important component of the "salvage pathways" that are necessary for the heart to recover from I/R injury. We have also demonstrated that administration of PAMAM dendrimers can block EGFR signaling in vivo and in vitro [8,48]. Thus, it is tempting to speculate that impaired cardiac function resulting from PAMAM exposure, especially that induced by high generation cationic PAMAMs, is likely mediated through a blockade of EGFR signaling—a key salvage pathway known to be involved in recovery of hearts post-I/R injury. Alternatively, cardiac function impairment, especially in CF and CVR, might occur via dendrimer-induced clot formation and subsequent occlusion of the coronary vasculature, as it has been shown that rapid i.v. administration of cationic PAMAM nanoparticles can induce hemolysis and blood coagulation [60]. However, this phenomenon is thought to be less likely when there is a slower biodistribution of dendrimer into the blood such as following i.p. administration [3,8,61]. Given the fact from our previous studies that even i.p administration of a cationic G6 PAMAM, where blood coagulation should be minimal, impaired cardiac recovery from I/R injury [14] and PAMAMs actually had beneficial effects in blood vessels by preventing diabetes-induced vascular dysfunction and remodeling [8], implies that it is more likely that these dendrimers inhibit key cardiac survival or salvage signaling cascades. However, chronic i.p administration of a cationic PAMAM (G4) dendrimer was reported to attenuate cardiac mitochondrial function [62], implying that, mechanistically, these dendrimers may also impair heart function through a dysregulation of mitochondrial function. Although these hypotheses need further study, strategies that mitigate the toxicity of PAMAMs will be useful in the potential use of PAMAMs as drug delivery systems in cardiovascular medicine.

Our current study suggests that the cardiotoxicity of high generation cationic PAMAMs can be circumvented by using lower generation cationic PAMAMs (e.g., G3) or PAMAMs with a neutral surface charge as these had the least effect on cardiac function. However, higher generation PAMAMs may be more desirable in some applications, e.g., for potential drug targeting to the ischemic heart to take advantage of their higher and selective accumulation in the heart (see discussion above). PEGylation and partial masking of charges are other possible approaches to off-set PAMAM toxicity (see [6] for recent review). However, in this study, we sought to determine if the adjunct delivery of a cardioprotective agent, Ang-(1-7) might mitigate cardiotoxicity of a high generation (G7) cationic dendrimer. We have previously shown that Ang-(1-7) protects hearts from cardiac ischemia injury [36,63] and mediates the beneficial effects of pacing post-conditioning [37], most likely through multiple mechanisms including anti-inflammatory, anti-oxidative stress and pro-vasodilatory actions (for reviews see [29–31]). In the present study, adjunct administration of Ang-(1-7) largely ameliorated the detrimental cardiac effects of G7 PAMAM dendrimer, an effect that was, at least partially, revoked by selective Mas receptor inhibitors A-779 or D-Pro, confirming that Ang-(1-7)/Mas receptor axis was involved in mediating cardioprotection. As to the possible downstream effectors of Ang-(1-7)-mediated cardioprotection, likely candidates include the inhibition of the pro-inflammatory transcription factor NF-kB [33,64], the oxidative stress-inducing NADPH-oxidases [36] and increased NO synthesis [37]. The latter would also facilitate coronary vessel vasodilation that might reduce or prevent any vessel occlusion that might be occurring as part of PAMAM-mediated cardiotoxicity. Indeed, a NO-releasing drug conjugated to a G4 PAMAM dendrimer improved cardiac function post I/R injury in an isolated, perfused rat heart [11]. Furthermore, since PAMAMs are known to induce oxidative stress, apoptosis and in some cases proinflammatory responses (for review see [6]), it is possible that Ang-(1-7) rescues PAMAM-induced cardiac dysfunction through a correction or counter-regulation of the pathways negatively affected by PAMAM dendrimers. Alternatively, the cardioprotective effects of Ang-(1-7) may occur via pathways independent of those adversely impacted by PAMAMs, and clearly both possibilities require further experimental study. The concept that Ang-(1-7) may serve as a novel therapeutic agent in mitigating cardiovascular toxicity of xenobiotics is further supported by the recent finding that Ang-(1-7) could reduce rat aortic arch dysfunction induced by the anti-cancer agent doxorubicin [65]. Additionally, Ang-(1-7) mitigated renal injury induced by gentamicin, an aminoglycoside antibiotic [66]. Thus, we propose that co-administration of Ang-(1-7) may represent a novel strategy to mitigate cardiotoxicity of nanoparticles in general as well as PAMAM dendrimers as described in our present study. As Ang-(1-7) is a peptide drug, to improve its biological stability and delivery in vivo, it can be formulated with cyclodextrins or even PAMAM delivery systems, which have been shown to be effective [66–69]. Furthermore, in clinical trials, Ang-(1-7) appears to be well tolerated and safe to use in humans [70,71].

Though not studied here, other cardioprotective drugs entrapped within or conjugated to the outer surface of PAMAM dendrimer nanoparticles might afford similar cardioprotection to Ang-(1-7). For example, an agonist of the A3 adenosine receptor, an important player in post-I/R cardiac recovery pathways, when conjugated to a G4 PAMAM dendrimer, led to cardioprotective effects in isolated hearts subjected to I/R injury [13]. Similarly, polymer nanoparticles laden with the cargo of antioxidants or anti-inflammatory agents, including curcumin or resveratrol, were also cardioprotective in animal models [72,73]. Therefore, by careful selection of dendrimer-drug combinations, or simple adjunct administration of effective cardioprotective agents such as Ang-(1-7), PAMAM dendrimers could conceivably be converted from potentially cardiotoxic to cardio-safe or even cardioprotective agents. Indeed, such approaches might be essential for mitigating dendrimer toxicity and for PAMAM-containing nanomedicines to meet the required safety profile for use in the clinic.

5. Conclusions

Administration of G7 PAMAM dendrimer dose-dependently attenuated cardiac contractility and coronary vascular dynamic functions following I/R injury. Impairment of cardiac function recovery correlated with the physicochemical properties of dendrimers with a strong influence of both surface charge and molecular size or generation. Neutral PAMAMs and low generation cationic PAMAMs (e.g. G3) appeared to have little or no effect on cardiac function and appeared safe for potential pre-clinical and clinical applications. Importantly, Ang-(1-7) mitigated cationic G7 PAMAM-induced cardiac dysfunction via a pathway involving its Mas receptor. We therefore propose that the adjunct use of Ang-(1-7) may represent a novel strategy to mitigate cardiotoxicity of cationic PAMAM nanoparticles. Our findings are therefore deemed highly important in further understanding the toxicology of dendrimers in the mammalian heart and, by identifying a novel strategy for mitigating their cardiotoxicity, may facilitate a broader and safer use of cationic PAMAMs in clinical nanomedicine.

Author Contributions: Conceptualization, S.A.; Methodology, S.A. and F.B.; Validation, F.B.; Formal analysis, F.B. and U.A.A.; Investigation, F.B.; Resources, S.A., F.B. and I.F.B.; Data curation, F.B. and U.A.A.; Writing—original draft, S.A., F.B. and U.A.A.; Writing—review & editing, S.A., F.B. and I.F.B.; Visualization, U.A.A.; Supervision, S.A. and F.B.; Project administration, S.A.; Funding acquisition, S.A. and F.B. All authors have read and agreed to the published version of the manuscript.

Funding: Funding for the research laboratory of S.A. was provided by Qatar University grant QUCG-CMED-22/23-540 and general funding for the laboratory of F.B. was obtained from Kuwait University (KU).

Institutional Review Board Statement: The animal study protocol was approved by the Health Science Center, Kuwait University Animal Ethics Committee. The study was conducted as per the EU Directive 2010/63/EU for experiments in animals.

Informed Consent Statement: Not applicable.

Data Availability Statement: The data presented in this study are available on request from the corresponding author.

Acknowledgments: We thank the late Sajan Varghese for his technical support in this research project.

Conflicts of Interest: The authors declare no conflict of interest.

References

1. Abedi-Gaballu, F.; Dehghan, G.; Ghaffari, M.; Yekta, R.; Abbaspour-Ravasjani, S.; Baradaran, B.; Ezzati Nazhad Dolatabadi, J.; Hamblin, M.R. PAMAM dendrimers as efficient drug and gene delivery nanosystems for cancer therapy. *Appl. Mater. Today* **2018**, *12*, 177–190. [CrossRef] [PubMed]
2. Kannan, R.M.; Nance, E.; Kannan, S.; Tomalia, D.A. Emerging concepts in dendrimer-based nanomedicine: From design principles to clinical applications. *J. Intern. Med.* **2014**, *276*, 579–617. [CrossRef] [PubMed]
3. Kheraldine, H.; Rachid, O.; Habib, A.M.; Al Moustafa, A.-E.; Benter, I.F.; Akhtar, S. Emerging innate biological properties of nano-drug delivery systems: A focus on PAMAM dendrimers and their clinical potential. *Adv. Drug Deliv. Rev.* **2021**, *178*, 113908. [CrossRef]
4. Li, J.; Liang, H.; Liu, J.; Wang, Z. Poly (amidoamine) (PAMAM) dendrimer mediated delivery of drug and pDNA/siRNA for cancer therapy. *Int. J. Pharm.* **2018**, *546*, 215–225. [CrossRef] [PubMed]
5. Tomalia, D.; Reyna, L.; Svenson, S. Dendrimers as multi-purpose nanodevices for oncology drug delivery and diagnostic imaging. *Biochem. Soc. Trans.* **2007**, *35*, 61–67. [CrossRef]
6. Kheraldine, H.; Gupta, I.; Alhussain, H.; Jabeen, A.; Cyprian, F.S.; Akhtar, S.; Al Moustafa, A.-E.; Rachid, O. Substantial cell apoptosis provoked by naked PAMAM dendrimers in HER2-positive human breast cancer via JNK and ERK1/ERK2 signalling pathways. *Comput. Struct. Biotechnol. J.* **2021**, *19*, 2881–2890. [CrossRef]

7. Akhtar, S.; Al-Zaid, B.; El-Hashim, A.Z.; Chandrasekhar, B.; Attur, S.; Benter, I.F. Impact of PAMAM delivery systems on signal transduction pathways in vivo: Modulation of ERK1/2 and p38 MAP kinase signaling in the normal and diabetic kidney. *Int. J. Pharm.* **2016**, *514*, 353–363. [CrossRef]
8. Akhtar, S.; Chandrasekhar, B.; Yousif, M.H.; Renno, W.; Benter, I.F.; El-Hashim, A.Z. Chronic administration of nano-sized PAMAM dendrimers in vivo inhibits EGFR-ERK1/2-ROCK signaling pathway and attenuates diabetes-induced vascular remodeling and dysfunction. *Nanomed. Nanotechnol. Biol. Med.* **2019**, *18*, 78–89. [CrossRef]
9. Akhtar, S.; El-Hashim, A.Z.; Chandrasekhar, B.; Attur, S.; Benter, I.F. Naked Polyamidoamine Polymers Intrinsically Inhibit Angiotensin II-Mediated EGFR and ErbB2 Transactivation in a Dendrimer Generation- and Surface Chemistry-Dependent Manner. *Mol. Pharm.* **2016**, *13*, 1575–1586. [CrossRef]
10. Chanyshev, B.; Shainberg, A.; Isak, A.; Litinsky, A.; Chepurko, Y.; Tosh, D.K.; Phan, K.; Gao, Z.-G.; Hochhauser, E.; Jacobson, K.A. Anti-ischemic effects of multivalent dendrimeric A3 adenosine receptor agonists in cultured cardiomyocytes and in the isolated rat heart. *Pharmacol. Res.* **2012**, *65*, 338–346. [CrossRef]
11. Johnson, T.A.; Stasko, N.A.; Matthews, J.L.; Cascio, W.E.; Holmuhamedov, E.; Johnson, C.B.; Schoenfisch, M.H. Reduced ischemia/reperfusion injury via glutathione-initiated nitric oxide-releasing dendrimers. *Nitric Oxide* **2010**, *22*, 30–36. [CrossRef] [PubMed]
12. Sayed, N.; Tambe, P.; Kumar, P.; Jadhav, S.; Paknikar, K.M.; Gajbhiye, V. miRNA transfection via poly(amidoamine)-based delivery vector prevents hypoxia/reperfusion-induced cardiomyocyte apoptosis. *Nanomedicine* **2020**, *15*, 163–181. [CrossRef] [PubMed]
13. Wan, T.C.; Tosh, D.K.; Du, L.; Gizewski, E.T.; Jacobson, A.K.; Auchampach, A.J. Polyamidoamine (PAMAM) dendrimer conjugate specifically activates the A3 adenosine receptor to improve post-ischemic/reperfusion function in isolated mouse hearts. *BMC Pharmacol.* **2011**, *11*, 11. [CrossRef] [PubMed]
14. Babiker, F.; Benter, I.F.; Akhtar, S. Nanotoxicology of Dendrimers in the Mammalian Heart: Ex vivo and in vivo Administration of G6 PAMAM Nanoparticles Impairs Recovery of Cardiac Function Following Ischemia-Reperfusion Injury. *Int. J. Nanomed.* **2020**, *15*, 4393–4405. [CrossRef]
15. Hausenloy, D.J.; Baxter, G.; Bell, R.; Bøtker, H.E.; Davidson, S.M.; Downey, J.; Heusch, G.; Kitakaze, M.; Lecour, S.; Mentzer, R.; et al. Translating novel strategies for cardioprotection: The Hatter Workshop Recommendations. *Basic Res. Cardiol.* **2010**, *105*, 677–686. [CrossRef]
16. Wereski, R.; Kimenai, D.M.; Bularga, A.; Taggart, C.; Lowe, D.J.; Mills, N.L.; Chapman, A.R. Risk factors for type 1 and type 2 myocardial infarction. *Eur. Heart J.* **2021**, *43*, 127–135. [CrossRef]
17. Zhang, Q.; Wang, L.; Wang, S.; Cheng, H.; Xu, L.; Pei, G.; Wang, Y.; Fu, C.; Jiang, Y.; He, C.; et al. Signaling pathways and targeted therapy for myocardial infarction. *Signal Transduct. Target. Ther.* **2022**, *7*, 78. [CrossRef]
18. Schäfer, A.; König, T.; Bauersachs, J.; Akin, M. Novel Therapeutic Strategies to Reduce Reperfusion Injury After Acute Myocardial Infarction. *Curr. Probl. Cardiol.* **2022**, *47*, 101398. [CrossRef]
19. Li, Y.; Gao, Y.; Li, G. Preclinical multi-target strategies for myocardial ischemia-reperfusion injury. *Front. Cardiovasc. Med.* **2022**, *9*. [CrossRef]
20. Babiker, A.F.; Elkhalifa, A.L.; Moukhyer, E.M. Awareness of hypertension and factors associated with uncontrolled hypertension in Sudanese adults: Cardiovascular topic. *Cardiovasc. J. Afr.* **2013**, *24*, 208–212. [CrossRef]
21. Ribichini, F. ACUTE MYOCARDIAL INFARCTION: REPERFUSION TREATMENT. *Heart* **2002**, *88*, 298–305. [CrossRef] [PubMed]
22. Saleh, M.; Ambrose, A.J. Understanding myocardial infarction. *F1000Research* **2018**, *7*, 1378. [CrossRef] [PubMed]
23. Vanagt, W.Y.; Cornelussen, R.N.; Poulina, Q.P.; Blaauw, E.; Vernooy, K.; Cleutjens, J.P.; van Bilsen, M.; Delhaas, T.; Prinzen, F.W. Pacing-Induced Dys-Synchrony Preconditions Rabbit Myocardium Against Ischemia/Reperfusion Injury. *Circulation* **2006**, *114*, I-264–I-269. [CrossRef] [PubMed]
24. Zhao, Z.-Q.; Corvera, J.S.; Halkos, M.E.; Kerendi, F.; Wang, N.-P.; Guyton, R.A.; Vinten-Johansen, J. Inhibition of myocardial injury by ischemic postconditioning during reperfusion: Comparison with ischemic preconditioning. *Am. J. Physiol. Heart Circ. Physiol.* **2003**, *285*, H579–H588. [CrossRef]
25. Reed, G.W.; Rossi, E.J.; Cannon, C.P. Acute myocardial infarction. *Lancet* **2016**, *389*, 197–210. [CrossRef]
26. Babiker, F.; Al-Jarallah, A.; Al-Awadi, M. Effects of Cardiac Hypertrophy, Diabetes, Aging, and Pregnancy on the Cardioprotective Effects of Postconditioning in Male and Female Rats. *Cardiol. Res. Pract.* **2019**, *2019*, 3403959. [CrossRef]
27. Babiker, F.A.; Al-Jarallah, A.; Joseph, S. Understanding pacing postconditioning-mediated cardiac protection: A role of oxidative stress and a synergistic effect of adenosine. *J. Physiol. Biochem.* **2016**, *73*, 175–185. [CrossRef]
28. Hausenloy, D.J.; Yellon, D.M. Preconditioning and postconditioning: Underlying mechanisms and clinical application. *Atherosclerosis* **2009**, *204*, 334–341. [CrossRef]
29. Akhtar, S.; Benter, I.F.; Danjuma, M.; Doi, S.A.R.; Hasan, S.S.; Habib, A.M. Pharmacotherapy in COVID-19 patients: A review of ACE2-raising drugs and their clinical safety. *J. Drug Target.* **2020**, *28*, 683–699. [CrossRef]
30. Shraim, B.A.; Moursi, M.O.; Benter, I.F.; Habib, A.M.; Akhtar, S. The Role of Epidermal Growth Factor Receptor Family of Receptor Tyrosine Kinases in Mediating Diabetes-Induced Cardiovascular Complications. *Front. Pharmacol.* **2021**, *12*. [CrossRef]
31. Xie, J.X.; Hu, J.; Cheng, J.; Liu, C.; Wei, X. The function of the ACE2/Ang(1-7)/Mas receptor axis of the renin-angiotensin system in myocardial ischemia reperfusion injury. *Eur Rev Med Pharmacol Sci. Mar* **2022**, *26*, 1852–1859. [CrossRef]

32. Vickers, C.; Hales, P.; Kaushik, V.; Dick, L.; Gavin, J.; Tang, J.; Godbout, K.; Parsons, T.; Baronas, E.; Hsieh, F.; et al. Hydrolysis of Biological Peptides by Human Angiotensin-converting Enzyme-related Carboxypeptidase. *J. Biol. Chem.* **2002**, *277*, 14838–14843. [CrossRef] [PubMed]
33. Al-Maghrebi, M.; Benter, I.F.; Diz, D.I. Endogenous angiotensin-(1-7) reduces cardiac ischemia-induced dysfunction in diabetic hypertensive rats. *Pharmacol. Res.* **2009**, *59*, 263–268. [CrossRef] [PubMed]
34. Benter, I.F.; Yousif, M.; Al-Saleh, F.M.; Raghupathy, R.; Chappell, R.R.M.C.; Diz, D.I. Angiotensin-(1-7) Blockade Attenuates Captopril- or Hydralazine-induced Cardiovascular Protection in Spontaneously Hypertensive Rats Treated With NG-nitro-l-Arginine Methyl Ester. *J. Cardiovasc. Pharmacol.* **2011**, *57*, 559–567. [CrossRef] [PubMed]
35. Benter, I.F.; Yousif, M.; Anim, J.T.; Cojocel, C.; Diz, D.I. Angiotensin-(1-7) prevents development of severe hypertension and end-organ damage in spontaneously hypertensive rats treated with l-NAME. *Am. J. Physiol. Circ. Physiol.* **2006**, *290*, H684–H691. [CrossRef]
36. Yousif, M.; Dhaunsi, G.S.; Makki, B.M.; Qabazard, B.A.; Akhtar, S.; Benter, I.F. Characterization of Angiotensin-(1-7) effects on the cardiovascular system in an experimental model of Type-1 diabetes. *Pharmacol. Res.* **2012**, *66*, 269–275. [CrossRef]
37. Abwainy, A.; Babiker, F.; Akhtar, S.; Benter, I.F. Endogenous angiotensin-(1-7)/Mas receptor/NO pathway mediates the cardioprotective effects of pacing postconditioning. *Am. J. Physiol. Circ. Physiol.* **2016**, *310*, H104–H112. [CrossRef]
38. Khalaf, A.; Babiker, F. Discrepancy in calcium release from the sarcoplasmic reticulum and intracellular acidic stores for the protection of the heart against ischemia/reperfusion injury. *J. Physiol. Biochem.* **2016**, *72*, 495–508. [CrossRef]
39. Babiker, F.A.; Joseph, S.; Juggi, J. The protective effects of 17beta-estradiol against ischemia–reperfusion injury and its effect on pacing postconditioning protection to the heart. *J. Physiol. Biochem.* **2013**, *70*, 151–162. [CrossRef]
40. Babiker, A.F.; Hoteit, L.J.; Joseph, S.; Mustafa, A.S.; Juggi, J.S. The role of 17-beta estradiol in ischemic preconditioning protection of the heart. *Exp. Clin. Cardiol.* **2012**, *17*, 95–100.
41. Babiker, F.; Al-Kouh, A.; Kilarkaje, N. Lead exposure induces oxidative stress, apoptosis, and attenuates protection of cardiac myocytes against ischemia–reperfusion injury. *Drug Chem. Toxicol.* **2018**, *42*, 147–156. [CrossRef] [PubMed]
42. Al-Herz, W.; Babiker, F. Acute Intravenous Infusion of Immunoglobulins Protects Against Myocardial Ischemia-Reperfusion Injury Through Inhibition of Caspase-3. *Cell. Physiol. Biochem.* **2017**, *42*, 2295–2306. [CrossRef] [PubMed]
43. Nigavekar, S.S.; Sung, L.Y.; Llanes, M.; El-Jawahri, A.; Lawrence, T.S.; Becker, C.W.; Balogh, L.; Khan, M.K. ^{3}H Dendrimer Nanoparticle Organ/Tumor Distribution. *Pharm. Res.* **2004**, *21*, 476–483. [CrossRef] [PubMed]
44. Magruder, J.T.; Crawford, T.C.; Lin, Y.-A.; Zhang, F.; Grimm, J.C.; Kannan, R.M.; Kannan, S.; Sciortino, C.M. Selective Localization of a Novel Dendrimer Nanoparticle in Myocardial Ischemia-Reperfusion Injury. *Ann. Thorac. Surg.* **2017**, *104*, 891–898. [CrossRef]
45. Shcharbin, D.; Janaszewska, A.; Klajnert-Maculewicz, B.; Ziemba, B.; Dzmitruk, V.; Halets, I.; Loznikova, S.; Shcharbina, N.; Milowska, K.; Ionov, M.; et al. How to study dendrimers and dendriplexes III. Biodistribution, pharmacokinetics and toxicity in vivo. *J. Control. Release* **2014**, *181*, 40–52. [CrossRef]
46. Akhtar, S. Cationic nanosystems for the delivery of small interfering ribonucleic acid therapeutics: A focus on toxicogenomics. *Expert Opin. Drug Metab. Toxicol.* **2010**, *6*, 1347–1362. [CrossRef]
47. Akhtar, S.; Benter, I. Toxicogenomics of non-viral drug delivery systems for RNAi: Potential impact on siRNA-mediated gene silencing activity and specificity. *Adv. Drug Deliv. Rev.* **2007**, *59*, 164–182. [CrossRef]
48. Akhtar, S.; Chandrasekhar, B.; Attur, S.; Dhaunsi, G.S.; Yousif, M.H.M.; Benter, I.F. Transactivation of ErbB Family of Receptor Tyrosine Kinases Is Inhibited by Angiotensin-(1-7) via Its Mas Receptor. *PLoS ONE* **2015**, *10*, e0141657. [CrossRef]
49. Akhtar, S.; Chandrasekhar, B.; Attur, S.; Yousif, M.; Benter, I.F. On the nanotoxicity of PAMAM dendrimers: Superfect®stimulates the EGFR–ERK1/2 signal transduction pathway via an oxidative stress-dependent mechanism in HEK 293 cells. *Int. J. Pharm.* **2013**, *448*, 239–246. [CrossRef]
50. Hotta, H.; Miura, T.; Miki, T.; Togashi, N.; Maeda, T.; Kim, S.J.; Tanno, M.; Yano, T.; Kuno, A.; Itoh, T.; et al. Short Communication: Angiotensin II Type 1 Receptor–Mediated Upregulation of Calcineurin Activity Underlies Impairment of Cardioprotective Signaling in Diabetic Hearts. *Circ. Res.* **2010**, *106*, 129–132. [CrossRef]
51. Omidi, Y.; Barar, J.; Heidari, H.R.; Ahmadian, S.; Yazdi, H.A.; Akhtar, S. Microarray Analysis of the Toxicogenomics and the Genotoxic Potential of a Cationic Lipid-Based Gene Delivery Nanosystem in Human Alveolar Epithelial A549 Cells. *Toxicol. Mech. Methods* **2008**, *18*, 369–378. [CrossRef]
52. Omidi, Y.; Hollins, A.J.; Benboubetra, M.; Drayton, R.; Benter, I.F.; Akhtar, S. Toxicogenomics of Non-viral Vectors for Gene Therapy: A Microarray Study of Lipofectin- and Oligofectamine-induced Gene Expression Changes in Human Epithelial Cells. *J. Drug Target.* **2003**, *11*, 311–323. [CrossRef]
53. Omidi, Y.; Hollins, A.; Drayton, R.; Akhtar, S. Polypropylenimine dendrimer-induced gene expression changes: The effect of complexation with DNA, dendrimer generation and cell type. *J. Drug Target.* **2005**, *13*, 431–443. [CrossRef]
54. Kumagai, S.; Koyama, S.; Nishikawa, H. Antitumour immunity regulated by aberrant ERBB family signalling. *Nat. Rev. Cancer* **2021**, *21*, 181–197. [CrossRef]
55. Hajjo, R.; Sweidan, K. Review on Epidermal Growth Factor Receptor (EGFR) Structure, Signaling Pathways, Interactions, and Recent Updates of EGFR Inhibitors. *Curr. Top. Med. Chem.* **2020**, *20*, 815–834. [CrossRef]
56. Sharifi, J.; Khirehgesh, M.R.; Safari, F.; Akbari, B. EGFR and anti-EGFR nanobodies: Review and update. *J. Drug Target.* **2020**, *29*, 387–402. [CrossRef]

57. Benter, I.F.; Juggi, J.S.; Khan, I.; Yousif, M.; Canatan, H.; Akhtar, S. Signal transduction mechanisms involved in cardiac preconditioning: Role of Ras-GTPase, Ca2 +/calmodulin-dependent protein kinase II and epidermal growth factor receptor. *Mol Cell. Biochem.* **2005**, *268*, 175–183. [CrossRef]
58. Akhtar, S.; Yousif, M.H.M.; Chandrasekhar, B.; Benter, I.F. Activation of EGFR/ERBB2 via Pathways Involving ERK1/2, P38 MAPK, AKT and FOXO Enhances Recovery of Diabetic Hearts from Ischemia-Reperfusion Injury. *PLoS ONE* **2012**, *7*, e39066. [CrossRef]
59. Benter, I.F.; Juggi, J.S.; Khan, I.; Akhtar, S. Inhibition of Ras-GTPase, but not tyrosine kinases or Ca2+/calmodulin-dependent protein kinase II, improves recovery of cardiac function in the globally ischemic heart. *Mol. Cell. Biochem.* **2004**, *259*, 35–42. [CrossRef]
60. Jones, C.F.; Campbell, R.A.; Brooks, A.E.; Assemi, S.; Tadjiki, S.; Thiagarajan, G.; Mulcock, C.; Weyrich, A.S.; Brooks, B.D. Ghandehari, H.; et al. Cationic PAMAM Dendrimers Aggressively Initiate Blood Clot Formation. *ACS Nano* **2012**, *6*, 9900–9910. [CrossRef]
61. Chauhan, A.S.; Diwan, P.V.; Jain, N.K.; Tomalia, D.A. Unexpected In Vivo Anti-Inflammatory Activity Observed for Simple Surface Functionalized Poly(amidoamine) Dendrimers. *Biomacromolecules* **2009**, *10*, 1195–1202. [CrossRef]
62. Labieniec-Watala, M.; Watala, C. PAMAM Dendrimers: Destined for Success or Doomed to Fail? Plain and Modified PAMAM Dendrimers in the Context of Biomedical Applications. *J. Pharm. Sci.* **2015**, *104*, 2–14. [CrossRef]
63. Benter, I.F.; Yousif, M.; Cojocel, C.; Al-Maghrebi, M.; Diz, D.I. Angiotensin-(1-7) prevents diabetes-induced cardiovascular dysfunction. *Am. J. Physiol. Circ. Physiol.* **2007**, *292*, H666–H672. [CrossRef]
64. El-Hashim, A.Z.; Renno, W.M.; Raghupathy, R.; Abduo, H.T.; Akhtar, S.; Benter, I.F. Angiotensin-(1-7) inhibits allergic inflammation, via the MAS1 receptor, through suppression of ERK1/2- and NF-κB-dependent pathways. *J. Cereb. Blood Flow Metab.* **2012** *166*, 1964–1976. [CrossRef]
65. Rahimi, O.; Melo, A.C.; Westwood, B.; Grier, R.D.; Tallant, E.A.; Gallagher, P.E. Angiotensin-(1-7) reduces doxorubicin-induced aortic arch dysfunction in male and female juvenile Sprague Dawley rats through pleiotropic mechanisms. *Peptides* **2022**, *152* 170784. [CrossRef]
66. Pacheco, L.F.; de Castro, C.H.; Dutra, J.B.R.; Lino, R.D.S.; Ferreira, P.M.; dos Santos, R.A.S.; Ulhoa, C.J. Oral Treatment with Angiotensin-(1-7) Attenuates the Kidney Injury Induced by Gentamicin in Wistar Rats. *Protein Pept. Lett.* **2021**, *28*, 1425–1433. [CrossRef]
67. Chi, L.A.; Asgharpour, S.; Correa-Basurto, J.; Bandala, C.R.; Martínez-Archundia, M. Unveiling the G4-PAMAM capacity to bind and protect Ang-(1-7) bioactive peptide by molecular dynamics simulations. *J. Comput. Mol. Des.* **2022**, *36*, 653–675. [CrossRef]
68. Magalhães, G.S.; Gregório, J.F.; Ramos, K.E.; Cançado-Ribeiro, A.T.P.; Baroni, I.F.; Barcelos, L.S.; Pinho, V.; Teixeira, M.M. Santos, R.A.S.; Rodrigues-Machado, M.G.; et al. Treatment with inhaled formulation of angiotensin-(1-7) reverses inflammation and pulmonary remodeling in a model of chronic asthma. *Immunobiology* **2020**, *225*, 151957. [CrossRef]
69. Márquez-Miranda, V.; Abrigo, J.; Rivera, J.C.; Araya-Duran, I.; Aravena, J.; Simon, F.; Pacheco, N.; Gonzalez-Nilo, F.D.; Cabello-Verrugio, C. The complex of PAMAM-OH dendrimer with Angiotensin (1-7) prevented the disuse-induced skeletal muscle atrophy in mice. *Int. J. Nanomed.* **2017**, *12*, 1985–1999. [CrossRef]
70. Rodgers, K.E.; Oliver, J.; Dizerega, G.S. Phase I/II dose escalation study of angiotensin 1-7 [A(1-7)] administered before and after chemotherapy in patients with newly diagnosed breast cancer. *Cancer Chemother. Pharmacol.* **2005**, *57*, 559–568. [CrossRef]
71. Savage, P.D.; Lovato, J.; Brosnihan, K.B.; Miller, A.A.; Petty, W.J. Phase II Trial of Angiotensin-(1-7) for the Treatment of Patients with Metastatic Sarcoma. *Sarcoma* **2016**, *2016*, 4592768. [CrossRef] [PubMed]
72. Boarescu, P.M.; Boarescu, I.; Bocșan, I.C.; Gheban, D.; Bulboacă, A.E.; Nicula, C.; Pop, R.M.; Râjnoveanu, R.-M.; Bolboacă, S.D. Antioxidant and Anti-Inflammatory Effects of Curcumin Nanoparticles on Drug-Induced Acute Myocardial Infarction in Diabetic Rats. *Antioxidants* **2019**, *8*, 504. [CrossRef] [PubMed]
73. Bulboacă, A.E.; Boarescu, P.M.; Bolboacă, S.D.; Blidaru, M.; Feștilă, D.; Dogaru, G.; Nicula, C.A. Comparative effect of curcumin versus liposomal curcumin on systemic pro-inflammatory cytokines profile, MCP-1 and RANTES in experimental diabetes mellitus. *Int. J. Nanomed.* **2019**, *14*, 8961–8972. [CrossRef] [PubMed]

pharmaceutics

MDPI

Article

Critical Analysis and Quality Assessment of Nanomedicines and Nanocarriers in Clinical Trials: Three Years of Activity at the Clinical Trials Office

Diego Alejandro Dri [1,2,*], Elisa Gaucci [1], Ilaria Torrieri [2], Maria Carafa [2], Carlotta Marianecci [2,*] and Donatella Gramaglia [1]

1 Clinical Trials Office, Italian Medicines Agency (AIFA), Via del Tritone 181, 00187 Rome, Italy; e.gaucci@aifa.gov.it (E.G.); d.gramaglia@aifa.gov.it (D.G.)

2 Department Drug Chemistry and Technologies (DCTF), Sapienza, University of Rome, Piazzale Aldo Moro 5, 00185 Rome, Italy; torrieri.1748856@studenti.uniroma1.it (I.T.); maria.carafa@uniroma1.it (M.C.)

* Correspondence: da.dri@aifa.gov.it (D.A.D.); carlotta.marianecci@uniroma1.it (C.M.); Tel.: +39-065-978-4118 (D.A.D.); +39-064-991-3970 (C.M.)

Abstract: Investigational medicinal products submitted over the course of 3 years and authorized at the Clinical Trials Office of the Italian Medicines Agency as part of a request for authorization of clinical trials were scrutinized to identify those encompassing nanomedicines. The quality assessment reports performed on the documentation submitted were analyzed, classifying and discussing the most frequently detected issues. The identification of nanomedicines retrieved and the information on their quality profiles are shared to increase the transparency and availability of information, providing feedback that can support sponsors in optimizing the quality part of the documentation and of the information submitted. Results confirm that nanomedicines tested as investigational medicinal products in clinical trials are developed and authorized in agreement with the highest standards of quality, meeting safety profiles according to the strong regulatory requirements in the European Union. Some key points are highlighted and indicate that the regulatory approach to innovation in a clinical trial setting could potentially be renewed to ride the wave of innovation, particularly in the nanotechnology field, capitalizing on lessons learned and still ensuring a strong and effective framework.

Keywords: clinical trials; investigational medicinal products; nanocarrier; nanomedicine; quality; regulatory

Citation: Dri, D.A.; Gaucci, E.; Torrieri, I.; Carafa, M.; Marianecci, C.; Gramaglia, D. Critical Analysis and Quality Assessment of Nanomedicines and Nanocarriers in Clinical Trials: Three Years of Activity at the Clinical Trials Office. *Pharmaceutics* **2022**, *14*, 1438. https://doi.org/10.3390/pharmaceutics14071438

Academic Editors: Raquel Fernández García, Francisco Bolás-Fernández and Ana Isabel Fraguas-Sánchez

Received: 21 June 2022
Accepted: 7 July 2022
Published: 9 July 2022

1. Introduction

Drug delivery systems can usually be categorized into organic nanostructures, mainly used in clinical treatment, or inorganic nanostructures, which find their application particularly in the diagnostic field. Depending on the active molecule to enclose, on the desired formulation and administration route, on the safety profile, and on the therapeutic rather than the diagnostic purpose, a different approach to the synthesis and selection of starting materials may apply [1,2]. Reviews and publications show how nanomedicines and nanocarrier-based delivery systems for drugs have future prospects in both therapeutic and diagnostic fields [3]. Nanomedicines, nanocarriers, and drug delivery systems are definitely an emerging and promising field of innovation in healthcare [4,5]. The excellent results achieved, with an increasing number of formulations reaching the market in the preceding decades [6,7], ultimately demonstrate that some of the challenges that this field of innovation is facing can be overcome when there is a common intent among the various stakeholders. In the case of the COVID-19 pandemic, the confluence of know-how, technological, economic, and regulatory efforts has supported the authorization of nanovaccines by regulatory bodies worldwide [8,9], even if in an emergency situation. However, there are still challenges ahead [10], and any further development in the field may suffer from the unavailability of dedicated regulatory guidelines or from non-standardized approaches to innovation. It is therefore crucial to identify those difficulties that hinder the clinical translation of nanomedicines and encourage high-quality and value, potentially low-cost, fast approachable nanotechnology innovation to address unmet medical needs [11].

There are publications and reviews illustrating how challenging is the translation from bench to the clinic [12–14]; however, there is limited information on the actual clinical application of innovation in the nanotechnology field when it comes to nanomedicines in clinical trials (CTs). It is our intent to provide valuable information to nanomedicines' developers and sponsors of CTs to help identify some of the potential areas of difficulty, with considerations in terms of good manufacturing practice (GMP) and chemistry, manufacturing, and controls (CMC). A medicinal product can be authorized in the European Union (EU) only after its efficacy and safety are investigated in CTs [15–19]; the assessors of the national competent authorities (NCAs) ensure a positive benefit–risk profile assessing the protocols and the investigational medicinal products (IMPs). In this article, we retrieve, critically analyze, and discuss the quality documentation and data provided by the sponsors in the clinical trial applications (CTA) with a nanomedicine, submitted to the Clinical Trials Office (CTO) of the Italian Medicines Agency (AIFA) and authorized from 2018 to 2020. The total number of CTs authorized during the 3 years of this research is 2021, slightly increasing each year during the period, as shown in Figure 1.

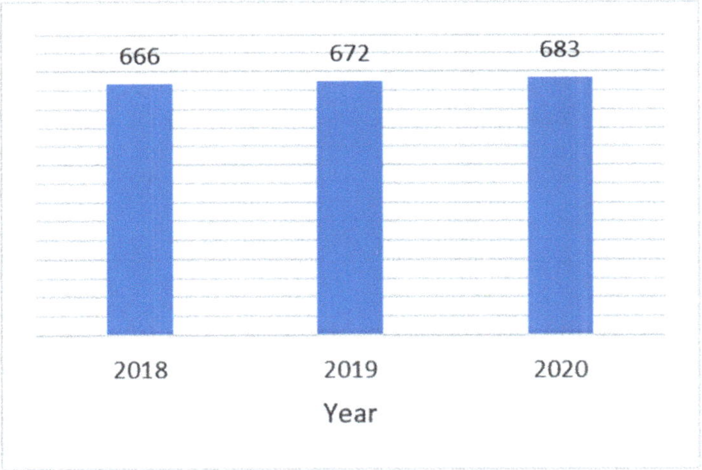

Figure 1. Number of CTs authorized per year at the CTO from 2018 to 2020.

Applications submitted through the Osservatorio Nazionale delle Sperimentazioni Cliniche (OsSC) [20], a national system, are assessed from different points of view, including regulatory, administrative, non-clinical, clinical, statistical, and of course quality perspective. The safety profile of IMPs can be confirmed only after the critical quality attributes are controlled and a suitable characterization is made available. Most of the information analyzed is commercially confidential, therefore data cannot be fully disclosed; however, results provided as aggregated data represent useful information, particularly for sponsors, and increase transparency for all stakeholders, triggering also regulatory reflections and highlighting critical key points to be further elaborated by the entire network.

2. Materials and Methods

Interventional CTs submitted and authorized from 2018 to 2020 at the CTO in AIFA were scrutinized to retrieve those involving IMPs that may be classified as nanomedicines. Structured data in the OsSC national system do not contain information on the presence of a nanotherapeutic tested as an IMP in a CT. Therefore, a manual process had to be implemented to assess, for every CT application, if the CMC quality documentation available in the Investigational Medicinal Product Dossier (IMPD) mentioned nanomedicine- or nanocarrier-related terms or if it contained information, descriptions, and analytical data suggesting the presence of a nanostructure, taking into consideration the terms of the JRC technical report [21].

The information managed is commercially confidential. Therefore, full open data cannot be disclosed. The number of CTs submitted every year to the CTO and authorized after the assessment is available through the national report on CTs in Italy [22]. For the purpose of our analysis, the list of CTs authorized in the period 2018–2020 has been further narrowed down to only those CTs testing an IMP without a marketing authorization, because we wanted to retrieve and analyze those new nanotherapeutics that had not yet received a marketing authorization and for whom complete information was not available. However, we included those IMPs declared in the CTA form as not having a marketing authorization because they were investigated with a different indication or formulation from the one already authorized. Reference products tested as comparators, placebos, and Phase IV CTs were also excluded. For a given CT, we did not retrieve more than one IMP involving a nanomedicine and a nanocarrier tested in the same study and we did not find that in the same CT any IMP was tested multiple times because of multiple pharmaceutical forms or strengths involved. We are reporting in Table 1 the number of CTs submitted between 2018 and 2020, the number of CTs authorized by the CTO, and the number of CTs within the scope of this research. During 2020, the first year of the COVID-19 pandemic, the number of IMPs without a marketing authorization tested in a CT dropped dramatically, in favor of testing-authorized medicinal products with a repurposing scope.

Table 1. CTs submitted, authorized, and within the scope of this research.

Year	CTs Submitted	CTs Authorized	CTs in Scope
2018	716	666	**433**
2019	722	672	**449**
2020	815	683	**359**

We analyzed the quality documentation available in the CMC section of the IMPDs and the quality-assessment outcome for all those 1241 CTs in scope according to the information declared by the sponsors in the CTA form. For the purpose of identifying the overall number of issues raised in the context of those CTs involving a nanomedicine as an IMP, we included in the list a few IMPs as duplicated when they were tested multiple times in different CTs, considering that a separate quality assessment was indeed performed for each CT.

After the quality assessment is completed by the assessor at the CTO, should any issue be identified during the assessment process, requests for clarification, additional data, or information are sent to the sponsors as grounds for non-acceptance. The sponsor has then the possibility to review the issues raised and to reply to the NCA. Only if the responses are considered acceptable, a final positive conclusion on the quality part is adopted, complementing the conclusion on the other parts of the dossier (regulatory, statistical, clinical, non-clinical) and contributing to the definition of a benefit–risk profile for the CTs and, in the end, to set a final decision on the application.

3. Results

In all, 22 IMPs that may be classified into categories attributed to nanomedicines were identified in CTs authorized in 2018 as a result of previously conducted research [23]. We are hereby capitalizing on those data, adding the CTs authorized during the following 2 years, 2019 and 2020, to the 2018 database. A total of 23 IMPs were further identified among CTs authorized in 2019, and the list is reported in Table A1. Among those, four contained an IMP already detected the previous year (N7 and 3 × N17) and three contained the same IMP (N28) but were included in the analysis because the IMP was evaluated in the context of a new CT. Instead, 19 IMPs were identified among CTs authorized in 2020 and the list is reported in Table A2. Among those, one contained an IMP already detected in 2018 and 2019 (N7), one already detected in 2019 (N34), and two detected twice in the same year (N42 and N53). As said above, they were included in the analysis. A total of 64 (3.17%) out of 2021 authorized CTs during the 3 years (2018–2020) included IMPs that may be classified as nanomedicines. Only 3 (4.69%) out of the 64 CTs were declared not to have a commercial nature. The vast majority (95.31%) were instead declared to be commercial, as reported in Figure 2.

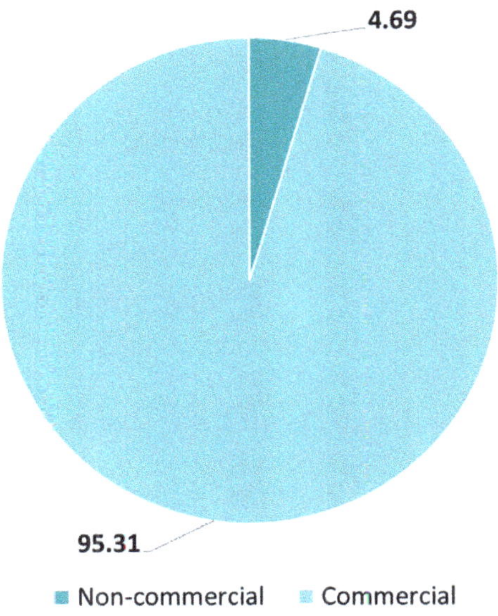

Figure 2. Percentage of commercial and non-commercial CTs assessed and authorized from 2018 to 2020, including a nanomedicine tested as an IMP.

3.1. Type of Nanomedicines

We are reporting all the IMPs that may be classified as nanomedicines, both those with a confirmed dimension in the nano-range and also those, the majority, without confirmation of the dimension but detected as having description, characteristics, or critical parameters that make them fit into one potential type of nanomedicine, as already reported for the analysis of the 2018 database.

IMPs were not declared as nanomedicines in the CTA form [24] nor in the IMPD; however, we classified them into a few types: nanocarriers (viral vectors, vaccine carriers, and adjuvants [25]), antibody–drug conjugates (ADC), polymer therapeutics (polymer–protein conjugates or chemically modified proteins [26]), and liposomes, in line with some of the terms used in the JRC technical report [21]. Two "nanobodies" were in addition declared in two CTs and were included in a standalone classification, even if they are single-domain antibody fragments and nanoscale dimensions were not confirmed in the dossier. In Figure 3, we are reporting the categories attributable to nanomedicines identified across the 3 years investigated.

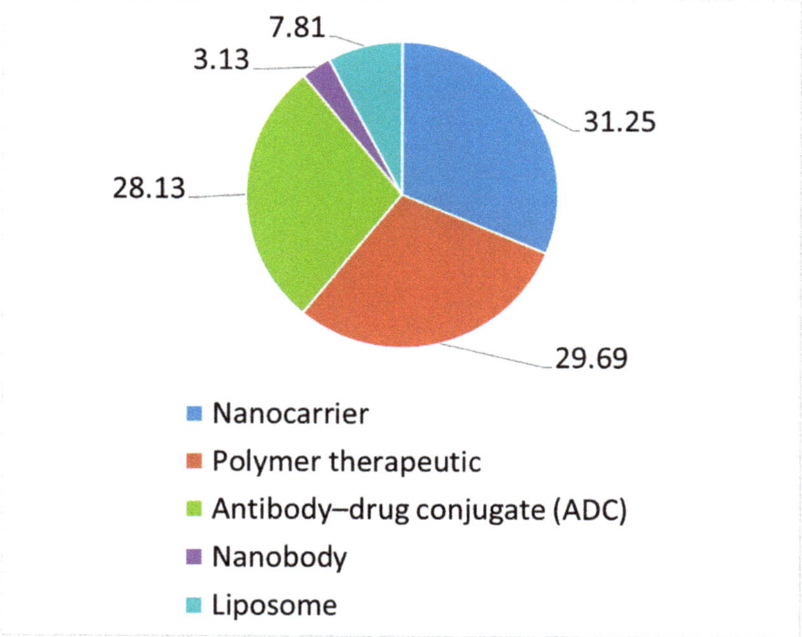

Figure 3. Categories attributable to nanomedicines identified in CTs assessed and authorized from 2018 to 2020.

Monoclonal antibodies, fusion proteins, and other recombinant products were not included in the scope because they are considered single biological molecules, even if their structural complexity is acknowledged. The same rationale applies for the three recombinant proteins that were not included, although dimensions in the nanoscale were confirmed by dynamic light scattering. CAR-T cells [27], and any other kind of cell therapy, were also not considered because their size was out of the nanoscale range. Although characterization data were provided for all IMPs, the nanoscale dimension has only been confirmed for 14 (21.88%) IMPs, while for the remaining 50 (78.12%) IMPs, the confirmation of the average size could not be retrieved. Nanocarriers, polymer therapeutics, antibody–drug conjugates, and nanobodies had already been retrieved in the analysis of the 2018 database, while in the analysis of the CTs authorized in the years 2019 and 2020, we also found IMPs that may be classified as liposomes. Liposomes are versatile drug delivery systems, developed for various routes of administration, that have the advantage of protecting the active substance enclosed in the vesicles, prolonging its half-life in the bloodstream and enhancing bioavailability. Several liposomal products have been authorized over the course of the last two decades by the European Medicines Agency (EMA) and the Food and Drug Administration (FDA) [28]. The distribution reported in Figure 4 shows that the vast majority of nanomedicines is tested in the therapeutic area of cancer, followed by eye disease, blood and lymphatic disease, virus disease, and respiratory tract disease therapeutic areas.

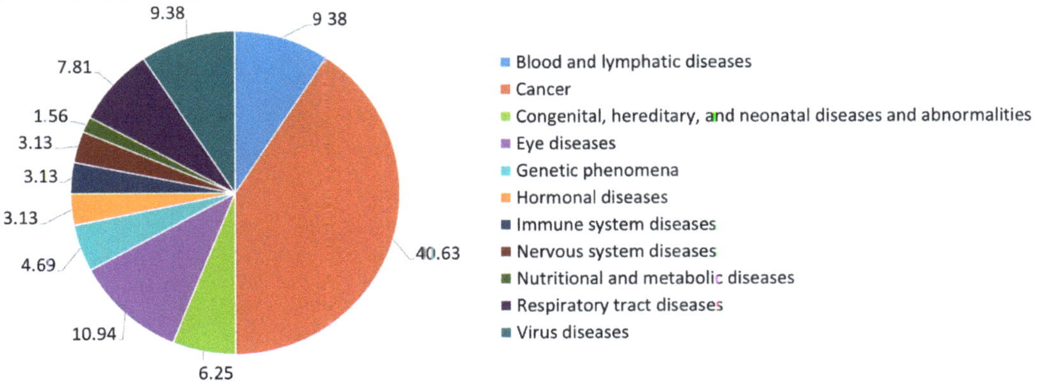

Figure 4. Distribution of therapeutic areas of CTs, including a nanomedicine tested as an IMP, assessed and authorized from 2018 to 2020.

3.2. Quality Issues

Quality issues were detected in 51 (79.69%) out of the 64 authorized CTs. The number of quality issues identified from 2018 to 2020 and their classification, according to the current applicable guidelines on the requirements concerning IMPs in CTs [29,30], are reported in Table A3.

Globally, 822 quality issues were detected, with an average of 16.12 issues per CT, considering only those with objections. In the enumeration of issues, we included requests to update documents, data and information, clarifications, conditions, and recommendations on quality aspects of the application. All categories are impacted, with the only exception being the nomenclature of the drug substance.

The greatest number of issues detected concerns stability, both of the drug substance and of the drug product, representing cumulatively 17.15% of the overall number of issues. Specifications is the second area with regard to the number of issues detected, representing 11.07% of all issues. If we add issues regarding GMP compliance, description of the manufacturing process and process control, batch analyses, and control of materials, these first six classification labels together represent 56.33% of all issues. The subsequent types of issues impacting the quality profile in terms of numerical relevance are: quality documentation compliance, process validation and/or evaluation, pharmaceutical development, controls of critical steps and intermediates, reference standards or materials, container closure system, and impurities. Figure 5 provides details of the number of issues detected for each classification label.

3.2.1. Stability

Considering the manufacturing date of batches reported in the IMPD, or the stability study start date, a request to provide updated stability data is often needed, whenever updated stability data should have been available but are not provided by the sponsor. In many other cases, stability data provided in the IMPD are limited and do not support the proposed retest or shelf life, particularly when an extrapolation is adopted. Other frequent requests are to investigate accelerated or stress conditions in order to identify potential degradation pathways or to justify out of specifications registered under normal conditions. It is also noted that a summary of results (including the description of the conditions tested, methods, and acceptance criteria) of the in-use stability and compatibility studies, which should support the product quality during clinical use, is not always provided, or, when it is provided, microbial parameters are sometimes missing. Another frequent issue is that product-related impurities are not tested at release and in stability studies.

Concerning biological IMPs, the control of purity is mandatory and should be included in the release and stability testing. Subvisible particles is instead a test required by *Ph. Eur.* for parenteral preparations and should be controlled in the drug product both at release and during stability.

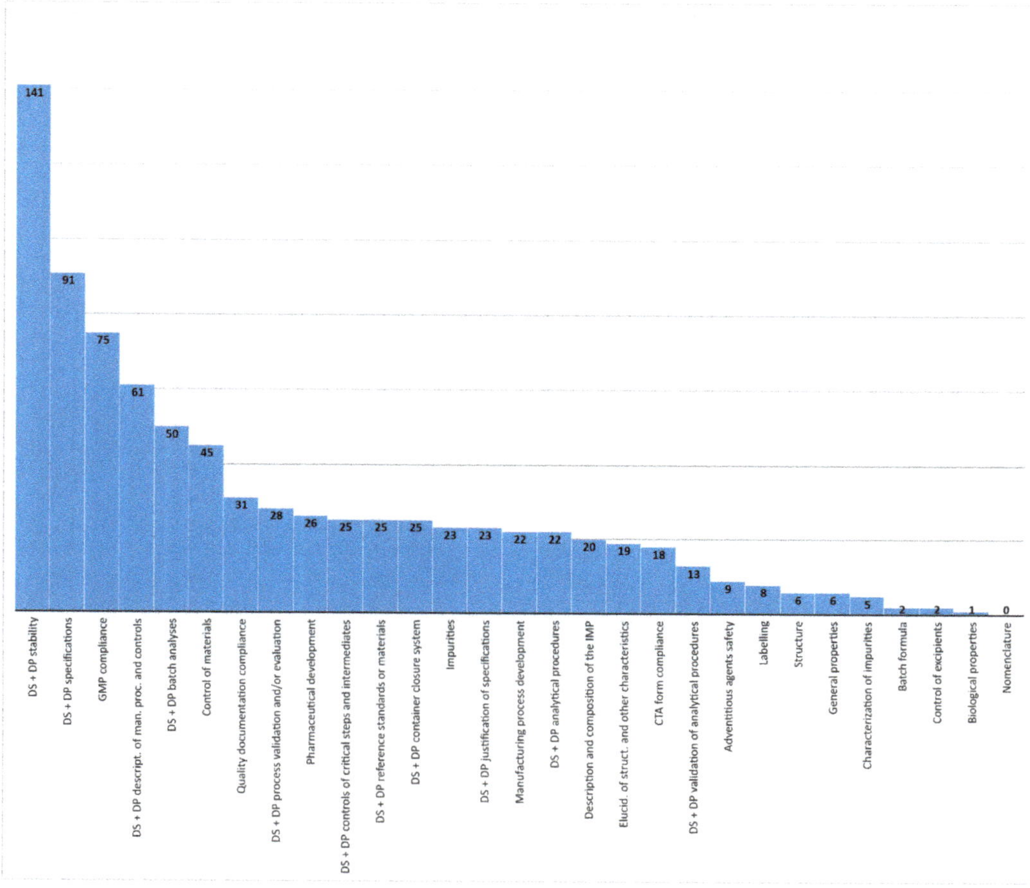

Figure 5. Number of quality issues combining drug substance (DS) and drug product (DP) classification label in CTs involving nanomedicines, assessed and authorized from 2018 to 2020.

3.2.2. Specifications

Drug substance and drug product batches intended to be used in CTs should be controlled with proper specifications and relevant tests, specifying the acceptance criteria. Depending on the type of drug substance or formulation of the drug product, a varied number of issues were detected. As an example, we report a non-exhaustive list of some of the significant criticalities encountered: solvents used in the last step of the synthesis (e.g., dichloromethane, heptane, and THF) not adequately controlled or amounts of these residual solvents not within ICH guideline limits; in parenteral preparations, subvisible particles or extractable volume not controlled; in suspensions or powders for injection, the uniformity of dosage units not controlled; for drug–device combinations, such as prefilled syringes, break loose and glide force, critical test parameters related to the functionality of the syringe, are not included in the specifications; the content of polysorbates, which are key excipients in biotechnological IMPs, not tested at release or during stability; for gene therapy products, transgene expression, vector aggregates, and genomic integrity of the vector not controlled at release by suitable methods.

3.2.3. GMP Compliance

Manufacturing licenses (MIA), GMP certificates, and qualified person's (QP) declaration of equivalence to EU GMP for IMPs manufactured in third countries (QP declaration) are frequently objects of non-compliance issues. Submitted MIAs sometimes do not cover IMPs but only authorized medicinal products. However, most of the issues are related to missing evidence that a manufacturer involved in the CT has a proper authorization to carry out the specific activities stated in the IMPD, such as batch certification of imported sterile biological medicinal products, quality control testing, primary or secondary packaging, and, in a few cases, also manufacturing activities. Concerning the QP declaration the document is often requested to be updated because the list of EEA manufacturers reported therein is not matching the information provided in the IMPD or, less frequently because the date of the audit to verify the EU GMP equivalence of the manufacturing sites is not recent.

3.2.4. Description of the Manufacturing Process and Process Controls

Issues are generally related to the lack of details or information on the manufacturing process and on its control, and these may vary according to the specificity of the process However, the most critical findings are noted on aseptic and sterilizing processes: the type and number of filters used per batch are not specified, data are not provided to demonstrate the compatibility with the filtered solution, and justification is not provided when the filter integrity test is conducted only after use. In addition, for the production of sterile medicinal products, it is necessary to provide information on the control of critical steps, such as the controls conducted to ascertain the efficiency of the production line in asepsis (e.g., media fill). Additional recurrent issues are noted when process intermediates are involved, and hold times and storage conditions are not justified and supported by data. In addition, when reprocessing is involved, it is not specified for which steps it is envisaged and in which cases. In this context, it is important to highlight that reprocessing could only be considered in exceptional circumstances, restricting these situations for biological products to certain re-filtration and re-concentration steps only, following a technical or mechanical failure of the equipment.

3.2.5. Batch Analyses

The most recurrent issue is the submission of data that are not recent or are incomplete (e.g., missing manufacturing date or manufacturing site). In addition, data of clinical batches are sometimes not provided. Batches considered representative of the ones to be used in the CT, including batches of all relevant manufacturing processes and manufacturing sites, should be provided. Certificates of analysis (CoAs) for batches intended for use in the CT are often requested.

3.2.6. Control of Materials

It is often necessary to request in-house specifications, including test methods and acceptance criteria, for non-compendial materials. Little information is usually submitted on the quality control of non-compendial raw materials, and representative CoAs, including specifications from suppliers and/or the in-house specifications for any testing performed on each non-compendial chemical raw materials, have to be requested. Sometimes, specifications provided do not include all the necessary controls, such as residual solvents or heavy metals. In general, a brief summary of the control of any critical attribute should be provided (e.g., if control is required to limit an impurity in the drug substance, or chiral control, metal catalyst control, or control of a precursor to a potential genotoxic impurity).

In addition, the information provided should be representative of the process employed for the manufacture of the clinical supplies intended to be used in the CT.

3.2.7. Quality Documentation Compliance

Most of the issues emerged from the need to update an IMPD that was not complete with all the required information and data. When updated documents are provided, substantial modifications should be listed and an updated version of the documents including track changes, as well as a clean version of the same documents, are expected to be submitted. An IMPD that was not representative of the IMP was rarely presented; more often instead, a cross-reference letter to an authorized version of the IMPD was not applicable because a more recent version had been authorized by the NCA or because the formulation of the referenced drug product was not deemed representative.

3.2.8. Process Validation and/or Evaluation

Issues concerned missing information in the IMPD, able to confirm that process validation was performed. Usually, data should not be required during the development phases, except for non-standard sterilization processes. In particular, although the manufacturing process may be at an early stage of development, for sterile, aseptic manufacturing and lyophilization, the state of the validation should be briefly described, as well as the in-process controls applied. In this regard, it should be taken into consideration that the validation of sterilizing processes should be of the same standard as for products authorized for marketing. Therefore, justification of missing validation of sterilizing processes is requested, e.g., in the case of a sterilizing filtration. Clarifications are also usually requested on how the bioburden control is performed prior to the sterilizing filtration. When batch formula may vary according to clinical needs, information should be provided on the batch size that has been validated by media fill.

3.2.9. Pharmaceutical Development

Development is still undergoing during CTs, and additional information is progressively collected on the manufacturing process, which is refined and optimized in due course. However, changes that occurred in the drug product manufacturing process during development are not always reported. When several process changes have been introduced (manufacturing scale, filter size, analytical methods for drug substance quantification, etc.) that could impact relevant quality attributes of the drug product, such as purity, the sponsor should support these changes with a comparability exercise, unless properly justified. The sponsor should provide a summary of the compatibility studies (including the description of the conditions tested, methods, acceptance criteria, and results) to support the product quality during clinical use. Discussion on leachable/extractable studies is expected for Phase III CTs.

3.2.10. Controls of Critical Steps and Intermediates

If hold times are foreseen in the manufacturing process, the maximum hold time should be indicated for each step and a summary of data supporting each hold time should be provided. Hold times and storage conditions for intermediates should be justified and supported by data. Critical process parameters should be identified and stated (e.g., bioburden prior to sterile filtration, filters integrity, and fill weight) and, depending on the stage of development (e.g., Phase III), at least preliminary acceptance criteria should be established. The maximum acceptable bioburden prior to sterile filtration should be reported, and test volumes of less than 100 mL should be justified.

3.2.11. Reference Standards or Materials

A reference standard should be established to ensure consistency between batches and comparability after process changes have been introduced. Adequate information on the reference standard and on its re-qualification is sometimes missing, and a request to clarify storage conditions and tests performed to confirm its stability over time is sometimes needed.

3.2.12. Container Closure System

Analytical procedures used to control the container closure and any validations should be specified if the methods are not compendial. Specifications for all the container closure components are usually not provided. Release specifications for the packaging material is sometimes requested and so are data on compatibility between the solution and the stopper. The quality standard of the stopper should be indicated. In case non-compendial materials are used, description and specifications should be provided.

3.2.13. Impurities

It is acknowledged that in the course of the development phase of an IMP, more in-depth knowledge is acquired and that at an early stage, less information may be available. However, the control of the impurity profile should always be present and upper limits taking safety considerations into account, should be set; limits may then be reviewed and adjusted during development. Quantitative information on impurities should be provided, including the maximum amount for the highest clinical dose. Sometimes, not all types of impurities are taken into consideration (e.g., organic, inorganic, process-related product-related, residual solvent, starting material, and potential mutagenic impurities). An inadequate control strategy is also a recurrent issue, e.g., not providing a justification based on a risk assessment for the proposed acceptance criteria. Data on the clearance of impurities and a safety assessment of the maximum amount per maximum dose in worst-case conditions are often requested and should be provided. Characterization of impurities was often found to be missing; at least the chemical structure should be provided in order to verify a potential toxicity profile. In connection with the setting and justification of specifications, particular focus on the limits set for process-related impurities and contaminants (e.g., bioburden and endotoxin) is needed. Impurities that are above the qualification threshold should be properly qualified by toxicological studies. Where a class 1 solvent might be present in another solvent (e.g., toluene and methanol containing benzene), a routine test for this class 1 solvent, on a suitable intermediate or on the final active substance, is required, unless an appropriate justification for residual levels is provided.

4. Discussion

This research is taking into account CTs authorized over a period of 3 years in Italy. For the 2018, a previous analysis [23] was conducted on the use of surfactants, nanomedicines, and nanocarriers in the context of CTs. We are now also investigating the quality issues and are adding those data to the databases of the following 2 years, 2019 and 2020, to provide a picture of the nanomedicine-related IMPs involved in CTs and the extent and type of quality issues detected across 3 years of cumulative activity at the CTO. CTs that were submitted to the CTO from 2018 to 2020 were quantified to be >22% of all those available in the EudraCT [31] system and therefore submitted in the EU in those years [22]. This pool of data can therefore represent a first estimate, even if partial, of the status in the overall EU.

Documentation submitted by the sponsors and information provided as structured data in the CTA form are not of help with the immediate identification of the presence of nanostructures tested as IMPs. In a few cases, a nanostructure is declared in the IMPD, but even in these cases, limited or no information is provided on dimension characterization. The nanoscale dimension has only been confirmed for 21.88% of the nanomedicine-related IMPs assessed. This issue is leading to a potential non-standardization in the characterization of nanotherapeutics. The CTO reacted by updating the draft submission cover letter [32] requesting sponsors to acknowledge if the CT involves the use of systems specially designed for clinical applications with at least one component in the nanometer scale from which specific and defined properties and characteristics derive, such as nanomedicines (nanocrystals, therapeutic polymers, albumin-bound nanoparticles, etc.), nanocarriers (e.g., liposomes, niosomes, nanoemulsions, micelles, and self-nanoemulsifying drug delivery systems (SNEDDs)), or nanodevices. Should a nanostructure be present, and should related information not be available within the IMPD, the sponsors are required to prepare an assessment of the benefit–risk associated with the nanomedicine, nanocarrier, or nanodevice to confirm the dimensions and to present a discussion of the nanotechnology used of the properties that may influence the kinetics and in vivo distribution, including a description of the analytical methods used for the characterization. These may include dynamic light scattering for hydrodynamic radius or polydispersion measurements; electron microscopy for morphology, purity, or core size; zeta potential, etc. This is a key point that should be taken up by the regulatory network to streamline and standardize the submission and assessment process of CTs involving nanotechnology, capitalizing on the sharing of best practices across NCAs.

In terms of nanomedicines' classification, results show that only a few categories were detected, as reported in Figure 3, and that these do not include any non-ionic surfactant-based nanocarriers (e.g., micelles, nanoemulsions, and niosomes) or more complex structures or nanodevices. Reasons cannot be identified from the data in our possession, but we can easily imagine that some types of nanomedicines and/or formulations in the nanoscale may be more complex, facing additional difficulties. During the development phase, physicochemical properties and biological functions should be elucidated and adequate analytical methods and techniques should be implemented in order to define the safety and efficacy profile of the product under investigation in CTs. During the manufacturing scale-up phase, producibility and costs are crucial. These are other key points to address, as far as possible, also from a regulatory standpoint, by envisaging dedicated support to the development of specific kinds of nanomedicines that are acknowledged to require additional efforts. An expert working group on nanomedicines, a number of specific guidelines, and an innovation task force have been set by the EMA in the EU. However, additional approaches in a clinical trial setting could take the form of a detailed, standardized guideline for the submission of nanomedicines in CTs or could foresee additional opportunities for a structured and accessible early interaction between the regulatory framework and those stakeholders in or owners of innovative nanotechnology, such as researchers and academia, medium-sized enterprises (SMEs) or start-ups, and pharmaceutical companies that are bringing along with innovation potential new scientific and regulatory challenges not yet coded in any already known clinical trial framework (nanopharmaceuticals, complex trials, decentralized CTs, use of machine learning or artificial intelligence in CTs, big data and real-world evidence for regulatory decision purposes in CTs, etc.). In our analysis, CTs including an IMP that may be classified as a nanomedicine were distributed across 11 therapeutic areas: more than 1/3 (40.63%) were tested in cancer therapy, and the other most impacted therapeutic areas were eye disease (10.94%), blood and lymphatic disease (9.38%), virus disease (9.38%), and respiratory tract disease (7.81%).

Quality issues were detected in 51 (79.69%) out of 64 CTs. The average is 16.12 issues per CT, considering only those with objections. This result denotes that, in general, more attention needs to be paid to compiling quality data for IMPs in CTs. All sections of the IMPD, with the exception of nomenclature, were impacted by quality issues. Therefore, it is evident that additional efforts should be pursued by sponsors when preparing quality documentation. As an example, the sponsors could contract a specialized company that may aid in the elaboration of the dossier or that may perform an evaluation of the documentation before its submission to the regulatory agencies. Considering both the drug substance and the drug product sections of the IMPDs, most of the quality issues were retrieved in the areas of stability, which alone accounts for 17.15% of all issues; specifications (11.07%), GMP compliance (9.12%), and the description of the manufacturing processes and processes control (7.42%) are the three other labels with the greatest number of issues detected. Batch analyses and control of materials slightly differ from each other, accounting, respectively, for 6.08% and 5.47% of the issues. Then follows a cluster of labels with a lower impact in terms of the number of issues detected but significant because it covers a large area of parameters and characteristics impacting the quality profile of the IMP: quality documentation compliance, process validation and/or evaluation, pharmaceutical development, controls of critical steps and intermediates, reference standards or materials, container closure system, and impurities.

CTs are regulated by strict standards to guarantee the rights, safety, and well-being of subjects and the quality and integrity of data, and it is necessary to have the required know-how to be able to test an IMP, resources, and regulatory knowledge. However, even when all these requirements are accomplished, further efforts may be needed to ensure full compliance during the assessment process of a CT, especially for specific types of innovative products. However, a re-evaluation of the regulatory approach to innovation in the health sector, with particular reference to the use of nanotechnology in CTs, should be envisaged by the regulatory network, with the highest priority, in order to support the translation of innovation in a safe but also effective and faster way. Training programs, development of dedicated guidelines, an earlier confrontation with small realities that generate innovation, researchers and academia, dedicated funding for SMEs, and non-commercial (academic) sponsors are just a few examples of potential interventions that the regulatory network in collaboration with all the stakeholders could and should consider in the interests of public health protection and support of technological innovation.

5. Conclusions

A critical analysis on the quality documentation and information provided by sponsors, along with the submission of CTs, authorized at the CTO from 2018 to 2020, shows that only 3.17% of the authorized CTs are impacted by the use of nanomedicines. This confirms that nanotechnology innovation does not progress as fast as standard formulations when it comes to the clinical development of an IMP. The categories detected were: nanobody (3.13%); liposomes (7.81%), tested in five CTs; polymer therapeutics (29.69%); antibody–drug conjugates (28.13%); and nanocarriers (31.25%). Nanocarriers mainly include viral vectors; there is no evidence of the use of other structured delivery systems, such as non-ionic surfactant-based nanocarriers. Even if CTs are spread across 11 therapeutic areas, more than 1/3 (40.63%) of IMPs that may be classified as nanomedicines are tested in cancer therapy, followed by other therapeutic areas, such as eye disease (10.94%), blood and lymphatic disease (9.38%), virus disease (9.38%), and respiratory tract disease (7.81%). Almost all (95.31%) CTs have a commercial nature, and this reflects how difficult it may be to translate nanotechnology innovation into clinical development in the absence of adequate funding, know-how, resources, and regulatory expertise. This is a critical point that should be tackled, envisaging additional strategies to provide at least regulatory support to those academia and SMEs driving research in the nanotechnology innovation field. The use of systems appropriately designed for clinical applications with at least one component in the nanometric scale, from which specific and definite properties and characteristics may derive, is not properly coded as structured data in the CTA form, and it is not explicitly reported by the sponsors in the quality information of the CMC section of the IMPDs. As a consequence, their characterization may not be always standardized. In addition, when a nanostructure is mentioned, no adequate characterization in terms of dimension confirmation could be retrieved in the majority of cases. This is another crucial regulatory point to be addressed, suggesting the need for a dedicated guideline on the assessment of nanotechnology-enabled IMPs in CTs.

The quality issues detected during the assessment of IMPs that may be classified as nanomedicines are shared, discussing for the first time the results of the assessment reports elaborated by the quality assessors at the CTO. For this research, we focused on CTs assessed and authorized from 2018 to 2020, which included a nanomedicine tested as an IMP, as explained above. Results confirm that the highest quality standards are guaranteed by the assessment process and are ensured before the authorization of a CT. Quality issues were detected for almost all sections of the IMPDs submitted, outlining that, in general, the quality of applications and related quality documentation should definitely be improved. In quantitative terms, considering both the drug substance and the drug product, the definition of the stability profile is the criticality with the greatest impact on the clinical development process of IMPs involving nanostructures. Other areas of major impact, both for the substance and the product, are specifications, compliance with GMPs, description of the manufacturing processes and process controls, batch analysis, and control of materials during manufacture. The compliance of quality documentation, process validation and/or evaluation, the pharmaceutical development, the controls of critical steps and intermediates, the reference standards or materials, the container closure system, and the impurity profile during the characterization of the active substance are additional sectors to which more attention needs to be paid. Findings provide valuable information to sponsors of CTs and developers of nanomedicines to focus on those areas of potential difficulty. Results should be capitalized on, leading to the development of a regulatory approach to innovation that takes into account the criticalities that emerge in due course of the investigations and the scientific evidence, suggesting improvements to the translation of innovation, continuing to guarantee the highest level of safety but at the same time supporting a more rapid, smooth, and effective application in a CT setting.

Author Contributions: Conceptualization, D.A.D.; methodology, D.A.D.; formal analysis, D.A.D., E.G. and D.G.; investigation, D.A.D., C.M., E.G. and D.G.; data curation, D.A.D., I.T. and E.G.; writing—original draft preparation, D.A.D.; writing—review and editing, D.A.D., I.T., M.C., C.M., E.G. and D.G. All authors have read and agreed to the published version of the manuscript.

Funding: This research received no external funding.

Institutional Review Board Statement: Not applicable.

Informed Consent Statement: Not applicable.

Data Availability Statement: Additional information on the data presented in this study is available on request from the corresponding author. The data are not publicly available due to the protection of commercially confidential information.

Acknowledgments: Italian Medicines Agency (AIFA). The quality assessors at the Clinical Trial Office and Pre-Authorization Department of AIFA.

Conflicts of Interest: The authors declare no conflict of interest. The conflict-of-interest declaration of the authors [1] is in accordance with the conflict-of-interest regulations approved by the AIFA Board of Directors (Resolution n. 37 dated 13 October 2020). The view and opinions expressed are those of the individual authors [1] and should not be attributed to the AIFA.

Appendix A

Table A1. Nanomedicines detected in CTs authorized in 2019.

Code	Description	Nanomedicine-Related Term	Analytical Method Confirming Nanoscale Dimension	Pharmaceutical Form	Study Phase	Therapeutic Area	Active Substance of Chemical Origin	Active Substance of Biological/Biotechnological Origin	Gene Therapy Medicinal Product
N23	RNA–peptide complex	Polymer therapeutic	Yes	Solution for injection	I	Cancer	No	Yes	No
N24	Recombinant type 5 adenovirus vector	Nanocarrier	Yes	Concentrate for solution for infusion ev	III	Cancer	No	No	Yes
N25	Pegylated protein	Polymer therapeutic	No	Solution for injection	I/II	Cancer	No	Yes	No
N17	Pegylated peptide	Polymer therapeutic	No	Solution for infusion	III	Blood and lymphatic diseases	Yes	No	No
N26	Recombinant adeno-associated virus vector serotype 5	Nanocarrier	No	Solution for infusion ev	III	Blood and lymphatic diseases	No	No	Yes
N27	Monoclonal antibody conjugated to a fluorochrome through a linker	Antibody–drug conjugate (ADC)	No	Concentrate for solution for injection	III	Cancer	No	Yes	No
N28	Monoclonal antibody conjugated to a cytotoxic agent through a linker	Antibody drug conjugate (ADC)	No	Powder for concentrate for solution for infusion	III	Cancer	No	Yes	No
N29	Recombinant protein attached to an albumin binding moiety	Nanocarrier	No	Solution for injection	III	Hormonal diseases	No	Yes	No
N30	Recombinant adenovirus serotype 155 viral vector	Nanocarrier	No	Suspension for injection	I	Respiratory tract diseases	No	Yes	No
N17	Pegylated peptide	Polymer therapeutic	No	Solution for injection	III	Eye diseases	Yes	No	No
N17	Pegylated peptide	Polymer therapeutic	No	Solution for injection	III	Eye diseases	Yes	No	No
N7	Pegylated enzyme	Polymer therapeutic	No	Concentrate for solution for infusion	III	Body processes—genetic phenomena	No	Yes	No
N31	Recombinant adeno-associated viral vector	Nanocarrier	Yes	Concentrate for solution for infusion	I/II	Congenital, hereditary, and neonatal diseases and abnormalities	No	No	Yes
N32	Liposomal adjuvant	Liposome	Yes	Powder for solution for injection	II	Respiratory tract diseases	No	Yes	No

Table A1. *Cont.*

Code	Description	Nanomedicine-Related Term	Analytical Method Confirming Nanoscale Dimension	Pharmaceutical Form	Study Phase	Therapeutic Area	Active Substance of Chemical Origin	Active Substance of Biological/Biotechnological Origin	Gene Therapy Medicinal Product
N33	Beads coated with the active ingredient	Nanocarrier	No	Soft capsule	II	Immune system diseases	No	Yes	No
N34	Pegylated recombinant protein	Polymer therapeutic	No	Powder for solution for injection	II	Cancer	No	Yes	No
N35	Recombinant adeno virus vector serotype 26	Nanocarrier	Yes	Solution for injection	III	Virus diseases	No	Yes	No
N36	Recombinant adeno-associated virus vector serotype 2	Nanocarrier	No	Solution for injection	I/II	Blood and lymphatic diseases	No	No	Yes
N37	Pegylated peptide	Polymer therapeutic	No	Solution for injection	II	Hormonal diseases	Yes	No	No
N38	Pegylated enzyme	Polymer Therapeutic	No	Concentrate for solution for infusion ev	III	Congenital, hereditary, and neonatal diseases and abnormalities	No	Yes	No
N39	Liposome-based adjuvant	Liposome	Yes	Powder for solution for injection	II	Virus diseases	No	Yes	No
N28	Monoclonal antibody conjugated to a cytotoxic agent through a linker	Antibody–drug conjugate (ADC)	No	Powder for concentrate for solution for infusion	III	Cancer	No	Yes	No
N28	Monoclonal antibody conjugated to a cytotoxic agent through a linker	Antibody–drug conjugate (ADC)	No	Powder for concentrate for solution for infusion	III	Cancer	No	Yes	No

Table A2. Nanomedicines detected in CTs authorized in 2020.

Code	Description	Nanomedicine-Related Term	Analytical Method Confirming Nanoscale Dimension	Pharmaceutical Form	Study Phase	Therapeutic Area	Active Substance of Chemical Origin	Active Substance of Biological/Biotechnological Origin	Gene Therapy Medicinal Product
N40	Monoclonal antibody conjugated to a cytotoxic agent through a linker	Antibody–drug conjugate (ADC)	No	Powder for solution for injection	II	Cancer	No	Yes	No
N41	Plasmid vector	Nanocarrier	No	Solution for injection	II	Cancer	No	Yes	No

Table A2. *Cont.*

Code	Description	Nanomedicine-Related Term	Analytical Method Confirming Nanoscale Dimension	Pharmaceutical Form	Study Phase	Therapeutic Area	Active Substance of Chemical Origin	Active Substance of Biological/Biotechnological Origin	Gene Therapy Medicinal Product
N42	Antibody conjugated with a biopolymer	Polymer therapeutic	No	Solution for injection	II	Eye diseases	No	Yes	No
N43	Adeno-associated virus serotype 9 vector	Nanocarrier	No	Concentrate for solution for infusion ev	III	Nervous system diseases	No	No	Yes
N44	Monoclonal antibody conjugated to a cytotoxic agent through a linker	Antibody–drug conjugate (ADC)	Yes	Concentrate for solution for infusion	III	Cancer	No	Yes	No
N45	Monoclonal antibody conjugated to a cytotoxic agent through a linker	Antibody–drug conjugate (ADC)	No	Powder for solution for infusion	I	Cancer	No	Yes	No
N46	Monoclonal antibody conjugated to a cytotoxic agent through a linker	Antibody–drug conjugate (ADC)	No	Concentrate for solution for infusion	III	Cancer	No	Yes	No
N7	Pegylated enzyme	Polymer therapeutic	No	Concentrate for solution for infusion	III	Body processes—genetic phenomena	No	Yes	No
N47	Pegylated oligonucleotide	Polymer therapeutic	No	Solution for injection	III	Eye diseases	Yes	No	No
N48	Adenoviral vector	Nanocarrier	No	Suspension for injection	I	Virus diseases	Yes	Yes	No
N34	Pegylated recombinant protein	Polymer therapeutic	No	Powder for solution for injection	III	Cancer	No	Yes	No
N49	Trivalent nanobody	Nanobody	No	Solution for infusion ev	II	Cancer	No	Yes	No
N50	Pegylated monoclonal antibody	Polymer therapeutic	No	Powder for solution for infusion ev	III	Immune system processes	No	Yes	No
N51	Liposomal formulation	Liposome	Yes	Powder for nebulization solution	II	Virus diseases	Yes	No	No
N52	Monoclonal antibody conjugated to a cytotoxic agent through a linker	Antibody–drug conjugate (ADC)	No	Powder for solution for infusion ev	II	Cancer	No	Yes	No
N53	Liposome suspension	Liposome	No	Inhalation suspension	III	Respiratory tract diseases	Yes	No	No
N54	Adenoviral vector	Nanocarrier	Yes	Solution for injection	III	Respiratory tract diseases	No	Yes	No
N42	Antibody conjugated with a biopolymer	Polymer therapeutic	No	Solution for injection	III	Eye diseases	No	Yes	No
N53	Liposome suspension	Liposome	No	Inhalation suspension	III	Respiratory tract diseases	Yes	No	No

Table A3. Number of quality issues and their classification for CTs assessed and authorized from 2018 to 2020.

Classification Label of Quality Issues		Totals Per Classification
CTA Form Compliance		18
Quality documentation compliance (IMPD, S-IMPD, SmPC, CE mark)		31
GMP compliance: information about all manufacturers involved (drug substance, drug product) and evidence of GMP (manufacturing licenses/GMP certificates, QP declarations, CEPs provided)		75
Drug Substance (DS)		
General information	Nomenclature	0
	Structure	6
	General properties	6
	Biological properties	1
Manufacture	Description of manufacturing process and process controls	42
	Control of materials	45
	Control of critical steps and intermediates	15
	Process validation and/or evaluation	6
	Manufacturing process development	22
Characterization	Elucidation of structure and other characteristics	19
	Impurities	23
Control of drug substance	Specifications	44
	Analytical procedures	13
	Validation of analytical procedures	9
	Batch analyses	33
	Justification of specification(s)	12
Reference standards or materials		20
Container closure system		9
Stability		57
Drug Product (DP)		
Description and composition of the investigational medicinal product		20
Pharmaceutical development		26
Manufacture	Batch formula	2
	Description of manufacturing process and process controls	19
	Controls of critical steps and intermediates	10
	Process validation and/or evaluation	22
Control of excipients		2
Control of drug product	Specifications	47
	Analytical procedures	9
	Validation of analytical procedures	4
	Batch analyses	17
	Characterization of impurities	5
	Justification of specification(s)	11

Table A3. *Cont.*

Classification Label of Quality Issues	Totals Per Classification
Reference standards or materials	5
Container closure system	16
Stability	84
Labeling	8
Adventitious agents' safety	9
TOTAL	822

References

1. Samrot, A.V.; Sean, T.C.; Kudaiyappan, T.; Bisyarah, U.; Mirarmandi, A.; Faradjeva, E.; Abubakar, A.; Ali, H.H.; Angalene, J.L.A.; Kumar, S.S. Production, characterization and application of nanocarriers made of polysaccharides, proteins, bio-polyesters and other biopolymers: A review. *Int. J. Biol. Macromol.* **2020**, *165*, 3088–3105. [CrossRef] [PubMed]
2. Aminu, N.; Bello, I.; Umar, N.M.; Tanko, N.; Aminu, A.; Audu, M.M. The influence of nanoparticulate drug delivery systems in drug therapy. *J. Drug Deliv. Sci. Technol.* **2020**, *60*, 101961. [CrossRef]
3. Patra, J.K.; Das, G.; Fraceto, L.F.; Campos, E.V.R.; del Pilar Rodriguez-Torres, M.; Acosta-Torres, L.S.; Diaz-Torres, L.A.; Grillo, R.; Swamy, M.K.; Sharma, S.; et al. Nano based drug delivery systems: Recent developments and future prospects. *J. Nanobiotechnol.* **2018**, *16*, 71. [CrossRef] [PubMed]
4. Longo, J.P.F.; Muehlmann, L.A.; Calderón, M.; Stockmann, C.; Azevedo, R.B. Editorial: Nanomedicine in Cancer Targeting and Therapy. *Front. Oncol.* **2021**, *11*, 4393. [CrossRef] [PubMed]
5. Prasad, M.; Lambe, U.P.; Brar, B.; Shah, I.; Manimegalaj, J.; Ranjan, K.; Rao, R.; Kumar, S.; Mahant, S.; Khurana, S.K.; et al. Nanotherapeutics: An insight into healthcare and multi-dimensional applications in medical sector of the modern world. *Biomed. Pharmacother.* **2017**, *97*, 1521–1537. [CrossRef] [PubMed]
6. Ventola, C.L. Progress in Nanomedicine: Approved and Investigational Nanodrugs. *Pharm. Ther.* **2017**, *42*, 742–755.
7. Farjadian, F.; Ghasemi, A.; Gohari, O.; Roointan, A.; Karimi, M.; Hamblin, M.R. Nanopharmaceuticals and nanomedicines currently on the market: Challenges and opportunities. *Nanomedicine* **2019**, *14*, 93–126. [CrossRef] [PubMed]
8. Sa-Nguanmoo, N.; Namdee, K.; Khongkow, M.; Ruktanonchai, U.; Zhao, Y.; Liang, X.-J. Review: Development of SARS-CoV-2 immuno-enhanced COVID-19 vaccines with nano-platform. *Nano Res.* **2021**, *15*, 2196–2225. [CrossRef] [PubMed]
9. Longo, J.P.F.; Muehlmann, L.A. How has nanomedical innovation contributed to the COVID-19 vaccine development? *Nanomedicine* **2021**, *16*, 1179–1181. [CrossRef] [PubMed]
10. Bhattacharjee, S.; Brayden, D.J. Addressing the challenges to increase the efficiency of translating nanomedicine formulations to patients. *Expert Opin. Drug Discov.* **2021**, *16*, 235–254. [CrossRef] [PubMed]
11. Germain, M.; Caputo, F.; Metcalfe, S.; Tosi, G.; Spring, K.; Åslund, A.K.; Pottier, A.; Schiffelers, R.; Ceccaldi, A.; Schmid, R. Delivering the power of nanomedicine to patients today. *J. Control. Release* **2020**, *326*, 164–171. [CrossRef] [PubMed]
12. Đorđević, S.; Gonzalez, M.M.; Conejos-Sánchez, I.; Carreira, B.; Pozzi, S.; Acúrcio, R.C.; Satchi-Fainaro, R.; Florindo, H.F.; Vicent, M.J. Current hurdles to the translation of nanomedicines from bench to the clinic. *Drug Deliv. Transl. Res.* **2022**, *12*, 500–525. [CrossRef] [PubMed]
13. Halwani, A.A. Development of Pharmaceutical Nanomedicines: From the Bench to the Market. *Pharmaceutics* **2022**, *14*, 106. [CrossRef] [PubMed]
14. Kapoor, B.; Gupta, R.; Gulati, M.; Singh, S.K.; Khursheed, R.; Gupta, M. The Why, Where, Who, How, and What of the vesicular delivery systems. *Adv. Colloid Interface Sci.* **2019**, *271*, 101985. [CrossRef] [PubMed]
15. European Commission. EudraLex—Volume 10—Clinical Trials Guidelines. 2010. Available online: https://ec.europa.eu/health/documents/eudralex/vol-10_en (accessed on 30 April 2022).
16. Directive 2001/20/EC of the European Parliament and of the Council of 4 April 2001 on the Approximation of the Laws, Regulations and Administrative Provisions of the Member States Relating to the Implementation of Good Clinical Practice in the Conduct of Clinical Trials on Medicinal Products for Human Use. Available online: https://eurlex.europa.eu/LexUriServ/LexUriServ.do?uri=OJ:L:2001:121:0034:0044:en:PDF (accessed on 30 April 2022).
17. European Commission. Annex 13 to Volume 4, EU Guidelines to Good Manufacturing Practice, Medicinal Products for Human and Veterinary Use. 2010. Available online: https://ec.europa.eu/health/sites/default/files/files/eudralex/vol-4/2009_06_annex13.pdf (accessed on 30 April 2022).
18. Regulation (EU) No 536/2014 of the European Parliament and of the Council of 16 April 2014 on Clinical Trials on Medicinal Products for Human Use, and Repealing Directive 2001/20/EC. Available online: https://ec.europa.eu/health/sites/default/files/files/eudralex/vol-1/reg_2014_536/reg_2014_536_en.pdf (accessed on 30 April 2022).

19. Italian Minister of Health Decree Dated 21 December 2007. Available online: https://www.gazzettaufficiale.it/atto/serie_generale/caricaDettaglioAtto/originario?atto.dataPubblicazioneGazzetta=2008-03-03&atto.codiceRedazionale=08A01360&elenco30giorni=false (accessed on 30 April 2022).
20. AIFA. Osservatorio Nazionale Sperimentazione Clinica. 2022. Available online: https://www.aifa.gov.it/osservatorio-nazionale-sperimentazione-clinica (accessed on 30 April 2022).
21. Quirós Pesudo, L.; Balahur, A.; Gottardo, S.; Rasmussen, K.; Wagner, G.; Joanny, G.; Bremer-Hoffmann, S. *Mapping Nano-medicine Terminology in the Regulatory Landscape*; Publications Office of the European Union: Luxembourg, 2018; ISBN 978-92-79-89872-3.
22. AIFA. Rapporto Sulla Sperimentazione Clinica dei Medicinali in Italia. 2022. Available online: https://www.aifa.gov.it/rapporto-sulla-sperimentazione-clinica-dei-medicinali-in-italia (accessed on 30 April 2022).
23. Dri, D.A.; Marianecci, C.; Carafa, M.; Gaucci, E.; Gramaglia, D. Surfactants, Nanomedicines and Nanocarriers: A Critical Evaluation on Clinical Trials. *Pharmaceutics* **2021**, *13*, 381. [CrossRef] [PubMed]
24. European Commission. Annex 1: Clinical trial Application Form Request for Authorisation of a Clinical Trial on a Medicinal Product for Human Use to the Competent Authorities and for Opinion of the Ethics Committees in the Community. Revision 4 November 2009; Updated on 22 November 2019. Available online: https://ec.europa.eu/health/system/files/2019-11/application-form_en_0.pdf (accessed on 30 April 2022).
25. Van Kan-Davelaar, H.E.; Van Hest, J.C.M.; Cornelissen, J.J.L.M.; Koay, M.S.T. Using viruses as nanomedicines. *J. Cereb. Blood Flow Metab.* **2014**, *171*, 4001–4009. [CrossRef] [PubMed]
26. Choi, Y.H.; Han, H.-K. Nanomedicines: Current status and future perspectives in aspect of drug delivery and pharmacokinetics. *J. Pharm. Investig.* **2019**, *48*, 43–60, Correction in *J. Pharm. Investig.* **2019**, *49*, 201. [CrossRef] [PubMed]
27. Titov, A.; Zmievskaya, E.; Ganeeva, I.; Valiullina, A.; Petukhov, A.; Rakhmatullina, A.; Miftakhova, R.; Fainshtein, M.; Rizvanov, A.; Bulatov, E. Adoptive Immunotherapy beyond CAR T-Cells. *Cancers* **2021**, *13*, 743. [CrossRef] [PubMed]
28. Liu, P.; Chen, G.; Zhang, J. A Review of Liposomes as a Drug Delivery System: Current Status of Approved Products, Regulatory Environments, and Future Perspectives. *Molecules* **2022**, *27*, 1372. [CrossRef] [PubMed]
29. European Medicines Agency. Committee for Medicinal Products for Human Use (CHMP)-Guideline on the Requirements for the Chemical and Pharmaceutical Quality Documentation Concerning Investigational Medicinal Products in Clinical Trials. 27 January 2022. EMA/CHMP/QWP/545525/2017 Rev. 2. Available online: https://www.ema.europa.eu/en/documents/scientific-guideline/guideline-requirements-chemical-pharmaceutical-quality-documentation-concerning-investigational_en-1.pdf (accessed on 30 April 2022).
30. European Medicines Agency. Committee for Medicinal Products for Human Use (CHMP)-Guideline on the Requirements for Quality Documentation Concerning Biological Investigational Medicinal Products in Clinical Trials. 27 January 2022. EMA/CHMP/BWP/534898/2008 Rev. 2. Available online: https://www.ema.europa.eu/en/documents/scientific-guideline/guideline-requirements-quality-documentation-concerning-biological-investigational-medicinal_en-2.pdf (accessed on 30 April 2022).
31. EudraCT. Available online: https://eudract.ema.europa.eu (accessed on 30 April 2022).
32. AIFA. Aggiornamento dei Modelli Delle Lettere di Ttrasmissione e Della Documentazione da Sottomettere per l'Autorizzazione di Sperimentazioni Cliniche e Relativi Emendamenti Sostanziali. 2019. Available online: https://www.aifa.gov.it/documents/20142/0/comunicazione_agg_mod_SC-ES_2019_08_01.pdf (accessed on 30 April 2022).

pharmaceutics

MDPI

Review

Microfluidic Manufacture of Lipid-Based Nanomedicines

Karim Osouli-Bostanabad [1,2], Sara Puliga [1], Dolores R. Serrano [3,4,*], Andrea Bucchi [5], Gavin Halbert [6] and Aikaterini Lalatsa [1,2,6,*]

1 Biomaterials, Bio-Engineering and Nanomedicine (BioN) Lab, Institute of Biomedical and Biomolecular Sciences, School of Pharmacy and Biomedical Sciences, University of Portsmouth, White Swan Road, Portsmouth PO1 2DT, UK
2 School of Pharmacy and Biomedical Sciences, Robertson Wing, University of Strathclyde, 161, Cathedral Street, Glasgow G4 0RE, UK
3 Pharmaceutics and Food Technology Department, School of Pharmacy, Universidad Complutense de Madrid, Plaza Ramón y Cajal s/n, 28040 Madrid, Spain
4 Facultad de Farmacia, Instituto Universitario de Farmacia Industrial, Universidad Complutense de Madrid, 28040 Madrid, Spain
5 School of Mechanical and Design Engineering, Faculty of Technology, University of Portsmouth, Portsmouth PO1 3DJ, UK
6 CRUK Formulation Unit, School of Pharmacy and Biomedical Sciences, Robertson Wing, University of Strathclyde, 161, Cathedral Street, Glasgow G4 0RE, UK
* Correspondence: dr.serrano@farm.ucm.es (D.R.S.); aikaterini.lalatsa@strath.ac.uk (A.L.); Tel.: +44-141-548-2675 (A.L.)

Abstract: Nanoparticulate technologies have revolutionized drug delivery allowing for passive and active targeting, altered biodistribution, controlled drug release (temporospatial or triggered), enhanced stability, improved solubilization capacity, and a reduction in dose and adverse effects. However, their manufacture remains immature, and challenges exist on an industrial scale due to high batch-to-batch variability hindering their clinical translation. Lipid-based nanomedicines remain the most widely approved nanomedicines, and their current manufacturing methods remain discontinuous and face several problems such as high batch-to-batch variability affecting the critical quality attributes (CQAs) of the product, laborious multistep processes, need for an expert workforce, and not being easily amenable to industrial scale-up involving typically a complex process control. Several techniques have emerged in recent years for nanomedicine manufacture, but a paradigm shift occurred when microfluidic strategies able to mix fluids in channels with dimensions of tens of micrometers and small volumes of liquid reagents in a highly controlled manner to form nanoparticles with tunable and reproducible structure were employed. In this review, we summarize the recent advancements in the manufacturing of lipid-based nanomedicines using microfluidics with particular emphasis on the parameters that govern the control of CQAs of final nanomedicines. The impact of microfluidic environments on formation dynamics of nanomaterials, and the application of microdevices as platforms for nanomaterial screening are also discussed.

Keywords: nanomedicine; microfluidics; liposomes; manufacture; engineering; scale-up

Citation: Osouli-Bostanabad, K.; Puliga, S.; Serrano, D.R.; Bucchi, A.; Halbert, G.; Lalatsa, A. Microfluidic Manufacture of Lipid-Based Nanomedicines. *Pharmaceutics* **2022**, *14*, 1940. https://doi.org/10.3390/pharmaceutics14091940

Academic Editor: Yusuke Sato

Received: 5 August 2022
Accepted: 2 September 2022
Published: 14 September 2022

1. The Nanomedicine Market and Bottlenecks to Market Entry

Nanomedicine is the application of nanotechnology in the medical field with important advances in terms of drug delivery, in vitro and in vivo diagnostics and imaging, regenerative medicine, and local implanted devices [1,2]. Nanoparticulate technologies have revolutionized drug delivery, allowing for passive and active targeting, altered biodistribution, controlled drug release (temporospatial or triggered), enhanced stability, improved solubilization capacity, and a reduction in dose and adverse effects. Nanomedicines can employ hard (inorganic) or soft nanomaterials and are disease-centered, while they combine a molecular understanding of cellular processes with capabilities to produce nanoscale material in a controlled manner for the diagnosis and treatment of diseases [3]. Nanopharmaceuticals can be developed either as drug delivery systems of biologically active drug products consisting of at least two components, one of which is the active ingredient [4].

The nanomedicine market is currently worth more than 150 billion USD, and this value is expected to rise to 334 billion USD by 2025 [5,6]. The market has considerably expanded in recent years due to numerous applications for the treatment of cancer, pain, and infections, as well as due to advances in drug delivery, and the increasing global incidence of cancer is estimated to be a key factor influencing industry growth. More than 50 nanomedicines have been clinically approved [3,4,7–19] after the initial approval of liposomal doxorubicin (Doxil®) for myeloma (multiple myeloma) due to the reduced cardiotoxicity of this formulation compared to unentrapped doxorubicin hydrochloride aqueous solutions [3], while more than 15 are in clinical trials and 75 are in the preclinical phase[9] Additionally, new applications in vaccinations as demonstrated by the formulation of mRNA vaccines in the recent COVID-19 pandemic are also currently contributing to the growth of the market [1,20]. Although data on the use of nanomedicines indicate that, in recent years, applications of nanomedicines have achieved considerable success, time their commercialization simultaneously suffers from many challenges and obstacles [21,22].

The current regulatory framework of the European Medicine Agency (EMA) focuses on the risk/benefit ratio, requiring that nanomedicines are subjected to toxicology and ecotoxicology studies, as well as remain under pharmacovigilance once marketed [23]. The Food and Drug Administration (FDA) has no specific regulatory framework for nanomedicines, but has recently published draft guidance for industry and special guidance for liposomal nanomedicines that are leading the entry into the market [24]. Although the FDA does not clearly separate biological products on the nanometer scale from nanoparticles, when considering whether a product involves the application of nanotechnology, it assesses whether a material or end product is engineered to exhibit properties or phenomena (physical, chemical, or biological) that are attributable to its dimensions, even if one of these dimensions falls outside the nanoscale range and is up to 1 μm [1,3].

The major bottlenecks in the uptake of nano-enabling technologies in the market involve difficulties in achieving relevant physiological test results in conventional prescreening platforms (in vitro), technical issues, including reliance on batch manufacturing to control of manufacturing qualities, the lack of a clear legislative framework, and economic risks as R&D is carried out mainly by small and medium-sized enterprises as big industries do not want to take risk on projects that have not yet been validated [25,26]. Once their potential and feasibility are demonstrated, big pharma is likely to buy the small–medium enterprises (SMEs) or license the products. Thus, to facilitate their technology readiness and scale-up to human studies, successful fabrication of nanomedicines with processes that can be continuous and able to match high-quality standards under GMP is critical.

2. Lipid-Based Nanomedicines

Lipid-based nanomedicines are prepared by bottom-up self-assembly methodologies and can be divided into the following broad categories on the basis of their physicochemical characteristics and fabrication methods such as liposomes, micelles, transferosomes, ethosomes, solid lipid nanoparticles, cochleates, and nanostructured lipid carriers (Figure 1, Table 1) [27], although others exist. Most of these nanoparticulate carriers result in spherical particles that possess at least one internal aqueous compartment surrounded by a single or double lipid layer and offer advantages in terms of high bioavailability, biocompatibility, drug loading, and permeability enhancement [28,29]. Most of the FDA-approved nanomedicines fall under this class of lipid-based nanomedicines [9,30].

Liposomes are the most widely approved lipid-based medicines and are typically prepared using phospholipids and cholesterol in multi- or unilamellar vesicles able to entrap lipophilic drugs in the bilayer and hydrophilic drugs in the aqueous internal compartment [31]. Their in vitro and in vivo stability, efficacy, and toxicity can be tuned by manipulating their surface charge, size, lipid composition, number of lamellas in the vesicles, and surface decoration with polymers such as polyethylene glycol or ligands, which allows for a versatile carrier for a range of clinical applications for passively or actively targeted strategies [29,32]. As the reticuloendothelial system can promptly take up liposomes, they often have surface modifications with polymers to improve their circulation half-life on the basis of the clinical application intended [28,33].

Transferosomes are lipid-based vesicular carriers that, compared to the rigid lipid bilayers (liposomes) or nonionic surfactant single layer vesicles (niosomes), are elastic, ultra-deformable, and stress-responsive [34]. Transferosomes are composed by four key elements: (i) phospholipids (such as phosphatidylcholine, dipalmitylphosphatidylcholine, distearylphosphatidylcholine), (ii) an edge activator such as a surfactant or bile salt ranging from 10% to 25% (e.g., sodium cholate, sodium deoxycholate, Tween® 80, Span® 80, and dipotassium glycyrrhizinate) [35], (iii) ethanol in a lower percentage usually below 10% (as higher concentrations are described as ethosomes), and (iv) water as a vehicle. In addition to phospholipids, they contain cholesterol or another edge activator such as bile salts and, in some cases, a small quantity of ethanol, typically below 10% [34,36]. The word transferosome is a registered trademark by the German company IDEA AG and the name derives from the Latin word "transferre" meaning "to carry across" and the Greek word "soma" meaning "body". The technology was first described in 1991 by Çevc and Blume and has been the subject of several patents and research over the last 30 years [34]. Transferosomes are highly ultra-deformable and are able to squeeze through biological barriers such as the stratum corneum (SC) and penetrate as intact vesicles through the skin when their size is below 300 nm and when they are applied under nonocclusive conditions which maintains the trans-epidermal osmotic gradient that acts as the driving force for the elastic transport into the skin [35,37,38]. The edge activator plays a key role as it provides a high radius of curvature that can destabilize the lipid bilayer, increasing the deformability of the membrane. This allows transferosomes to spontaneously squeeze though channels in the SC that are less than one-tenth the diameter of the vesicles, preventing vesicle rupture when crossing through the different skin layers [37,38]. The concentration of the edge activator in the formulation (usually between 10% and 20%) is crucial and ideally included in sublytic concentrations, i.e., not able to cause destruction of vesicles [35,37,39]. The risk of formation of mixed micelles increases when amounts of edge activator greater than 15% are used [40].

Ethosomes are phospholipid bilayer particles that incorporate alcohols (<10%) to impart a high degree of flexibility to the vesicle membranes, allowing relatively large vesicles to traverse the small intercellular pores within the SC. Ethosomes are soft, malleable vesicles that can range between 30 nm and several microns. Their size is smaller than that of liposomes prepared under the same conditions without the need of a size reduction step due to the high concentration of ethanol employed (20–45% typically) [41,42]. Additionally, ethanol confers a strong negative charge on the vesicles [43]. However, for systemic delivery through the bloodstream, both transferosomes and ethosomes are not ideal since large and flexible lipid-based particles are subject to rapid opsonization and phagocytotic clearance.

Bilosomes, similar to transferosomes, but without incorporating the alcohol content, are bile-salt-stabilized vesicles (bilayers) that have been applied in the oral delivery of antigens, proteins, and peptides [44]. Inclusion of bile salts into the lipid bilayers makes them repulsive to the intestinal bile salts in the gastrointestinal tract and, thus, offer great oral stability [45]. Additionally, these bile salts such as sodium glycocholate (SGC), sodium deoxycholate (SDC), and sodium taurocholate (STC) are also used as intestinal penetration enhancers as they enhance the low aqueous solubility of drugs and enhance oral permeability [46]. Among these, SGC is used widely as it exhibits less toxicity, enhances protease enzyme-inhibiting potential in the gastrointestinal system, and improves the permeation effect [47,48].

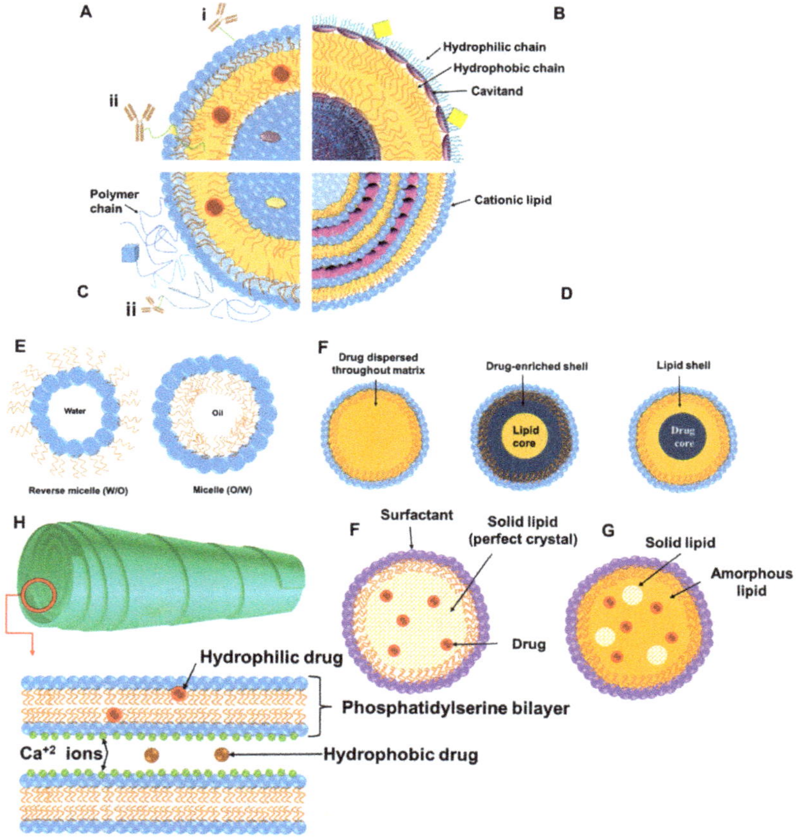

Figure 1. Schematic representation of lipid-based nanomedicines. Liposomes (**A–D**): Hydrophobic molecules up to few nm in diameter can be entrapped in the phospholipid bilayer (red spheres), while hydrophilic cargo can be loaded in the core (purple pentagon) and their surface can be modified antibodies (hydrophobically anchored (i) or conjugated via a linker or a hydrophilic polymer chain (immunoliposomes (ii)) (**A**). Liposomes with cavitands able to allow host–guest chemical reactions with molecules of complementary shape or size to allow loading in the bilayer, cavitands, and core (**B**). Stealth liposomes and targeted stealth liposomes where the liposome surface is decorated with hydrophilic polymer chains such as polyethylene glycol or a stimulus-responsive polymer, and a targeting moiety or diagnostic moiety (blue square) can be conjugated (peptides, cell-penetrating peptides, and antibodies). Drugs, genetic material, or diagnostic agents (gold, silver, or magnetic particles) can be loaded in the bilayer, core, or surface via conjugation, and lipids can be negatively or positively charged (preferred for complexation with DNA/RNA). **Micelles or inverse micelles** (**E**) are prepared via self-assembly of amphiphiles such as phospholipids and can load hydrophobic or hydrophilic molecules. **Solid lipid nanoparticles (SLNs)** (**F**) are colloidal carriers where liquid lipids have been substituted by a solid lipid, offering unique properties such as small size, large surface area, high drug loading, and the interaction of phases at the interfaces, and they are attractive for their potential to improve performance of pharmaceuticals, nutraceuticals, and other materials, appearing in three forms depending on where drug is loaded (homogeneous matrix (melting point of drug equal to that of lipid), lipid-enriched core (melting point of drug < lipid), and drug-enriched core (melting point of drug > lipid)). **Nanostructured lipid carriers (NLCs)** (**G**) are colloidal carriers prepared by blending of solid lipids with oils, but the matrix remains solid at body temperature to overcome problems of SLNs (low payload for drugs, drug expulsion during storage, and high water

content of SLN dispersions). **Cochleates** (**H**) are phospholipid–calcium precipitates derived from the interaction of anionic lipid vesicles with divalent cations such as calcium with a multilayered structure consisting of large and continuous lipid bilayer sheets rolled up in a spiral structure with no internal aqueous phases.

Solid lipid nanoparticles (SLNs) are colloidal carriers developed as an alternative system to other existing traditional carriers (emulsions, liposomes, and polymeric nanoparticles). They are a new generation of submicron-sized lipid emulsions where the liquid lipid (oil) has been substituted by a solid lipid. The drug-loading capacity of conventional SLNs is limited by the solubility of drug in the lipid melt, the miscibility of the drug melts and lipid melt, the chemical and physical structure of the lipid matrix, and the polymorphic state of the lipid matrix [49]. If the lipid matrix consists of especially similar molecules (i.e., tristearin or tripalmitin), a perfect crystal with few imperfections is formed. Since incorporated drugs are located between fatty acid chains, between the lipid layers, and also in crystal imperfections, a highly ordered crystal lattice cannot accommodate large amounts of drug. Therefore, the use of more complex lipids is more sensible for higher drug loading. Thus, potential disadvantages such as poor drug loading capacity, drug expulsion after polymeric transition during storage, and relatively high water content of the dispersions (70–99.9%) have been observed. Release can be controlled depending on where the drugs are incorporated within the particle (solid solution model and core–shell model with a drug-enriched shell or a drug-enriched core; Figure 1). When ionizable lipids are used, they can complex genes; moreover, as they are usually neutral at physiological pH and charged in acidic endosomes, they encourage endosomal escape for intracellular delivery of genes [50,51]. There is no need for organic solvents in the production of solid lipid nanoparticles, which excludes the toxicity risk resulting from solvent residues. Furthermore, the large-scale manufacturing and great reproducibility of lipid nanoparticles are vital characteristics for clinical applications [52] Sharing advantages with SLNs, nanostructured lipid carriers (NLCs) which are made with unstructured lipid blends of liquid and solid lipids able to form an imperfect crystal internally, as well as possess improved drug loading and enhanced stability over storage, as the liquid phase prevents the release of drugs during storage [53].

Cochleates are small-sized and stable lipid-based carriers comprising mainly of a negatively charged lipid (e.g., phosphatidylinositol, phosphatidylserine, phosphatidylcholine and diolylphosphatidylserine) and a divalent cation such as calcium with a cigar-shaped spiral multilayered structure [54–56]. Hydrophobic, amphiphilic, and negatively or positively charged molecules have been delivered by cochleates and are ideal candidates for oral and systemic delivery of hydrophobic and hydrophilic drugs prone to oxidation [56], enabling an enhancement in permeability and a reduction in the dose of drugs. Divalent cations are generally used for rolling of lipid sheets and interacting with the lipids which are present on the outer membrane of the cells [57]. Cochleates show many applications such as oral delivery of amphotericin B (AmB) for leishmaniasis, cochleates for antibiotic resistance, antigen transportation for treatment of meningitis B, encapsulation of volatile oil for leishmaniasis, and topical application for antifungal applications [56].

Lipid-based nanomedicines can enable passive (based on their size and enhanced permeation and retention effect observed in tumors as in the case of Doxil®) or active targeting by modifying their surface with ligands able to bind specific receptors (e.g., EGFR Transferrin, HER-2, and asialoglycoprotein receptors [58]), which allows beneficial biodistribution and tumor/tissue accumulation tailored to the indication [59,60]. Liposomes however, remain over the last three decades the nanomedicines that resulted in the majority of approved therapeutics [7,61–63] for multiple applications such as oncology, pain, and infection, while liposomes are well represented in current clinical trials for chemotherapy gene therapy, and vaccination (Table S1 [64–81]).

Recently, therapeutics based on nucleic acids, including small activating, interfering and messenger RNAs (saRNA, siRNA, and mRNA, respectively) have received interest for a broad range of diseases and infections [82,83]. However, there are some inherent drawbacks with using nucleic acids, such as low immunogenicity of DNA and the possibility of its integration with the human genome [84,85], rapid degradation of RNAs in physiological environments, and their excretion within a short time (<10 min) by glomerular filtration [86]. Lipid nanomedicines are emerging as formulations able to reduce serum endonuclease degradation, as well as to target the genetic medicines to the cells/tissues required [87]. Various lipids possess robust self-adjuvant activity, particularly cationic lipids (e.g., dimethyldioctadecylammonium bromide), which enables antigen deposition at the injection place, while improving intracellular delivery and complexation of antigens [88]. However, the level of immunogenicity is highly dependent on the formulation type (i.e., lipid nanoparticles showed high antigen complexation and cell uptake, while emulsion-based systems indicated elevated antibody responses) [88]. In another study, mRNA lipid nanoparticles with adjuvants (tri-palmitoyl-*S*-glyceryl-cysteine (Pam(3)Cys) bound to the pentapeptide) were able to elicit synergistic effects in cancer immunotherapy [89]. Various TLRs (Toll-like receptors) were triggered by this formulation to enhance the $CD8^+$ T-cell population required to limit tumor growth [89].

Table 1. Summary of main components, characteristics, methods of manufacture, and advantages and disadvantages of lipid-based nanosystems.

System	Components	Diameter (nm)/Shape	Manufacturing	Pros	Cons	Refs.
Transferosomes	Edge activators, phospholipids	Less than 300/spherical bilayer	Vortexing, sonication, rotary film, or reverse-phase evaporations	Good stability, higher penetration	Susceptible to oxidative degradation	[36,90]
Liposomes	Cholesterol, phospholipids, essential oils	10–1000/spherical bilayers	Solvent dispersion, mechanical dispersion, detergent removal	Controlled release, drug protection, solubility improvement for hydrophobic drugs, high biodistribution and bioavailability	Rigid structure, limited penetration across the stratum corneum	[28,29,32,33,62,90]
Nanostructured lipid carriers (NLCs)	Liquid and solid lipids, surfactants	50–1000/spherical single layer	Sonication, micro emulsification, high-pressure homogenization	High cell uptake, appropriate protection of therapeutics in acidic pH, biodegradable and biocompatible, simplicity of drug entrapment, long shelf-life, more sustainable drug dissolution, high payload, reduced loss of drug during storage	Solid/liquid lipid ratio optimization difficulties	[52,53,91–93]
Solid lipid nanoparticles (SLNs)	Surfactants, solid lipids	50–1000/spherical single layer	Sonication, micro emulsification, high-pressure homogenization	High cell uptake, appropriate protection of therapeutics in acidic pH, biodegradable and biocompatible ingredients, simplicity of drug entrapment, long shelf-life	Gelling tendency	[50–52,91–98]
Ethosomes	Phospholipids, edge activator, high concentration of a low-molecular-weight alcohol (ethanol ≤45% w/w), water	<200 or 300/spherical with diverse lamellarities	Solvent dispersion, ethanol injection–sonication, thin-film hydration, reverse-phase evaporation, transmembrane pH gradient, extrusion, and sonication	Increased efficacy and therapeutic index, reduce toxicity of API, improved permeation, entrapment of lipophilic, hydrophilic, and amphiphilic agents, simplicity of manufacturing, noninvasive, better solubility and stability, selective passive targeting	Low production yield, only for potent drugs, skin dermatitis or irritation may occur, drug leakage during transfer from organic to water media	[99,100]
Cochleates	Phospholipid–cation precipitates (formed by a continuous, solid, lipid bilayer sheet rolled up in a spiral)	100–1000/cylindrical shape	Trapping method (a bridging agent is mixed with an aqueous lipid suspension), hydrogel method, dialysis, emulsification–lyophilization, microfluidic method, solvent injection	Nonimmunogenic, noninflammatory, and nontoxic, a stable structure due to their tightly packed nature, less susceptible to oxidation of both the encapsulated drug and the phospholipids, sustained release is achievable, enhanced shelf-life, improvements in oral bioavailability of drugs	Aggregation on storage, high production cost	[56,101]

Since the outbreak of the COVID-19 pandemic, vaccines based on mRNAs have revolutionized vaccination, enabling shorter research and development cycles, simple manufacturing procedures, and the capability of intense immune response induction. Currently, most COVID-19 vaccine candidates based on mRNAs employ lipid-based nanoparticles (LNPs) as a delivery vehicle formed from four elements, including helper phospholipids (e.g., oleoylphosphatidylethanolamine or dioleoylphosphatidylcholine), cholesterol, PEGylated lipids, and ionizable lipids. More than 300 vaccine candidates for the COVID-19 pandemic were reported to be under development by the WHO, of which 47 were vaccines based on mRNAs, among which 23 have entered clinical trials [102,103]. Pfizer–BioNTech was the first officially approved COVID-19 vaccine on 23 August 2021 by the FDA for commercialization [104], being also the first-ever approved vaccine for emergency use in children 5 through 11 years old [105]. Additionally, liposomes have also been used for vaccination as adjuvants as in the case of Shingrix, Mosquirix, Epaxal, and Inflexal V, which are four approved and successfully commercialized liposomal vaccines [62,63,88]. These vaccines offer several advantages compared to vaccines based on conventional proteins, such as high safety, ease of synthesis, efficient manipulation of antigens, low cost, and having the capability for scaling up [85,106], while they offer advantages in terms of their pharmacokinetics, ability to protect the genetic material, and capability of targeted and intracellular delivery (macrophages and dendritic cells), as well as tissue distribution [81,84,107–109]. Similar results were also shown for anticancer vaccines [86,107,110].

2.1. *Current Methods for Lipid-Based Nanomedicine Manufacture*

Lipid-based nanomaterial fabrication can be categorized as organic solvent injection, hydration, reverse-phase evaporation, and detergent removal methods [111–115]. The classic manufacturing techniques for nanomedicines and in particular for liposomes are labor-intensive and suffer from a number of difficulties in their application at an industrial level, e.g., poor reproducibility and insufficient cost-effectiveness (Table 2) [116–118]. Batch synthetic methods for liposomes are generally based on specific parameters to guarantee the self-assembly [117]. Lipid-based nanoparticles using injection of organic solvents can be fabricated in a single step. In this method, lipid concentrations, mixing rate, injected volume, ratio of aqueous solution, and solvent/lipid ratios are the main variables to control the size of produced nanoparticles [119]. The hydration technique is the most conventional procedure for manufacturing of large multilamellar vesicles (100–1000 nm). Briefly, a lipid film is fabricated via an organic solvent evaporation from the lipid–solvent solution in a flask or tube; subsequently, an aqueous solution (e.g., phosphate-buffered saline) is added to form multilamellar vesicles. The vesicles fabricated by experiencing extra size tuning processes (e.g., sonication and extrusion) are turned to unilamellar small vesicles (<100 nm) [120,121]. The size of the vesicles is optimized in terms of applied power (sonication) and pore sizes of the employed membrane (extrusion). After fabrication of unilamellar small vesicles, a freeze/thaw method is used for drug loading in lipid-based nanoparticles [122]. The detergent removal technique works on the basis of vesicle formation (lipid molecules and detergents) and detergent elimination by dialysis [123]. As aforementioned, these fabrication approaches commonly contain three main steps: dissolution of lipids in organic solvents, lipidic phase dispersion in aqueous media/solution, and purification of the resulting samples (e.g., liposomes and nanoparticles) using some complex methods (i.e., centrifugation and/or gel permeation chromatography). These methods mainly yield large uni/multilamellar vesicles; hence, further steps (e.g., ultrasonication, high-pressure homogenization, or extrusion) are required to manufacture small unilamellar vesicles with low polydispersity index. The drawbacks of all these conventional manufacturing techniques are the use of volatile organic solvents in large quantities, the complexity scaling up, the heterogeneity of the prepared products, the high cost of excipients, and the need for multiple time-consuming steps.

Table 2. Summary of liposome preparation methods and their suitability for continuous manufacturing Reprinted/adapted with permission from [117] and used under the Creative Commons license permission (CC BY 4.0). Copyright 2018, John Wiley & Sons, Inc. All rights reserved.

Method	Mechanism	Suitability for Continuous Manufacturing
Bangham	Rehydration of thin lipid film	Not practical—needs continuous dehydration/rehydration steps
Sonication	Sonication of aqueous lipid suspensions	Requires small-scale batch operation to ensure sonication efficiency
Reverse-phase evaporation	Aqueous phase added to organic phase and evaporated to form liposomes	Very complex to regulate continuous solvent evaporation, sterile boundary hard to establish
Detergent depletion	Liposomes forms through detergent–lipid interaction	Slow process with difficult-to-establish sterile boundary, detergent use generally disadvantageous
Microfluidic channel	Intersection of lipid and API solutions in micromixers	Continuous but small/medium scale that can be upscaled in parallel
High-pressure homogenization	Liposome formation through high-pressure mixing	Very high pressures required, difficulty in sterilizing equipment
Heating	Heating of lipid aqueous/glycerol solution to form liposomes	Hydration step and high temperatures make continuous production impractical
Supercritical fluid methods	Use of supercritical fluids as solvent for lipids instead	High pressures required for feed vessels make resupply/continuous operation impractical
Dense gas	Use of dense gas as solvent for lipids	High pressures required for feed vessels make resupply/continuous operation impractical
Dual asymmetric centrifugation	Mechanical turbulence and cavitation	Only for batch sizes ~1 g or less
Ethanol/ether injection	Precipitation of liposome from organic phase into aqueous	Simple process with inherently continuous liposome formation step
Crossflow	In-line precipitation of liposome from organic phase into aqueous	Simple process with inherently continuous liposome formation step

2.2. Challenges with Lipid-Based Nanomedicine Manufacture and Clinical Translation

One of the main challenges in the field of nanotechnology has been the lack of continuous and easily scalable method for the controlled manufacture of nanomedicines with critical quality attributes (CQAs) such as size, size distribution, drug loading, surface charge, surface density of ligands or decorated polyethylene glycol chains, and stability able to ensure batch-to-batch reproducibility. Absence of protocols and access to facilities for product characterization, as well as challenges in scale-up and good manufacturing practice, along with lack of well-trained industrial staff, contribute to delays in uptake of these technologies by the pharmaceutical industry [17,124]. Although academics possess the necessary skills and knowledge to develop these systems, the lack of business management education at academic level contributes toward challenges in their industrial and clinical uptake. The absence of proper controls, inadequately outlined critical quality characteristics, and the lack of animal models with adequate clinical relevance to humans that actually mimic the action mechanisms of nanomedicines in the body have limited extensive clinical translations. The restrictions enforced by too complicated models or too simplistic procedures that impede reliable data interpretation emphasize that there is a need for stratification and standardization of methodologies [125]. Nanomedicines are not formally controlled and organized differently from conventional small therapeutics. To be effectively translated into the healthcare market, the EMA and FDA both ask that nanomedicines satisfy the same efficacy, safety, and pharmaceutical characteristic standards used for all therapeutic products [126]. However, because of the hybrid and unique nature of nanomedicines, the quality evaluation of these products shows considerable analytical challenges in comparison with small biological (e.g., antibodies) or molecular drugs. In addition to the identity, potency, strength, impurities, stability measurements, bioburden, and bacterial endotoxins of various chemical ingredients, further physicochemical characteristics and sterility must be evaluated for the final nanomedicine. These evaluated characteristics include size distribution, particle size, polydispersity, drug loading, surface charge, drug dissolution behavior, complex core/shell physical and chemical structure, size, and chemical stability while in storage or contact with biological environments [127]. Classical characterization approaches are usually not able to be used to assess nanomaterials, and more advanced methodological techniques are required to realize how nanomedicine characteristics could affect their efficacy and safety profiles (e.g., assessed by their biodistribution, pharmacokinetics, immunological effects, degradation profile, and metabolism) to identify the essential quality features of each system [128,129]. Thus, the lag with respect to regulatory guidance hinders the progression of nanomedicines in clinical development.

3. Microfluidic Manufacture and the Problem of Mixing

The current manufacturing methods for the majority of licensed nanomedicines remain discontinuous and face a number of problems such as high batch-to-batch variability affecting the CQAs of the product, laborious multistep processes, need for an expert workforce, and not being easily amenable to industrial scale-up involving typically a complex process control [1]. Inability to control the CQAs for nanomedicine is linked to poor control of bioequivalence that invariably results in poor therapeutic efficacy. The FDA also supports transforming batch to continuous manufacturing processes to improve product quality and reproducibility, which would also be less labor- and time-intensive [130].

Several techniques have emerged in recent years for nanomedicine manufacture; however, a paradigm shift occurred when microfluidic strategies were employed. Microfluidics is the technology of fluid manipulation in channels with dimensions of tens of micrometers [131,132], and small volumes of liquid reagents are rapidly mixed in a microchannel in a highly controlled manner to form nanoparticles with tunable and reproducible structure that can be tailored for drug delivery, resulting in a continuous and industrial amenable manufacturing process. Largely irrespective of the nature of the process, continuous flow conditions offer clear advantages over traditional batch processes, as quantity of the product scales directly with time but does not require different reactors (easy scalability), while fixed geometries allow for a precise control of mixing conditions (reproducibility) and enable lower size dispersity, as well as, in some cases, better drug loading; moreover, fine-tuning of particle properties such as a size is possible via control of the process parameters such as flow [133–136].

3.1. *Microfluidic Devices and Principles*

3.1.1. Principles of Mass Transfer and Fluid Mixing

Theoretically, in microfluidic environments, the fluid flow is controlled by the same rules governing the flow of a fluid at the macroscale. Microfluidic devices are not simply a miniaturized type of their macroscale versions, due to several physical features (e.g., high ratio of surface/volume and mass transfer based on diffusion) that do not linearly scale from macrodomains to microdomains. Microfluidic systems are described by the ubiquity of laminar flow, because of the controlling role applied by viscous forces [137–140]. It is important to remember that microfluidic mixing due to the small lateral dimension of the channels causes the flow to be laminar as the Reynolds number (*Re*, Equation (1)) is inevitably an order of magnitude lower than the minimum necessary to achieve turbulence ($Re >> 10^3$).

$$Re = \frac{Vdp}{\eta}. \tag{1}$$

where V is the flow rate, d is the diameter of the channel, p is the density of the fluid, and η is the viscosity. Increasing the *Re* cannot be only increased by a large increase in flow rate, as this would significantly increase the pressure and flow rate while decreasing channel diameter. Thus, where the flow is laminar in the fluidic domain, mass transfer is governed by passive molecular advection and diffusion [1,139,140]. Mixing at the macroscale is commonly obtained via the formation of turbulent flow, enabling it to separate fluid in small parts, thus resulting in a decrease and an increase in the mixing path and contact surface, respectively. Architecture of a micromixer is usually designed in such a manner to reduce the path of mixing and enhance the contact surface region. As mixing is based on diffusion, the mixing time (t_{mix}) is proportional to the square of the width of the fluid stream (d) and inversely proportional to the diffusion coefficient (D). The latter is inversely related to size (hydrodynamic radius of the particles), which means that it is slow for polymers, and this can lead to more thermodynamically stable products such as microparticles with lower interfacial energy than nanoparticles due to a slower nanoprecipitation process as shown by the Einstein–Stokes equation (Equation (2)).

$$D = \frac{kT}{6\pi\eta R}, \tag{2}$$

where D is the diffusion coefficient for a particle in a free volume, k is the Boltzmann constant, T is the absolute temperature, η is the viscosity of the solution, and R is the hydrodynamic radius of the particles. Considering the diffusion coefficient for poly(ethylene glycol) (PEG) 1 kDa polymer ($D \approx 3 \times 10^{-10}$ $m^2 \cdot s^{-1}$) in water, the solution would cover 100 μm in 30 s which would need a flow rate of 1 $mL \cdot min^{-1}$ in a channel that would be at least 15 cm long.

Often, materials and solvents are chosen to maximize the reciprocal diffusion coefficient and to minimize viscosity. Typically, the geometry and nature of the flow are designed to act on the area of convergence of the different fluids or the area immediately after (mixing region) (Figure 2). Hydrodynamic flow focusing (HFF) devices focus on the confluence point and control the width of a central flow that carries the material of interest and is enveloped by lateral flows. The second type aims to transition from a laminar to chaotic flow. Although this can be achieved by curvilinear channels, passive micromixers typically have paths with complex and tortuous shapes. Heterogeneity in the flow itself, e.g., by introducing high-molecular-weight polymers that alter microviscosity of the liquid, can also contribute toward achieving chaotic mixing [127,128]. Static mixer efficiency is usually compared via the Peclet number (length of channel) as it is indicative of the ratio between mass transport through convective (chaotic flow) and diffusive flux (laminar flow) and is calculated using Equation (3).

$$Pe = \frac{vl}{D}, \tag{3}$$

where v is the velocity of the fluid, l is the characteristic length of the fluid, and D is the diffusion coefficient. Micromixers are regularly categorized as being active or passive, subject to the used mechanism for the formation of mixing processes at the microscale. Active devices introduce chaotic features by exploiting exterior energy powers and energy of the fluid pumping, to make time-restrained perturbations of the flow field and expedite the mixing procedure (Figure 2) [129]. According to the type of external force used, micromixers can be subdivided as driven by ultrasound energy (acoustic/cavitation) [141], pressure field [142], or magneto-hydrodynamics [143], or induced by temperature [144].

These micromixers have typically higher mixing yield in comparison with passive micromixers [145]. However, the application of these devices in practical situations is limited due to the necessity of integrating the system with secondary equipment (i.e., actuators for an exterior energy source) and the expensive and laborious manufacturing processes. Additionally, the application of external energy powers (e.g., ultrasonic waves) may lead to the formation of high-temperature gradients, which can possibly destroy involved or loaded bioactive molecules. Therefore, these mixers are not a common option when using microfluidics to chemical, pharmaceutical, and biological applications [145]. Passive mixers are the leading microfluidic devices due to the ease of their manufacturing methods and associated cost-effectiveness in comparison with active micromixers. The mixing time reduction is obtained through various approaches, including focusing fluid flows using hydrodynamic principles [146], fluid stream splitting benefiting from parallel or serial lamination [147], increasing chaotic advection employing designed groves and ribs on walls of the channel [148,149], and introducing bubbles of liquid (droplet) or gas (slug) into the stream (Figure 2) [150,151]; these were previously summarized thoroughly [152]. Although the geometry of the channel is critical in the mixing and, thus, nanoprecipitation, the engineering of microfluidic devices remains complex and available to limited manufacturers for microfluidic devices. Recent attempts have utilized 3D printing to enable the production of easily tailored geometries toward the production of microfluidic devices for the manufacture of nanomedicines [1,153].

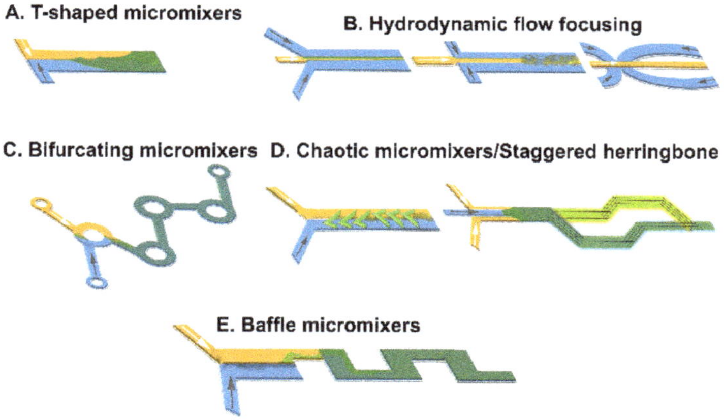

Figure 2. Summary of schematic designs of microfluidic mixers for lipid nanoparticle development: (**A**) T-shaped mixer, (**B**) hydrodynamic flow focusing, (**C**) bifurcating mixers, (**D**) chaotic, staggered micromixers, and (**E**) baffle mixers.

3.1.2. Microreactor Design and Mixing

A quick mass/heat transfer can significantly enhance the controllability of the mixing process that subsequently defines the physicochemical characteristics of the manufactured nanomaterials. Considering the mixing method and device features, microreactors for production of nanomaterials can be categorized into two types: segmented and continuous microreactors (Figure 2).

Microreactors with Continuous Flow

Microreactors with continuous flow in comparison with segmented flow are usually recognized by higher efficiency and the feasibility to continuously alter the composition of reactants through the reaction channel [154–156]. Accordingly, it is practicable to obtain multistep procedures by linking various reactors in series [157]. As the stream pattern is simple, scaling up can be obtained by easily enhancing the rate of used flow [158]. These microreactors can also be grouped into three main subtypes based on their microchannel network architecture (i.e., micromixer, coaxial flow, and capillary tube).

Capillary tube devices have the simplest configuration and are made of polymer [159], steel [160], or silica [161] capillary tubes with the lumen diameter of channels in the micron range, where an enhanced nanoparticle yield can be obtained through quick and precise temperature control. Their easy operation and production, along with the feasibility to employ robust materials, make them capable of tolerating the necessities of high-temperature applications, increasing the interest in capillary devices for manufacturing of nanocrystals of semiconductor and metallic nanomaterials. However, there are risks of chemical adhesion to the surface of channels, lumen blockage, and comparatively high polydispersity in products in the application of these devices [161,162]. To tackle these challenges, microreactors with coaxial stream have been designed [157,163]. Flögel et al. applied a silicon continuous flow microreactor for peptide synthesis and showed that the employed microreactor not only enables scanning the reaction conditions quickly, but also empowers the procurement of synthetically appropriate amounts of peptides [164]. It was demonstrated that coupling of peptide with 9-fluorenylmethoxycarbonyl (Fmoc)- and *tert*-butyloxycarbonyl (Boc)-protected amino acids was achieved at 120 °C in 1–5 min, and a further improvement in synthesis efficiency of β-peptides was also achieved via the application of a fluorous benzyl tag [164]. The ability to undertake couplings within the chips remains a desirable feature if functionalized particles are intended as similar chemistry is employed. In microreactors with coaxial flow, the direct contact of the reaction mixture with the channel walls are prevented by an ensheathing stream to minimize adhesion to the walls and clogging of the channels, while eliciting nanomaterials with reduced polydispersity, as the stream comprising the precipitating species is at the center of the channel center where the fluid velocity is more homogeneous compared to the flow near the channel walls. This results in a more homogeneous residence time distribution for the growing nanomaterials inside the microreactor, and various growing nanomaterials have a similar growth time within the process [157,163]. Lipid emulsions injected in flow-focusing microfluidic chips were also shown to be able to entrap microspheres, proteins, and cells [165]. A dispersed phase of aqueous solutions consisting of cells, microspheres, or proteins was sheared by the continuous phase of dissolved phospholipids in oleic acids to produce stable lipid emulsions. The prepared emulsions were injected into a mixture of ethanol and water that was an appropriate solvent for oleic acid. Forcing phospholipids in the acid resulted in rearrangement at the emulsion surface toward lipid particles due to rapid dissolution of the oleic acid into the ethanol. The encapsulated cells remained viable, and the efficiency of encapsulation depended on the flow rate of the continuous phase and on the ethanol concentration in the mixture to eliminate excess oleic acids [165]. In addition to lipidic particles, this was also applied to polymersomes [166]. Double emulsions with a core–shell structure (aqueous cores) were manufactured using a flow focusing chip and subsequently dispersed in a continuous phase of water containing glycerol (80% v/v). The emulsion shell was a layer of the cosolvent mixture of toluene and tetrahydrofuran containing the di-block copolymers of poly(n-butyl acrylate)/poly(acrylic acid). As tetrahydrofuran was exceedingly miscible with water, in the outer layer of the double emulsions, the cosolvent diffused into the continuous phase, resulting in the self-assembly of di-block copolymers on the double emulsion concentric interfaces [166]. Polymersomes with a stable membrane and a uniform size were formed when the evaporation step was completed. Evaluating membrane permeability revealed that the polymersomes with 1.5 μm thick walls were comparable in permeability to those with a thickness of ~10–20 nm. This finding showed the possibility of thickness inhomogeneities in the manufactured vesicles (membranes) [166]. A similar microfluidic approach was used to fabricate biocompatible monodisperse polymersomes with a membrane of poly(ethylene-glycol)-*b*-polylactic acid [167] that showed that the release of the encapsulated hydrophilic fluorescent solute could be affected by osmotic pressure differences. They studied the formation process of di-block copolymers with various molecular weight ratios of the hydrophobic and the hydrophilic blocks, such as PEG(5000)-*b*-PLA(1000), PEG(1000)-*b*-PLA(5000), and PEG(5000)-*b*-PLA(5000), which revealed that the properties of the polymersomes could be altered by incorporating various homopolymers and altering the hydrophobic and hydrophilic block ratio [167].

MHF microfluidic techniques have been shown to produce uniformly dispersed liposomes and allow for the direct control of liposome size via fine adjustments to either the flow rate ratio (FRR) or the total flow rate (TFR) [168]. A micromixer with basic channel configuration (i.e., Y-shaped) was applied to fabricate hydrocortisone (a drug with poor water solubility) nanosuspensions [169], boehmite and barium sulfate nanocrystals [158], and cadmium sulfide [170]. However, these have not been used for lipid-based nanoparticles apart from studies that utilized Y-shaped mixers incorporating staggered herringbone elements to induce chaotic advection [171,172], where the resulting liposome size correlated with the FRR in the microfluidics process (~50 nm), and high-throughput manufacturing of liposomes of similar CQAs was possible by increasing fourfold the volumetric flow rate [171]. Microfluidic hydrodynamic focusing (MHF) T-shaped chips and coaxial geometries were used for the one-pot synthesis of injectable size liposomes [173]. Narrowly distributed unilamellar nanoliposomes (~85 nm, polydispersity index of 0.13) with a composition similar to that of Doxil®/Caelyx® could be synthesized at production rates 15–20 times larger compared to T-shaped MHF chips, and the size depended on the Reynolds number (5–50) in the coaxial configuration due to viscosity-induced mixing dynamics at the water–ethanol interface [173].

Microreactors with Segmented Flow

Microreactors with segmented flows can be divided into multiphase (liquid–liquid) stream or slug (gas–liquid) stream microfluidic devices [174–176]. A significant variable, which impacts on the monodispersity of the synthesized nanomaterials is the residence time distribution (the average spent time in the reactor). In microfluidic reactors with a laminar flow, the parabolic stream profile (i.e., slower fluid movement near the walls of channel compared to that of the fluid in the center of the channel) and the accompanied axial dispersion result in a difference in residence time that subsequently causes a broader distribution in the size of the prepared nanomaterials [177]. This issue in reactors with a laminar flow can be addressed by employing microreactors with a segmented stream, which result in a proper control on the size and size distribution of nanoparticles. This is due to slugs (gas–liquid) or droplets (liquid–liquid) that can act as a microscale reactor and flow through the channel during the process time (this is only determined by the rate of the flow). In these microreactors, mixing is obtained by leveraging the microflow produced inside the droplet or slug while it is streaming through the winding and straight channels [177]. In other words, extremely short residence times can be established using this approach, and the point of particle formation can, therefore, be better defined. The principle of flow focusing in microchannels has been used to successfully precipitate organic nanoparticles [178–180]. An additional compartmentation in droplets or plugs can suppress the free convection, and particle growth is controlled by diffusion and convection within the nanoliter compartments [181]. The segmentation of the continuous flow by injection of gas creates Taylor flows with plugs in which a recirculating convection occurs [182]. Accordingly, the mixing is intensified. Different studies have investigated the enhanced mixing processes in these two-phase flows [183,184]. Nevertheless, Taylor flows in microfluidic systems with separated flow focusing and gas displacement can become unstable, and nonperiodic tear-off in the gas bubbles impedes the control of plug volumes and mixing. Furthermore, in continuous flow focusing systems, nanoparticles precipitate immediately and can stick to the channel walls, leading to fouling jeopardizing stable operation and small particle sizes. Slug-flow reactors have the advantage of easy gas separation from the final reaction medium. Thus, there is no need for further post-purification processes. However, the process should be conducted very carefully in limited volumes to obtain a steady pattern of the multiphase gas flow [158]. The first microfluidic system based on droplets for producing unilamellar liposomes was studied by Tan et al. [165]. This study showed that proteins, cells, and beads could be efficiently encapsulated in liposomes with 27 to 55 μm in diameters and could facilitate ion exchange between the external environment and inner compartment [165]. This approach was also used to fabricate size controlled segmented wormlike micelles by polystyrene-*block*-poly(4-vinyl pyridine) self-assembly [185]. Comparing the assembly of these micelles with off-chip assembled block copolymers at the same solution characteristics revealed that the prepared segmented wormlike micelles were thermodynamically metastable structures and kinetically controlled assemblies, which were created by the aggregation of preformed spherical micelles in an ordered manner due to the quick mixing procedure in microfluidic channels. Furthermore, by altering the total flow velocity or the flow velocity ratio of the block copolymer and water solution, both the sizes and the percentages of segmented wormlike micelles among the whole assemblies were effectively controlled [185]. Additionally, microfluidic approaches have been employed to produce lipid vesicles (layer-by-layer asymmetric). Matosevic et al. developed an assembly-line procedure with the capability to perform a completely reproducible and parameterized phospholipid vesicle manufacture [186]. The feasibility of a flow focusing device for the fabrication of droplets and the subsequent (phospholipid) stabilization was later demonstrated as multilamellar asymmetric vesicles were formed by droplets trapping within pockets and by gradually exchanging the continuous phase with a secondary phase, including various types of phospholipids that can be deposited on the formerly created bilayer [187]. A symmetric design of a segmented flow device with the capability to combine flow focusing and segmentation was also described in which the backflow of liquid into the gas channel is suppressed, avoiding destabilization of the injected gas bubble that causes premature precipitation [188]. Consequently, the symmetric design not only widened the range of stable Taylor flows, but also allowed operation for longer periods without severe fouling [188]. Tuning the time allowance for complete mixing down to 9 ms was achieved, and lipid nanodroplets with tunable sizes down to 74 nm were fabricated [188]. However, fouling was observed when an ethanolic Softisan© 100 was used as the mixture of triglycerides crystallized within the channel. Deposition of lipid material in a segmented flow micromixer could be reduced through a modification of the design [189]. The investigated segmented flow micromixer was fabricated from 700 μm thick glass wafers and had a symmetrical design with three inlets for the aqueous and ethanolic liquid phase, as well as for the gas phase, in diameters of 193 μm, 87 μm, and 146 μm, respectively. Castor oil and glycerol monooleate (monoolein) were used in this study due to their good solubility in ethanol (>100 mg·mL^{-1}) [189], resulting in nanoemulsions with a droplet size between 120 and 200 nm and polydispersity indices of 0.14, when the surfactant was included via the aqueous phase, or smaller sizes when the surfactant was included via the ethanolic phase.

Micromixer Channel Dimensions and Residence Time Effects

Microreactors, in addition to the ability to effectively control the characteristics of prepared nanomaterials dimensionally, can be used to control and study the fundamental reaction procedures in the formation of nanomaterials [155,190]. Several methods, including small-angle X-ray scattering, spectroscopy, and spatially resolved photoluminescence imaging, are employed to study the kinetics of nanoprecipitation [191–195]. Continuous flow in microscale channels allows precise temporal and spatial control of reactions via the addition of reagents at predetermined time intervals within the reaction process. These characteristics allow microfluidic devices to enable pre-/post-treatments, as well as multistep synthetic processes within the reactor. A stream of lipid mixture was hydrodynamically focused at a microchannel cross-junction between two aqueous buffer streams. The formation of liposomes was energetically favorable at points in the system where the concentration of the mixture of isopropyl alcohol and buffer solution reached a critical condition where lipid solubility was low [196], resulting in liposomes (100–300 nm). Furthermore, the effect of mixing performance on the size of lipid nanoparticles using microfluidic methods was studied by Maeki et al. [196] using chaotic micromixers with various depths (i.e., 11 and 31 μm). LNPs with the smallest size and a narrow particle distribution were formed in channels of 31 μm. The size of LNPs could be tuned within 10 nm by ensuring optimum residence time and critical ethanol concentration. The critical ethanol concentration range was estimated to be between 60% and 80% according to laser scanning confocal microscopy. The residence times at the critical concentration necessary to control the LNP size were 10, 15–25, and 50 ms timescales for 30, 40, and 50 nm-sized LNPs, respectively [196].

3.1.3. Heat Transfer and Temperature Control

Temperature is one of crucial factors that needs to be considered during nanomedicine fabrication as it can affect supersaturation, solubility, and kinetics. Microfluidic devices include channels with typical diameters around 10 to 1000 μm with an enhanced ratio of surface to volume (~ 10,000 to 50,000 $m^2 \cdot m^{-3}$) in comparison with macroscale channels (~100 to 2000 $m^2 \cdot m^{-3}$) [138,197]. Microfluidic devices usually show high efficiencies of thermal transfer, and this enables their use for high temperatures and/or exothermic reactions in a controllable and effective (isothermal) way [140,185,186], thus offering effective temperature control in chemical synthesis or functionalization reactions using continuous flow reactors [155,198]. The high surface-to-volume ratio speeds up heat exchange; for example, ~0.4 s is required for a channel of 200 μm diameter to increase the temperature of a liquid from 20 °C to 300 °C [199]. Temperature has multiple effects such as (i) by changing the free energy kT and the diffusion coefficients, (ii) by changing the viscosity, and (iii) by changing the membrane elasticity at or below the transition temperature and by changing the line tension. By modifying three parameters (i.e., volumetric flow rate ratio of the buffer to alcohol, phospholipid acyl chain length, and temperature) using a microfluidic hydrodynamic focusing approach, studies showed that liposomes formed at temperatures below the transition temperature of phospholipids had the largest size compared to those formed at a temperature closer to transition temperature of the lipids [200]. The larger size of liposomes at lower temperatures was due to the membranes having a much higher elastic modulus below the transition temperature. For the liposomes formed at temperatures lower than the transition temperature (e.g., ≤40 °C for 1,2-distearoyl-*sn*-glycero-3-phosphocholine or ≤10 °C for 1,2-dipalmitoyl-*sn*-glycero-3-phosphocholine), the stream of alcohol in the focusing region was not stable and slowly grew over time [200]. At these temperatures at the alcohol–buffer interfaces, large visible aggregates formed in the focusing region. At the bottom and top of the channel, these aggregates were likely the reason behind the unsteady focusing resulting in more polydisperse and larger liposomes at lower flow rate ratios. However, even at low temperatures, smaller liposomes were formed at higher flow rate ratios, although they were still bigger than the liposomes formed at higher temperatures at the same flow rates. Consequently, all tested liposome compositions through this work could produce liposomes using high flow rate ratios at or above room temperature; however, at room temperature, liposomes prepared with 1,2-distearoyl-*sn*-glycero-3-phosphocholine were less reproducible because of flow fluctuations and aggregations in the focusing region [200]. It was shown that the size of the liposomes was decreased in a microfluidic process with decrease in needle diameter (or increase in hydrodynamic pressure), decrease in lipid concentration in the alcohol solution, decrease in phase transition temperature (T_m) of the lipid bilayer, and absence of cholesterol (or decrease in membrane rigidity) [201].

3.2. *Materials for Microfluidic Chip Fabrication Applicable for Nanomaterial Production*

Initial materials for the manufacture of microfluidic devices were taken from microelectronics where silicon is widely used [1,202–204] due to its monocrystalline structure, availability, compatibility of its physicochemical properties with a broad range of applications, and feasibility of integration with electronic circuits. Glass is used due to its desired optical characteristics, low cost, efficient dissipation of heat capability, and high resistance to chemical and mechanical stress [202–205]; crown white, quartz, borosilicate, and soda–lime glasses are the most commonly used types [204,205]. However, the amorphous structure of glasses is the main drawback of these materials due to the possibility of nonparallel wall formation during isotropic wet etching of a glass with hydrofluoric acid. The etching procedure takes place on the exposed surfaces of the glass, and, as the etching process goes further in a channel, there is a simultaneous etching on side walls, also resulting in the formation of channel geometries with low aspect ratios. To achieve a channel with a deep length, dry etching approaches (e.g., deep reactive ion etching) can be used, but this requires costly instrumentation to be processed [204,205]. The prolonged process cycles and complex instruments accompanying the microfabrication of silicones and glasses create a necessity for the development of microfluidic devices using other substances. Polymers are emerging as materials for microfluidic devices [1,138,204,206], with poly(dimethylsiloxane) (PDMS) being a preferred material due to (i) its capability to be molded (elastomeric material), patterned easily into channels, and recreate features in micro-size with high accuracy, (ii) its low water permeability, and (iii) its appropriate optical transparency. PDMS is biocompatible, has low cost and low toxicity, and remains chemically inert, showing mechanical flexibility. The soft nature of the mold has several advantages such as optimal contact between the mold and the surface without the addition of external pressures, while the porous nature allows working both with polymeric solutions and gelling because the solvent can evaporate through the mold. The soft mold, like the PDMS mold, can be used in soft lithography (Figure 3 reproduced from [207]), originating from an original hard master mold generated with other techniques [208].

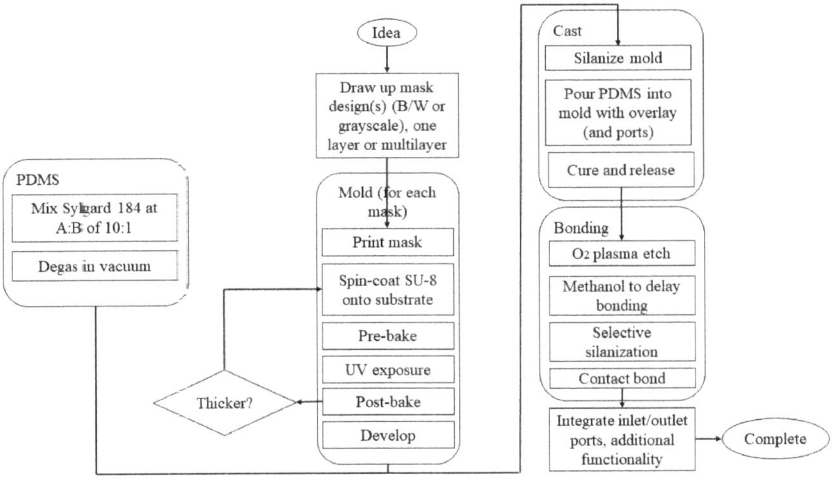

Figure 3. Process of making microfluidic devices using PDMS. Different materials are used to produce the mold, but SU-8 is usually chosen in the production of PDMS-based microfluidic devices. Once the mold has been prepared with the appropriate steps, the next step is casting, followed by hardening and release of PDMS from the mold. The PDMS is deposited on the mold; everything is placed in the oven for 24 h at 65 °C so that the PDMS cures and, once hardened, can be easily removed from the mold. Then, the bonding phase follows, where the surface of the PDMS is generally exposed to oxygen plasma for 10 min and then in contact with a layer of glass or another layer of PDMS to generate a bond. The process ends with the interfacing and integration phase where input and output zones are created with the help of needles, in the case of temporary applications, or with specific structures for longer applications. Reprinted with permission from [207]. Copyright 2022, AIP Publishing LLC.

However, the main drawback of using PDMS in the synthesis of organic nanoparticles is its poor resistance to organic solvents (it is swelled in the presence of organic solvents), including aromatic and aliphatic hydrocarbons, while it is dissolved in strong acids (e.g., trifluoroacetic and sulfuric acids) and amines [1,184,193,195]. PDMS chips require manual operations during manufacture and clean rooms, while manufacturing devices in series is not possible; thus, the process remains very costly with long manufacturing times [207].

For this reason, other manufacturing techniques have been developed that guarantee the production of microfluidic devices at the nanoscale with time and cost reduction, as well as the possibility to work with different materials. Alternative polymeric substances (i.e., acrylates, modified poly(dimethylsiloxane), polyether ether ketone, cyclic olefin polymer, cyclic olefin copolymer, polycarbonate, and poly(methyl methacrylate)) have recently been used in rapid prototyping approaches to create microfluidic reactors with high resistance to solvents, precise replication ability of micropatterns with high-quality surfaces, and suitability for mass production at a low cost [1,138,153,204,206]. Cyclic olefin copolymers are transparent, amorphous thermoplastics composed of linear olefins (ethene) and monomers of cyclic olefin (norbornene). In comparison with other thermoplastics, cyclic olefin copolymer has apparent advantages, such as low autofluorescence and water absorption, good optical transparency and thermal resistance, and high chemical resistance [209,210]. Due to these promising advantages, they are progressively employed as appropriate materials for the fabrication of microfluidic devices and microsystems [210]. Among the most recent manufacturing techniques, 3D printing is emerging as a low-cost and easily personalized manufacturing technique for prototypes of microfluidic devices without the need of molds and using existing materials such as cyclic olefin co-polymers and polylactic acid or photocurable resins. For instance, stereolithography 3D printers as one of the mostly used printing methods for manufacturing of microfluidic devices use photocurable polymers to fabricate a 3D structure layer by layer [153]. Objects with complex design and geometry, as well as intricate shape, can be printed using high-resolution stereolithography 3D printing [211]. Current stereolithography printing is mostly relies on photocurable resin formulations based on methacrylate or acrylate monomers and crosslinkers. These formulations quickly cure and can be affordably produced at low prices [212]. However, variable mechanical characteristics [213], shrinkage stress [214], and oxygen inhibition [215] because of their early gelation or incomplete cure are some of the potential drawbacks of this method. These challenges can be defeated using other types of resins such as epoxy resins [216], resins based on ring-opening spiro compounds [217], and composite resins [218] in the stereolithography 3D printing context. This has been extensively reviewed previously [1,138,204,206].

4. Microfluidic Manufacture of Lipid-Based Nanomedicines: Studies to Date

Microfluidic manufacture of lipid nanomedicines considering critical parameters such as the lipid concentration, transition temperature, total flow rate (TFR), flow rate ratio (FRR), chip geometry (chip-based or capillary-based), and purification or treatment after elution has yielded systems with controlled CQAs compared to conventional techniques [1,185,195,196,198,206,219–226]. Figure 4 summarizes the advantages and disadvantages of microfluidic and bulk techniques for manufacturing of LNPs [227].

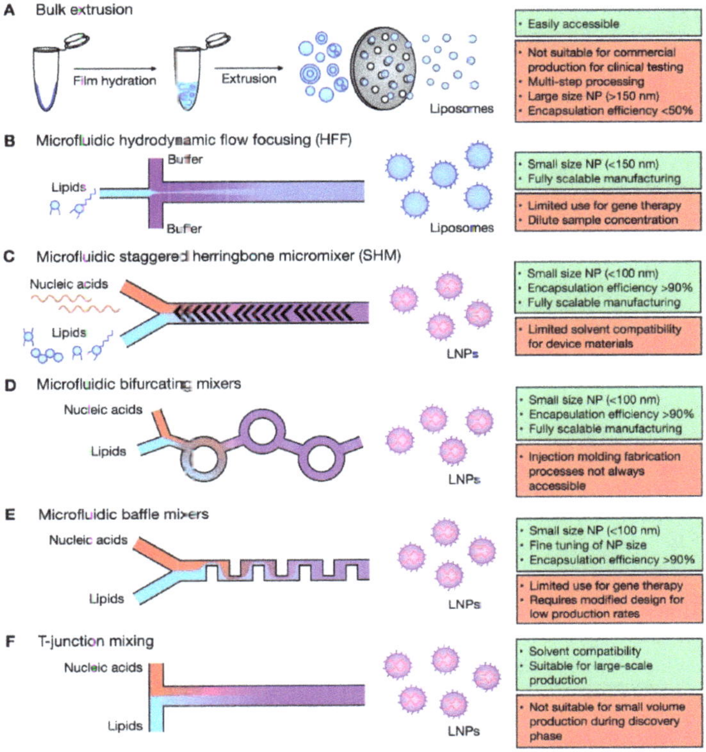

Figure 4. Microfluidic techniques for liposome and lipid nanoparticle (LNP) formulation. Summary of bulk and microfluidic techniques for production of liposomes (**A**,**B**) and lipid nanoparticles (**C**–**F**), highlighting advantages (green) and disadvantages (red) for each. Reproduced with permission from [227] and used under the Creative Commons license permission (CC BY 4.0). Copyright 2021, Elsevier Ltd. All rights reserved.

The size of lipid nanomedicines produced microfluidically is largely dependent on the TFF and FRR, while devices able to enable chaotic mixing are able to control better the size of the particles [228–230]. Rapid mixing has a significant effect on the size of the particle especially if small sizes are required, and 20 nm particles have been demonstrated under high flow rates [150,231]. However, mixing performance under high flow rates is decreased in chaotic mixers due to high *Re* [150,231]. However, recent studies have shown that the size and size distribution in microfluidic manufacture using chaotic mixers does not require complete mixing to control the size of lipid-based nanomedicines of small size. [230].

The formation of lipid-based nanomedicines such as liposomes is governed by the diffusion of different molecular species such as alcohol, water, and lipids at the liquid interface between the solvent (alcohol) and nonsolvent (water in buffer) phases and is dominated by the construction of intermediate disc-like constructs, their stability at the critical aggregate concentration, and their lifetime (Figure 5) [149,196,230]. Larger particle sizes are obtained when a large amount of bilayered phospholipid fragments fuse together, typically when the diffusion of the alcohol to the aqueous phase is slow [196]. Increasing the concentration of lipid is also likely to result in larger sizes [196]. Self-assembly of the hydrophobic chain of lipids occurred due to the solution polarity enhancement as the semi-stable bilayer phospholipid fragments grew until they transformed into thermodynamically stable vesicles (i.e., lipid nanoparticles) due to an enhancement of surface energy. Subsequently, the grown bilayer phospholipid fragments were transformed to lipid nanoparticles to reduce the surface energy in the system. However, if the solvent (e.g., ethanol) is diluted quickly, the phospholipid fragments cannot grow enough to produce lipid nanoparticles (Figure 5) [196].

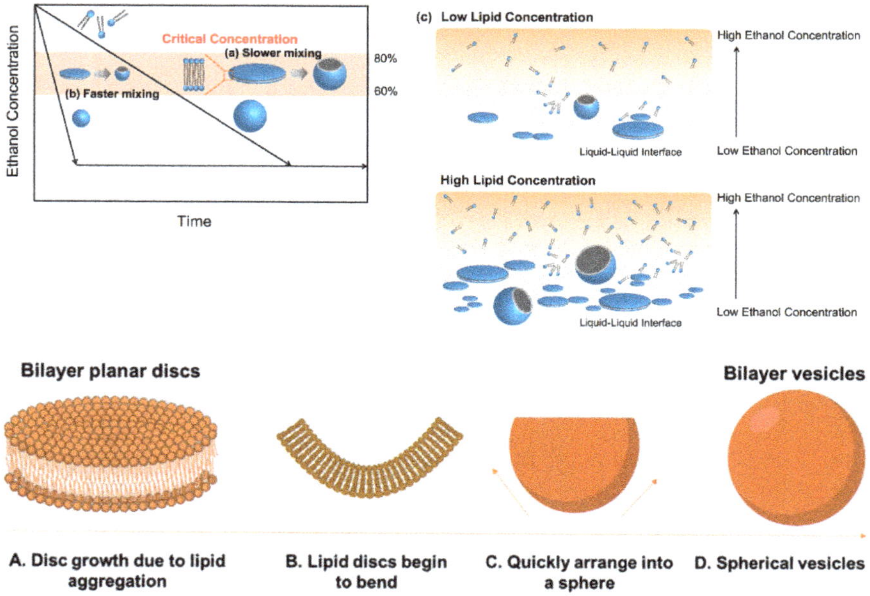

Figure 5. A Schematic diagram depicting a hypothesized LNP formation mechanism. The formation of LNPs in (**a**) slower and (**b**) faster mixing conditions. (**c**) Schematic representation of the formation of LNPs at the interface of ethanol–saline. The process starts with the aggregation of lipids in discs (**A**). The hydrophobic chains around the edges are stabilized by alcohol molecules and, as the alcohol concentration reduces, these lipid discs bend (**B**) and rapidly close (**C**) and form spherical vesicles (**D**). Thus, the polarity change during the liposome formation process is related to the initial polarity of the organic phase. The figure is adapted from **Copyright:** © 2017 Maeki et al. [196] under the terms of the Creative Commons Attribution License. All rights reserved.

4.1. Nanomedicines Prepared with T- or Y-Junction (Shaped) Mixers

These mixers are the simplest and earliest geometric designs (Figures 2A and 4) used for lipid based nanomedicines allowing for a fast mixing process [232], where an anti-solvent and solvent are combined under laminar flow, and diffusion-based mixing takes place at the interface of these two fluids [180]. In devices with Y-shaped geometry, the mixing takes place at the interface of the solvent/aqueous in the surface of the main channel, and the main factor that controls mixing is the rate of diffusion; the fluid mixing time tends to be long at quite low *Re* due to the dominating flow regime that is laminar. Consequently, by modifying the geometric design of these mixers, the capability of application of higher flow rates was created to produce perturbations that could enhance the efficiency of the mixing [233]. A broad range of mixing can be achieved using T-mixer designs with flow regimes from a laminar to a turbulent flow with *Re* in the range of 100 to 4000 [234] for nanomedicines. A segmented gas–liquid flow strategy has been proposed to improve the efficiency of mixing between two miscible liquids and to decrease mixing time, enabling mixing length shortening [150,235]. Recent studies have shown the ability to produce cannabidiol (CBD)-loaded liposomes after passive mixing using 3D fused deposition modeling (FDM)-printed polypropylene T-mixers with either a zigzag bas-relief (a 1 mm square section attached to the zigzag structure having a height of 500 μm and a total length of

60 mm) or a split-and-recombine channel shape (two square inlets at 1 mm to form a T-junction attached to main channel where circular splitting is repeated six times and kept unequal to allow a difference in the fluid velocities leading to unbalanced collisions of fluid streams with the major square sub-channel having a section of 600 μm while the minor sub-channel has a section of 400 μm) [236]. Liposomes were prepared using soya phosphatidylcholine (SPC) and cholesterol (3:1 w/w) and CBD in ethanol at two different lipid concentration (10 and 15 mg/mL) with FRR (1:3 or 1:5 ethanol/water) and a TFR of either 10 or 12 mL·min^{-1}. Mixing was more efficient with an FRR of 1:3 at a TFR of 10 mL·min^{-1} and resulted in liposomes with a size <150 nm and low polydispersity (<0.15) with high loading (~73%) (Table 3) [236]. However, T-mixers alone with no further medication allow for poor control of particle size of fabricated particles and typically require a high volume of starting solutions, which limits their use in pilot studies [237].

4.2. Microfluidic Hydrodynamic Flow (MHF) Focusing

This configuration involves a cross-shaped flattened pattern where laminar flow predominates, and an organic solution is flowed between two streams of aqueous liquids entering from two tubes perpendicular to the organic liquid tube (Figures 2B and 4) [130]. A stream of lipid in alcohol solution is forced to flow in the central channel of the device which is intersected and sheathed by two lateral or coaxial streams of aqueous phase (e.g., buffer), such that the lipid containing stream is hydrodynamically focused into a narrow sheet having a rectangular cross-section (chips with cross flow geometry) or a circular cross-section (3D annular coaxial chips) [168,180,238]. The size of the focused stream is tuned by adjusting the volumetric flow rate ratio (FRR) between the lipid- and water-phase streams and the total flow rate (TFR) [239].

The formation of lipid-based nanomedicines such as liposomes in MHF chips is governed by the diffusion of different molecular species such as alcohol, water, and lipids at the liquid interface between the solvent (alcohol) and nonsolvent (water in buffer) phases [238,240]. The reduction in alcohol concentration in which the lipids are initially solubilized by diffusion into the water and vice versa reaches a critical level below the solubility limit of the lipids, thus triggering the formation of intermediate structures (in the form of oblate micelles) that subsequently form liposomes (self-assembly, Figure 5) [200,238,241]. These devices can fabricate lipid nanoparticles with high encapsulation efficiency in a broad range of particle sizes (i.e., 30−250 nm) [242]. MHF microfluidic techniques produce uniformly dispersed lipid-based particles where the size is controlled by fine adjustments of the FRR and TFR. Decreasing the sample stream width to micrometer length can allow for controlled and reproducible mechanical and chemical conditions across the stream width that has no analogous protocol on the macroscale [243]. The microfluidic parameters that affect the particle characteristic are directly related to lipid concentration [244–246] and inversely related to FRR [238,239], and TFR has only a small effect on overall particle size [180,238,239]. A particle size of 30–250 nm can be obtained without the need for extrusion through the pores of polycarbonate membranes, treatment with ultrasound, homogenization, or repetitive freezing and thawing cycles [180,238].

In most studies, isopropanol (IPA) is used as the lipid solvent (Table 3); however, very few if any studies provide the residual IPA content, and few studies utilize ethanol, which is less toxic for medicinal applications [247,248]. The miscibility of the solvent with the aqueous buffer depends on its chemical structure but also on its surface tension, whereby a lower hydrocarbon chain of the solvent results in higher miscibility. Ethanol, which is almost always the solvent of choice, has a short carbon chain and is able to form hydrogen bonds with water [241]. Safe levels of the solvent in the final formulation and generally regarded as safe (GRAS) status are established according to the International Council for Harmonization guidelines (*ICH guideline Q3C (R8) on impurities: guideline for residual solvents)* [249], representing another parameter that needs to be considered (methanol; ICH class 2, limit: 3000 ppm, ethanol: ICH class 3, ICH limit: 5000 ppm, IPA: ICH Class 3, ICH limit: 3000 ppm) [241]. Studies have shown, however, that methanol–PBS (phosphate-buffered saline) results in smaller vesicles regardless of the lipid component used, while liposomes based on distearoylphosphatidylcholine (DSPC) showed an increase size in ethanol/PBS possibly due to the DSPC being more difficult to solubilize compared to other lipids [250]. Additionally, methanol and ethanol as solvents showed higher ability to load proteins compared to isopropanol [241].

The osmolarity of the buffer used and salt concentration can also affect the size of produced lipid vesicles. For cationic liposomes prepared with 1,2-dioleoyl-*sn*-3-phosphoethanolamine (DOPE) and 1,2-dioleoyl-3-trimethylammonium-propane (DOTAP), the vesicles showed an increased vesicle size from 40 to 600 nm when the Tris buffer concentration increased, while, for neutral liposomes prepared with DSPC and cholesterol, the particle size remained unchanged irrespective of the salt concentration of the buffer [251].

High drug loading can be obtained, and studies have demonstrated that, even for lipid–nucleic acid complexes, encapsulation efficiency can be improved by 20% compared to bulk mixing [242]. MHF mixers can enable the manufacture of stealth liposomes, as well as liposomes with surface modifications (e.g., folic acid as an active targeting ligand) [225]. In this work, a central flow of lipids in isopropanol that was focused using streams of PBS resulted in 55–200 nm liposomes with the size decreasing with increasing PBS-to-isopropanol flow rate ratios [225]. MHF microfluidic devices have been used for manufacturing dual-targeted liposomes functionalized with a cell-penetrating peptide and folic acid that resulted in improved targeting and extended retention in a xenograft ovarian adenocarcinoma tumor model (SK-OV-3) compared to single-functionalized or stealth liposomes alone [223]. The density of the ligands on the surface of these liposomes was independent of the FRR for the cell penetrating peptide and folic acid [223]. In particular for 3D annular coaxial chips, particles with an extremely low polydispersity (<0.05) were demonstrated along with even fourfold higher yield [252]. However, 3D annual coaxial chips require high FRR and, thus, high volumes, which can increase production costs for some therapeutics (e.g., nucleic acids) and can also lead to sample dilution that can require postprocessing to obtain desirable concentrations for preclinical or clinical studies [121]. The lipid concentration typically used for liposomes produced by MHF is relatively low with respect to liposomes present in commercial medicines (Table 3). For liposomes produced with an FRR of 10 or 30, the typical final total concentration of lipids ranges between 0.16 and 0.45 mM; however, in other techniques, this ranges between 0.1 and 2.0 mM according to FRR [168]. This limitation of MHF techniques is particularly critical when microfluidically produced liposomes are compared to liposomes for preclinical or clinical studies, where lipid concentrations range between 5 and 25 mM [253,254]. Even though MHF devices have not been employed as widely as other microfluidic platforms, they deliver remarkable benefits over traditional manufacturing methods (e.g., ethanol injection, extrusion) and can be cost-effective [168,252].

4.3. Microfluidic Staggered Herringbone (SHM) (Chaotic) Micromixers

SHMs are micromixer chips (Figure 2D) that induce chaotic mixing due to their asymmetric protrusions; consequently, they can process lipid nanoparticles with different sizes in a range of 20–140 nm by adjusting the FRR and TFR [149,229,255–257]. These chips are efficient with low-availability materials and have been used for efficient mixing, even of very low volumes of siRNAs (as low as 10 μL), which empowers screening strategies and, therefore, lipid composition identification for early preclinical studies [258]. It is important to note, however, that, as the concentration of lipids increases, the size of liposomes also increases [259]. The impact of the micromixer channel dimensions, FRR, and particle size is not as well characterized, considering that smaller particle size is achieved with higher FRR [228]. Although the micromixer channels need to have internal structure to produce sizes below 50 nm, for low FRR ($\leq$3), micromixer channels of at least 30 μm in diameter are required as smaller channels (~11 μm) were not able to control the size. However, for FRR ($\geq$9), both devices were able to control the size [196]. SHM cycle numbers of 10 were suggested as the limiting cycles to manufacture small-sized LNPs under all FRR conditions [230]. Increasing the contents of PEGylated lipids resulted in lipoplexes using SHM with sizes down to 20 nm and encapsulation efficiencies of siRNA above 95% [228]. Additionally, upscaling of the manufacture of these particles was shown to be feasible at a high rate by device architecture parallelization (six staggered herringbone micromixers into one chip to fabricate lipid-based nanoparticles at 72 mL/min) [228]. Lipid-based nanoparticles in smaller sizes with narrow polydispersity have been shown to be obtained by enhancing the staggered herringbone cycle number or increasing the FRR [230]; however, ten cycles have been shown to elicit particles of desired sizes with narrower polydispersity index and without the undesirable increase in FRR [230]. High pressures are associated with high FRR, and this usually adversely impacts both the chip and the pump used. When SHM strategies are combined with design-of-experiments methodologies, quick optimization of desired formulation for siRNA is possible and results in formulations that were reported to elicit to sevenfold higher expression compared to traditional preparation methods [260,261]. Studies have also demonstrated that an enhanced identification of hits is possible by combining molecular barcoding with SHM microfluidic preparation toward a library of lipid-based nanoparticles with encapsulated factor VII siRNA or identical DNA barcodes to investigate hepatic gene silencing and accumulation of particles [262,263]. SHM strategies have been used to formulate lipid-based particles loaded with poorly soluble drugs. Propofol-loaded liposomes prepared using phosphatidylcholine and cholesterol allowed aqueous dispersions of propofol of ~300 mg·mL^{-1} that were 2000-fold higher as a function of propofol's aqueous solubility (0.15 mg·mL^{-1}) [264]. These liposomes also surpassed the solubilization capacity of liposomes prepared using conventional sonication methods (120 mg·mL^{-1}) [264]. However, the major drawback of using chaotic mixer devices for the production of LNPs is the possibility of their groove's blockage by LNPs that leads to the sample flow stagnation [265].

4.4. Bifurcating Mixer

Although SHM micromixers have been effective in the manufacture of controlled lipid-based nanoparticles, their production rate is limited to a low TFR due to their microchannel design (Table 4), which might prove challenging in large-scale manufacture. As the recent pandemic has demonstrated, the pharmaceutical industry was only able to respond to the unmet societal needs by utilizing current technologies to rapidly optimize and enable large-scale manufacture of mRNA lipid-based vaccines as targeted and safe delivery carriers with acceptable toxicological profile. NxGen (Precision Nanosystems, San Francisco, CA, USA) has been proposed as a novel chip design based on bifurcating mixers in series (Figure 2C), also known as a toroidal mixer. The fluid flow in this device is divided and subsequently combined several times to create a rapidly mixed environment. NxGen technology is able to produce lipid-based nanomedicines at a high rate (up to 200 mL·min^{-1}), while maintaining the same effectiveness of SHM micromixers and control over the particle polydispersity and encapsulation efficiency [266]. GenVoy-ILM™, a proprietary ionizable lipid mix formulation loaded with PolyA (N/P 6), was produced using different microfluidic mixers: a staggered herringbone (SHM) and a toroidal mixer (TrM) (NanoAssemblr Classic and NxGen™ respectively; Precision NanoSystems Inc., Vancouver, BC, Canada). The produced GenVoy-ILM™-based Poly (A) iLNP nanoparticles were diluted to an ethanol concentration below 1% and ultracentrifuged at 3000 rpm using 10 kDa MWCO ultrafiltration units for the removal of solvent [266]. An in vitro and in vivo investigation of gene editing using the transthyretin gene (Cas9 mRNA and sgRNA) complexed with lipid-based nanoparticles for single guide RNA delivery in murine models demonstrated that the optimized editing formulation resulted in knockdown of transthyretin protein (>97%) for a year [267]. Other studies also showed that using this technology cholesterol can be substituted with other derivatives and that β-sitosterol enabled enhanced transfection in vitro for mRNA [268].

4.5. Baffle Mixers

In addition to bifurcating mixer platforms, another design of microfluidic devices has been applied for the controlled fabrication of lipid-based nanoparticles and liposomes. In baffle mixers, a series of perpendicular turns are designed in pathways of a fluid to mix components of lipid-based nanoparticles more rapidly (Figure 2E) [269]. To overcome the issue of sample flow stagnation observed with SHM, a two-dimensional baffle mixer (iLiNP) was developed [269]. Lipid nanoparticles with an average size of 20 nm to 100 nm were formulated, with 10 nm intervals, by adjusting the flow rate and its ratio, as well as the device dimensions. Thus, the size could be manipulated in 10 nm intervals by adjusting the TFR and FRR and device dimensions. However, a device with a chaotic mixer structure produced LNPs sized in the narrow range of 30 to 40 nm at the same flow rate conditions (FFR 9) [269]. The authors stated that the secondary flow generation in the iLiNP device was indispensable for tuning the size of LNPs and fabricating the small-sized LNPs [269]. Factor VII gene silencing in ICR mice was found to be more than 90% at a predetermined dose of lipid nanoparticles (YSK-5 and 1,2-dimuristoyl-*rac*-glycero-3-methoxypolyethylene glycol) of siRNA (0.1 mg/kg) manufactured using a baffle mixer [269]. In general, baffle and bifurcating mixers are both single-layer chips that have demonstrated feasibility for the production of lipid nanoparticles as alternative approaches to SHM and MHF, while they are capable of being used in screening with low availability of material.

Table 3. Summary of microfluidic manufactured lipid-based nanomedicines.

Delivery System/Lipids	Drug/API	Chip Design	FRR (aq:org)	TFR ($mL \cdot min^{-1}$)	In Vitro Findings	In Vivo Findings	Optimized Formula			Ref.
							Mean Diameter (nm)	PDI	LE%	
Lipoplex/ DOTAP:EPC:DOPE	pDNA	FF Patterned walls FF	10:1	140 $mm \cdot s^{-1}$	Transfection efficacy ~10 × 10^7 relative light units (RLU)·mg of protein^{-1} Transfection efficacy ~6 × 10^7 RLU·mg of protein^{-1}	NA	~135 ~115	~2.3 ~2.0	NA	[270]
Lipid nanoparticles/ mPEG-DSPC:POPC	AmB	NASHM T-junction	3:1	12 24	IC_{50}: 0.085 $\mu g \cdot mL^{-1}$, hemolytic at ≥25 $\mu g \cdot mL^{-1}$	NA	~39	~0.115	88	[271]
Liposomes/ SPC:Chol (3:1 *w/w*)	CBD	T-junction and zig zag or split and combine	1:5	10	NA	NA	~110	~0.13	~73	[236]
Lipoplex/ DOTAP:DOPE:DOPC:DSPE-PEG_{2000}-FolA or DOTAP:DOPE:DOPC:DSPE-PEG_{2000}	siRNA	HFF	9:1	0.0167	In vitro studies on wildtype epithelial carcinoma KB cells show endosomal uptake in the perinuclear region	NA	~40	NA	~60	[242]
Targeted Lipoplex/ DODMA:DOTMA or DCChol:EggPC:mPEG-DSPE) modified with Tf	siRNAs (LOR-1284)	HFF	5:1	0.025–2.000	siRNA complex was stable in serum for 8 h compared to 40% of free siRNA; no significant cytotoxicity in MV4-11 cells; 6.14-fold reduction in IC_{50} for siRNA complex (105.27 nM) and increased downregulation compared to free siRNA	20% of IV dose remained in plasma after 24 h ($t_{1/2}$: 10.2 h, AUC: 5.5 h $\mu g \cdot mL^{-1}$) compared to 1% for free siRNA. ($t_{1/2}$: 2.93 h); 3-fold increase in $t_{1/2}$ and decreased protein expression by 86%.	~80	NA	91.5 ± 4.5	[272]
Transferrin-conjugated Lipoplex (Tf-LNPs-MF)/ DOTMA:DODMA:EPC: Chol:mPEG-Cho	siRNAs	SHM	3 inlets: 3:1:1	NA	Increased permeability in HepG-2 cells by Tf receptor mediated uptake	Tf-LNPs-MF-siRNA in blood was >100 $ng \cdot mL^{-1}$ and $t_{1/2}$ was 25.6 h 48 h post IV vs. <10 $ng \cdot mL^{-1}$ and $t_{1/2}$ of 15.1 h for free siRNA	132.6	0.129	N/A	[224]
Lipoplex/ DLinKC2-DMA(cationic lipid):Chol:DSPC:PEG_{2000}-C-DMA	siRNAs	SHM	3:1	0.02–4.00	NA	50% silencing in hepatocytes at 10 $\mu g \cdot kg^{-1}$ in mice	28–54	<0.1	~100	[228]
Lipoplex/ DSPC:$mPEG_{2000}$-DMG:Chol:range of cationic lipids	siRNAs	SHM	1:1:2 (lipids: siRNA: buffer	1.2	NA	Gene silencing potency of >90% at 1.0 $mg \cdot kg^{-1}$ in mice	90.5	NA	~80	[258]

Table 3. *Cont.*

Delivery System/Lipids	Drug/API	Chip Design	FRR (aq:org)	TFR (mL·min^{-1})	In Vitro Findings	In Vivo Findings	Optimized Formula			Ref.
							Mean Diameter (nm)	PDI	LE%	
Cubosomes/ DOTAP:Glycerol monooleate (GMO):GMO-PEG_{2000}	siRNAs	SHM	6:1	4	Gene-knockdown efficiency of 73.6% for a $\rho = n_{DOTAP}/n_{NA}$ of 3 vs. Lipofectamine (45.8%) efficiency; Up to $\rho = 10$, no significant damage to cell membranes.	NA	77	0.06	>90%	[273]
Lipid nanoparticles/ YSK05 (cationic pH-sensitive lipid):Chol:mPEG2000-DMG	siRNA	SHM	3:1	1.5	Particles with 1%, 1.25%, and 1.5% *w*/*w* and <2% mPEG (67.1, 57.3, and 53.8 nm) show high and similar gene silencing efficiencies	FVII gene silencing activity of 50% Chol-rich 1% mPEG-LNPs was higher than 3% mPEG-LNPs	32−67	NA	~100	[274]
Lipid nanoparticles/ YSK05 (cationic pH-sensitive lipid):Chol:mPEG2000-DMG	siRNA	Baffle mixers	3:1	0.5	NA	YSK-LNPs showed high FVII gene-silencing activity with no dose dependency	80	0.1	>90%	[269]
Liposomes/ EPC:DMPC:DPPC:DSPC	Metformin (M) and glipizide (G)	NASHM	5:1	5–15	Sustained release was achieved	NA	80–90	0.11–0.22	~20 (M) ~40 (G)	[250]
Lipid nanoparticles/ DSPC:D-Lin-MC3-DMA:Chol:PEG-DMG	siRNA	NASHM	3:1	12	79% mRNA knockdown produced by 1 µg siRNA	15 mg·kg^{-1} (3 doses IV over 24 h) results in a 100% uptake in peripheral blood cells that remain positive until day 10; no liver toxicity or other biochemical alternation; after 10 IV doses over 35 days, luciferase signal decreased 0.75-fold, while it increased in control mice 1.6-fold; 60% knockdown efficiency of BCR-ABL by LNP-anti-BCR-ABL siRNA in sorted leukemia cells from the myelosarcoma mouse tissue	55.03	0.046	>90	[275]

Table 3. *Cont.*

Delivery System/Lipids	Drug/API	Chip Design	FRR (aq:org)	TFR (mL min^{-1})	In Vitro Findings	In Vivo Findings	Optimized Formula			Ref.
							Mean Diameter (nm)	PDI	LE%	
Liposomes/ DSPC:mPEG$_{2000}$-DSPE	Dox, ICU	SHM	10:1 and/or 16:1	5	After 48 h, ~90% of drug was released (first order); less cytotoxic to MCF-7, MDA-MB 231 and BT-474 breast cancer cells vs. free doxorubicin	NA	~100	0.2	>80	[276]
Liposomes/ DMPC:DPPC:DSPC	Curcumin	NASHM	5:1	17	Increased 700-fold the aqueous curcumin solubility	When co-administered with cisplatin, it enhances cisplatin's efficacy in multiple mouse tumor models with decreased nephrotoxicity	~125	<0.2	87.7	[277]
Nanoemulsions/ Cold pressed hempseed oil:lecithin:Poloxamer 188	Hempseed oil	NASHM	4:1	12	>98% Caco-2 cell viability; increased uptake by 38.2%	NA	62	0.032	> 99	[278]
Liposomes/ HSPC:DOPC:mPEG$_{2000}$-DSPE	Dox	NASHM	9:1	10	Burst release (20–30%) followed by <10% release over 7 days at 37 °C or during 3 weeks storage at 4 °C	Higher tumor accumulation (5–6% dose/g) at days 1 and 4.	~50	<0.2	> 80	[279]
Liposomes/ EPC or DMPC or DPPC or DSPC or PS:Chol	OVA	NASHM	3:1	15	Longer chain lipids have slower release rates; burst release observed within 12 h followed by a slower release rate	NA	60–100	<0.2	20–35	[280]
Liposomes/ EPC:Chol	Propofol	NASHM	3:1	2	Burst release (40%,1 h) reaching 90% within 8 h	NA	~40	0.4	85	[264]
Liposomes/DMPC:Chol:DEPE-PEG2000:DSPE-PEG$_{2000}$—FA or DSPE-PEG$_{2000}$-Cys-TAT(CYGRKKRRQRRR) 55:40:3:1 molar ratio	Folic acid (FA)	HFF	16:1	28.8 µL/min	FA and TAT liposomes have 37% and 98% increased targeting in SKOV3 cell spheroids compared to TAT liposomes and FA liposomes, respectively	Improved tumor targeting and longer tumor retention (up to 72 h); 140%, 136%, and 62% higher tumor accumulation than pegylated liposomes and FA or TAT targeted liposomes, respectively	~60	<0.3	NA	[223]
Lipoplex/DSPC:cholesterol: DOTAB or DDAB or D-Lin-MC3-DMA:DMG-PEG$_{2000}$,	mRNA or ssDNA, Poly A	NxGen	5:1–1:1	12–200	NA	NA	<100	<0.25	>90	[266]

Table 3. *Cont.*

Delivery System/Lipids	Drug/API	Chip Design	FRR (aq:org)	TFR (mL·min^{-1})	In Vitro Findings	In Vivo Findings	Optimized Formula			Ref.
							Mean Diameter (nm)	PDI	LE%	
Liposomes/HSPC:Chol:DSPE-PEG_{2000} 56:38:5 molar ratio and EPC:Chol 45:55 molar ratio	Dox	M110P Microfluidizer®	Pressures of 5–20 Kpsi	1–3 cycles	NA	NA	100–110	<0.2	97–98	[281]

Key: **AmB**: amphotericin B, **BT-474**: human ductal breast carcinoma cells, **Chol**: cholesterol, **DCChol**: 3β-[*N*-(*N*′,*N*′-dimethylaminoethane)carbamoyl] cholesterol, **DDAB**: DLin-MC3-DMA: (6Z,9Z,28Z,31Z)-heptatriacont-6,9,28,31-tetraene-19-yl 4-(dimethylamino)butanoate, **DLinKC2-DMA**: 2-[2,2-bis[(9Z,12Z)-octadeca-9,12-dienyl]-1,3-dioxolan-4-yl]-*N*,*N*-dimethylethanamine (ionizable cationic lipid), **DMPC**: 1,2-dimyristoyl-*sn*-glycero-3-phosphocholine, **DPPC**: 1,2-diplmitoylphosphatidylcholine, **DODMA**: 1,2-dioleyloxy-*N*,*N*-dimethyl-3-aminopropane, **DOL**: dolomite microfluidic system equipped with a 5-input chip (part: 3200735, Dolomite, Royston, UK), **DOPC**: DOPE: l-α-dioleoyl phosphatidylethanolamine, **DOTAP**: 1,2-dioleoyl-3-trimethylammonium propane, **DOTMA**: *N*-[1-(2,3-dioleyloxy)propyl]-*N*,*N*,*N*-trimethylammonium chloride, **DSPC**: 1,2-distearoyl-*sn*-glycero-3-phosphocholine, **DSPE-PEG$_{2000}$**: 1,2-distearoyl-*sn*-glycero-3-phosphoethanolamine-*N*-[methoxy(polyethylene glycol)-2000] (ammonium salt); **DSPE-PEG$_{2000}$-FolA**: 1,2-distearoyl-*sn*-glycero-3-phosphoethanolamine-*N*-[folate(polyethylene glycol)-2000] (ammonium salt), **DSPC**: 1,2-distearoyl-*sn*-glycero-3-phosphocholine, **DSPG**: 1,2-distearoyl-*sn*-glycero-3-phospho-(1′-*rac*-glycerol), **Dox**: doxorubicin, **EPC**: egg phosphatidylcholine, **FF**: flow focusing, **HFF**: hydrodynamic flow focusing, **HSPC**: hydrogenated soy l-α-phosphatidylcholine, **ICU**: isoprenylated coumarin umbelliprenin, **LE**: loading efficiency, **NxGen**: NxGen (Precision Nanosystems, CA, USA), **MCF-7**: human breast adenocarcinoma cells (hormone-positive), **MDA-MB 231**: human breast adenocarcinoma cells (triple-negative), **mPEG-CHO**: methoxy poly(ethylene glycol) aldehyde, **mPEG: DMG**: dimirystoyl-*sn*-glycero, methoxyethyleneglycol 2000 ether, **mPEG$_{2000}$-DSPC**:1,2-distearoyl-*sn*-glycero-3 phosphoethanolamine-*N*-[methoxy-(polyethylene glycol)-2000], **NASHM**: NanoAssemblr Benchtop with SHM, **OVA**: ovalbumin, **PDI**: polydispersity, **PEG$_{2000}$-C-DMA**: *N*-[(methoxy poly(ethylene glycol)$_{2000}$ carbamyl]-1,2-dimyristyloxlpropyl-3-amine, **POPC**: 1-palmitoyl-2-oleoyl-*sn*-glycero-3-phosphocholine, **PS**: L-α-phosphatidylserine, **SKOV-3** cells: human ovarian cancer cells, **SHM**: staggered herringbone micromixer, **SPC**: soy phosphatidylcholine, **TAT** cell-penetrating peptide sequence: CYGRKKRRQRRR, **TF**: transferrin, **YSK05**: 1-methyl-4,4-bis[(9Z,12Z)-9,12-octadecadien-1-yloxy]-piperidine (pH-sensitive cationic lipid).

Table 4. Summary of microfluidic purification techniques for nanoparticles. Adapted with permission from [282] and used under the Creative Commons license permission (CC BY 3.0). Copyright 2017, Royal Society of Chemistry. All rights reserved.

Techniques	Mechanism	Separation Marker	Sizes Separated (nm)	Efficiency (%)	Throughput (mL·min^{-1})	Pros	Cons
Field flow fractionation	Asymmetrical flow FFF	Size	5–250	87–88	0.4–1.1	Very high throughput with high separation efficiency	Specific sample/solvent systems and compatible membrane
Centrifugal	Centrifugal force	Size, density	50–200	-	0.0075	High throughput, density gradient, and dilution not required	Discontinuous
Optical	Optical force	Size, refractive index, polarizability	70–1000	-	0.010–0.375	High separation efficiency	Heating and photodamage, low throughput
Affinity capture	Surface interactions	Antigenic site, hydrophobicity, charge	100	-	0.010	High capture efficiency and purity	Expensive, multiple preparation steps
Electrophore-sis	Uniform electric field	Size, charge	<50	97	0.0004	Very high separation efficiency and resolution	Flow rate change with chemistry (buffers, wall effects)
Dielectropho-resis	Nonuniform electric field	Polarizability and size	30–60	85–100	0.000009	High throughput and separation efficiency	Requires high voltage, depends on medium conductivity, very low throughput
Magnetopho-resis	Magnetic field	Size, magnetic properties	5–200	90	0.300	Very high throughput, low cost	Long time for magnetic bead antibody labeling
Acoustopho-resis	Ultrasonic sound wave	Size, density, compressibility	<200	>90	0.00043–0.00081	High separation efficiency, controlled cut off separation	Complex fabrication, limited device material to transmit acoustic power efficiently
Ion concentration polarization	Electric field	Size, electrophoretic mobility	100–500	-	0.0005	Low voltage, no need for internal electrode	Low resolution on small size particles, low throughput
Electrohydro-dynamic vortices	Traveling waves, ohmic heating	Size, charge	200	~100	0.000033	High separation efficiency	Complex fabrication of microelectrode, low throughput
Deterministic lateral displacement	Laminar flow stream	Size, deformability	190–2000	~100	0.00001	Controllable cutoff size, simple and efficient, high separation efficiency (20 nm resolution)	Very low throughput, precise fabrication required, pillar clogging is possible
Hydrodyna-mic filtration	Hydrodynamic sieving	Size	100–1000	-	0.001	Simple, high separation efficiency, medium throughput	Prone to clogging
Spiral microfluidics	Dean vortices	Size, shape	590–7320	95	0.010	Very high separation efficiency, simple	Prone to particle-particle interactions and diffusion disruption
Inertial microfluidics	Shear and wall lift	Size, shape	590–1980	-	-	Very high throughput, separation efficiency, simple	Prone to particle–particle interactions and diffusion disruption

Table 4. *Cont.*

Techniques	Mechanism	Separation Marker	Sizes Separated (nm)	Efficiency (%)	Throughput (mL·min^{-1})	Pros	Cons
Electrostatic sieving	Electric double-layer force	Size, charge	19–50	97	0.0006	Very high separation efficiency, controllable cut-off size	Separation only possible in low ionic strength conditions, low throughput
Bacterial chemotaxis	Chemotaxis, diffusion, and bacterial motility	Selective adhesion on bacteria	320–390	81	0.000013	Simple, low cost	Requires antibody conjugation for selective adhesion to bacteria, very low throughput, and relatively medium separation efficiency

5. Further Application and Processes of Microfluidic Approaches

5.1. Purification Strategies

To ensure the high quality of final nanomedicines produced microfluidically, optimization and tailoring of the final purification strategy are required. The classic purification techniques are ultracentrifugation, electrophoresis, chromatography, filtration, size-selective precipitation, and the addition of solvent (Table 4). Despite being effective purification techniques, they depend on the properties of the sample such as purity, density, solubility, and hydrophobicity. Purification methods ideally need to be continuous to combine with microfluidic manufacture and be able to work efficiently with minimal sample volume; utilizing microfluidic separation methods is likely to guarantee a continuous separation, at low costs, which are especially suitable for products with reduced dimensions such as nanoparticles [282]. The parameters that play a role in the successful separation of nanometer samples are size, diffusion, conformational structure, surface forces, pH, and buffers. Surface forces decrease with decreasing particle size, while Brownian movement increases, making separation more complex. Thus, designing devices with internal microchannel structures such as membranes and obstacles such as pillars or pores that can separate particles according to their size by exploiting phenomena such as sieving or laminar flow are typically utilized [248]. The costs for the realization of these devices at nanoscale increase considerably, and it must be added that the separation process is made even more complex by the differences in terms of shapes, structures, and morphological characteristics of the nanoparticle. Nanoparticles have a high surface-to-volume ratio, and this results in a greater aggregation tendency due to the enhanced surface energy. Thus, selection of the appropriate surface microfluidic interactions is critical in the design of a microfluidic purification process and can be achieved by tailoring parameters such as composition, solvents, pH, and temperature. Microfluid separation techniques can be classified into active and passive (Table 4), where external energy sources are used in active techniques; although these techniques guarantee an effective and controlled purification, they are dependent on association with other equipment. Passive techniques are based purely on the device design and action parameters, as it is the hydrodynamic and surface forces that guarantee the separation [248].

5.2. Analysis on a Chip and Production with a High Throughput

Integrated and miniaturized analysis on a chip in nanomedicine fabrication can play a crucial role in efficient characterization of different nanomedicines, broadening knowledge about the effect of process parameters and roles of their optimization in final products. On-chip diagnostic and analysis devices can be located at the nanoprecipitation downstream site to enable in situ measurements. Placement of these devices for in situ measurements at other locations through the channel also provides information about the temporal and spatial characteristics of the reaction process [283,284]. An example of this is a microfluidic system based on electrowetting on dielectric coupled to a silicon nanowire-based surface-assisted laser ionization–desorption interface applicable in analysis (mass spectrometry) of small biomolecules [285]. Here, analytes transfer was attained on particular locations on the surface-assisted laser desorption–ionization interface, and their subsequent mass spectrometry evaluations without the application of an organic matrix were performed. To do so, a device comprising a patterned interface of superhydrophilic/superhydrophobic silicon nanowire and a microfluidic system was developed. For the analyte displacement (droplets containing analytes) inside the superhydrophilic patterns via an electrowetting actuation the microfluidic system was served. The nanopatterned silicon interface acted as an inorganic target for the dried analyte matrix-free mass spectrometry analysis. It was demonstrated that the evaluation of compounds with a low molecular weight (700 m/z) could be attained with a very high sensitivity (down to 10 fmol·μL^{-1}) [285]. Furthermore, a tumor-on-a-chip model based on a microfluidic approach was designed for evaluating efficacy and targeting capability of multifunctional liposomes for cancer therapy [286]. The device contained three groups of hemispheric wells with various sizes for the formation of tumor spheroids and assessing of liposomes under a controlled flow regime. There was a good conformity between the tumor targeting capability of fluorescent liposomes during the test in the tumor-on-a-chip model and in in vivo mouse models. In comparison with 3D tumor spheroid models and 2D cell monolayers, the anticancer efficacy evaluation of four paclitaxel-loaded liposome formulations revealed that the developed microfluidic model could better predict the anticancer efficacy (in vivo) of targeted liposomes. Lastly, to study the correlation between treatment efficacy and flow rates, the cytotoxicity of PTX-loaded formulations was evaluated under three flow rates (i.e., 0.25, 1, and 4 $\mu L \cdot min^{-1}$). The highest cytotoxicity or the lowest spheroid viability using the smallest flow rate was 43.7% and the viability of the tumor spheroid was increased to 60.9% and 69.5% by increasing the flow rate to 1 and 4 $\mu L \cdot min^{-1}$, respectively, revealing reduced cytotoxicity. The growth curve of the tumor spheroid also showed that lower flow rates resulted in better capability of tumor inhibition. At a flow rate of 0.25 $\mu L \cdot min^{-1}$, the PTX-loaded liposomes could obviously reduce the volume of tumor spheroids, while the tumor suppression effect was much weaker at the highest flow rate. To further study the influence of the flow rates on the efficacy of tumor inhibitions, the liposome accumulation at the spheroids was evaluated under various flow rates. Quantitative and qualitative results all depicted that higher flow rates resulted in a lower uptake efficiency, showing a reduced liposome accumulation in the tumor spheroid, which might clarify the weaker effect of the tumor suppression at high flow rates. This study demonstrated that the tumor-on-a-chip model could provide a convenient and feasible platform for reliable and rapid cancer drug study [286].

5.3. Scale-Up Manufacture

Microreactor application for nanomaterial production on an industrial scale relies extensively on reactor parallelization, where each unit individually process only a small part of a total reaction volume. Scaling up the size of a microfluidic device represents an obvious rise in the used liquid volumetric flow rate that is streamed along the microreactor according to $Q = U \times A$ (Q, U, and A are the volumetric flow rate, average fluid velocity, microchannel cumulative cross-sectional area, respectively) [154]. A scaling up scheme generally includes the cumulative flow enhancement using the microchannel cross-section via increasing the microreactor numbers. Generally, a considerable increase in average velocity of the fluid leads to unwanted drops in pressure over the microchannel. Commonly, a scaling up strategy has three levels: (i) increasing the channel numbers providing channels identically in the same lamina, (ii) increasing the layer numbers, which create multiple layers with arrays of the channel, and (iii) increasing the device numbers by employing devices with identical structure and function linked in parallel. To obtain an effective microfluidic device with the ability of scaling up the production of nanomaterials, the flow rate must be the same in all the arrayed microchannels. As aforementioned, the flow rate throughout the channel is a key parameter in controlling the characteristics affecting reactions (e.g., mass and heat transfer, particle residence time) and, subsequently, the prepared nanomaterials [1,138,206]. Heterogeneity and large particle size can be improved by enhancing the FRR using HFF devices, but this will also decrease the concentration of LNPs in the product; thus, HFF devices may not be a suitable choice for LNP mass production using a lipid solution with a high concentration [245,265,287,288]. Pumps for each individual channel can satisfy the necessity of a uniform flow distribution across the arrayed channels but increases manufacturing costs. A more practical approach is distributing the flow from a main joint reservoir along microchannels to a common reservoir for the prepared product. However, achieving a uniform flow rate for all the distributed flows in each channel is not an easy task [289]. Comparing the conventional extrusion method with microfluidics for liposome (sphingomyelin/cholesterol) production and scale-up [290] showed that an increase in mixing ratio and higher flow rate ratio led to smaller liposomes, resulting in liposomes with a lipid concentration and size appropriate for clinical translation. The cellular efficacy data indicated that the vinblastine-*N*-oxide-loaded liposomes prepared using the microfluidic method and microfluidically prepared/freeze-dried vinblastine-*N*-oxide-loaded liposomes achieved similar efficacy to vinblastine-*N*-oxide-loaded liposomes prepared using the extrusion method. The maximum tolerated dose and pharmacokinetic studies further demonstrated that there was no difference between the in vivo properties of the vinblastine-*N*-oxide-loaded liposome manufactured using the extrusion or microfluidics methods [290]. In another study, PEGylated liposomal doxorubicin was prepared microfluidically followed by tangential flow filtration allowed for scalable production [291] of liposomes with critical quality attributes comparable to those of Caelyx®/Doxil®. High encapsulation efficiencies (EE% $\geq$ 90) were attained for all three assessed drugs (doxorubicin, acridine orange, and vincristine). Thus, these microfluidically doxorubicin-loaded liposomes demonstrated comparable physicochemical behavior and pharmaceutical quality criteria correlation to Doxil®/Caelyx® in terms of liposomal size, zeta potential, size distribution, drug loading, product sterilization, particle stability, and drug release, while the control of CQAs was possible in a scale-independent manner [291].

The lipid concentration typically used for microfluidically prepared lipid-based nanomedicines is low; for example, in the case of liposomes produced with an FRR of 10 or 30, the lipid concentration varied between 0.16 and 0.45 mM, respectively [168]. Even at studies where the lipid concentration was higher (0.1–2 mM depending on FRR) using MHF mixers, the concentration was far lower than the clinical liposomal formulation (5–25 mM) [35]. One way to overcome this is by feeding a highly concentrated lipid solution into microfluidic devices to boost productivity. The advantage of using a solution with high lipid concentrations is the capability of fabricating concentrated LNPs in a short run time, which allows for dilution to obtain a sample with desired concentration. The feasibility of mass production of highly concentrated LNPs is more desirable than their concentration using tangential flow filtration or ultracentrifugation. This can also prevent alterations in the particle characteristics of the LNPs within concentration steps. However, the use of high lipid concentrations is at the expense of control of particle size (polydispersity) and results in larger particle sizes [86,292–298]. Matsuura-Sawada et al. studied the controllability of LNP production with low-to-high lipid concentrations using iLiNP baffle mixes (microchannels with a height and width of 100 and 200 μm, respectively) [299]. The interval, length, and width of each baffle were 100, 100, and 150 μm (a total of 20 baffles) (Figure 6) [299], and the FRR was fixed to 3. They fixed the FRR of the lipid phase to the aqueous phase at 3. At a lipid (POPC) concentration of 10 mg/mL, LNPs smaller than 100 nm were produced; however, when the concentration increased 10-fold, even at high flow rate conditions, the LNPs size was in the range of 130–140 nm (PDI < 0.2) [299].

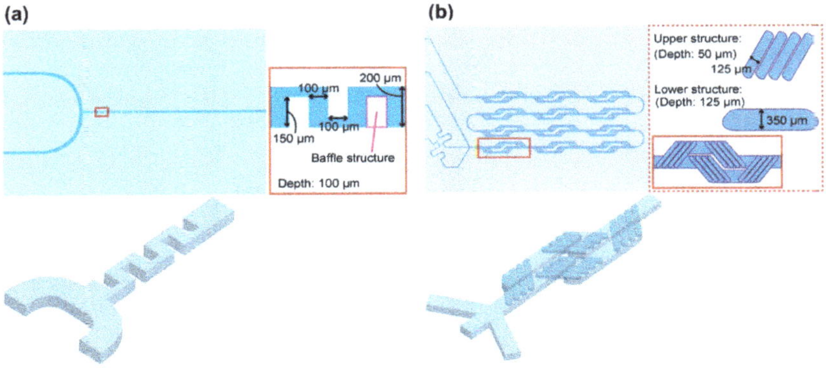

Figure 6. Schematic of (a) iLiNP (two inlets) and (b) micromixer device. Modified from [299] and used under the Creative Commons license permission (CC BY 4.0). Copyright 2022, American Chemical Society. All rights reserved.

The lipid concentration effects on the size of LNPs produced using iLiNP at a TFR of 1000 μL/min (POPC concentration 10–50 mg/mL) resulted in LNPs < 100 nm. Applying the same conditions in the micromixer device (Figure 6) led to LNPs at least 1.4 times bigger than those fabricated by iLiNP [299]. It was found that iLiNP at a TFR of 500 μL/min (FRRs of 3 and 9) could attain a complete mixing state within 3 ms [269], where, at a TFR of 500 μL/min (FRR of 1), approximately 192 ms was required for the micromixer device to attain a complete mixing state [300]. In the range of 10–50 mg/mL for POPC this was comparable to the differences in the size of LNPs [299]. The LNPs manufactured at a concentration of 100 mg/mL POPC using iLiNP represented a roughly similar size reduction trend to those fabricated using the micromixer device. By increasing TFR from 500 to 1000 μL/min, the size of the produced LNPs using iLiNP remained at 130 nm, but LNPs prepared using the micromixer device showed a reduction in size upon increasing TFR. These results depicted that the threshold concentration of POPC is between 50 and 100 mg/mL for various size decrement tendencies using the micromixer and iLiNP devices [299]. It also showed that higher concentration of LNPs can be manufactured using iLiNP per unit volume, which suggests that microfluidic devices have the feasibility for mass production of size-controlled LNPs.

Acoustically (ultrasound) driven microfluidic micromixers can potentially allow for feeding higher lipid concentrations; however, this has still not been demonstrated [301] The acoustic microstreaming reinforced by integrating sharp edges and bubbles in the devices can trigger higher throughput of liposomes with lower polydispersity, along with a controlled size at lower FRR, which can enable higher lipid concentrations, avoiding large nanoparticle aggregates and clogging of the channel [302]. However, the vibrational amplitude of sharp edges rapidly diminished as the flow rate increased, limiting the throughput.

Thus, to prepare lipid nanomedicines for drug delivery, micromixers may generally be a better choice because of their relatively high encapsulation efficiency, easy usability, and full use of encapsulated materials. The throughput of micromixers was exponentially scaled up by incorporating an array of numerous mixing channels that operate simultaneously [303]. In fact, commercial devices based on micromixers such as NanoAssemblr™ platforms have been universally used in many studies to prepare lipid particles for different applications, such as CRISPR/Cas9 genome editing for cancer therapy [304] and in utero mRNA delivery for monogenic fetal diseases [305] Notably, COVID-19 vaccine nanoparticles manufactured by Pfizer were scaled up using parallel microfluidic mixers [295,306].

6. Future Perspectives and Challenges

Microfluidic approaches enable the continuous manufacture of lipid-based nanomedicines for preclinical and clinical administration with controlled properties, efficacy, and safety profiles, as the latter are linked to particle properties. Developing continuous and scalable approaches to the manufacture of nanomedicines will allow for the translation of novel technologies and enhance the likelihood of uptake of these technologies by the pharmaceutical industry. Knowledge transfer among academic institutions, industrial partners, and clinicians creates the ideal environment for innovation needed to enable nanomedicine translation to overcome societal challenges as shown in the case of COVID-19 vaccines. Current advances in 3D printing technologies enable facile generation of tailored systems for pilot studies that can make initial optimization a facile and cost-effective process compared to planar micromachining approaches such as soft lithography. Continuous flow microfluidic fabrication methods are amenable to scale-up processes, while digital microfluidics with liquid marbles and droplets can address the issue of cumbersome-to-manufacture constructs.

Supplementary Materials: The following supporting information can be downloaded at https://www.mdpi.com/article/10.3390/pharmaceutics14091940/s1: Table S1. Lipid-based formulations in clinical trials.

Author Contributions: Conceptualization, K.O.-B., S.P. and A.L.; methodology, K.O.-B., S.P. and A.L.; formal analysis, K.O.-B., S.P. and A.L.; investigation, K.O.-B., S.P. and A.L.; resources, D.R.S. and A.L.; data curation, K.O.-B., S.P. and A.L.; writing—original draft preparation, K.O.-B., S.P. and A.L.; writing—review and editing, K.O.-B., S.P., D.R.S., A.B., G.H. and A.L.; visualization, K.O.-B., D.R.S. and A.L.; supervision, A.B. and A.L.; project administration, A.L.; funding acquisition, A.L. All authors have read and agreed to the published version of the manuscript.

Funding: K.O.-B. is funded by the Global Bursary, University of Portsmouth.

Institutional Review Board Statement: Not applicable.

Informed Consent Statement: Not applicable.

Data Availability Statement: Not applicable.

Conflicts of Interest: The authors declare no conflict of interest. The funders had no role in the design of the study; in the collection, analyses, or interpretation of data; in the writing of the manuscript, or in the decision to publish the results.

References

1. Kara, A.; Vassiliadou, A.; Ongoren, B.; Keeble, W.; Hing, R.; Lalatsa, A.; Serrano, D.R. Engineering 3D Printed Microfluidic Chips for the Fabrication of Nanomedicines. *Pharmaceutics* **2021**, *13*, 2134. [CrossRef] [PubMed]
2. Abedinoghli, D.; Charkhpour, M.; Osouli-Bostanabad, K.; Selselehjonban, S.; Emami, S.; Barzegar-Jalali, M.; Adibkia, K. Electrosprayed Nanosystems of Carbamazepine—PVP K30 for Enhancing Its Pharmacologic Effects. *Iran. J. Pharm. Res.* **2018**, *17*, 1431–1443. [PubMed]
3. Barenholz, Y. Doxil®—The first FDA-approved nano-drug: Lessons learned. *J. Control. Release* **2012**, *160*, 117–134. [CrossRef] [PubMed]
4. Specification, P.A. *Terminology for Nanomaterials*; British Standards Institute: London, UK, 2007.
5. Bosetti, R.; Jones, S.L. Cost–effectiveness of nanomedicine: Estimating the real size of nano-costs. *Nanomedicine* **2019**, *14*, 1367–1370. [CrossRef]
6. Peptide Therapeutics Market. Reports and Data. 2020, p. 294. Available online: https://www.reportsanddata.com/report-detail/peptide-therapeutics-market (accessed on 5 August 2022).
7. Bobo, D.; Robinson, K.J.; Islam, J.; Thurecht, K.J.; Corrie, S.R. Nanoparticle-Based Medicines: A Review of FDA-Approved Materials and Clinical Trials to Date. *Pharm. Res.* **2016**, *33*, 2373–2387. [CrossRef]
8. Germain, M.; Caputo, F.; Metcalfe, S.; Tosi, G.; Spring, K.; Åslund, A.K.O.; Pottier, A.; Schiffelers, R.; Ceccaldi, A.; Schmid, R. Delivering the power of nanomedicine to patients today. *J. Control. Release* **2020**, *326*, 164–171. [CrossRef]
9. Anselmo, A.C.; Mitragotri, S. Nanoparticles in the clinic: An update. *Bioeng. Transl. Med.* **2019**, *4*, e10143. [CrossRef]
10. Forssen, E.A. The design and development of DaunoXome®for solid tumor targeting in vivo. *Adv. Drug Deliv. Rev.* **1997**, *24*, 133–150. [CrossRef]

11. Boswell, G.W.; Buell, D.; Bekersky, I. AmBisome (Liposomal Amphotericin B): A Comparative Review. *J. Clin. Pharmacol.* **1998**, *38*, 583–592. [CrossRef]
12. Bulbake, U.; Doppalapudi, S.; Kommineni, N.; Khan, W. Liposomal Formulations in Clinical Use: An Updated Review. *Pharmaceutics* **2017**, *9*, 12. [CrossRef]
13. Silverman, J.A.; Deitcher, S.R. Marqibo® (vincristine sulfate liposome injection) improves the pharmacokinetics and pharmacodynamics of vincristine. *Cancer Chemother. Pharmacol.* **2013**, *71*, 555–564. [CrossRef] [PubMed]
14. Liu, X.; Jiang, J.; Chan, R.; Ji, Y.; Lu, J.; Liao, Y.-P.; Okene, M.; Lin, J.; Lin, P.; Chang, C.H.; et al. Improved Efficacy and Reduced Toxicity Using a Custom-Designed Irinotecan-Delivering Silicasome for Orthotopic Colon Cancer. *ACS Nano* **2019**, *13*, 38–53. [CrossRef] [PubMed]
15. Akinc, A.; Maier, M.A.; Manoharan, M.; Fitzgerald, K.; Jayaraman, M.; Barros, S.; Ansell, S.; Du, X.; Hope, M.J.; Madden, T.D.; et al. The Onpattro story and the clinical translation of nanomedicines containing nucleic acid-based drugs. *Nat. Nanotechnol.* **2019**, *14*, 1084–1087. [CrossRef] [PubMed]
16. Choi, Y.H.; Han, H.-K. Nanomedicines: Current status and future perspectives in aspect of drug delivery and pharmacokinetics. *J. Pharm. Investig.* **2018**, *48*, 43–60. [CrossRef]
17. Martins, J.P.; das Neves, J.; de la Fuente, M.; Celia, C.; Florindo, H.; Günday-Türeli, N.; Popat, A.; Santos, J.L.; Sousa, F.; Schmid, R.; et al. The solid progress of nanomedicine. *Drug Deliv. Transl. Res.* **2020**, *10*, 726–729. [CrossRef]
18. Thi, T.T.H.; Suys, E.J.A.; Lee, J.S.; Nguyen, D.H.; Park, K.D.; Truong, N.P. Lipid-Based Nanoparticles in the Clinic and Clinical Trials: From Cancer Nanomedicine to COVID-19 Vaccines. *Vaccines* **2021**, *9*, 359. [CrossRef]
19. Mitchell, M.J.; Billingsley, M.M.; Haley, R.M.; Wechsler, M.E.; Peppas, N.A.; Langer, R. Engineering precision nanoparticles for drug delivery. *Nat. Rev. Drug Discov.* **2021**, *20*, 101–124. [CrossRef]
20. Shin, M.D.; Shukla, S.; Chung, Y.H.; Beiss, V.; Chan, S.K.; Ortega-Rivera, O.A.; Wirth, D.M.; Chen, A.; Sack, M.; Pokorski, J.K.; et al. COVID-19 vaccine development and a potential nanomaterial path forward. *Nat. Nanotechnol.* **2020**, *15*, 646–655. [CrossRef]
21. Soares, S.; Sousa, J.; Pais, A.; Vitorino, C. Nanomedicine: Principles, Properties, and Regulatory Issues. *Front. Chem.* **2018**, *6*, 360. [CrossRef]
22. Selselehjonban, S.; Garjani, A.; Osouli-Bostanabad, K.; Tanhaei, A.; Emami, S.; Adibkia, K.; Barzegar-Jalali, M. Physicochemical and pharmacological evaluation of carvedilol-eudragit(®) RS100 electrosprayed nanostructures. *Iran. J. Basic Med. Sci.* **2019**, *22* 547–556. [CrossRef]
23. Kim, B.Y.S.; Rutka, J.T.; Chan, W.C.W. Nanomedicine. *N. Engl. J. Med.* **2010**, *363*, 2434–2443. [CrossRef] [PubMed]
24. Khurana, A.; Allawadhi, P.; Khurana, I.; Allwadhi, S.; Weiskirchen, R.; Banothu, A.K.; Chhabra, D.; Joshi, K.; Bharani, K.K. Role of nanotechnology behind the success of mRNA vaccines for COVID-19. *Nano Today* **2021**, *38*, 101142. [CrossRef] [PubMed]
25. Ahn, J.; Ko, J.; Lee, S.; Yu, J.; Kim, Y.; Jeon, N.L. Microfluidics in nanoparticle drug delivery; From synthesis to pre-clinical screening. *Adv. Drug Deliv. Rev.* **2018**, *128*, 29–53. [CrossRef] [PubMed]
26. Fornaguera, C.; García-Celma, M.J. Personalized Nanomedicine: A Revolution at the Nanoscale. *J. Pers. Med.* **2017**, *7*, 12. [CrossRef]
27. Tapeinos, C.; Battaglini, M.; Ciofani, G. Advances in the design of solid lipid nanoparticles and nanostructured lipid carriers for targeting brain diseases. *J. Control. Release* **2017**, *264*, 306–332. [CrossRef]
28. Fonseca-Santos, B.; Gremião, M.P.D.; Chorilli, M. Nanotechnology-based drug delivery systems for the treatment of Alzheimer's disease. *Int. J. Nanomed.* **2015**, *10*, 4981–5003. [CrossRef]
29. Sercombe, L.; Veerati, T.; Moheimani, F.; Wu, S.Y.; Sood, A.K.; Hua, S. Advances and Challenges of Liposome Assisted Drug Delivery. *Front. Pharmacol.* **2015**, *6*, 286. [CrossRef]
30. Fenton, O.S.; Olafson, K.N.; Pillai, P.S.; Mitchell, M.J.; Langer, R. Advances in Biomaterials for Drug Delivery. *Adv. Mater.* **2018**, *30*, 1705328. [CrossRef]
31. Sarfraz, M.; Afzal, A.; Yang, T.; Gai, Y.; Raza, S.M.; Khan, M.W.; Cheng, Y.; Ma, X.; Xiang, G. Development of Dual Drug Loaded Nanosized Liposomal Formulation by A Reengineered Ethanolic Injection Method and Its Pre-Clinical Pharmacokinetic Studies. *Pharmaceutics* **2018**, *10*, 151. [CrossRef]
32. Sedighi, M.; Sieber, S.; Rahimi, F.; Shahbazi, M.-A.; Rezayan, A.H.; Huwyler, J.; Witzigmann, D. Rapid optimization of liposome characteristics using a combined microfluidics and design-of-experiment approach. *Drug Deliv. Transl. Res.* **2019**, *9*, 404–413. [CrossRef]
33. Lalatsa, A.; Schätzlein, A.G.; Uchegbu, I.F. Drug delivery across the blood-brain barrier. In *Comprehensive Biotechnology*; Elsevier: Amsterdam, The Netherlands, 2019; pp. 628–637.
34. Fernández-García, R.; Lalatsa, A.; Statts, L.; Bolás-Fernández, F.; Ballesteros, M.P.; Serrano, D.R. Transferosomes as nanocarriers for drugs across the skin: Quality by design from lab to industrial scale. *Int J. Pharm* **2020**, *573*, 118817. [CrossRef]
35. Rai, S.; Pandey, V.; Rai, G. Transfersomes as versatile and flexible nano-vesicular carriers in skin cancer therapy: The state of the art. *Nano Rev. Exp.* **2017**, *8*, 1325708. [CrossRef] [PubMed]
36. Opatha, S.A.T.; Titapiwatanakun, V.; Chutoprapat, R. Transfersomes: A Promising Nanoencapsulation Technique for Transdermal Drug Delivery. *Pharmaceutics* **2020**, *12*, 855. [CrossRef] [PubMed]
37. Naik, U.S. The Synthesis and Characterisation of Novel Ultra-Flexible Lipidic Vesicles Using Propanol. Ph.D. Thesis, University of Central Lancashire, Preston, UK, 2013.

38. Rane, B.R.; Gujarathi, N.A. Transfersomes and Protransfersome: Ultradeformable Vesicular System. In *Novel Approaches for Drug Delivery*; Keservani, R.K., Sharma, A.K., Kesharwani, R.K., Eds.; IGI Global: Hershey, PA, USA, 2017; pp. 149–169.
39. Rajan, R.; Jose, S.; Biju Mukund, V.; Vasudevan, D. Transferosomes—A vesicular transdermal delivery system for enhanced drug permeation. *J. Adv. Pharm. Technol. Res.* **2011**, *2*, 138–143. [CrossRef] [PubMed]
40. Jangdey, M.S.; Gupta, A.; Saraf, S.; Saraf, S. Development and optimization of apigenin-loaded transfersomal system for skin cancer delivery: In vitro evaluation. *Artif. Cells Nanomed. Biotechnol.* **2017**, *45*, 1452–1462. [CrossRef] [PubMed]
41. Touitou, E. Compositions for Applying Active Substances to or through the Skin. U.S. Patent No. 5,540,934, 30 July 1996.
42. Touitou, E.; Dayan, N.; Bergelson, L.; Godin, B.; Eliaz, M. Ethosomes—Novel vesicular carriers for enhanced delivery: Characterization and skin penetration properties. *J. Control. Release* **2000**, *65*, 403–418. [CrossRef]
43. Touitou, E. Composition for Applying Active Substances to or through the Skin. U.S. Patent No. 5,716,638, 10 February 1998.
44. Saifi, Z.; Rizwanullah, M.; Mir, S.R.; Amin, S. Bilosomes nanocarriers for improved oral bioavailability of acyclovir: A complete characterization through in vitro, ex-vivo and in vivo assessment. *J. Drug Deliv. Sci. Technol.* **2020**, *57*, 101634. [CrossRef]
45. Conacher, M.; Alexander, J.; Brewer, J.M. Oral immunisation with peptide and protein antigens by formulation in lipid vesicles incorporating bile salts (bilosomes). *Vaccine* **2001**, *19*, 2965–2974. [CrossRef]
46. Pavlović, N.; Goločorbin-Kon, S.; Đanić, M.; Stanimirov, B.; Al-Salami, H.; Stankov, K.; Mikov, M. Bile Acids and Their Derivatives as Potential Modifiers of Drug Release and Pharmacokinetic Profiles. *Front. Pharmacol.* **2018**, *9*, 1283. [CrossRef]
47. Niu, M.; Lu, Y.; Hovgaard, L.; Guan, P.; Tan, Y.; Lian, R.; Qi, J.; Wu, W. Hypoglycemic activity and oral bioavailability of insulin-loaded liposomes containing bile salts in rats: The effect of cholate type, particle size and administered dose. *Eur. J. Pharm. Biopharm.* **2012**, *81*, 265–272. [CrossRef]
48. Aburahma, M.H. Bile salts-containing vesicles: Promising pharmaceutical carriers for oral delivery of poorly water-soluble drugs and peptide/protein-based therapeutics or vaccines. *Drug Deliv.* **2016**, *23*, 1847–1867. [CrossRef] [PubMed]
49. Müller, R.H.; Mäder, K.; Gohla, S. Solid lipid nanoparticles (SLN) for controlled drug delivery—A review of the state of the art. *Eur. J. Pharm. Biopharm.* **2000**, *50*, 161–177. [CrossRef]
50. Patel, S.; Ryals, R.C.; Weller, K.K.; Pennesi, M.E.; Sahay, G. Lipid nanoparticles for delivery of messenger RNA to the back of the eye. *J. Control. Release* **2019**, *303*, 91–100. [CrossRef] [PubMed]
51. Vhora, I.; Lalani, R.; Bhatt, P.; Patil, S.; Misra, A. Lipid-nucleic acid nanoparticles of novel ionizable lipids for systemic BMP-9 gene delivery to bone-marrow mesenchymal stem cells for osteoinduction. *Int. J. Pharm.* **2019**, *563*, 324–336. [CrossRef]
52. Duan, Y.; Dhar, A.; Patel, C.; Khimani, M.; Neogi, S.; Sharma, P.; Kumar, N.S.; Vekariya, R.L. A brief review on solid lipid nanoparticles: Part and parcel of contemporary drug delivery systems. *RSC Adv.* **2020**, *10*, 26777–26791. [CrossRef]
53. Laffleur, F.; Keckeis, V. Advances in drug delivery systems: Work in progress still needed? *Int. J. Pharm. X* **2020**, *2*, 100050. [CrossRef]
54. Zarif, L.; Graybill, J.R.; Perlin, D.; Mannino, R.J. Cochleates: New Lipid-Based Drug Delivery System. *J. Liposome Res.* **2000**, *10*, 523–538. [CrossRef]
55. Zarif, L. Elongated supramolecular assemblies in drug delivery. *J. Control. Release* **2002**, *81*, 7–23. [CrossRef]
56. Shende, P.; Khair, R.; Gaud, R.S. Nanostructured cochleates: A multi-layered platform for cellular transportation of therapeutics. *Drug Dev. Ind. Pharm.* **2019**, *45*, 869–881. [CrossRef]
57. Talke, S.; Salunkhe, K.; Chavan, M. A Review on nanocochleates novel approach for drug delivery. *World J. Pharm. Pharm. Sci.* **2018**, *7*, 284–294.
58. Shi, J.; Kantoff, P.W.; Wooster, R.; Farokhzad, O.C. Cancer nanomedicine: Progress, challenges and opportunities. *Nat. Rev. Cancer* **2017**, *17*, 20–37. [CrossRef] [PubMed]
59. Xu, X.; Ho, W.; Zhang, X.; Bertrand, N.; Farokhzad, O. Cancer nanomedicine: From targeted delivery to combination therapy. *Trends Mol. Med.* **2015**, *21*, 223–232. [CrossRef] [PubMed]
60. Yingchoncharoen, P.; Kalinowski, D.S.; Richardson, D.R. Lipid-Based Drug Delivery Systems in Cancer Therapy: What Is Available and What Is Yet to Come. *Pharmacol. Rev.* **2016**, *68*, 701–787. [CrossRef]
61. Ventola, C.L. Progress in Nanomedicine: Approved and Investigational Nanodrugs. *Pharm. Ther.* **2017**, *42*, 742–755.
62. Shah, S.; Dhawan, V.; Holm, R.; Nagarsenker, M.S.; Perrie, Y. Liposomes: Advancements and innovation in the manufacturing process. *Adv. Drug Deliv. Rev.* **2020**, *154–155*, 102–122. [CrossRef]
63. Fan, Y.; Marioli, M.; Zhang, K. Analytical characterization of liposomes and other lipid nanoparticles for drug delivery. *J. Pharm. Biomed. Anal.* **2021**, *192*, 113642. [CrossRef]
64. Lamichhane, N.; Udayakumar, T.S.; D'Souza, W.D.; Simone II, C.B.; Raghavan, S.R.; Polf, J.; Mahmood, J. Liposomes: Clinical Applications and Potential for Image-Guided Drug Delivery. *Molecules* **2018**, *23*, 288. [CrossRef]
65. Spectrum Pharmaceuticals, Inc. Topotecan Liposomes Injection for Small Cell Lung Cancer (SCLC), Ovarian Cancer and Other Advanced Solid Tumors. Available online: https://clinicaltrials.gov/ct2/show/NCT00765973 (accessed on 13 November 2020).
66. Swiss Group for Clinical Cancer Research. TLD-1, a Novel Liposomal Doxorubicin, in Patients with Advanced Solid Tumors. Available online: https://clinicaltrials.gov/ct2/show/NCT03387917 (accessed on 7 September 2022).
67. Mebiopharm Co., Ltd. Safety Study of MBP-426 (Liposomal Oxaliplatin Suspension for Injection) to Treat Advanced or Metastatic Solid Tumors. Available online: https://clinicaltrials.gov/ct2/show/NCT00355888 (accessed on 2 December 2014).
68. Mebiopharm Co., Ltd. Study of MBP-426 in Patients with Second Line Gastric, Gastroesophageal, or Esophageal Adenocarcinoma. Available online: https://www.clinicaltrials.gov/ct2/show/NCT00964080 (accessed on 2 December 2014).

69. Munster, P.; Krop, I.E.; LoRusso, P.; Ma, C.; Siegel, B.A.; Shields, A.F.; Molnár, I.; Wickham, T.J.; Reynolds, J.; Campbell, K.; et al. Safety and pharmacokinetics of MM-302, a HER2-targeted antibody–liposomal doxorubicin conjugate, in patients with advanced HER2-positive breast cancer: A phase 1 dose-escalation study. *Br. J. Cancer* **2018**, *119*, 1086–1093. [CrossRef]
70. Celsion. Study of ThermoDox with Standardized Radiofrequency Ablation (RFA) for Treatment of Hepatocellular Carcinoma (HCC) (OPTIMA). Available online: https://clinicaltrials.gov/ct2/show/NCT02112656 (accessed on 24 October 2018).
71. Mebiopharm Co., Ltd. Active Targeting Drug Delivery System. Available online: http://www.mebiopharm.com/english/pro.html (accessed on 4 August 2021).
72. Yonezawa, S.; Koide, H.; Asai, T. Recent advances in siRNA delivery mediated by lipid-based nanoparticles. *Adv. Drug Deliv. Rev.* **2020**, *154–155*, 64–78. [CrossRef]
73. Ely, A.; Singh, P.; Smith, T.S.; Arbuthnot, P. In vitro transcribed mRNA for expression of designer nucleases: Advantages as a novel therapeutic for the management of chronic HBV infection. *Adv. Drug Deliv. Rev.* **2021**, *168*, 134–146. [CrossRef]
74. McGoron, A.J. Perspectives on the Future of Nanomedicine to Impact Patients: An Analysis of US Federal Funding and Interventional Clinical Trials. *Bioconj. Chem.* **2020**, *31*, 436–447. [CrossRef] [PubMed]
75. ModernaTX, Inc.; AstraZeneca. Dose Escalation Study of mRNA-2752 for Intratumoral Injection to Participants in Advanced Malignancies. Available online: https://clinicaltrials.gov/ct2/show/NCT03739931 (accessed on 18 July 2022).
76. ModernaTX, Inc. Dose Escalation and Efficacy Study of mRNA-2416 for Intratumoral Injection Alone and in Combination with Durvalumab for Participants with Advanced Malignancies. Available online: https://clinicaltrials.gov/ct2/show/NCT03323398 (accessed on 11 July 2022).
77. National Cancer Institute (NCI). T4N5 Liposomal Lotion in Preventing The Recurrence of Nonmelanoma Skin Cancer in Patients Who Have Undergone a Kidney Transplant. Available online: https://clinicaltrials.gov/ct2/show/NCT00089180 (accessed on 4 December 2015).
78. BioNTech, SE. Evaluation of the Safety and Tolerability of i.v. Administration of a Cancer Vaccine in Patients with Advanced Melanoma (Lipo-MERIT). Available online: https://clinicaltrials.gov/ct2/show/NCT02410733 (accessed on 24 August 2022).
79. ModernaTX, Inc.; Merck Sharp & Dohme Corp. An Efficacy Study of Adjuvant Treatment with the Personalized Cancer Vaccine mRNA-4157 and Pembrolizumab in Participants with High-Risk Melanoma (KEYNOTE-942). Available online: https://clinicaltrials.gov/ct2/show/NCT03897881 (accessed on 24 August 2022).
80. Ebinger, J.E.; Fert-Bober, J.; Printsev, I.; Wu, M.; Sun, N.; Prostko, J.C.; Frias, E.C.; Stewart, J.L.; Van Eyk, J.E.; Braun, J.G.; et al. Antibody responses to the BNT162b2 mRNA vaccine in individuals previously infected with SARS-CoV-2. *Nat. Med.* **2021**, *27*, 981–984. [CrossRef] [PubMed]
81. Weiss, C.; Carriere, M.; Fusco, L.; Capua, I.; Regla-Nava, J.A.; Pasquali, M.; Scott, J.A.; Vitale, F.; Unal, M.A.; Mattevi, C.; et al. Toward Nanotechnology-Enabled Approaches against the COVID-19 Pandemic. *ACS Nano* **2020**, *14*, 6383–6406. [CrossRef]
82. Kulkarni, J.A.; Cullis, P.R.; van der Meel, R. Lipid Nanoparticles Enabling Gene Therapies: From Concepts to Clinical Utility. *Nucleic Acid Ther.* **2018**, *28*, 146–157. [CrossRef] [PubMed]
83. Rudra, A.; Li, J.; Shakur, R.; Bhagchandani, S.; Langer, R. Trends in Therapeutic Conjugates: Bench to Clinic. *Bioconj. Chem.* **2020**, *31*, 462–473. [CrossRef]
84. Van Riel, D.; de Wit, E. Next-generation vaccine platforms for COVID-19. *Nat. Mater.* **2020**, *19*, 810–812. [CrossRef] [PubMed]
85. Ng, W.H.; Liu, X.; Mahalingam, S. Development of vaccines for SARS-CoV-2. *F1000Res* **2020**, *9*, 991. [CrossRef]
86. Ickenstein, L.M.; Garidel, P. Lipid-based nanoparticle formulations for small molecules and RNA drugs. *Expert Opin. Drug Deliv.* **2019**, *16*, 1205–1226. [CrossRef]
87. Hu, B.; Zhong, L.; Weng, Y.; Peng, L.; Huang, Y.; Zhao, Y.; Liang, X.-J. Therapeutic siRNA: State of the art. *Signal Transduct. Target Ther.* **2020**, *5*, 101. [CrossRef]
88. Anderluzzi, G.; Schmidt, S.T.; Cunliffe, R.; Woods, S.; Roberts, C.W.; Veggi, D.; Ferlenghi, I.; O'Hagan, D.T.; Baudner, B.C.; Perrie, Y. Rational design of adjuvants for subunit vaccines: The format of cationic adjuvants affects the induction of antigen-specific antibody responses. *J. Control. Release* **2021**, *330*, 933–944. [CrossRef]
89. Lee, K.; Kim, S.Y.; Seo, Y.; Kim, M.H.; Chang, J.; Lee, H. Adjuvant incorporated lipid nanoparticles for enhanced mRNA-mediated cancer immunotherapy. *Biomater. Sci.* **2020**, *8*, 1101–1105. [CrossRef] [PubMed]
90. Jain, S.; Tripathi, S.; Tripathi, P.K. Invasomes: Potential vesicular systems for transdermal delivery of drug molecules. *J. Drug Deliv. Sci. Technol.* **2021**, *61*, 102166. [CrossRef]
91. Nasirizadeh, S.; Malaekeh-Nikouei, B. Solid lipid nanoparticles and nanostructured lipid carriers in oral cancer drug delivery. *J. Drug Deliv. Sci. Technol.* **2020**, *55*, 101458. [CrossRef]
92. Chacko, I.A.; Ghate, V.M.; Dsouza, L.; Lewis, S.A. Lipid vesicles: A versatile drug delivery platform for dermal and transdermal applications. *Colloids Surf. B Biointerfaces* **2020**, *195*, 111262. [CrossRef] [PubMed]
93. Xu, Y.; Michalowski, C.B.; Beloqui, A. Advances in lipid carriers for drug delivery to the gastrointestinal tract. *Curr. Opin. Colloid Interface Sci.* **2021**, *52*, 101414. [CrossRef]
94. Leung, A.K.K.; Tam, Y.Y.C.; Chen, S.; Hafez, I.M.; Cullis, P.R. Microfluidic Mixing: A General Method for Encapsulating Macromolecules in Lipid Nanoparticle Systems. *J. Phys. Chem. B* **2015**, *119*, 8698–8706. [CrossRef]
95. Kulkarni, J.A.; Witzigmann, D.; Leung, J.; Tam, Y.Y.C.; Cullis, P.R. On the role of helper lipids in lipid nanoparticle formulations of siRNA. *Nanoscale* **2019**, *11*, 21733–21739. [CrossRef]

96. Cheng, X.; Lee, R.J. The role of helper lipids in lipid nanoparticles (LNPs) designed for oligonucleotide delivery. *Adv. Drug Deliv. Rev.* **2016**, *99*, 129–137. [CrossRef]
97. Cheng, Q.; Wei, T.; Farbiak, L.; Johnson, L.T.; Dilliard, S.A.; Siegwart, D.J. Selective organ targeting (SORT) nanoparticles for tissue-specific mRNA delivery and CRISPR–Cas gene editing. *Nat. Nanotechnol.* **2020**, *15*, 313–320. [CrossRef]
98. Berraondo, P.; Martini, P.G.V.; Avila, M.A.; Fontanellas, A. Messenger RNA therapy for rare genetic metabolic diseases. *Gut* **2019**, *68*, 1323–1330. [CrossRef]
99. Razavi, H.; Janfaza, S. Ethosome: A nanocarrier for transdermal drug delivery. *Arch. Adv. Biosci.* **2015**, *6*, 38–43. [CrossRef]
100. Abdulbaqi, I.M.; Darwis, Y.; Khan, N.A.K.; Abou Assi, R.; Khan, A.A. Ethosomal nanocarriers: The impact of constituents and formulation techniques on ethosomal properties, in vivo studies, and clinical trials. *Int. J. Nanomed.* **2016**, *11*, 2279. [CrossRef] [PubMed]
101. Lipa-Castro, A.; Legrand, F.-X.; Barratt, G. Cochleate drug delivery systems: An approach to their characterization. *Int. J. Pharm.* **2021**, *610*, 121225. [CrossRef] [PubMed]
102. World Health Organisation. COVID-19 Vaccine Tracker and Landscape. 2021. Available online: https://www.who.int/publications/m/item/draft-landscape-of-covid-19-candidate-vaccines (accessed on 6 September 2022).
103. Fang, E.; Liu, X.; Li, M.; Zhang, Z.; Song, L.; Zhu, B.; Wu, X.; Liu, J.; Zhao, D.; Li, Y. Advances in COVID-19 mRNA vaccine development. *Signal Transduct. Target. Ther.* **2022**, *7*, 94. [CrossRef]
104. FDA News Release, Food and Drug Administration. FDA Approves First COVID-19 Vaccine. 2021. Available online: https://www.fda.gov/news-events/press-announcements/fda-approves-first-covid-19-vaccine (accessed on 5 August 2022).
105. FDA News Release, Food and Drug Administration. FDA Authorizes Pfizer-BioNTech COVID-19 Vaccine for Emergency Use in Children 5 through 11 Years of Age. 2021. Available online: https://www.fda.gov/news-events/press-announcements/fda-authorizes-pfizer-biontech-covid-19-vaccine-emergency-use-children-5-through-11-years-age (accessed on 5 August 2022).
106. Koirala, A.; Joo, Y.J.; Khatami, A.; Chiu, C.; Britton, P.N. Vaccines for COVID-19: The current state of play. *Paediatr. Respir. Rev.* **2020**, *35*, 43–49. [CrossRef]
107. Samaridou, E.; Heyes, J.; Lutwyche, P. Lipid nanoparticles for nucleic acid delivery: Current perspectives. *Adv. Drug Deliv. Rev.* **2020**, *154–155*, 37–63. [CrossRef]
108. Theobald, N. Emerging vaccine delivery systems for COVID-19: Functionalised silica nanoparticles offer a potentially safe and effective alternative delivery system for DNA/RNA vaccines and may be useful in the hunt for a COVID-19 vaccine. *Drug Discov. Today* **2020**, *25*, 1556–1558. [CrossRef]
109. Shih, H.-I.; Wu, C.-J.; Tu, Y.-F.; Chi, C.-Y. Fighting COVID-19: A quick review of diagnoses, therapies, and vaccines. *Biomed. J.* **2020**, *43*, 341–354. [CrossRef]
110. Nakamura, T.; Harashima, H. Dawn of lipid nanoparticles in lymph node targeting: Potential in cancer immunotherapy. *Adv. Drug Deliv. Rev.* **2020**, *167*, 78–88. [CrossRef]
111. Bangham, A.D.; Standish, M.M.; Watkins, J.C. Diffusion of univalent ions across the lamellae of swollen phospholipids. *J. Mol. Biol.* **1965**, *13*, 238–252, IN26–IN27. [CrossRef]
112. Batzri, S.; Korn, E.D. Single bilayer liposomes prepared without sonication. *Biochim. Biophys. Acta* **1973**, *298*, 1015–1019. [CrossRef]
113. Zumbuehl, O.; Weder, H.G. Liposomes of controllable size in the range of 40 to 180 nm by defined dialysis of lipid/detergent mixed micelles. *Biochim. Biophys. Acta* **1981**, *640*, 252–262. [CrossRef]
114. Smith, L.; Serrano, D.R.; Mauger, M.; Bolás-Fernández, F.; Dea-Ayuela, M.A.; Lalatsa, A. Orally Bioavailable and Effective Buparvaquone Lipid-Based Nanomedicines for Visceral Leishmaniasis. *Mol. Pharm.* **2018**, *15*, 2570–2583. [CrossRef]
115. Fernández- García, R.; Statts, L.; de Jesus, J.A.; Dea-Ayuela, M.A.; Bautista, L.; Simão, R.; Bolás-Fernández, F.; Ballesteros, M.P.; Laurenti, M.D.; Passero, L.F.D.; et al. Ultradeformable Lipid Vesicles Localize Amphotericin B in the Dermis for the Treatment of Infectious Skin Diseases. *ACS Infect. Dis.* **2020**, *6*, 2647–2660. [CrossRef] [PubMed]
116. Colombo, S.; Beck-Broichsitter, M.; Bøtker, J.P.; Malmsten, M.; Rantanen, J.; Bohr, A. Transforming nanomedicine manufacturing toward Quality by Design and microfluidics. *Adv. Drug Deliv. Rev.* **2018**, *128*, 115–131. [CrossRef]
117. Worsham, R.D.; Thomas, V.; Farid, S.S. Potential of Continuous Manufacturing for Liposomal Drug Products. *Biotechnol. J.* **2019**, *14*, 1700740. [CrossRef] [PubMed]
118. Maherani, B.; Arab-Tehrany, E.; Mozafari, R.M.; Gaiani, C.; Linder, M. Liposomes: A Review of Manufacturing Techniques and Targeting Strategies. *Curr. Nanosci.* **2011**, *7*, 436–452. [CrossRef]
119. Pandita, D.; Ahuja, A.; Lather, V.; Benjamin, B.; Dutta, T.; Velpandian, T.; Khar, R.K. Development of Lipid-Based Nanoparticles for Enhancing the Oral Bioavailability of Paclitaxel. *AAPS PharmSciTech* **2011**, *12*, 712–722. [CrossRef]
120. Aditya, N.P.; Patankar, S.; Madhusudhan, B.; Murthy, R.S.R.; Souto, E.B. Arthemeter-loaded lipid nanoparticles produced by modified thin-film hydration: Pharmacokinetics, toxicological and in vivo anti-malarial activity. *Eur. J. Pharm. Sci.* **2010**, *40*, 448–455. [CrossRef]
121. Evers, M.J.W.; Kulkarni, J.A.; van der Meel, R.; Cullis, P.R.; Vader, P.; Schiffelers, R.M. State-of-the-Art Design and Rapid-Mixing Production Techniques of Lipid Nanoparticles for Nucleic Acid Delivery. *Small Methods* **2018**, *2*, 1700375. [CrossRef]
122. Pick, U. Liposomes with a large trapping capacity prepared by freezing and thawing of sonicated phospholipid mixtures. *Arch. Biochem. Biophys.* **1981**, *212*, 186–194. [CrossRef]
123. Obeid, M.A.; Tate, R.J.; Mullen, A.B.; Ferro, V.A. Chapter 8—Lipid-based nanoparticles for cancer treatment. In *Lipid Nanocarriers for Drug Targeting*; Grumezescu, A.M., Ed.; William Andrew Publishing: Oxford, UK, 2018; pp. 313–359. [CrossRef]

124. Richardson, J.; Caruso, F. Nanomedicine toward 2040. *Nano Lett.* **2020**, *20*, 1481–1482. [CrossRef] [PubMed]
125. Kamb, A. What's wrong with our cancer models? *Nat. Rev. Drug Discov.* **2005**, *4*, 161–165. [CrossRef]
126. Tyner, K.M.; Zou, P.; Yang, X.; Zhang, H.; Cruz, C.N.; Lee, S.L. Product quality for nanomaterials: Current U.S. experience and perspective. *WIREs Nanomed. Nanobiotechnol.* **2015**, *7*, 640–654. [CrossRef]
127. Burghelea, T.; Segre, E.; Bar-Joseph, I.; Groisman, A.; Steinberg, V. Chaotic flow and efficient mixing in a microchannel with a polymer solution. *Phys. Rev. E* **2004**, *69*, 066305. [CrossRef] [PubMed]
128. Lee, C.-Y.; Wang, W.-T.; Liu, C.-C.; Fu, L.-M. Passive mixers in microfluidic systems: A review. *Chem. Eng. J.* **2016**, *288*, 146–160. [CrossRef]
129. Yaralioglu, G.G.; Wygant, I.O.; Marentis, T.C.; Khuri-Yakub, B.T. Ultrasonic Mixing in Microfluidic Channels Using Integrated Transducers. *Anal. Chem.* **2004**, *76*, 3694–3698. [CrossRef]
130. Lee, S.L.; O'Connor, T.F.; Yang, X.; Cruz, C.N.; Chatterjee, S.; Madurawe, R.D.; Moore, C.M.V.; Yu, L.X.; Woodcock, J. Modernizing Pharmaceutical Manufacturing: From Batch to Continuous Production. *J. Pharm. Innov.* **2015**, *10*, 191–199. [CrossRef]
131. Whitesides, G.M. The origins and the future of microfluidics. *Nature* **2006**, *442*, 368–373. [CrossRef]
132. Tokeshi, M.; Sato, K. Micro/Nano Devices for Chemical Analysis. *Micromachines* **2016**, *7*, 164. [CrossRef]
133. Karnik, R.; Gu, F.; Basto, P.; Cannizzaro, C.; Dean, L.; Kyei-Manu, W.; Langer, R.; Farokhzad, O.C. Microfluidic Platform for Controlled Synthesis of Polymeric Nanoparticles. *Nano Lett.* **2008**, *8*, 2906–2912. [CrossRef] [PubMed]
134. Donno, R.; Gennari, A.; Lallana, E.; De La Rosa, J.M.R.; d'Arcy, R.; Treacher, K.; Hill, K.; Ashford, M.; Tirelli, N. Nanomanufacturing through microfluidic-assisted nanoprecipitation: Advanced analytics and structure-activity relationships. *Int. J. Pharm.* **2017**, *534*, 97–107. [CrossRef] [PubMed]
135. Bramosanti, M.; Chronopoulou, L.; Grillo, F.; Valletta, A.; Palocci, C. Microfluidic-assisted nanoprecipitation of antiviral-loaded polymeric nanoparticles. *Colloids Surf. A Physicochem. Eng. Asp.* **2017**, *532*, 369–376. [CrossRef]
136. Jaradat, E.; Weaver, E.; Meziane, A.; Lamprou, D.A. Microfluidics Technology for the Design and Formulation of Nanomedicines. *Nanomaterials* **2021**, *11*, 3440. [CrossRef]
137. Beebe, D.J.; Mensing, G.A.; Walker, G.M. Physics and Applications of Microfluidics in Biology. *Annu. Rev. Biomed. Eng.* **2002**, *4*, 261–286. [CrossRef]
138. Nguyen, N.-T.; Wereley, S.T.; Shaegh, S.A.M. *Fundamentals and Applications of Microfluidics*; Artech House: Norwood, MA, USA, 2019.
139. Zhang, Z.; Zhao, P.; Xiao, G.; Lin, M.; Cao, X. Focusing-enhanced mixing in microfluidic channels. *Biomicrofluidics* **2008**, *2*, 014101. [CrossRef]
140. Kumar, V.; Paraschivoiu, M.; Nigam, K.D.P. Single-phase fluid flow and mixing in microchannels. *Chem. Eng. Sci.* **2011**, *66*, 1329–1373. [CrossRef]
141. Yang, Z.; Matsumoto, S.; Goto, H.; Matsumoto, M.; Maeda, R. Ultrasonic micromixer for microfluidic systems. *Sens. Actuators A Phys.* **2001**, *93*, 266–272. [CrossRef]
142. Glasgow, I.; Aubry, N. Enhancement of microfluidic mixing using time pulsing. *Lab Chip* **2003**, *3*, 114–120. [CrossRef]
143. Turkyilmazoglu, M. Magnetohydrodynamic Moving Liquid Plug Within a Microchannel: Analytical Solutions. *J. Biomech. Eng.* **2020**, *143*, 011012. [CrossRef]
144. Tsai, J.-H.; Lin, L. Active microfluidic mixer and gas bubble filter driven by thermal bubble micropump. *Sens. Actuators A Phys.* **2002**, *97–98*, 665–671. [CrossRef]
145. Wu, Z.; Nguyen, N.-T. Convective–diffusive transport in parallel lamination micromixers. *Microfluid. Nanofluidics* **2005**, *1*, 208–217. [CrossRef]
146. Knight, J.B.; Vishwanath, A.; Brody, J.P.; Austin, R.H. Hydrodynamic Focusing on a Silicon Chip: Mixing Nanoliters in Microseconds. *Phys. Rev. Lett.* **1998**, *80*, 3863–3866. [CrossRef]
147. Kamholz, A.E.; Yager, P. Molecular diffusive scaling laws in pressure-driven microfluidic channels: Deviation from one-dimensional Einstein approximations. *Sens. Actuators B Chem.* **2002**, *82*, 117–121. [CrossRef]
148. Johnson, T.J.; Ross, D.; Locascio, L.E. Rapid Microfluidic Mixing. *Anal. Chem.* **2002**, *74*, 45–51. [CrossRef]
149. Stroock, A.D.; Dertinger, S.K.W.; Ajdari, A.; Mezić, I.; Stone, H.A.; Whitesides, G.M. Chaotic Mixer for Microchannels. *Science* **2002**, *295*, 647–651. [CrossRef]
150. Günther, A.; Jhunjhunwala, M.; Thalmann, M.; Schmidt, M.A.; Jensen, K.F. Micromixing of Miscible Liquids in Segmented Gas−Liquid Flow. *Langmuir* **2005**, *21*, 1547–1555. [CrossRef]
151. Song, H.; Tice, J.D.; Ismagilov, R.F. A microfluidic system for controlling reaction networks in time. *Angew. Chem.* **2003**, *115*, 792–796. [CrossRef]
152. Capretto, L.; Cheng, W.; Hill, M.; Zhang, X. Micromixing Within Microfluidic Devices. In *Microfluidics: Technologies and Applications*; Lin, B., Ed.; Springer: Berlin/Heidelberg, Germany, 2011; pp. 27–68.
153. Osouli-Bostanabad, K.; Masalehdan, T.; Kapsa, R.M.I.; Quigley, A.; Lalatsa, A.; Bruggeman, K.F.; Franks, S.J.; Williams, R.J.; Nisbet, D.R. Traction of 3D and 4D Printing in the Healthcare Industry: From Drug Delivery and Analysis to Regenerative Medicine. *ACS Biomater. Sci. Eng.* **2022**, *8*, 2764–2797. [CrossRef]
154. Chang, C.-H.; Paul, B.K.; Remcho, V.T.; Atre, S.; Hutchison, J.E. Synthesis and post-processing of nanomaterials using microreaction technology. *J. Nanopart. Res.* **2008**, *10*, 965–980. [CrossRef]

155. Bertuit, E.; Neveu, S.; Abou-Hassan, A. High Temperature Continuous Flow Syntheses of Iron Oxide Nanoflowers Using the Polyol Route in a Multi-Parametric Millifluidic Device. *Nanomaterials* **2022**, *12*, 119. [CrossRef] [PubMed]
156. Liu, Y.; Yang, G.; Hui, Y.; Ranaweera, S.; Zhao, C.-X. Microfluidic Nanoparticles for Drug Delivery. *Small* **2022**, *18*, 2106580. [CrossRef] [PubMed]
157. Abou-Hassan, A.; Bazzi, R.; Cabuil, V. Multistep continuous-flow microsynthesis of magnetic and fluorescent γ-Fe_2O_3@ SiO_2 core/shell nanoparticles. *Angew. Chem.* **2009**, *121*, 7316–7319. [CrossRef]
158. Ying, Y.; Chen, G.; Zhao, Y.; Li, S.; Yuan, Q. A high throughput methodology for continuous preparation of monodispersed nanocrystals in microfluidic reactors. *Chem. Eng. J.* **2008**, *135*, 209–215. [CrossRef]
159. Boleininger, J.; Kurz, A.; Reuss, V.; Sönnichsen, C. Microfluidic continuous flow synthesis of rod-shaped gold and silver nanocrystals. *Phys. Chem. Chem. Phys.* **2006**, *8*, 3824–3827. [CrossRef]
160. Ju, J.; Zeng, C.; Zhang, L.; Xu, N. Continuous synthesis of zeolite NaA in a microchannel reactor. *Chem. Eng. J.* **2006**, *116*, 115–121. [CrossRef]
161. She, Q.M.; Liu, J.H.; Aymonier, C.; Zhou, C.H. In situ fabrication of layered double hydroxide film immobilizing gold nanoparticles in capillary microreactor for efficient catalytic carbonylation of glycerol. *Mol. Catal.* **2021**, *513*, 111825. [CrossRef]
162. Takagi, M.; Maki, T.; Miyahara, M.; Mae, K. Production of titania nanoparticles by using a new microreactor assembled with same axle dual pipe. *Chem. Eng. J.* **2004**, *101*, 269–276. [CrossRef]
163. Liu, Z.; Lu, Y.; Yang, B.; Luo, G. Controllable Preparation of Poly(butyl acrylate) by Suspension Polymerization in a Coaxial Capillary Microreactor. *Ind. Eng. Chem. Res.* **2011**, *50*, 11853–11862. [CrossRef]
164. Flögel, O.; Codée, J.D.C.; Seebach, D.; Seeberger, P.H. Microreactor Synthesis of β-Peptides. *Angew. Chem. Int. Ed.* **2006**, *45*, 7000–7003. [CrossRef]
165. Tan, Y.-C.; Hettiarachchi, K.; Siu, M.; Pan, Y.-R.; Lee, A.P. Controlled Microfluidic Encapsulation of Cells, Proteins, and Microbeads in Lipid Vesicles. *J. Am. Chem. Soc.* **2006**, *128*, 5656–5658. [CrossRef] [PubMed]
166. Lorenceau, E.; Utada, A.S.; Link, D.R.; Cristobal, G.; Joanicot, M.; Weitz, D.A. Generation of Polymerosomes from Double-Emulsions. *Langmuir* **2005**, *21*, 9183–9186. [CrossRef] [PubMed]
167. Shum, H.C.; Kim, J.-W.; Weitz, D.A. Microfluidic Fabrication of Monodisperse Biocompatible and Biodegradable Polymersomes with Controlled Permeability. *J. Am. Chem. Soc.* **2008**, *130*, 9543–9549. [CrossRef]
168. Carugo, D.; Bottaro, E.; Owen, J.; Stride, E.; Nastruzzi, C. Liposome production by microfluidics: Potential and limiting factors. *Sci. Rep.* **2016**, *6*, 25876. [CrossRef] [PubMed]
169. Ali, H.S.M.; York, P.; Blagden, N. Preparation of hydrocortisone nanosuspension through a bottom-up nanoprecipitation technique using microfluidic reactors. *Int. J. Pharm.* **2009**, *375*, 107–113. [CrossRef]
170. Edel, J.B.; Fortt, R.; deMello, J.C.; deMello, A.J. Microfluidic routes to the controlled production of nanoparticles. *Chem. Commun.* **2002**, *10*, 1136–1137. [CrossRef]
171. Kastner, E.; Kaur, R.; Lowry, D.; Moghaddam, B.; Wilkinson, A.; Perrie, Y. High-throughput manufacturing of size-tuned liposomes by a new microfluidics method using enhanced statistical tools for characterization. *Int. J. Pharm.* **2014**, *477*, 361–368. [CrossRef]
172. Aranguren, A.; Torres, C.E.; Munoz-Camargo, C.; Osma, J.F.; Cruz, J.C. Synthesis of Nanoscale Liposomes via Low-Cost Microfluidic Systems. *Micromachines* **2020**, *11*, 1050. [CrossRef]
173. Zizzari, A.; Carbone, L.; Cesaria, M.; Bianco, M.; Perrone, E.; Rendina, F.; Arima, V. Continuous flow scalable production of injectable size-monodisperse nanoliposomes in easy-fabrication milli-fluidic reactors. *Chem. Eng. Sci.* **2021**, *235*, 116481. [CrossRef]
174. Shestopalov, I.; Tice, J.D.; Ismagilov, R.F. Multi-step synthesis of nanoparticles performed on millisecond time scale in a microfluidic droplet-based system. *Lab Chip* **2004**, *4*, 316–321. [CrossRef]
175. Chan, E.M.; Alivisatos, A.P.; Mathies, R.A. High-Temperature Microfluidic Synthesis of CdSe Nanocrystals in Nanoliter Droplets. *J. Am. Chem. Soc.* **2005**, *127*, 13854–13861. [CrossRef] [PubMed]
176. Prakash, G.; Shokr, A.; Willemen, N.; Bashir, S.M.; Shin, S.R.; Hassan, S. Microfluidic fabrication of lipid nanoparticles for the delivery of nucleic acids. *Adv. Drug Deliv. Rev.* **2022**, *184*, 114197. [CrossRef] [PubMed]
177. Khan, S.A.; Günther, A.; Schmidt, M.A.; Jensen, K.F. Microfluidic Synthesis of Colloidal Silica. *Langmuir* **2004**, *20*, 8604–8611. [CrossRef] [PubMed]
178. Zhang, S.-H.; Shen, S.-C.; Chen, Z.; Yun, J.-X.; Yao, K.-J.; Chen, B.-B.; Chen, J.-Z. Preparation of solid lipid nanoparticles in co-flowing microchannels. *Chem. Eng. J.* **2008**, *144*, 324–328. [CrossRef]
179. Génot, V.; Desportes, S.; Croushore, C.; Lefèvre, J.-P.; Pansu, R.B.; Delaire, J.A.; von Rohr, P.R. Synthesis of organic nanoparticles in a 3D flow focusing microreactor. *Chem. Eng. J.* **2010**, *161*, 234–239. [CrossRef]
180. Jahn, A.; Vreeland, W.N.; Gaitan, M.; Locascio, L.E. Controlled Vesicle Self-Assembly in Microfluidic Channels with Hydrodynamic Focusing. *J. Am. Chem. Soc.* **2004**, *126*, 2674–2675. [CrossRef]
181. Yun, J.; Zhang, S.; Shen, S.; Chen, Z.; Yao, K.; Chen, J. Continuous production of solid lipid nanoparticles by liquid flow-focusing and gas displacing method in microchannels. *Chem. Eng. Sci.* **2009**, *64*, 4115–4122. [CrossRef]
182. Gupta, R.; Fletcher, D.F.; Haynes, B.S. Taylor Flow in Microchannels: A Review of Experimental and Computational Work. *J. Comput. Multiph. Flows* **2010**, *2*, 1–31. [CrossRef]

183. Tice, J.D.; Song, H.; Lyon, A.D.; Ismagilov, R.F. Formation of Droplets and Mixing in Multiphase Microfluidics at Low Values of the Reynolds and the Capillary Numbers. *Langmuir* **2003**, *19*, 9127–9133. [CrossRef]
184. Kreutzer, M.T.; Kapteijn, F.; Moulijn, J.A.; Heiszwolf, J.J. Multiphase monolith reactors: Chemical reaction engineering of segmented flow in microchannels. *Chem. Eng. Sci.* **2005**, *60*, 5895–5916. [CrossRef]
185. Tan, Z.; Lan, W.; Liu, Q.; Wang, K.; Hussain, M.; Ren, M.; Geng, Z.; Zhang, L.; Luo, X.; Zhang, L.; et al. Kinetically Controlled Self-Assembly of Block Copolymers into Segmented Wormlike Micelles in Microfluidic Chips. *Langmuir* **2019**, *35*, 141–149. [CrossRef] [PubMed]
186. Matosevic, S.; Paegel, B.M. Stepwise Synthesis of Giant Unilamellar Vesicles on a Microfluidic Assembly Line. *J. Am. Chem. Soc.* **2011**, *133*, 2798–2800. [CrossRef]
187. Matosevic, S.; Paegel, B.M. Layer-by-layer cell membrane assembly. *Nat. Chem.* **2013**, *5*, 958–963. [CrossRef] [PubMed]
188. Erfle, P.; Riewe, J.; Bunjes, H.; Dietzel, A. Optically monitored segmented flow for controlled ultra-fast mixing and nanoparticle precipitation. *Microfluid. Nanofluidics* **2017**, *21*, 179. [CrossRef]
189. Riewe, J.; Erfle, P.; Melzig, S.; Kwade, A.; Dietzel, A.; Bunjes, H. Antisolvent precipitation of lipid nanoparticles in microfluidic systems—A comparative study. *Int. J. Pharm.* **2020**, *579*, 119167. [CrossRef]
190. Zinoveva, S.; De Silva, R.; Louis, R.D.; Datta, P.; Kumar, C.S.; Goettert, J.; Hormes, J. The wet chemical synthesis of Co nanoparticles in a microreactor system: A time-resolved investigation by X-ray absorption spectroscopy. *Nucl. Instrum. Methods Phys. Res. Sect. A: Accel. Spectrometers Detect. Assoc. Equip.* **2007**, *582*, 239–241. [CrossRef]
191. Erfan, M.; Gnambodoe-Capochichi, M.; Sabry, Y.M.; Khalil, D.; Leprince-Wang, Y.; Bourouina, T. Spatiotemporal dynamics of nanowire growth in a microfluidic reactor. *Microsyst. Nanoeng.* **2021**, *7*, 77. [CrossRef]
192. Li, J.; Šimek, H.; Ilioae, D.; Jung, N.; Braese, S.; Zappe, H.; Dittmeyer, R.; Ladewig, B.P. In Situ Sensors for Flow Reactors—A Review. *React. Chem. Eng.* **2021**, *6*, 1497–1507. [CrossRef]
193. Sounart, T.L.; Safier, P.A.; Voigt, J.A.; Hoyt, J.; Tallant, D.R.; Matzke, C.M.; Michalske, T.A. Spatially-resolved analysis of nanoparticle nucleation and growth in a microfluidic reactor. *Lab Chip* **2007**, *7*, 908–915. [CrossRef]
194. Just, J.; Coughlan, C.; Singh, S.; Ren, H.; Müller, O.; Becker, P.; Unold, T.; Ryan, K.M. Insights into Nucleation and Growth of Colloidal Quaternary Nanocrystals by Multimodal X-ray Analysis. *ACS Nano* **2021**, *15*, 6439–6447. [CrossRef]
195. Herbst, M. *Microfluidic and X-ray Techniques for Investigations of Nanoparticle Nucleation and Growth*; ProQuest Dissertations Publishing: Bayreuth, Germany, 2021; p. 28485697.
196. Maeki, M.; Fujishima, Y.; Sato, Y.; Yasui, T.; Kaji, N.; Ishida, A.; Tani, H.; Baba, Y.; Harashima, H.; Tokeshi, M. Understanding the formation mechanism of lipid nanoparticles in microfluidic devices with chaotic micromixers. *PLoS ONE* **2017**, *12*, e0187962. [CrossRef] [PubMed]
197. Wilms, D.; Klos, J.; Frey, H. Microstructured Reactors for Polymer Synthesis: A Renaissance of Continuous Flow Processes for Tailor-Made Macromolecules? *Macromol. Chem. Phys.* **2008**, *209*, 343–356. [CrossRef]
198. Yu, W.; Chen, H.; Wu, H.; Lin, P.; Xu, H.; Xie, Q.; Shi, K.; Xie, G.; Chen, Y. Continuous-flow rapid synthesis of wavelength-tunable luminescent lanthanide metal-organic framework nanorods by a microfluidic reactor. *J. Alloys Compd.* **2022**, *890*, 161860. [CrossRef]
199. Nakamura, H.; Yamaguchi, Y.; Miyazaki, M.; Maeda, H.; Uehara, M.; Mulvaney, P. Preparation of CdSe nanocrystals in a micro-flow-reactor. *Chem. Commun.* **2002**, *1*, 2844–2845. [CrossRef] [PubMed]
200. Zook, J.M.; Vreeland, W.N. Effects of temperature, acyl chain length, and flow-rate ratio on liposome formation and size in a microfluidic hydrodynamic focusing device. *Soft Matter* **2010**, *6*, 1352–1360. [CrossRef]
201. Pradhan, P.; Guan, J.; Lu, D.; Wang, P.G.; Lee, L.J.; Lee, R.J. A Facile Microfluidic Method for Production of Liposomes. *Anticancer Res.* **2008**, *28*, 943.
202. Miranda, I.; Souza, A.; Sousa, P.; Ribeiro, J.; Castanheira, E.M.S.; Lima, R.; Minas, G. Properties and Applications of PDMS for Biomedical Engineering: A Review. *J. Funct. Biomater.* **2022**, *13*, 2. [CrossRef]
203. Zhang, H.; Huang, L.; Tan, M.; Zhao, S.; Liu, H.; Lu, Z.; Li, J.; Liang, Z. Overview of 3D-Printed Silica Glass. *Micromachines* **2022**, *13*, 81. [CrossRef]
204. Damodara, S.; Shahriari, S.; Wu, W.-I.; Rezai, P.; Hsu, H.-H.; Selvaganapathy, R. 1—Materials and methods for microfabrication of microfluidic devices. In *Microfluidic Devices for Biomedical Applications*, 2nd ed.; Li, X., Zhou, Y., Eds.; Woodhead Publishing: Cambridge, UK, 2021; pp. 1–78. [CrossRef]
205. Shubhava; Jayarama, A.; Kannarpady, G.K.; Kale, S.; Prabhu, S.; Pinto, R. Chemical etching of glasses in hydrofluoric Acid: A brief review. *Mater. Today Proc.* **2021**, *55*, 46–51. [CrossRef]
206. Bahrani, S.; Ghalamfarsa, F.; Nekoi, S.; Ghaedi, M.; Hashemi, S.A.; Mousavi, S.M. Chapter 17—Microfluidics technology: Past, present, and future prospects for biomarker diagnostics. In *The Detection of Biomarkers*; Ozkan, S.A., Bakirhan, N.K., Mollarasouli, F., Eds.; Academic Press: Cambridge, MA, USA, 2022; pp. 457–485. [CrossRef]
207. Friend, J.; Yeo, L. Fabrication of microfluidic devices using polydimethylsiloxane. *Biomicrofluidics* **2010**, *4*, 026502. [CrossRef]
208. Kim, P.; Kwon, K.W.; Park, M.C.; Lee, S.H.; Kim, S.M.; Suh, K.Y. Soft Lithography for Microfluidics: A Review. *Biochip J.* **2008**, *2*, 1–11.
209. Perez-Toralla, K.; Champ, J.; Mohamadi, M.R.; Braun, O.; Malaquin, L.; Viovy, J.-L.; Descroix, S. New non-covalent strategies for stable surface treatment of thermoplastic chips. *Lab Chip* **2013**, *13*, 4409–4418. [CrossRef] [PubMed]

210. Agha, A.; Waheed, W.; Alamoodi, N.; Mathew, B.; Alnaimat, F.; Abu-Nada, E.; Abderrahmane, A.; Alazzam, A. A Review of Cyclic Olefin Copolymer Applications in Microfluidics and Microdevices. *Macromol. Mater. Eng.* **2022**, *307*, 2200053. [CrossRef]
211. Garcia-Rey, S.; Nielsen, J.B.; Nordin, G.P.; Woolley, A.T.; Basabe-Desmonts, L.; Benito-Lopez, F. High-Resolution 3D Printing Fabrication of a Microfluidic Platform for Blood Plasma Separation. *Polymers* **2022**, *14*, 2537. [CrossRef] [PubMed]
212. Stansbury, J.J.W.; Idacavage, M.J. 3D printing with polymers: Challenges among expanding options and opportunities. *Dent. Mater.* **2016**, *32*, 54–64. [CrossRef]
213. Dizon, J.R.C.; Espera, A.H.; Chen, Q.; Advincula, R.C. Mechanical characterization of 3D-printed polymers. *Addit. Manuf.* **2018**, *20*, 44–67. [CrossRef]
214. Schoerpf, S.; Catel, Y.; Moszner, N.; Gorsche, C.; Liska, R. Enhanced reduction of polymerization-induced shrinkage stress via combination of radical ring opening and addition fragmentation chain transfer. *Polym. Chem.* **2019**, *10*, 1357–1366. [CrossRef]
215. Iedema, P.D.; Schamböck, V.; Boonen, H.; van der Linden, M.N.; Willemse, R. Photocuring of di-acrylate in presence of oxygen. *Chem. Eng. Sci.* **2019**, *207*, 130–144. [CrossRef]
216. Peerzada, M.; Abbasi, S.; Lau, K.T.; Hameed, N. Additive Manufacturing of Epoxy Resins: Materials, Methods, and Latest Trends. *Ind. Eng. Chem. Res.* **2020**, *59*, 6375–6390. [CrossRef]
217. Li, S.; Sun, D.; Li, A.; Cui, Y. Study on curing shrinkage and mechanism of DHOM-modified epoxy-acrylate-based UV-curing 3D printing materials. *J. Appl. Polym. Sci.* **2021**, *138*, 49859. [CrossRef]
218. Mohan, D.; Sajab, M.S.; Bakarudin, S.B.; Roslan, R.; Kaco, H. 3D Printed Polyurethane Reinforced Graphene Nanoplatelets. *Mater. Sci. Forum* **2021**, *1025*, 47–52. [CrossRef]
219. Sun, B.; Jiang, J.; Shi, N.; Xu, W. Application of microfluidics technology in chemical engineering for enhanced safety. *Process Saf. Prog.* **2016**, *35*, 365–373. [CrossRef]
220. Zhang, H.; Anoop, K.; Huang, C.; Sadr, R.; Gupte, R.; Dai, J.; Han, A. A circular gradient-width crossflow microfluidic platform for high-efficiency blood plasma separation. *Sens. Actuators B Chem.* **2022**, *354*, 131180. [CrossRef]
221. Nix, C.; Fillet, M. Chapter 10—Microfluidics in three key aspects of the drug-development process: Biomarker discovery, preclinical studies, and drug delivery systems. In *Multidisciplinary Microfluidic and Nanofluidic Lab-on-a-Chip*; Li, X., Yang, C., Li, P.C.H., Eds.; Elsevier: Amsterdam, The Netherlands, 2022; pp. 275–295. [CrossRef]
222. Luo, X.; Su, P.; Zhang, W.; Raston, C.L. Microfluidic Devices in Fabricating Nano or Micromaterials for Biomedical Applications. *Adv. Mater. Technol.* **2019**, *4*, 1900488. [CrossRef]
223. Ran, R.; Wang, H.; Liu, Y.; Hui, Y.; Sun, Q.; Seth, A.; Wibowo, D.; Chen, D.; Zhao, C.-X. Microfluidic self-assembly of a combinatorial library of single- and dual-ligand liposomes for in vitro and in vivo tumor targeting. *Eur. J. Pharm. Biopharm.* **2018**, *130*, 1–10. [CrossRef]
224. Li, Y.; Lee, R.J.; Huang, X.; Li, Y.; Lv, B.; Wang, T.; Qi, Y.; Hao, F.; Lu, J.; Meng, Q.; et al. Single-step microfluidic synthesis of transferrin-conjugated lipid nanoparticles for siRNA delivery. *Nanomed. Nanotechnol. Biol. Med.* **2017**, *13*, 371–381. [CrossRef]
225. Ran, R.; Middelberg, A.P.J.; Zhao, C.-X. Microfluidic synthesis of multifunctional liposomes for tumour targeting. *Colloids Surf. B Biointerfaces* **2016**, *148*, 402–410. [CrossRef]
226. Maeki, M.; Uno, S.; Niwa, A.; Okada, Y.; Tokeshi, M. Microfluidic technologies and devices for lipid nanoparticle-based RNA delivery. *J. Control. Release* **2022**, *344*, 80–96. [CrossRef]
227. Shepherd, S.J.; Issadore, D.; Mitchell, M.J. Microfluidic formulation of nanoparticles for biomedical applications. *Biomaterials* **2021**, *274*, 120826. [CrossRef]
228. Belliveau, N.M.; Huft, J.; Lin, P.J.C.; Chen, S.; Leung, A.K.K.; Leaver, T.J.; Wild, A.W.; Lee, J.B.; Taylor, R.J.; Tam, Y.K.; et al. Microfluidic Synthesis of Highly Potent Limit-size Lipid Nanoparticles for In Vivo Delivery of siRNA. *Mol. Ther. Nucleic Acids* **2012**, *1*, e37. [CrossRef]
229. Zhigaltsev, I.V.; Belliveau, N.; Hafez, I.; Leung, A.K.K.; Huft, J.; Hansen, C.; Cullis, P.R. Bottom-Up Design and Synthesis of Limit Size Lipid Nanoparticle Systems with Aqueous and Triglyceride Cores Using Millisecond Microfluidic Mixing. *Langmuir* **2012**, *28*, 3633–3640. [CrossRef] [PubMed]
230. Maeki, M.; Saito, T.; Sato, Y.; Yasui, T.; Kaji, N.; Ishida, A.; Tani, H.; Baba, Y.; Harashima, H.; Tokeshi, M. A strategy for synthesis of lipid nanoparticles using microfluidic devices with a mixer structure. *RSC Adv.* **2015**, *5*, 46181–46185. [CrossRef]
231. Nguyen, D.P.; Kloosterman, F.; Barbieri, R.; Brown, E.N.; Wilson, M.A.; Klausberger, T.Z. Micromixers—A review. *J. Micromech. Microeng.* **2005**, *15*, R1–R16. [CrossRef]
232. Zimmermann, T.S.; Lee, A.C.; Akinc, A.; Bramlage, B.; Bumcrot, D.; Fedoruk, M.N.; Harborth, J.; Heyes, J.A.; Jeffs, L.B.; John, M.; et al. RNAi-mediated gene silencing in non-human primates. *Nature* **2006**, *441*, 111–114. [CrossRef] [PubMed]
233. Liu, D.; Zhang, H.; Fontana, F.; Hirvonen, J.T.; Santos, H.A. Current developments and applications of microfluidic technology toward clinical translation of nanomedicines. *Adv. Drug Deliv. Rev.* **2018**, *128*, 54–83. [CrossRef] [PubMed]
234. Schikarski, T.; Trzenschiok, H.; Peukert, W.; Avila, M. Inflow boundary conditions determine T-mixer efficiency. *React. Chem. Eng.* **2019**, *4*, 559–568. [CrossRef]
235. Günther, A.; Khan, S.A.; Thalmann, M.; Trachsel, F.; Jensen, K.F. Transport and reaction in microscale segmented gas–liquid flow. *Lab Chip* **2004**, *4*, 278–286. [CrossRef]
236. Tiboni, M.; Tiboni, M.; Pierro, A.; Del Papa, M.; Sparaventi, S.; Cespi, M.; Casettari, L. Microfluidics for nanomedicines manufacturing: An affordable and low-cost 3D printing approach. *Int. J. Pharm.* **2021**, *599*, 120464. [CrossRef]

237. Camarri, S.; Mariotti, A.; Galletti, C.; Brunazzi, E.; Mauri, R.; Salvetti, M.V. An Overview of Flow Features and Mixing in Micro T and Arrow Mixers. *Ind. Eng. Chem. Res.* **2020**, *59*, 3669–3686. [CrossRef]
238. Jahn, A.; Stavis, S.M.; Hong, J.S.; Vreeland, W.N.; DeVoe, D.L.; Gaitan, M. Microfluidic Mixing and the Formation of Nanoscale Lipid Vesicles. *ACS Nano* **2010**, *4*, 2077–2087. [CrossRef]
239. Jahn, A.; Vreeland, W.N.; DeVoe, D.L.; Locascio, L.E.; Gaitan, M. Microfluidic Directed Formation of Liposomes of Controlled Size. *Langmuir* **2007**, *23*, 6289–6293. [CrossRef] [PubMed]
240. Capretto, L.; Carugo, D.; Mazzitelli, S.; Nastruzzi, C.; Zhang, X. Microfluidic and lab-on-a-chip preparation routes for organic nanoparticles and vesicular systems for nanomedicine applications. *Adv. Drug Deliv. Rev.* **2013**, *65*, 1496–1532. [CrossRef]
241. Webb, C.; Khadke, S.; Tandrup Schmidt, S.; Roces, C.B.; Forbes, N.; Berrie, G.; Perrie, Y. The Impact of Solvent Selection: Strategies to Guide the Manufacturing of Liposomes Using Microfluidics. *Pharmaceutics* **2019**, *11*, 653. [CrossRef] [PubMed]
242. Krzysztoń, R.; Salem, B.; Lee, D.J.; Schwake, G.; Wagner, E.; Rädler, J.O. Microfluidic self-assembly of folate-targeted monomolecular siRNA-lipid nanoparticles. *Nanoscale* **2017**, *9*, 7442–7453. [CrossRef]
243. van Swaay, D.; DeMello, A. Microfluidic methods for forming liposomes. *Lab Chip* **2013**, *13*, 752–767. [CrossRef]
244. Mijajlovic, M.; Wright, D.; Zivkovic, V.; Bi, J.X.; Biggs, M.J. Microfluidic hydrodynamic focusing based synthesis of POPC liposomes for model biological systems. *Colloids Surf. B Biointerfaces* **2013**, *104*, 276–281. [CrossRef] [PubMed]
245. Balbino, T.T.A.; Aoki, N.T.; Gasperini, A.A.M.; Oliveira, C.L.P.; Azzoni, A.R.; Cavalcanti, L.P.; de la Torre, L.G. Continuous flow production of cationic liposomes at high lipid concentration in microfluidic devices for gene delivery applications. *Chem. Eng. J.* **2013**, *226*, 423–433. [CrossRef]
246. Hood, R.R.; Shao, C.; Omiatek, D.M.; Vreeland, W.N.; DeVoe, D.L. Microfluidic Synthesis of PEG- and Folate-Conjugated Liposomes for One-Step Formation of Targeted Stealth Nanocarriers. *Pharm. Res.* **2013**, *30*, 1597–1607. [CrossRef]
247. Church, A.S.; Witting, M.D. Laboratory testing in ethanol, methanol, ethylene glycol, and isopropanol toxicities. *J. Emerg. Med.* **1997**, *15*, 687–692. [CrossRef]
248. Wu, N.; Zhu, Y.; Leech, P.; Sexton, B.; Brown, S.; Easton, C. Effects of Surfactants on the Formation of Microdroplets in the Flow Focusing Microfluidic Device. In Proceedings of the BioMEMS and Nanotechnology III, Canberra, ACT, Australia, 4–7 December 2007; Volume 6799.
249. ICH. Guideline Q3C (R8) on Impurities: Guideline for Residual Solvents. *European Medicines Agency. EMA/CHMP/ICH/82260/2006* 2021. Available online: https://www.ema.europa.eu/en/ich-q3c-r8-residual-solvents (accessed on 4 August 2022).
250. Joshi, S.; Hussain, M.T.; Roces, C.B.; Anderluzzi, G.; Kastner, E.; Salmaso, S.; Kirby, D.J.; Perrie, Y. Microfluidics based manufacture of liposomes simultaneously entrapping hydrophilic and lipophilic drugs. *Int. J. Pharm.* **2016**, *514*, 160–168. [CrossRef]
251. Lou, G.; Anderluzzi, G.; Woods, S.; Roberts, C.W.; Perrie, Y. A novel microfluidic-based approach to formulate size-tuneable large unilamellar cationic liposomes: Formulation, cellular uptake and biodistribution investigations. *Eur. J. Pharm. Biopharm.* **2019**, *143*, 51–60. [CrossRef] [PubMed]
252. Hood, R.R.; DeVoe, D.L.; Atencia, J.; Vreeland, W.N.; Omiatek, D.M. A facile route to the synthesis of monodisperse nanoscale liposomes using 3D microfluidic hydrodynamic focusing in a concentric capillary array. *Lab Chip* **2014**, *14*, 2403–2409. [CrossRef] [PubMed]
253. Allen, T.M.; Cullis, P.R. Liposomal drug delivery systems: From concept to clinical applications. *Adv. Drug Deliv. Rev.* **2013**, *65*, 36–48. [CrossRef]
254. Chang, H.I.; Yeh, M.K. Clinical development of liposome-based drugs: Formulation, characterization, and therapeutic efficacy. *Int. J. Nanomed.* **2012**, *7*, 49–60. [CrossRef]
255. Yang, J.-T.; Fang, W.-F.; Tung, K.-Y. Fluids mixing in devices with connected-groove channels. *Chem. Eng. Sci.* **2008**, *63*, 1871–1881. [CrossRef]
256. van Schijndel, T.; Singh, M.K.; Gillies, M.; Kahya, N.; Kharin, A.; den Toonder, J.M.J. Toward Gradient Formation in Microfluidic Devices by using Slanted Ridges. *Macromol. Mater. Eng.* **2011**, *296*, 373–379. [CrossRef]
257. Lin, D.; He, F.; Liao, Y.; Lin, J.; Liu, C.; Song, J.; Cheng, Y. Three-dimensional staggered herringbone mixer fabricated by femtosecond laser direct writing. *J. Opt.* **2013**, *15*, 025601. [CrossRef]
258. Chen, D.; Love, K.T.; Chen, Y.; Eltoukhy, A.A.; Kastrup, C.; Sahay, G.; Jeon, A.; Dong, Y.; Whitehead, K.A.; Anderson, D.G. Rapid Discovery of Potent siRNA-Containing Lipid Nanoparticles Enabled by Controlled Microfluidic Formulation. *J. Am. Chem. Soc.* **2012**, *134*, 6948–6951. [CrossRef] [PubMed]
259. Ianovska, M. Microfluidic Tools for Multidimensional Liquid Chromatography. Ph.D. Thesis, University of Groningen, Groningen, The Netherlands, 2018.
260. Kauffman, K.J.; Dorkin, J.R.; Yang, J.H.; Heartlein, M.W.; DeRosa, F.; Mir, F.F.; Fenton, O.S.; Anderson, D.G. Optimization of Lipid Nanoparticle Formulations for mRNA Delivery in Vivo with Fractional Factorial and Definitive Screening Designs. *Nano Lett.* **2015**, *15*, 7300–7306. [CrossRef]
261. Gooding, O.W. Process optimization using combinatorial design principles: Parallel synthesis and design of experiment methods. *Curr. Opin. Chem. Biol.* **2004**, *8*, 297–304. [CrossRef]
262. Dahlman, J.E.; Kauffman, K.J.; Xing, Y.; Shaw, T.E.; Mir, F.F.; Dlott, C.C.; Langer, R.; Anderson, D.G.; Wang, E.T. Barcoded nanoparticles for high throughput in vivo discovery of targeted therapeutics. *Proc. Natl. Acad. Sci. USA* **2017**, *114*, 2060–2065. [CrossRef]

263. Guimaraes, P.P.G.; Zhang, R.; Spektor, R.; Tan, M.; Chung, A.; Billingsley, M.M.; El-Mayta, R.; Riley, R.S.; Wang, L.; Wilson, J.M.; et al. Ionizable lipid nanoparticles encapsulating barcoded mRNA for accelerated in vivo delivery screening. *J. Control. Release* **2019**, *316*, 404–417. [CrossRef]
264. Kastner, E.; Verma, V.; Lowry, D.; Perrie, Y. Microfluidic-controlled manufacture of liposomes for the solubilisation of a poorly water soluble drug. *Int. J. Pharm.* **2015**, *485*, 122–130. [CrossRef]
265. Hood, R.R.; DeVoe, D.L. High-Throughput Continuous Flow Production of Nanoscale Liposomes by Microfluidic Vertical Flow Focusing. *Small* **2015**, *11*, 5790–5799. [CrossRef]
266. Roces, C.B.; Lou, G.; Jain, N.; Abraham, S.; Thomas, A.; Halbert, G.W.; Perrie, Y. Manufacturing Considerations for the Development of Lipid Nanoparticles Using Microfluidics. *Pharmaceutics* **2020**, *12*, 1095. [CrossRef]
267. Finn, J.D.; Smith, A.R.; Patel, M.C.; Shaw, L.; Youniss, M.R.; van Heteren, J.; Dirstine, T.; Ciullo, C.; Lescarbeau, R.; Seitzer, J.; et al. A Single Administration of CRISPR/Cas9 Lipid Nanoparticles Achieves Robust and Persistent In Vivo Genome Editing. *Cell Rep.* **2018**, *22*, 2227–2235. [CrossRef]
268. Patel, S.; Ashwanikumar, N.; Robinson, E.; Xia, Y.; Mihai, C.; Griffith, J.P.; Hou, S.; Esposito, A.A.; Ketova, T.; Welsher, K.; et al. Naturally-occurring cholesterol analogues in lipid nanoparticles induce polymorphic shape and enhance intracellular delivery of mRNA. *Nat. Commun.* **2020**, *11*, 983. [CrossRef]
269. Kimura, N.; Maeki, M.; Sato, Y.; Note, Y.; Ishida, A.; Tani, H.; Harashima, H.; Tokeshi, M. Development of the iLiNP Device: Fine Tuning the Lipid Nanoparticle Size within 10 nm for Drug Delivery. *ACS Omega* **2018**, *3*, 5044–5051. [CrossRef]
270. Balbino, T.A.; Azzoni, A.R.; de la Torre, L.G. Microfluidic devices for continuous production of pDNA/cationic liposome complexes for gene delivery and vaccine therapy. *Colloids Surf. B Biointerfaces* **2013**, *111*, 203–210. [CrossRef]
271. Kulkarni, J.A.; Chen, S.; Tam, Y.Y.C. Scalable Production of Lipid Nanoparticles Containing Amphotericin B. *Langmuir* **2021**, *37*, 7312–7319. [CrossRef]
272. Yang, Z.; Yu, B.; Zhu, J.; Huang, X.; Xie, J.; Xu, S.; Yang, X.; Wang, X.; Yung, B.C.; Lee, L.J.; et al. A microfluidic method to synthesize transferrin-lipid nanoparticles loaded with siRNA LOR-1284 for therapy of acute myeloid leukemia. *Nanoscale* **2014**, *6*, 9742–9751. [CrossRef]
273. Kim, H.; Sung, J.; Chang, Y.; Alfeche, A.; Leal, C. Microfluidics Synthesis of Gene Silencing Cubosomes. *ACS Nano* **2018**, *12*, 9196–9205. [CrossRef]
274. Sato, Y.; Note, Y.; Maeki, M.; Kaji, N.; Baba, Y.; Tokeshi, M.; Harashima, H. Elucidation of the physicochemical properties and potency of siRNA-loaded small-sized lipid nanoparticles for siRNA delivery. *J. Control. Release* **2016**, *229*, 48–57. [CrossRef]
275. Jyotsana, N.; Sharma, A.; Chaturvedi, A.; Budida, R.; Scherr, M.; Kuchenbauer, F.; Lindner, R.; Noyan, F.; Sühs, K.-W.; Stangel, M.; et al. Lipid nanoparticle-mediated siRNA delivery for safe targeting of human CML in vivo. *Ann. Hematol.* **2019**, *98*, 1905–1918. [CrossRef]
276. Gkionis, L.; Campbell, R.A.; Aojula, H.; Harris, L.K.; Tirella, A. Manufacturing drug co-loaded liposomal formulations targeting breast cancer: Influence of preparative method on liposomes characteristics and in vitro toxicity. *Int. J. Pharm.* **2020**, *590*, 119926. [CrossRef]
277. Hamano, N.; Böttger, R.; Lee, S.E.; Yang, Y.; Kulkarni, J.A.; Ip, S.; Cullis, P.R.; Li, S.-D. Robust Microfluidic Technology and New Lipid Composition for Fabrication of Curcumin-Loaded Liposomes: Effect on the Anticancer Activity and Safety of Cisplatin. *Mol. Pharm.* **2019**, *16*, 3957–3967. [CrossRef]
278. Fathordoobady, F.; Sannikova, N.; Guo, Y.; Singh, A.; Kitts, D.D.; Pratap-Singh, A. Comparing microfluidics and ultrasonication as formulation methods for developing hempseed oil nanoemulsions for oral delivery applications. *Sci. Rep.* **2021**, *11*, 72. [CrossRef]
279. Dong, Y.-D.; Tchung, E.; Nowell, C.; Kaga, S.; Leong, N.; Mehta, D.; Kaminskas, L.M.; Boyd, B.J. Microfluidic preparation of drug-loaded PEGylated liposomes, and the impact of liposome size on tumour retention and penetration. *J. Liposome Res.* **2019**, *29*, 1–9. [CrossRef]
280. Forbes, N.; Hussain, M.T.; Briuglia, M.L.; Edwards, D.P.; Horst, J.H.t.; Szita, N.; Perrie, Y. Rapid and scale-independent microfluidic manufacture of liposomes entrapping protein incorporating in-line purification and at-line size monitoring. *Int. J. Pharm.* **2019**, *556*, 68–81. [CrossRef]
281. Khadke, S.; Roces, C.B.; Donaghey, R.; Giacobbo, V.; Su, Y.; Perrie, Y. Scalable solvent-free production of liposomes. *J. Pharm. Pharmacol.* **2020**, *72*, 1328–1340. [CrossRef]
282. Salafi, T.; Zeming, K.K.; Zhang, Y. Advancements in microfluidics for nanoparticle separation. *Lab Chip* **2017**, *17*, 11–33. [CrossRef]
283. Petreus, T.; Cadogan, E.; Hughes, G.; Smith, A.; Pilla Reddy, V.; Lau, A.; O'Connor, M.J.; Critchlow, S.; Ashford, M.; Oplustil O'Connor, L. Tumour-on-chip microfluidic platform for assessment of drug pharmacokinetics and treatment response. *Commun. Biol.* **2021**, *4*, 1001. [CrossRef] [PubMed]
284. Sharma, S.; Bhatia, V. Magnetic nanoparticles in microfluidics-based diagnostics: An appraisal. *Nanomedicine* **2021**, *16*, 1329–1342. [CrossRef]
285. Lapierre, F.; Piret, G.; Drobecq, H.; Melnyk, O.; Coffinier, Y.; Thomy, V.; Boukherroub, R. High sensitive matrix-free mass spectrometry analysis of peptides using silicon nanowires-based digital microfluidic device. *Lab Chip* **2011**, *11*, 1620–1628. [CrossRef] [PubMed]
286. Ran, R.; Wang, H.-F.; Hou, F.; Liu, Y.; Hui, Y.; Petrovsky, N.; Zhang, F.; Zhao, C.-X. A Microfluidic Tumor-on-a-Chip for Assessing Multifunctional Liposomes' Tumor Targeting and Anticancer Efficacy. *Adv. Healthc. Mater.* **2019**, *8*, 1900015. [CrossRef] [PubMed]

287. Zizzari, A.; Bianco, M.; Carbone, L.; Perrone, E.; Amato, F.; Maruccio, G.; Rendina, F.; Arima, V. Continuous-Flow Production of Injectable Liposomes via a Microfluidic Approach. *Materials* **2017**, *10*, 1411. [CrossRef]
288. Yanar, F.; Mosayyebi, A.; Nastruzzi, C.; Carugo, D.; Zhang, X. Continuous-Flow Production of Liposomes with a Millireactor under Varying Fluidic Conditions. *Pharmaceutics* **2020**, *12*, 1001. [CrossRef]
289. Amador, C.; Gavriilidis, A.; Angeli, P. Flow distribution in different microreactor scale-out geometries and the effect of manufacturing tolerances and channel blockage. *Chem. Eng. J.* **2004**, *101*, 379–390. [CrossRef]
290. Shah, V.M.; Nguyen, D.X.; Patel, P.; Cote, B.; Al-Fatease, A.; Pham, Y.; Huynh, M.G.; Woo, Y.; Alani, A.W.G. Liposomes produced by microfluidics and extrusion: A comparison for scale-up purposes. *Nanomed. Nanotechnol. Biol. Med.* **2019**, *18*, 146–156. [CrossRef]
291. Roces, C.B.; Port, E.C.; Daskalakis, N.N.; Watts, J.A.; Aylott, J.W.; Halbert, G.W.; Perrie, Y. Rapid scale-up and production of active-loaded PEGylated liposomes. *Int. J. Pharm.* **2020**, *586*, 119566. [CrossRef]
292. Lamb, Y.N. BNT162b2 mRNA COVID-19 Vaccine: First Approval. *Drugs* **2021**, *81*, 495–501. [CrossRef]
293. Schoenmaker, L.; Witzigmann, D.; Kulkarni, J.A.; Verbeke, R.; Kersten, G.; Jiskoot, W.; Crommelin, D.J.A. mRNA-lipid nanoparticle COVID-19 vaccines: Structure and stability. *Int. J. Pharm.* **2021**, *601*, 120586. [CrossRef] [PubMed]
294. Roberts, S.A.; Parikh, N.; Blower, R.J.; Agrawal, N. SPIN: Rapid synthesis, purification, and concentration of small drug-loaded liposomes. *J. Liposome Res.* **2018**, *28*, 331–340. [CrossRef] [PubMed]
295. Tenchov, R.; Bird, R.; Curtze, A.E.; Zhou, Q. Lipid Nanoparticles–From Liposomes to mRNA Vaccine Delivery, a Landscape of Research Diversity and Advancement. *ACS Nano* **2021**, *15*, 16982–17015. [CrossRef] [PubMed]
296. Stone, N.R.H.; Bicanic, T.; Salim, R.; Hope, W. Liposomal Amphotericin B (AmBisome®): A Review of the Pharmacokinetics, Pharmacodynamics, Clinical Experience and Future Directions. *Drugs* **2016**, *76*, 485–500. [CrossRef]
297. O'Brien, M.E.R.; Wigler, N.; Inbar, M.; Rosso, R.; Grischke, E.; Santoro, A.; Catane, R.; Kieback, D.G.; Tomczak, P.; Ackland, S.P.; et al. Reduced cardiotoxicity and comparable efficacy in a phase IIItrial of pegylated liposomal doxorubicin HCl(CAELYX™/Doxil®) versus conventional doxorubicin forfirst-line treatment of metastatic breast cancer. *Ann. Oncol.* **2004**, *15*, 440–449. [CrossRef]
298. Zhang, X.; Goel, V.; Robbie, G.J. Pharmacokinetics of Patisiran, the First Approved RNA Interference Therapy in Patients With Hereditary Transthyretin-Mediated Amyloidosis. *J. Clin. Pharmacol.* **2020**, *60*, 573–585. [CrossRef] [PubMed]
299. Matsuura-Sawada, Y.; Maeki, M.; Nishioka, T.; Niwa, A.; Yamauchi, J.; Mizoguchi, M.; Wada, K.; Tokeshi, M. Microfluidic Device-Enabled Mass Production of Lipid-Based Nanoparticles for Applications in Nanomedicine and Cosmetics. *ACS Appl. Nano Mater.* **2022**, *5*, 7867–7876. [CrossRef]
300. Bresseleers, J.; Bagheri, M.; Lebleu, C.; Lecommandoux, S.; Sandre, O.; Pijpers, I.A.B.; Mason, A.F.; Meeuwissen, S.; Nostrum, C.F.v.; Hennink, W.E.; et al. Tuning Size and Morphology of mPEG-b-p(HPMA-Bz) Copolymer Self-Assemblies Using Microfluidics. *Polymers* **2020**, *12*, 2572. [CrossRef]
301. Giraldo, K.A.; Bermudez, J.S.; Torres, C.E.; Reyes, L.H.; Osma, J.F.; Cruz, J.C. Microfluidics for Multiphase Mixing and Liposomal Encapsulation of Nanobioconjugates: Passive vs. Acoustic Systems. *Fluids* **2021**, *6*, 309. [CrossRef]
302. Rasouli, M.R.; Tabrizian, M. An ultra-rapid acoustic micromixer for synthesis of organic nanoparticles. *Lab Chip* **2019**, *19*, 3316–3325. [CrossRef] [PubMed]
303. Shepherd, S.J.; Warzecha, C.C.; Yadavali, S.; El-Mayta, R.; Alameh, M.G.; Wang, L.; Weissman, D.; Wilson, J.M.; Issadore, D.; Mitchell, M.J. Scalable mRNA and siRNA Lipid Nanoparticle Production Using a Parallelized Microfluidic Device. *Nano Lett.* **2021**, *21*, 5671–5680. [CrossRef] [PubMed]
304. Rosenblum, D.; Gutkin, A.; Kedmi, R.; Ramishetti, S.; Veiga, N.; Jacobi, A.M.; Schubert, M.S.; Friedmann-Morvinski, D.; Cohen, Z.R.; Behlke, M.A.; et al. CRISPR-Cas9 genome editing using targeted lipid nanoparticles for cancer therapy. *Sci Adv.* **2020**, *6*, eabc9450. [CrossRef] [PubMed]
305. Riley, R.S.; Kashyap, M.V.; Billingsley, M.M.; White, B.; Alameh, M.G.; Bose, S.K.; Zoltick, P.W.; Li, H.; Zhang, R.; Cheng, A.Y.; et al. Ionizable lipid nanoparticles for in utero mRNA delivery. *Sci Adv.* **2021**, *7*, eaba1028. [CrossRef]
306. Sealy, A. How Pfizer Makes Its Millions of COVID-19 Vaccine Doses. Available online: https://edition.cnn.com/2021/03/31/health/pfizer-vaccine-manufacturing/index.html (accessed on 2 April 2021).

MDPI
St. Alban-Anlage 66
4052 Basel
Switzerland
www.mdpi.com

Pharmaceutics Editorial Office
E-mail: pharmaceutics@mdpi.com
www.mdpi.com/journal/pharmaceutics

www.ingramcontent.com/pod-product-compliance
Lightning Source LLC
LaVergne TN
LVHW070502100526
838202LV00014B/1775
* 9 7 8 3 7 2 5 8 1 0 9 6 3 *